COMPREHENSIVE PERIODONTICS

FOR THE DENTAL HYGIENIST

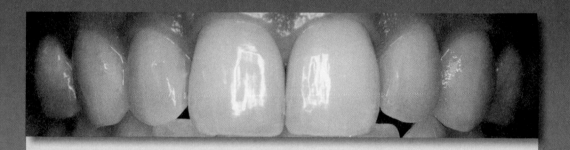

FOURTH EDITION

Mea A. Weinberg, D.M.D., M.S.D., R.Ph.

Cheryl M. Westphal Theile, Ed.D., R.D.H.

Stuart J. Froum, D.D.S.

Stuart L. Segelnick, D.D.S., M.S.

New York University College of Dentistry
New York, New York

Pearson

Boston Columbus Indianapolis New York San Francisco Upper Saddle River Amsterdam
Cape Town Dubai London Madrid Milan Munich Paris Montreal Toronto Delhi Mexico City Sao Paulo
Sydney Hong Kong Seoul Singapore Taipei Tokyo

Publisher: Julie Levin Alexander
Assistant to Publisher: Regina Bruno
Editor-in-Chief: Marlene McHugh Pratt
Executive Acquisitions Editor: John Goucher
Program Manager: Nicole Ragonese
Editorial Assistant: Erica Viviani
Director of Marketing: David Gesell
Executive Marketing Manager: Katrin Beacom
Senior Marketing Coordinator: Alicia Wozniak
Media Program Manager: Amy Peltier
Media Project Manager: Lorena Cerisano

Project Management Lead: Cynthia Zonneveld
Project Manager: Christina Zingone-Luethje
Production Editor: Patty Donovan, Laserwords
Operations Specialist: Nancy Maneri-Miller
Senior Art Director/Interior: Maria Guglielmo
Creative Director: Jayne Conte
Art Director/Cover: Bruce Kenselaar
Composition: Laserwords Private Limited
Printer/Binder: Courier/Kendallville
Cover Printer: Moore Langen
Cover Image: © DrHitch / Fotolia

Credits and acknowledgments for content borrowed from other sources and reproduced, with permissions, appear on page of this textbook.

Library of Congress Cataloging-in-Publication Data

Weinberg, Mea A., author.
Comprehensive periodontics for the dental hygienist /
Mea A. Weinberg, Cheryl Westphal Theile, Stuart J. Froum,
Stuart L. Segelnick.—Fourth edition.
    p. ; cm.
Preceded by Comprehensive periodontics for the dental hygienist /
Mea A. Weinberg . . . [et al.] ; consulting editor, James Burke Fine.
3rd ed. c2010.
    Includes bibliographical references and index.
    ISBN-13: 978-0-13-307772-8
    ISBN-10: 0-13-307772-1
    I. Theile, Cheryl M. Westphal, author. II. Froum, Stuart J., author.
III. Segelnick, Stuart L., author. IV. Title.
[DNLM: 1. Periodontal Diseases. WU 240]
RK361
617.6'32--dc23

                                2013035040

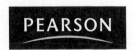
www.pearsonhighered.com

10 9 8 7 6 5 4 3 2 1
ISBN-13: 978-0-13-307772-8
ISBN-10: 0-13-307772-1

CONTENTS

FOREWORD

There is no subject of greater importance to the practice of dental hygiene than periodontology. *Comprehensive Periodontics for the Dental Hygienist* by Weinberg and colleagues offers an exceptional opportunity to learn this pivotal aspect of clinical practice at its best. This text accomplishes several important goals in thoughtful and compelling ways: It fosters an evidence-based approach—one that has become central to all clinical disciplines. It cultivates in the practitioner an identity as a person of science—that is, as a sophisticated *consumer* of research. Whereas scientists are assigned the responsibility of generating new knowledge, every practitioner must see him- or herself as a consumer of such information, capable of assessing and critiquing it for him- or herself. The text also underscores the interrelationship between oral disease and systemic health while helping prepare the dental hygienist to cope with increasingly complex technologies and innovations.

The attentive student has much to gain from the text's format, including the convenient use of outlines, goals, statements of educational objectives, inclusion of key words, reference to relevant websites, and use of self-assessment quizzes. Extraordinary knowledge of the field is available to the student of dental hygiene who is willing to invest time and effort exploiting the opportunities this text affords.

Periodontology is a discipline with a strong scientific base. A flavor of the richness of the underlying literature is reflected in the citations at the end of each chapter. Thus students and practitioners have at their disposal the means to secure a more in-depth treatment of specific topic areas by accessing the foundational literature on which the text is based. Those who do so can become adept at interpreting that literature for themselves, developing in the process the tools they will need to think independently and to remain current in their discipline with the passage of time.

Charles N. Bertolami
Professor and Herman Robert Fox Dean
College of Dentistry
New York University

PREFACE

There is a significant body of knowledge about the risk factors, pathogenesis, treatment, and prevention of periodontal diseases. This knowledge is rarely applied as an evidence-based approach to the difficult problem of deciding when specific treatments or examination methods are appropriate. Classic and current references are included in each chapter, along with applicable websites so the reader can supplement information in the textbook with information from other sources.

This basic text has been written in an attempt to make the professions' understanding of periodontal diseases accessible to the dental hygiene student, the practicing dental hygienist, and the dentist needing to update their knowledge through a concise synopsis of clinical periodontics.

Part I deals with the anatomy of the periodontium, risk (markers) factors (e.g., dental biofilm, smoking, and diabetes mellitus) for periodontal discases, and periodontal disease as a potential risk factor for systemic conditions (the periodontal–medicine relationship) such as stroke, cardiovascular disease, and respiratory conditions. This interrelationship between medicine and periodontology has opened new insights into the concept of oral health being an integral part of the overall general and systemic health of an individual. Oral and intravenous bisphosphonates are discussed as they relate to osteonecrosis of the jaw (ONJ).

Part I also reviews the etiology of periodontal diseases including oral biofilm, the bacterial and host response, and periodontal–systemic connection.

Part II discusses in detail the different periodontal diseases according to the most current Classification System of the Periodontal Diseases (American Academy of Periodontology).

Part III deals with the clinical assessment phase of the dental hygiene process of care. This part discusses the various assessment tools that are required to be performed on a patient for the development of a dental hygiene diagnosis.

Part IV discusses the treatment planning, implementation, and evaluation process of dental hygiene care. Nonsurgical and surgical therapy through problem-based learning (PBL) are discussed in detail. A problem-based system with basic concepts of treatment planning will be introduced to the student. A comprehensive review of halitosis is presented. In this section is an extensive review of drugs used in periodontal therapy, including various controlled-release drug devices (e.g., Arestin®) and enzyme suppression drugs (e.g., doxycycline 20 mg). An expanded section on surgery and implants is included with many color images.

Part V reviews four in-depth periodontal cases with extensive discussion of answers.

The appendices include a comprehensive listing of periodontic informatics, how to critically assess the periodontal literature, and smoking cessation therapy.

At the end of each chapter are board-type questions including new item type formats such as multiple correct answers, extended matching, and ordering which have now been introduced on the National Board Dental Hygiene Examinations. Included in the textbook are four problem-oriented, evidence-based case studies. Each case details the problem, followed by a discussion of the questions and answers to the problem. "Rapid Dental Hints" remind students about key information or a task that should be performed related to the topic discussed. In addition, there are "Did You Know?" comments found within all chapters that provide whimsical information on the topic at hand.

We hope this book will serve as a helpful text for all dental practitioners.

Mea A. Weinberg, D.M.D., M.S.D., R.Ph.

CONTRIBUTORS

Mary Elizabeth Aichelmann-Reidy, D.D.S.
Assistant Professor, Department of Periodontics
University of Maryland
Baltimore, Maryland

Khalid Almas, B.D.S., M.Sc.
Associate Professor, Division of Periodontology, School of Dental Medicine
University of Connecticut
Farmington, Connecticut

Sangeetha Chandrasekaran, B.D.S., Masters Biomedical Sciences, Masters in Oral Sciences
Assistant Professor
Department of Surgical Dentistry
University of Colorado School of Dental Medicine
Aurora, Colorado

Denise Estafan, D.D.S, M.S.
Associate Professor and Director of Clinical Esthetics
Department of Cariology and Comprehensive Care
New York University College of Dentistry
New York, New York

James Burke Fine, D.M.D
Associate Dean of Postgraduate Studies
Associate Professor of Clinical Dentistry
Director of Postgraduate Periodontics
Columbia University College of Dental Medicine
New York, New York

Cynthia Fong, R.D.H., M.S.
Lecturer/Instructor in Periodontics
Department of Dental Hygiene
Pierce College
Tacoma, Washington

Herbert Frommer, D.D.S.
Professor and Director of Radiology
New York University College of Dentistry
New York, New York

Stuart J. Froum, D.D.S.
Clinical Professor, Director of Research
Department of Periodontology and Implant Dentistry
New York University College of Dentistry
New York, New York

Rosemary DeRosa Hays, R.D.H., M.S.
Clinical Associate Professor, Dental Hygiene Program
New York University College of Dentistry
New York, New York

Debra Jacobowitz, D.D.S.
(Candidate 2014)
New York University College of Dentistry
New York, New York

Judith Kreismann, R.D.H., B.S., M.S.
Clinical Associate Professor, Dental Hygiene Program
New York University College of Dentistry
New York, New York

Josephine Lomangino-Cheung, D.D.S., M.S.
Clinical Assistant Professor
Department of Cariology and Comprehensive Care
New York University College of Dental Medicine
New York, New York

Eva M. Lupovici, R.D.H., M.S.
Clinical Associate Professor, Dental Hygiene Program
New York University College of Dentistry
New York, New York

Deborah M. Lyle, R.D.H., B.S., M.S.
Director of Professional & Clinical Affairs
Water Pik, Inc.
Morris Plains, New Jersey

John D. Mason, B.A., D.D.S.
Associate Professor, Department of Periodontics
Director of Predoctoral Periodontics
Louisiana State University School of Dentistry
New Orleans, Louisiana

Trisha E. O'Hehir, R.D.H., B.S.
Editor of Perio Reports
Senior Consulting Editor, RHD Magazine
Vice President, Perio-Data™ Company
Assistant Visiting Professor Northern Arizona University
Flagstaff, Arizona

Toula A. Palaiologou, D.D.S., M.S.
Director of Postgraduate Periodontics
Louisiana State University School of Dentistry
New Orleans, Louisiana

Scott W. Podell, D.M.D., M.P.H.
Group Practice Director
Clinical Assistant Professor
Department of Cariology and Comprehensive Care
New York University College of Dentistry
New York, New York

Charles A. Powell, D.D.S., M.S.
Chair, Division of Periodontics and Director of Postgraduate Periodontics
University of Colorado School of Dental Medicine
Aurora, Colorado

Jill Rethman, R.D.H., B.A.
Visiting Clinical Instructor, Department of Dental Hygiene
Editorial Director Dimensions of Dental Hygiene
University of Pittsburgh
Pittsburgh, Pennsylvania
2012 President Hawaii's Dental Hygienists' Association

Michael P. Rethman, D.D.S., M.S.
Past President of the American Academy of Periodontology
Former Chief of Periodontics
Tripler Medical Center
Honolulu, Hawaii

Paul S. Rosen, D.M.D., M.S.
Full-time Periodontic Practice, Yardley, Pennsylvania
Clinical Associate Professor of Periodontics
University of Maryland Dental School
Baltimore, Maryland

Stuart L. Segelnick, D.D.S., M.S.
Clinical Associate Professor
Department of Periodontology and Implant Dentistry
New York University College of Dentistry
New York, New York

Surendra Singh, D.D.S., M.S.
Professor, Department of Periodontics
University of Medicine and Dentistry of New Jersey School of Dentistry
Newark, New Jersey

Jeanine Stabulas-Savage, R.D.H., B.S., M.P.H.
Clinical Assistant Professor
Oral and Maxillofacial Pathology, Radiology and Medicine
New York University College of Dentistry
New York, New York

Mea A. Weinberg, D.M.D., M.S.D., R.Ph.
Clinical Associate Professor and Director of Second Year Periodontics
Department of Periodontology and Implant Dentistry
New York University College of Dentistry
New York, New York

Cheryl M. Westphal Theile, Ed.D., R.D.H.
Clinical Associate Professor and Assistant Dean for Allied Health Programs
Director, Dental Hygiene Program
New York University College of Dentistry
New York, New York

Pinelopi Xenoudi, D.D.S., M.S.
Assistant Professor
Surgical Dentistry
University of Colorado School of Dental Medicine
Aurora, Colorado

Raymond A. Yukna, D.M.D., M.S.
Professor, Directory Periodontic Residency Program
University of Colorado School of Dental Medicine Aurora, Colorado

Selected Illustrations by Jesse Doscher, D.D.S.

Selected Photographs Courtesy of Dr. John Eum, Dr. James Fine, Dr. Xiu Yan Li, Dr. Jacqueline Plemmons, Dr. Jesse Sorrentino, Dr. Michael Turner, and Dr. Harvey Wishe.

REVIEWERS

Karmen Aplanalp, R.D.H., B.S.D.H., M.Ed.
College of Southern Nevada
Henderson, Nevada

Catherine Boos, D.M.D.
Camden Community College
Camden. New Jersey

Barbara Bush, R.D.H., M.S.Ed.
Western Kentucky University
Bowling Green, Kentucky

Paula E. Covert, C.D.A., R.D.H., B.S.D.H.
Asheville-Buncombe Technical Community College
Asheville, North Carolina

Sheree Duff, R.D.H., M.S.
Baker College of Auburn Hills
Auburn Hills, Michigan

Laura Joseph, R.D.H., M.S., Ed.D.
State University of New York at Farmingdale
Farmingdale, New York

Tricia Moore, R.D.H.
Northern Arizona University
Flagstaff, Arizona

Kemaly Parr, R.D.H., M.D.H.
Columbus Technical College
Columbus, Georgia

Shelly A. Purtell, R.D.H., Ph.D.
Broome Community College
Binghamton, New York

Rebecca Smith, R.D.H., A.S.D.H., B.H.S.A., M.P.H., Ed.D.
Miami Dade College
Miami, Florida

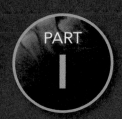

Periodontal Diseases: Introduction and Background

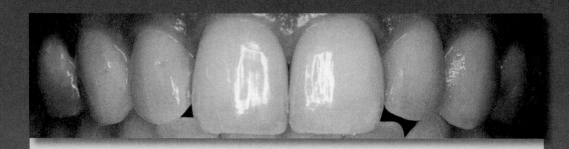

OUTLINE

Anatomy of the Periodontal Structures: The Healthy State

Mea A. Weinberg and Debra Jacobowitz

OUTLINE

Clinical Anatomy of the Gingival
Unit
Microscopic Anatomy of the
Gingival Unit
Attachment Apparatus
Physiology of the Periodontium
Changes with Aging
Dental Hygiene Application
Key Points
Self-Quiz
Case Study
References

EDUCATIONAL OBJECTIVES

Upon completion of this chapter, the reader should be able to:

* Illustrate and discuss the clinical anatomy of the periodontium.
* Illustrate and describe the microscopic anatomy of the periodontium.
* List and describe the functions of the periodontium.
* Discuss the importance of the dentogingival unit.
* Describe the lymphatic, blood, and nerve supply to the gingiva and the attachment apparatus.

GOAL: To provide knowledge of the structures and functions of the periodontium in health.

KEY WORDS

Introduction

The **periodontium**, translated in Latin to mean "around the tooth," consists of the **gingiva**, periodontal ligament, cementum, and alveolar and supporting bone of the teeth (Figure 1–1a ■). The **attachment apparatus** consists of periodontal tissues involved in the attachment and support of the root in the tooth socket, specifically the periodontal ligament, cementum, and alveolar bone (Hassell, 1993). A working knowledge of the ultrastructural anatomy and biology of the periodontal tissues is an important prerequisite for practitioners to recognize and treat periodontal diseases.

To understand the different stages of diseases in the periodontium, it is necessary to recognize the structures and functions of the periodontium in health (Bartold, 2006). This chapter describes the clinical and microscopic features of the periodontium in health and will be the foundation for ensuing discussions in this text.

Clinical Anatomy of the Gingival Unit

The oral mucosa is divided into three types: (1) masticatory mucosa, which includes the gingiva and hard palate; (2) lining mucosa, which consists of the alveolar mucosa, soft palate, lining of lips, cheeks, and sublingual area; and (3) specialized mucosa, which is found on the dorsum of the tongue.

Masticatory Mucosa (Gingiva)

The gingiva forms a protective covering over the other components of the periodontium and is well adapted to protect against mechanical insults (e.g., toothbrushing and chewing). The gingiva encircles the cervical portion of the teeth and covers the alveolar process. Anatomically, the gingiva is subdivided into the free gingiva, attached gingiva, and interdental gingiva or papilla (Figure 1–1b). The outer surface of the gingiva consists of stratified squamous epithelium.

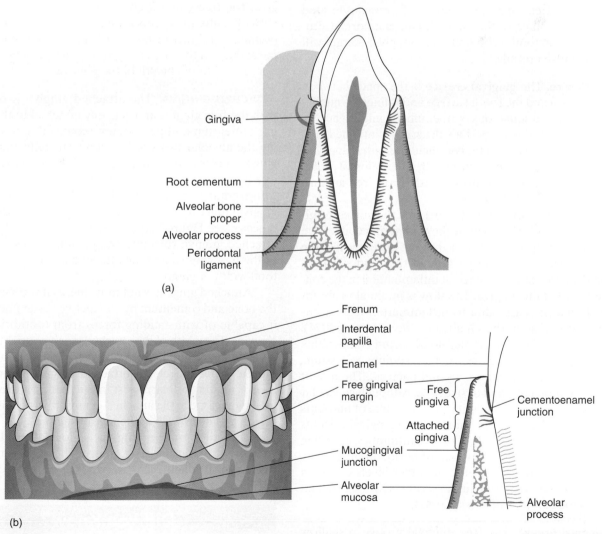

FIGURE 1–1 (a) Schematic drawing of a tooth with its periodontium. (b) Landmarks of the gingival unit. (*Left*) The gingiva is salmon pink, whereas the alveolar mucosa is thinner and redder in color. (*Right*) Schematic drawing of a cross-section of the periodontium.

Underneath the epithelium is gingival connective tissue, which is termed the lamina propria.

FREE GINGIVA (MARGINAL GINGIVA) The free gingiva, or marginal gingiva, surrounds the neck of the tooth. Its boundaries are, coronally, the free gingival margin; apically, the free gingival groove; and laterally, the gingival crevice and the tooth (see Figure 1–1b). The free gingiva is approximately 1.5 mm wide and has a smooth surface. The free gingiva lies on and adapts to the enamel and can be separated from the tooth with a periodontal instrument (Schroeder & Listgarten, 1997).

In health, the free gingival margin is the edge or the most coronal part of the free gingiva and in a fully erupted tooth is located on the enamel approximately 0.5 to 2 mm coronal to the cementoenamel junction (CEJ). In health and if teeth contact in the anterior region, the free gingival margin usually has a scalloped outline following the contour of the cementoenamel junction (see Figure 1–1b). If there is an open contact, the free gingival margin becomes blunted. In the posterior region, the architecture becomes less scalloped. Prior to the completed eruption of permanent teeth in children, the free gingival margin usually remains located on the cervical bulge of the enamel. This is a normal situation, and as the tooth erupts the free gingival margin will ultimately move apically.

Gingival Crevice. The **gingival crevice** is the space between the free gingiva and the tooth surface and is lined by nonkeratinized stratified squamous epithelium. In gingival health, the gingival crevice is termed a sulcus; once inflamed, it is termed a pocket. Healthy gingiva sulcular depth is approximately 1 to 3 mm when measured with a periodontal probe. Only in experimental conditions with germ-free animals can the sulcular depth be zero.

Gingival crevicular fluid (GCF) fills the sulcus, originates from blood vessels within the underlying connective tissue (lamina propria), and flows through the tissue into the gingival crevice. The rate of passage of this fluid is dependent on the absence or presence of inflammation in the connective tissue of the gingiva. The flow is minimal to absent in health, but increases due to inflammation from accumulation of plaque in the gingival crevice (Alfano, 1974). Components of GCF resemble blood serum components and include elements such as calcium, sodium, potassium, and phosphorus, along with cells and bacteria. The role of GCF is both protective and destructive. Although crevicular fluid flow cleanses the sulcus, it is also a source of nutrients for subgingival bacteria and supports subgingival calculus formation (Mukherjee, 1985). Certain antibiotics, including tetracyclines used in the treatment of periodontal diseases, have been found to concentrate in higher levels locally in the GCF (pocket area) than in the serum (Gordon, Walker, Murphy, Goodson, & Socransky, 1981).

Free Gingival Groove. The free gingival groove, a shallow depression on the outer surface of the gingiva, is about 1 to 2 mm apical from the margin of the gingiva and is slightly

Did You Know?

The gingival crevicular fluid (GCF), which bathes the gingival crevice subgingivally, contains many minerals and substances. Subgingival calculus is usually a dark color, such as black, due to the influence of GCF.

Rapid Dental Hint

It is important to transpose the patient's free gingival margin and mucogingival junction to the periodontal chart because this will help you determine if there is a soft tissue defect present and to monitor the attachment level and gingival recession.

apical to the level of the cementoenamel junction. This groove separates the free gingiva from the attached gingiva. The free gingival groove is present in about 30% to 40% of adults and occurs most frequently in the mandibular premolar and incisor areas. It is more pronounced on the facial than on the lingual regions. Its absence or presence is not related to the health of the gingiva.

ATTACHED GINGIVA The attached gingiva is continuous with the free gingiva and is firmly attached to the underlying cementum and periosteum (connective tissue) covering the alveolar process. It extends apically from the free gingival groove to the mucogingival junction (MGJ). If the free gingival groove is not present, then the landmark is at a horizontal plane placed at the level of the CEJ. The mucogingival junction joins the attached gingiva to the alveolar mucosa (see Figure 1–1b) except on the palate because the attached gingiva runs into the palatal mucosa. The width of the free gingiva and the attached gingiva consists of the total width of gingiva.

Attached gingiva is not movable, as it is bound down to the bone and cementum by connective tissue fibers, making it capable of withstanding forces from toothbrushing and chewing. The width of the attached gingiva varies in different areas of the mouth and between individuals (Figure 1–2 ■). On the facial aspect, the attached gingiva is widest in the incisor region and narrowest in the first premolar area. On the lingual aspect, the attached gingiva is widest in the molar region and narrowest in the incisor region.

The color of the gingiva is normally salmon pink with slight variations. The gingiva shows varying degrees of brownish-black color depending on ethnic variation

Did You Know?

Dogs, cats, and other animals also have gingiva, just like us.

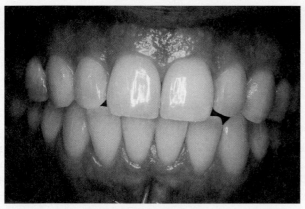

FIGURE 1–2 Varying amounts of attached gingiva; the narrowest width is on the mandibular premolars, and the widest is on the maxillary incisors.

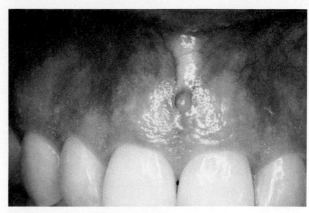

FIGURE 1–4 Surface stippling of the attached gingiva and the interdental gingiva. Note the dimpling or depressions on the surface. The surface of the free gingiva is not stippled.

(Figure 1–3 ■), which is considered to be normal gingival coloring and is referred to as melanin pigmentation.

Stippling. Clinically, the outer surface of the attached gingiva has an appearance similar to an orange peel with shallow depressions between elevations. The free gingiva has a

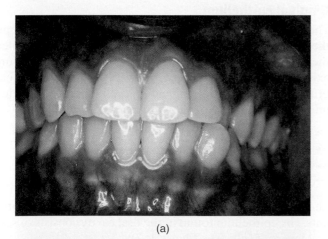

(a)

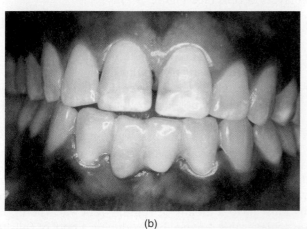

(b)

FIGURE 1–3 (a) Physiological gingival pigmentation varies: light pigmentation. (b) darker, more pronounced pigmentation.

smooth surface and is not stippled (Figure 1–4 ■). A histologic description of stippling is discussed in the following section.

Stippling may be present in health or disease. The absence of stippling does not necessarily indicate the presence of disease. On the other hand, the presence of inflammation with the loss of stippling can be considered part of the disease process, assuming stippling was present initially.

Stippling is present in only about 40% of adults and varies in different individuals, ages, and sexes. Stippling of the attached gingiva is absent in children under 5 years of age and may be more evident in men than women. It is more prominent in the anterior than the posterior region and may even be absent in the molar areas. The facial gingiva shows more prominent stippling than the lingual.

INTERDENTAL GINGIVA (INTERDENTAL PAPILLA) In health the interdental gingiva tightly fills the gingival embrasure, which is the space between the contact point and alveolar bone of two adjacent teeth. The margin and lateral borders of the interdental gingiva are an extension of the free gingiva, whereas the remaining parts are attached gingiva (Figure 1–5 ■).

The size and shape of the papillae are determined by tooth-to-tooth contact, the curvature of the cementoenamel junction, and the width (faciolingually) of the interproximal tooth surfaces. When teeth are crowded, often seen in mandibular incisors, the papillae may be slender and narrow. Anterior papillae are pyramidal in shape whereas posterior papillae are rounder and slightly flatter. An anterior papilla forms a single pyramidal structure because there is only one papilla. The papillae of posterior teeth (premolars and molars) are wedge shaped, with one vestibular (facial) and one oral (lingual) papilla connected by a concave area called the **col** (Figure 1–5). The col is directly apical to the contact area, representing the fusion of the interproximal junctional epithelia of two adjacent teeth. Although an anterior papilla can form a col shape, it is more prominent

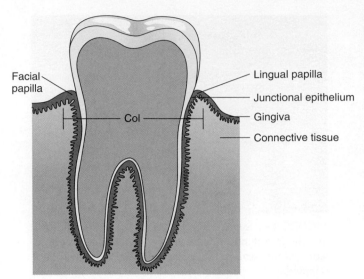

FIGURE 1–5 Features of the interdental gingiva. The col is directly under the contact area of the teeth.

Rapid Dental Hint

Remember that anterior teeth may have a small col or it may not be detectable.

in posterior papillae. When a diastema (loss of contact between two adjacent teeth) is present, the interdental papilla is absent, and there is no col. Because the shape of a col is concave and may not be keratinized, it may predispose the interproximal area to the accumulation of dental plaque.

Lining Mucosa

ALVEOLAR MUCOSA Although not actually part of the periodontium, the alveolar mucosa is an important periodontal structure and deserves discussion. The alveolar mucosa extends apically from the mucogingival junction to the mucous membrane of the cheek, lip, and floor of the mouth (see Figure 1–1b). In comparison to the attached gingiva, alveolar mucosa is thinner and redder in color, has a smooth surface, is movable, and is not keratinized.

FRENUM ATTACHMENTS Frenum (plural: frena) attachments are folds of alveolar mucosa. They are not concentrations of muscle, having no more muscle fibers than alveolar mucosa. The function of a frenum is to attach lips and cheeks to the maxillary and mandibular mucosa and to limit the movement of the lips and cheeks. There are usually seven frena located in the canine/premolar area, between the central incisors and in the mandibular anterior lingual area.

Did You Know?

Gingiva is salmon pink in color due to keratin. Keratin is a protein that is also involved in forming hair, skin, and fingernails.

Specialized Mucosa

The mucosa of the dorsum of the tongue contains numerous papillae of three types: filiform, fungiform, and circumvallate. The circumvallate papillae are located along the V-shaped groove on the back of the tongue. Each papilla is surrounded by a circular groove. The taste buds are located mainly on the sides of these papillae. The filiform papillae are slender ones and the most abundant, covering the entire top or dorsal surface of the tongue. No taste buds are associated with these papillae; they respond only to heat and mechanical stimuli. The fungiform papillae, which are broad and flat, are found chiefly at the edges of the tongue and are provided with taste buds.

Microscopic Anatomy of the Gingival Unit

Gingival Epithelium

The gingiva is covered by a layer of stratified squamous epithelium with an underlying core of connective tissue called the lamina propria (Figure 1–6 ■). The gingival epithelium exists as structurally different forms specific to certain areas of the teeth. Thus, the gingival epithelium can be divided into (Figure 1–7 ■) the following elements:

- The oral epithelium (OE)
- The sulcular or crevicular epithelium (SE)
- The junctional epithelium (JE)

The gingival epithelium is avascular and relies on the underlying lamina propria for its blood supply and nutrients. The epithelium found in the oral cavity consists of several layers of cells (see Figure 1–7):

- Stratum basale or stratum germinativum (basal cell layer); deepest layer next to the lamina propria.
- Stratum spinosum (spinous cell layer).
- Stratum granulosum (granular layer).
- Stratum corneum (keratinized/cornified cell layer; also called the superficial cell layer); this outermost layer serves as a barrier membrane protecting the underlying periodontal tissues from invasion by foreign substances.

CELL RENEWAL Just like the epithelium of the skin, the gingival epithelium is also subject to considerable insult and thus must have a means of regular renewal. The epithelium achieves this renewal by producing a pool of cells that migrate from the basal layer to the oral environment. This process by which epithelial cells differentiate or mature is

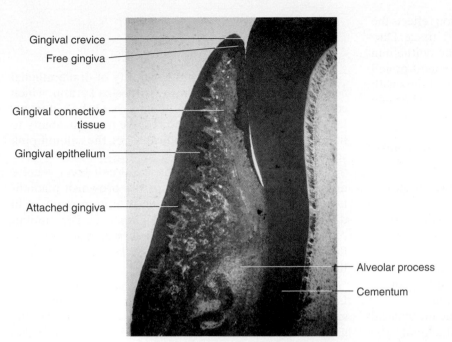

Gingival crevice

Free gingiva

Gingival connective tissue

Gingival epithelium

Attached gingiva

Alveolar process

Cementum

FIGURE 1–6 Photomicrograph of the gingival epithelium. (Courtesy of Dr. Harvey Wishe, New York University College of Dentistry.)

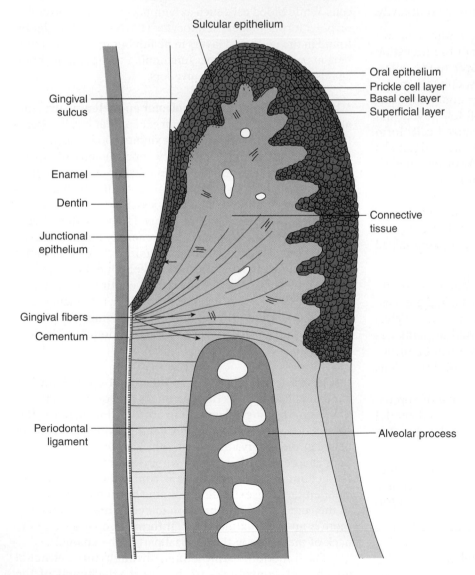

Sulcular epithelium

Oral epithelium

Prickle cell layer

Basal cell layer

Superficial layer

Gingival sulcus

Enamel

Dentin

Junctional epithelium

Connective tissue

Gingival fibers

Cementum

Periodontal ligament

Alveolar process

FIGURE 1–7 Diagram of the layers of the gingival epithelium. Underlying the epithelium is the gingival connective tissue (lamina propria).

called keratinization. The type of differentiation reflects the functional demands or stimulus placed on the tissue. During keratinization, the entire thickness of the epithelium is replaced. The time it takes for this replacement or cell renewal is called the turnover time. This time differs with the various types of epithelium. Such differences become important during tissue healing after periodontal surgery or tissue damage.

The keratinization process occurs as follows (Moss-Salentijn & Hendricks-Klyvert, 1990):

- Basal cells in the basal cell layer divide and produce new cells.
- The "older" basal cells travel or move into the next layer, the spinous cell layer, on their way to the most outer epithelial cell layer.
- Once in the spinous cell layer, the basal cells become keratinocytes. On their way to the outer surface, the keratinocytes synthesize or produce keratin.
- Keratin is a protein that contributes to the mechanical toughness of the outer surface of the epithelium.
- When the keratinocytes reach the outer epithelial surface, they are shed from the surface into the oral cavity.

Three grades of keratinization or maturation are identified according to the completeness of the transition of the keratinocyte from the basal cell layer to the outermost, superficial cell layer. Consequently, epithelium can be (ortho) keratinized, parakeratinized, or nonkeratinized. Keratinized epithelium is composed of all four layers and is primarily seen in the skin. Fully keratinized cells form keratin and lose their nuclei by the time they migrate to the outer surface. Findings show that 76% of the gingival exhibit parakeratin cells, which retain their nuclei but show some signs of being keratinized. The stratum granulosum is usually difficult to recognize, and a surface parakeratinized outer layer is present. Epithelial cells found in the junctional epithelium and alveolar mucosas are nonkeratinized and do not undergo keratinization.

ORAL EPITHELIUM The **oral epithelium** faces the oral cavity on the outer surface of the free and attached gingivae extending from the free gingival margin to the mucogingival junction. The gingiva is generally composed of parakeratinized stratified squamous epithelium, but can be orthokeratinized in small patches and in other species such as monkeys.

The gingiva has an epithelial turnover time of approximately 10 days as demonstrated in an animal model (Schroeder & Listgarten, 1997), whereas in the skin it is approximately 28 days.

Cells in the Oral Epithelium. The function of the oral epithelium is to protect the underlying structures and act as a mechanical barrier. The oral epithelium contains the following types of cells:

- Keratinocytes
- Nonkeratinocytes (also called clear cells)
- Melanocytes
- Langerhans cells
- Merkel cells
- Inflammatory cells (e.g., neutrophils)

Keratinocytes make up the majority of oral epithelial cells. Keratinocytes function to synthesize keratin, which contributes to the mechanical toughness of the outer surface of the oral epithelium and relative impermeability to fluids and cells. It is also responsible for the salmon pink color of the gingiva.

Melanocytes located in the basal cell layer secrete melanin, which is responsible for the brownish pigmentation in the gingiva. Pigmentation is more prominent in darker-skinned individuals (see Figure 1–3). The amount of pigmentation is genetically predetermined according to the potential of the cells to produce melanin, rather than to the number of cells present.

Other cell types in the gingival epithelium are the Langerhans cells, which are located in the stratum spinosum and are involved in the early defense mechanism of the gingiva. Merkel cells are found in the basal cell layer and are associated with nerve endings acting as touch-sensory cells. White blood cells such as lymphocytes and neutrophils or polymorphonuclear leukocytes (PMNs) are transiently found in the epithelial layers in health but increase in numbers in periodontal disease, functioning to defend the body against bacteria and other invaders.

SULCULAR EPITHELIUM The **sulcular epithelium** is structurally similar to the oral epithelium except that it is less keratinized. The sulcular epithelium exhibits good resistance to mechanical forces and is relatively impermeable (resistant) to the flow of fluids and cells. The sulcular epithelium may have epithelial ridges, or rete pegs, in health or disease, as does the oral epithelium, but to a lesser extent. Sulcular or crevicular epithelium lines the gingival sulcus without being attached to the tooth surface. It is generally nonkeratinized and thin but can become parakeratinized if exposed to the oral environment. The sulcular epithelium exhibits two or three cell layers, but a definitive and continuous cornified layer is absent. At the free gingival margin, the sulcular epithelium is continuous with the oral epithelium. Apically, it overlaps the coronal surface of the junctional epithelium (see Figure 1–7).

JUNCTIONAL EPITHELIUM The **junctional epithelium** is a band of epithelial cells that surrounds the tooth and creates a "seal" at the gingival crevice to hold it firmly in place. It is continuous with the free gingiva and provides the contact between the gingiva and the tooth. The junctional epithelium can be regarded as a down growth of the squamous epithelium of the gingiva and is continuous with the sulcular epithelium, extending from the bottom of the crevice to the cementoenamel junction in health and in gingivitis; there is no loss of attachment. It forms a collar around the neck of the tooth on the cervical part of the enamel.

The junctional epithelium, through the epithelial attachment, contributes to the direct attachment of the gingiva to the tooth surface and thus serves a significant role in periodontal health and disease when this attachment to the tooth is lost.

The junctional epithelium is composed of nonkeratinized stratified squamous epithelium. It is composed of only two epithelial layers, either an active basal cell layer and an inactive suprabasal cell layer or a basal cell and spinous cell layer (Hassell, 1993; Schroeder & Listgarten, 1997). The junctional epithelium in health has no rete ridges. When inflammation sets in, the junctional epithelium develops epithelial projections into the adjacent inflamed connective tissue.

At the coronal portion, the thickness of the junctional epithelium is about 15 to 30 cells, whereas apically, near the cementoenamel junction, there may be only 1 to 2 cells (see Figure 1–7). Interproximally, the junctional epithelium of adjacent teeth fuses coronally to form the lining of the col area (Schroeder & Listgarten, 1997).

Semipermeable Membrane. The junctional epithelium is more permeable than the oral or sulcular epithelium. Thus, the junctional epithelium is referred to as a semipermeable structure, allowing the movement of bacterial products, fluids, and cells of certain sizes (Kornman, Page, & Tonetti, 1997). There are fewer intercellular junctions and thus wider spaces between the cells than in the oral or sulcular epithelium, and the cells are arranged in a parallel fashion. This allows for easy passage of cells and tissue fluid from the lamina propria into the sulcus and for passage of bacteria and its by-products from the gingival sulcus into the lamina propria. It is also more permeable because the cells do not keratinize. The coronal part of the junctional epithelium that is closest to the bottom of the sulcus is the most permeable part, whereas the apical part is where cell division for tissue renewal occurs.

Cells in the Junctional Epithelium. In addition to keratinocytes, the junctional epithelium may contain clear cells. In health, small numbers of PMNs are transiently seen in the junctional epithelium (Tonetti, Imboden, Gerber, & Lang, 1995). They will usually pass through the junctional epithelium into the gingival sulcus, where they play a role in the defense of the host (body) against bacteria and other microorganisms.

Cellular Turnover. A unique characteristic of the junctional epithelium is its high rate of cellular turnover. As demonstrated in an animal model, the cells of the junctional epithelium undergo constant turnover every 4 to 7 days,

whereby the basal cells migrate coronally out through the sulcus where the old cells are shed into the oral cavity.

Alveolar Mucosa

The alveolar mucosa is compressible and movable due to the presence of a submucosa between the thin lamina propria and the underlying tissue, usually muscle. The presence of elastic fibers, and an underlying loose connective tissue that is attached to the underlying periosteum of the alveolar process, also allows for movement.

The epithelium of the alveolar mucosa has about the same thickness as that of the gingiva, but its structure is completely different (Schroeder, 1991; Schroeder & Listgarten, 1997). A granular layer is not present, and the superficial layer does not histologically stain, as does the surface of parakeratinized epithelium (Squier & Hill, 1998). The epithelium contains melanocytes, Langerhans cells, Merkel cells, and small lymphocytes.

Epithelial ridges are usually not present; if present, they are indistinct because they are shorter and wider than in the gingiva, giving a smoother surface texture. The color is darker red than the gingiva because of its highly vascular underlying connective tissue. The point where there is a marked increase in elastic fibers within the underlying connective tissue demarcates the mucogingival junction.

Gingival Connective Tissue

Underlying the stratified squamous epithelium and encircling the tooth is the gingival connective tissue or lamina propria (Nanci & Bosshardt, 2006).

CONNECTIVE TISSUE/EPITHELIUM INTERFACE The interface between the connective tissue and oral epithelium is through connecting epithelial ridges that extend into the connective tissue (Figure 1–8 ■). At the intersection of epithelial ridges are pits or depressions that contain connective tissue extensions called connective tissue papillae. Clinically, these depressions may be evident on the surface of the gingiva, creating a stippled appearance. Stippling is established at the areas of fusion between adjacent epithelial ridges. In periodontal health the epithelial ridges are absent from the junctional epithelium and are not well developed in the sulcular epithelium. The main purposes of stippling are to aid in the increased strength between the epithelium and connective tissue and to enable the epithelium to obtain its blood supply from the connective tissue papillae in the shortest distance possible (Nanci & Bosshardt, 2006).

GINGIVAL CONNECTIVE TISSUE The main component of the gingival connective tissue, as with all connective tissue, is collagen fibers, accounting for about 60% of the total volume. Collagen is a protein composed of amino acids. There are many different types of collagen, with Types I (95%) and III (5%) found in gingival connective tissues. Type I collagen fibers give the gingiva its firmness and resiliency. The lamina propria provides mechanical support and nutrients

---

Did You Know?

The junctional epithelium is only three to four layers thick in early life but its thickness increases with age. The length of junctional epithelium is only about 0.25 to 1.35 mm. Just think about this—only about 1 mm long!

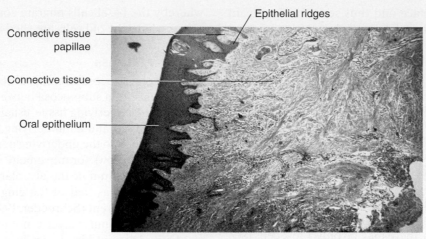

Connective tissue papillae

Epithelial ridges

Connective tissue

Oral epithelium

FIGURE 1–8 A photomicrograph of the gingival oral epithelium/connective tissue interface. Note prominent epithelial ridges. Intersections between the epithelial ridges under the epithelial surface correspond to depressions seen on the surface of the gingiva. Fingerlike projections termed connective tissue papillae extend into the depressions on the undersurface of the epithelium. This produces the characteristic stippled appearance of the attached gingiva. (Courtesy of Dr. Harvey Wishe, New York University College of Dentistry.)

for the avascular epithelium. The remainder of gingival connective tissue consists of ground substance, which is composed of proteins termed proteoglycans, in which the collagen fibers, cells (5%), nerves, and blood vessels (65%) are embedded. Proteoglycans have a protein core with carbohydrate side chains (glycosaminoglycans) of chondroitin sulphate, heparin sulphate, and hyaluronic acid. The ground substance also allows for the transportation of water and nutrients through the tissue.

Gingival Fibers. The free and attached gingivae are attached to the tooth surface through a **connective tissue attachment**. Collagen fibers in the gingiva are arranged so that they maintain the gingiva against the tooth and bone. The collagen fibers are organized in bundles or groups according to their origin and insertion (Schroeder & Listgarten, 1997). The collagen fibers embedded on one end in the cementum are termed Sharpey's fibers (Goldman, 1951). Collectively, the gingival fiber bundles are called the gingival fibers, the supracrestal fiber apparatus (because they are located coronal to the crest of alveolar bone), or the gingival connective tissue attachment. These three terms will be used interchangeably throughout the text. Table 1–1 ■ reviews the primary collagen fiber groups in the gingiva (Figure 1–9 ■), including the circular, dentogingival, dentoperiosteal, alveologingival, and transseptal fibers. Secondary gingival fiber groups include periostogingival, interpapillary, transgingival, intercrevicular, semicircular, and intergingival fibers. Their function is to support and give contour to the free and attached gingivae and firmly connect the attached gingiva to the underlying cementum and alveolar bone. The free gingiva is not actually free nor is it attached to the tooth, but rather it is held in close proximity to the tooth by the

gingival fibers, which prevent the free gingiva from being deflected from the tooth during mastication.

COLLAGEN ORGANIZATION Collagen fibers are either densely or loosely organized. Dense connective tissue that is found in the lamina propria of the gingiva consists of heavy, tightly packed fibers that function to resist tension. Loose connective tissue, as exemplified by alveolar mucosa, is composed of the collagen fibers that are thin and delicate and do not have a mechanical protective function. Collagen is constantly being synthesized and degraded as part of the normal remodeling or turnover of gingival connective tissue.

Cellular and Vascular Elements

The cellular part of the lamina propria predominately consists of the following:

- Fibroblasts
- Macrophages
- Mast cells
- Plasma cells, lymphocytes, and neutrophils

Fibroblasts synthesize ground substance, collagen, and collagenase. Collagenase is an enzyme responsible for the breakdown of collagen during remodeling. Thus, fibroblasts play a chief role in the maintenance and remodeling of connective tissue. Other cells in the lamina propria include red blood cells, PMNs, macrophages, lymphocytes, and mast cells, which are involved in the defense of the host against toxins.

A rich vascular complex is found in the lamina propria. Because there is no submucosa, as is found in the alveolar mucosa, the blood supply passes directly to the lamina propria.

Table 1–1 Classification of the Gingival Fibers

Name of Fiber	Origin and Distribution	Function
Circular	Encircles the tooth within the free gingiva	Provides support and contour to the free gingiva
Dentogingival	From the cementum at the base of the gingival sulcus, flares coronally into the free gingiva (group A), laterally into the attached gingiva (group B), and apically into the periosteum (group C); found on the facial, lingual, and interproximal surfaces	Contributes to the support of the gingiva
Dentoperiosteal	Extends from the cementum apically over the alveolar crest into the periosteum	Anchors the tooth to the bone
Alveologingival	Extends from the periosteum of the alveolar crestal bone coronally into the connective tissue	Attaches the gingiva to the alveolar bone
Transseptal	Runs from the Cementum of one tooth interproximal to the cementum of the adjacent tooth	Keeps teeth in alignment and protects the interproximal bone from the inflammatory infiltrate; resistant to inflammation and will continuously reform when bone and fibers are destroyed

Cell-to-Cell Tissue Junction

EPITHELIAL CELL-TO-CELL ATTACHMENT Electron microscopy has demonstrated that epithelial cells are held together by intercellular bridges or desmosomes. A desmosome consists of two adjacent attachment plaques, which are continuous with the innermost leaflet of the cell membrane (Figure 1–10 ■). A space exists between adjacent desmosomes, allowing passage of material and fluid through the tissue while holding together epithelial cells. Junctional epithelium has four times fewer desmosomes than oral epithelium, so the intercellular spaces are wider.

EPITHELIUM-TOOTH SURFACE/CONNECTIVE TISSUE INTERFACE The junctional epithelium adheres to the tooth surface (e.g., enamel) through the epithelial attachment. The basal cells of the junctional epithelium do not contact the enamel or the connective tissue directly. Instead, between the junctional epithelium and the tooth and connective tissue is a basal lamina and hemidesmosomes (Stern, 1965; see also Figure 1–10). The basal lamina and the hemidesmosomes are referred to as the epithelial attachment, and it provides the attachment of the junctional epithelium to the tooth surface as seen under the electron microscope.

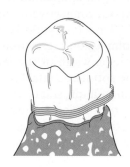
(a) Circular fibers

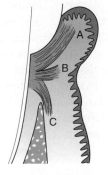
(b) Dentogingival fibers

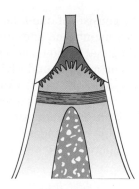
(c) Transseptal fibers

FIGURE 1–9 The major component of the connective tissue of the free and attached gingivae is composed of collagen fibers that are arranged in groups or bundles. The name indicates the origin and insertion of the fibers: circular fibers, dentogingival fibers, dentoperiosteal fibers, and transseptal fibers.

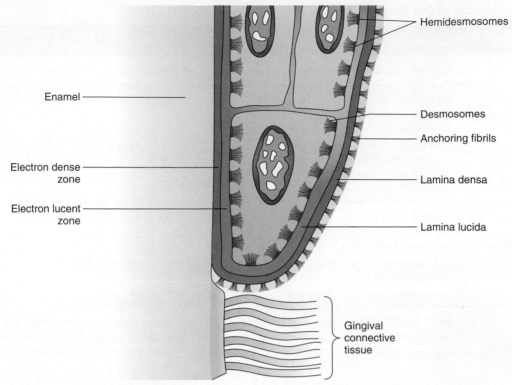

Enamel

Electron dense zone

Electron lucent zone

Hemidesmosomes

Desmosomes

Anchoring fibrils

Lamina densa

Lamina lucida

Gingival connective tissue

FIGURE 1–10 Schematic illustration showing the attachment of the junctional epithelium to the tooth surface and the underlying connective tissue and enamel. The electron-dense zone is a continuation of the lamina densa; the electron-lucent zone is a continuation of the lamina lucida; anchoring fibrils radiate out into the lamina propria. The cell membrane of the epithelial cells harbor hemidesmosomes toward the enamel and the connective tissue. Adjacent epithelial cell membranes also harbor desmosomes, which hold epithelial cells together.

The epithelial attachment is not synonymous with junctional epithelium, which refers to the entire epithelium. The basal lamina has an outer electron-lucent (lighter) zone called the lamina lucida and an inner electron-dense (darker) zone called the lamina densa. The basal lamina is continuous around the base of the junctional epithelium. These structures lie in a sandwich-like arrangement, one on top of the other.

A hemidesmosome consists of one attachment plaque continuous with the cell membrane and attaches the epithelial (basal) cell to the basal lamina. This in turn attaches to the enamel on one side and the underlying connective tissue on the other side (see Figure 1–10). Connective tissue fibers called anchoring fibrils attach the lamina densa to the underlying connective tissue. This same structural relationship also exists between the oral and sulcular epithelium, where a basal lamina separates the epithelium from the connective tissue.

Dentogingival Unit

The **dentogingival unit** collectively refers to the epithelial attachment and the gingival connective tissue attachment (gingival fibers) to the cementum, both of which are involved in the stabilization of the gingiva to the tooth. Of the two types of attachment, the gingival connective tissue (gingival fibers) forms a firmer one, supporting the epithelium and probably inhibiting movement of the epithelium apically (Bartold & Narayana, 2006).

The combined length of the dentogingival unit has been described in the literature as the **biologic width** (Figure 1–11 ■). A study using human cadaver models determined that the components of the biologic width included the junctional epithelium with a mean length of 0.97 mm and gingival connective tissue attachment with a mean length of 1.07 mm (Gargiulo, Wentz, & Orban, 1961). This soft-tissue dimension is essential to maintaining gingival health. Biologic width or the length (coronalapical dimension) of the soft tissue attachments becomes important during periodontal-prosthetic (restorative) treatment. The margin of a restoration should not disturb the biologic width. Thus, the margin of a restoration should not be closer than 2 mm to the alveolar bone crest.

FORMATION OF THE DENTOGINGIVAL UNIT The formation of the dentogingival unit has important clinical implications during the periodontal evaluation and in the healing of the gingiva after periodontal treatment. After completion of the enamel, the ameloblasts produce the primary enamel cuticle

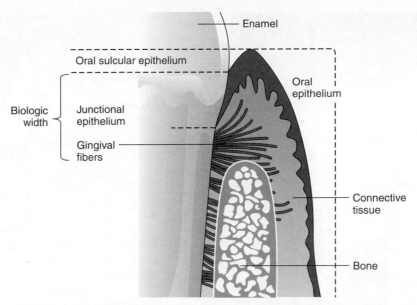

FIGURE 1–11 Schematic illustration of the biologic width includes the length of the junctional epithelium (0.97 mm) and the gingival connective tissue attachment (1.07 mm).

Rapid Dental Hint

Biologic width is important when evaluating a tooth for a crown. There must be an adequate amount of biologic width (soft tissue attachment) for periodontal health. Look at the radiograph to determine the amount of space between the CEJ and the crest of bone.

as their last function before they degenerate and become part of the reduced enamel epithelium. It disappears as the reduced ameloblasts are replaced by the junctional epithelium (secondary epithelial attachment). At the time of tooth eruption, the enamel is still covered with reduced enamel epithelium, which is connected to the enamel by the primary enamel cuticle. As tooth eruption occurs, the reduced enamel epithelium fuses with the oral epithelium at the base of the sulcus, forming the junctional epithelium. The reduced enamel epithelium forms the lining of the gingival sulcus. The junctional epithelium produces another cuticle between itself and the enamel called the secondary cuticle, which holds the junctional epithelium in close proximity to the tooth. While the tooth erupts into occlusion, the junctional epithelium gradually moves apically down the crown exposing it. Several stages occur during this passive eruption process. Eventually, the junctional epithelium ends at the cementoenamel junction. With gingival inflammation, the junctional epithelium also migrates onto the cementum, while the *base of the sulcus remains located on the enamel*, at the cementoenamel junction or on the root surface. In other words, the base of the epithelial attachment of the gingiva is at the cementoenamel junction in health and gingivitis. This situation changes in periodontitis, where the junctional epithelium migrates apically along the root surface. This concept of attachment level is important when performing periodontal probing and monitoring periodontal disease progression.

Attachment Apparatus

The periodontal ligament, cementum, and alveolar and supporting bone constitute the attachment apparatus (Figure 1–12 ■). The function of these tissues is to support and anchor the teeth within the alveolar process (Hassell, 1993).

Rapid Dental Hint

Attachment level refers to the level of attachment of the junctional epithelium to the tooth surface. When probing, this attachment level is what is actually being measured. In periodontal disease, this attachment of the junctional epithelium is "lost" or moves laterally away from the tooth and apically onto the root surface (the term for this is "attachment loss"), thus creating a periodontal pocket where the probing depth will be deeper.

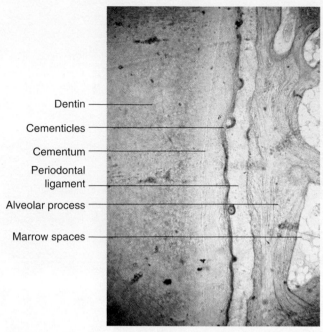

Dentin

Cementicles

Cementum

Periodontal ligament

Alveolar process

Marrow spaces

FIGURE 1–12 Photomicrograph of the attachment apparatus. (Courtesy of Dr. Harvey Wishe, New York University College of Dentistry.)

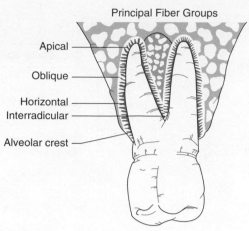

Principal Fiber Groups

Apical

Oblique

Horizontal
Interradicular

Alveolar crest

FIGURE 1–13 Schematic diagram showing the location of the periodontal ligament between the alveolar bone proper and the root cementum. The tooth is joined to the bone by bundles of collagen fibers, which can be divided into the following main groups: alveolar crest fibers, horizontal fibers, oblique fibers, interradicular fibers, and apical fibers.

Periodontal Ligament

The connective tissue that extends from the cementum covering the root surface to the alveolar bone is termed the periodontal ligament. This connective tissue is continuous with the gingival connective tissue. The periodontal ligament is primarily composed of collagen fibers and islands of loose connective tissue, creating interstitial spaces where blood vessels, nerves, lymphatics, and cells are embedded in a ground substance (Beertsen, McCulloch, & Sodek, 1997). The primary cell of the periodontal ligament is the fibroblast, which synthesizes collagen, collagenase, and ground substance. On one side of the periodontal ligament is the alveolar bone, where osteoblasts reside and are involved in bone formation. The other side of the periodontal ligament is the cementum, where cementoblasts reside and are involved in the formation of cementum.

CONNECTIVE TISSUE ATTACHMENT: PERIODONTAL LIGA-MENT The primary component of the periodontal ligament is collagen fibers. The fibers are arranged in groups or bundles that blend into one another and are collectively called the principal fibers (see Figure 1–13 ■). This constitutes the second type of connective tissue. The principal fibers are a continuation of the gingival fibers or gingival connective tissue attachment (the other type of connective tissue attachment) in the gingiva and are also named according to their direction of insertion and location. Table 1–2 ■ reviews the principal fiber groups (Hassell, 1993). The ends of the fibers, which are embedded into alveolar bone and cementum, are termed Sharpey's fibers. The first principal fibers formed before the tooth erupts are the alveolar crest fibers. With definitive tooth-to-tooth contact, the oblique fibers mature.

Eventually, with the formation of the apical fibers, the periodontal ligament is established. Because the periodontal ligament contains few elastic fibers, it is the wavy configuration of the principal fibers that permits slight movement of the tooth under function (tooth-to-tooth contact).

Collagen turnover time is five times faster in the periodontal ligament than in bone or gingiva because of the greater functional demands placed on it. Besides containing collagen, different types of cells are also present in the periodontal ligament, including fibroblasts (make and resorb collagen), cementoblasts (make cementum), cementoclasts (cementum resorption), osteoblasts (make bone), and osteoclasts (resorb bone).

PERIODONTAL LIGAMENT SPACE Although the width of the periodontal ligament varies from tooth to tooth and from different areas on the same tooth, the average width is approximately 0.25 mm. Seen radiographically, a tooth that has heavy occlusal loads placed on it for long periods of time will have a thicker periodontal ligament space. A tooth that is not in function, such as a tooth without an antagonist, will have a narrower periodontal ligament space.

Functions of the Periodontal Ligament

The periodontal ligament functions include the following:

- Suspensory: Acts like a suspensory mechanism attaching the tooth to the alveolar bone.
- Shock absorption: Acts as a shock absorber transmitting occlusal forces to the alveolar bone. Axial-placed forces, which are parallel to the long axis of the tooth, are more easily absorbed than lateral or rotational forces.

Table 1–2 Classification of the Principal Fiber Groups of the Periodontal Ligament

Name of Fiber Bundle	Direction	Function	Features
Alveolar crest	Originates from the cementum and runs apically to insert into the alveolar crest	Resists lateral movement of the tooth and keeps tooth in its socket	The first fibers to be formed before tooth eruption has occurred
Horizontal	Originates from cementum and runs at right angles and inserts into bone	Opposes lateral forces	The second fibers to be formed as soon as the first tooth-to-tooth contact has occurred
Oblique	Found in the middle third of the root apical to the horizontal fibers; originates from cementum and runs coronally and diagonally into bone	Absorbs occlusal forces	The most abundant and thus the principal attachment of the tooth
Apical	Originates from cementum of the apex of the root, spreading out apically and laterally into bone	Resists tipping of the tooth	One of the last fibers to form
Interradicular	From the crest of the interradicular septum extending to the cementum in the furcation area	Resists the forces of luxation (pulling out) and tipping	Lost when bone is destroyed in the furcation area in disease

- Remodeling: Serves a remodeling function by providing cells that are involved in the formation and resorption of cementum and bone and itself.
- Formative: Carries a blood supply to the rest of the periodontium for nutrition.
- Sensory: Transmits tactile pressure and pain perception via the trigeminal nerve.
- Proprioceptive: Allows the feeling of localization of pain and pressure to be transmitted through proprioceptive nerve endings (e.g., trigeminal nerve) found in the periodontal ligament. For example, when biting into a hard object, the mouth quickly opens. This quick reflex sensation is a function of the periodontal ligament. The greatest amount of sensory receptors is found in the apical area.

ABNORMALITIES   Histologically, besides collagen fibers, clusters of epithelial cells are found within the periodontal ligament. These clusters are called epithelial rests of Malassez. Epithelial rests of Malassez are considered to be remains of epithelium of Hertwig's epithelial root sheath, which plays an important role in the development of the cementum and the shape of the roots. Their presence and function are controversial, but they may play a role in the formation of dental cysts.

Cementicles are calcified bodies of cementum seen in the periodontal ligament of older adults (see Figure 1–12). Either they are attached to the cementum, embedded within the cementum, or not associated with the root. It is unknown if cementicles present any clinical significance.

Cementum

The cementum is a layer of mineralized tissue covering the root of the tooth and is composed of collagen, ground substance, cells, and calcium and phosphate in the form of hydroxyapatite. The primary function of the cementum is to attach the principal fibers to the root surface.

The cementum is a product of the periodontal ligament and forms in layers or increments. As a layer of uncalcified cementoid forms, adjacent cementoblasts found in the periodontal ligament stop producing. When the layer of cementoid becomes 80% to 90% calcified, more cementoid is laid down. Therefore, the cementum is never fully calcified. Cementoid serves a protective function, resisting resorption. Sharpey's fibers are embedded into cementoid allowing for repositioning of the tooth in response to biting forces.

Did You Know?

The periodontal ligament is like a shock absorber on a car. It takes the bumps and pressure from biting and chewing.

Rapid Dental Hint

Remember that cementum does not contain nerves or blood vessels. When a patient complains of sensitivity to cold, take a look at the tooth. Usually, there is gingival recession, and the exposed tooth structure is not cementum, but dentin.

The surface of the cementum is soft and relatively permeable, allowing bacterial by-products and toxins to easily penetrate the cemental surface. However, it is now recognized that the toxins are actually not as deeply penetrated into the root surface as was once thought (Nakib, Bissada, Simmelink, & Goldstine, 1982). The cementum is avascular and does not contain lymph vessels or nerves.

RELATIONSHIP OF CEMENTUM AND ENAMEL The relationship of the cementum to the enamel margin varies (Figure 1–14 ■). In 60% to 65% of the population, the cementum overlaps the enamel. In 30% of the population, the cementum meets exactly with the enamel in an edge-to-edge relationship, and in 5% to 10% of the population, the cementum and enamel do not meet, and the dentin is exposed, leaving an area of possible sensitivity.

TYPES OF CEMENTUM Two kinds of cementum are identified under the light microscope. Acellular cementum, which is formed before tooth eruption, is found on the coronal two-thirds of the root and is approximately 0.1 mm in thickness, with the cementoenamel junction being the thinnest area. Because a cellular cementum does not contain cementocytes, it is not involved in the laying down of new cementum. Cellular cementum, which covers the apical third of the root and furcations, has a thickness of about 0.5 mm and is formed much faster than acellular cementum. Cellular cementum can be laid down on top of acellular cementum, or it can comprise the entire thickness of the cementum.

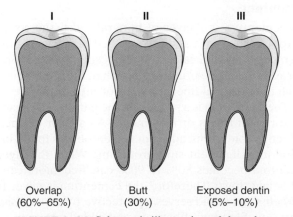

I	II	III
Overlap (60%–65%)	Butt (30%)	Exposed dentin (5%–10%)

FIGURE 1–14 Schematic illustration of the relationships of the cementum to the enamel at the cementoenamel junction.

PHYSIOLOGIC FEATURES As teeth wear down (attrition) on either the occlusal surface or incisal edge, there is a compensatory deposition of cellular cementum in the apical area in addition to deposition of bone at the alveolar crest and in the socket. This acts to maintain the vertical dimension of the face and maintain the length of the root. Instead of remodeling (resorption and deposition) like bone, cementum is deposited continuously. Cementum thickens with increasing age, but the production of cementum slows.

Cementum does not resorb as readily as bone due to its avascularity and protective layer of cementoid. This property makes orthodontic movement possible without normally resorbing the roots. However, cementum can be resorbed under certain circumstances such as inappropriate orthodontic movement, cysts, tumors, trauma, replanted teeth, periapical disease, and periodontal disease or for no known reason. Therefore, instead of resorption followed by deposition, a new layer of cementum is formed on the most superficial or oldest layer.

ABNORMALITIES Hypercementosis is a condition characterized by an atypical thickening of the cementum. It may be localized to one tooth due to factors such as excessive and rapid orthodontic movement, or it may result from excessive occlusal force placed on a tooth.

Alveolar Process

The alveolar process constitutes that part of the maxilla and mandible that forms and supports the sockets or alveoli of the teeth. Periosteum is connective tissue that covers the outer surface of the alveolar process and is well supplied with blood vessels and nerves, some of which enter the bone. Endosteum covers the inner surface of the alveolar process facing the tooth surface.

PARTS OF THE ALVEOLAR PROCESS There are two parts to the alveolar process: the alveolar bone proper and the supporting bone. It is important to distinguish between the alveolar process and the alveolar bone proper. The alveolar bone proper or cribriform plate is hard compact bone that lines the tooth socket, which is contained within the alveolar process (Figure 1–15 ■). Radiographically, it is referred to as the lamina dura (Figure 1–16 ■). The bone where Sharpey's fibers terminate is called bundle bone and is found at the inner surface of the tooth socket. The cribriform plates are thin plates of bone that is perforated by numerous openings that carry blood, nerves, and lymphatics from the bone to the periodontal ligament.

The supporting bone is composed of two parts: compact bone and cancellous bone (also called spongy or trabecular bone). Compact bone, which covers the alveolar process, consists of buccal (outer) and lingual (inner) cortical plates that are continuous with the cribriform plate. The buccal and lingual cortical plates vary in thickness. Generally, the cortical plate is thicker in the mandible than in the maxilla. In the maxilla, the compact bone is thicker

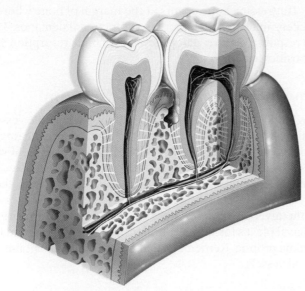

FIGURE 1–15 A section through the mandible after removal of all teeth. The thin bone lining the tooth socket (cribriform plate or alveolar bone proper) is clearly seen. (Source: BSIP SA / Alamy).

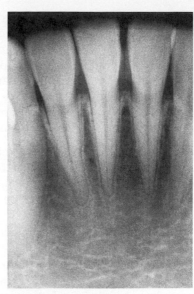

FIGURE 1–16 Radiographic appearance of the lamina dura. The lamina dura is a radiopaque (white) line around the roots of the teeth and the alveolar crest.

on the palatal than on the buccal surfaces. In the mandible, the bone is thicker in the buccal area of the premolar and molar areas and thinnest in the incisor area.

Cancellous bone fills the area between the buccal and lingual cortical plates and between the alveolar bone proper of adjacent teeth. There may be little or no cancellous bone when there is close root proximity of adjacent teeth. In these cases, the interdental septum is thin and the alveolar bone proper is fused with the cortical plate of bone.

MORPHOLOGY The cortical plate of bone covering the roots of the teeth is called radicular bone. Interradicular bone is found between roots of the same teeth (e.g., bi- and trifurcation areas of multirooted teeth). The interdental septum or interproximal bone consists of the cribriform plate of two adjacent teeth and some cancellous bone. The alveolar bone crest is the most coronal part of the alveolar bone. It is where the outer cortical plate is continuous with and fuses with the cribriform plate. At this area cancellous bone is absent.

Alveolar Bone Crest. The shape of the alveolar bone crest is influenced by the width of the interdental space, stage of eruption, position of the teeth in the arch, and shape of the cementoenamel junction. By following the contour of the cementoenamel junction, the alveolar bone crest is relatively flat in the posterior and more convex and pointed in the anterior. In health, the shape of bone takes on a form where the alveolar bone crest is more coronal than the radicular bone. The slope of the alveolar bone crest follows an imaginary parallel line connecting the cementoenamel junction of adjacent teeth (Ritchey & Orban, 1953) and is approximately 2 mm apical to it if the biologic width is taken into consideration (Figure 1–17 ▪), but this relationship may vary.

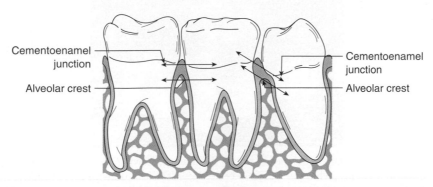

Cementoenamel junction

Alveolar crest

Cementoenamel junction

Alveolar crest

FIGURE 1–17 The alveolar crest is parallel to a line connecting the cemento-enamel junctions of adjacent teeth, even when a tooth is tilted and the cementoenamel junction on one tooth may be lower than the adjacent tooth.

COMPOSITION OF BONE The alveolar process is primarily composed of collagen fibers and cells embedded in a ground substance (proteoglycans), which make up the organic component. The inorganic salts of bone are principally calcium and phosphate. The salts allow bone to withstand compression. The combination of fibers and salts makes bone exceptionally strong without being brittle. The cells present in the alveolar and supporting bone are the following:

- Osteoblasts, which synthesize and secrete bone
- Osteocytes, which are osteoblasts that are embedded within lacunae as bone is being laid down
- Osteoclasts, which destroy or resorb bone

METABOLISM Despite its rigid physical characteristic, bone is a vascular tissue and the least stable of all the periodontal tissues. There is a constant remodeling with formation and resorption of bone due to the functional demand placed on it. This occurs more rapidly in cancellous than compact bone. The normal remodeling of bone occurs by resorption by osteoclasts followed by deposition by osteoblasts. During orthodontic movement, bone is resorbed on the pressure side and laid down on the tension side.

VARIATIONS IN ANATOMY Roots of teeth are usually contained entirely within the alveolar bony plates. Frequently, the bone may not completely encircle prominent roots of teeth that are rotated, in facioversion, in lingoversion, tipped, or crowded. The resulting defects take the form of windows (fenestrations) where the radicular cortical bone is lost except for the most coronal edge or clefts (dehiscences) where the cortical bone, including the marginal bone (most coronal edge of bone), is lost over the root (Figure 1–18 ■). The etiology of these defects is not definitive. These defects occur more frequently on facial bone than on lingual bone.

Buttressing bone occurs at the margin of bone where it thickens in response to increased functional demands. This is a response to the repair process, with bone resorption and deposition occurring.

Physiology of the Periodontium

The blood to the gingiva is primarily supplied by the vessels of the periosteum (supraperiosteal), periodontal ligament, and alveolar bone (Figure 1–19 ■). The supraperiosteal vessels run along the facial and lingual surfaces of the alveolar bone and give off many little branches as they make their way toward the gingiva. These finally join with blood vessels of the alveolar bone and periodontal ligament to form a gingival plexus located just under the oral epithelium in the laminia propria. Remember that the epithelium contains no blood vessels.

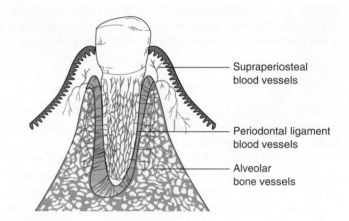

Supraperiosteal blood vessels

Periodontal ligament blood vessels

Alveolar bone vessels

FIGURE 1–19 The blood supply to the periodontium comes from three sources: (1) supraperiosteal blood vessels, (2) blood vessels from the periodontal ligament, and (3) blood vessels of the alveolar process.

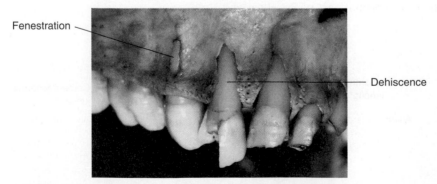

Fenestration

Dehiscence

FIGURE 1–18 Dry skull specimen of a dehiscence showing loss of radicular cortical bone involving the marginal bone and a fenestration with loss of radicular bone but not involving the marginal bone.

The inferior and superior alveolar arteries supplying the periodontal ligament originate from the apical foramen, the alveolar bone, and the gingiva.

The blood supply to the cortical bone is via branches of the supraperiosteal blood vessels. The vessels that enter the interdental septum, in addition to the vessels that supply the remainder of the alveolar bone, supply blood to the cancellous bone.

Lymphatic drainage from the gingiva starts in the papillae of the connective tissue and drains into the regional lymph nodes, primarily the submandibular nodes. The lymphatic vessels follow the course of the blood vessels. The submandibular lymph nodes also drain lymph fluid from the tongue, submaxillary salivary gland, lips, and mouth. The submental lymph nodes drain lymph fluid from the tip of the tongue, incisor teeth, central part of the lower lip, and floor of the mouth.

The nerves supplying the periodontium branch off from the trigeminal nerve (fifth cranial nerve). The nerves follow the course of the blood vessels that supply blood to the periodontium. Gingival branches of the anterior superior alveolar nerve innervate the gingiva overlying the maxillary incisors and canines. The gingival branches of the middle superior alveolar nerve supply the gingiva around the maxillary premolars. The posterior superior alveolar nerve supplies the gingiva around the maxillary molars.

The gingival branches of the inferior alveolar nerve supply the facial gingiva of the mandibular incisors, canines, premolars, and molars. The mental nerve supplies the mandibular facial gingiva of the incisors, canines, and premolars. The gingival branches of the buccal nerve supply the facial gingiva of the mandibular molars. The lingual nerve supplies the mandibular lingual gingiva.

Changes with Aging

With increasing age, certain changes in the hard- and soft-tissue components of the periodontium occur, as well as a thinning of the gingiva with reduced keratinization. The amount of stippling is either reduced or unchanged. Within the lamina propria, there is a decrease in the number of cells, and the gingival fibers become less dense. Cementum increases in thickness throughout life, with a greater deposition in the apical area in response to the continuing tooth eruption that compensates for tooth attrition. Cells within the periodontal ligament decrease in number, whereas the number of elastic fibers increases. The width of the periodontal ligament can be either increased or decreased. Changes in the alveolar bone occur with aging just as in any other bone in the body. There may be a decrease in vascularity and healing. A physiologic tendency with increasing age is for the proximal surface contacts of teeth to wear down (attrition), causing the teeth to migrate in a mesial direction (mesial drifting) while retaining tooth-to-tooth contact. Accordingly, bone is laid down on the distal surface, which is the tension side, and bone is resorbed on the mesial surface, which is the pressure side.

Dental Hygiene Application

This chapter reviewed the structure and functions of the periodontal soft and hard tissues including the gingiva, periodontal ligament, cementum, and supporting and alveolar bone. The periodontium is a dynamic, highly specialized structure that is constantly changing with the demands placed on it. Knowing the macro- and microstructure of the periodontium in health will help the hygienist to understand the process that leads to pathological destruction and subsequent treatment of the periodontal patient.

Key Points

- The attachment of the soft and hard tissues to the tooth surface contributes to the stability and health of the periodontium.
- The junctional epithelium is a semipermeable structure involved in the movement of fluids, cells, and substances from the lamina propria into the gingival crevice and vice versa.
- The dentogingival unit is involved in the attachment of the gingiva to the tooth.

- The biologic width comprises the length of the junctional epithelium and the gingival fibers.
- The biologic width is important during prosthetic treatment. There must be an adequate amount of bone from the finish line of the crown to the crest of the bone to not invade the biologic width. If the biologic width is not adequate, inflammation may occur.

Self-Quiz

1. From the following list, select the items associated with the attachment apparatus.
   a. gingiva
   b. cementum
   c. alveolar and supporting bone
   d. periodontal ligament
   e. dental pulp
   f. minor salivary glands
   g. submandibular lymph nodes

2. At which one of the following areas is the width of attached gingiva greatest?
   a. mandibular second premolars
   b. mandibular canines
   c. maxillary lateral incisors
   d. maxillary first premolars
   e. maxillary second molars

3. Which one of the following substances is the primary component of the connective tissue of the periodontium?
   a. gingival crevicular fluid
   b. calcium
   c. collagen
   d. proteoglycans

4. Which one of the following structures directly attaches the junctional epithelium to the enamel?
   a. desmosomes
   b. hemidesmosomes
   c. basal lamina
   d. gingival fibers

5. Which one of the following structures is involved in the attachment of the gingiva to the tooth surface?
   a. alveolar mucosa
   b. dentogingival unit
   c. mucogingival junction
   d. desmosomes

6. From the following list, select the items associated with biologic width.
   a. gingival sulcus
   b. sulcular epithelium
   c. junctional epithelium
   d. gingival connective tissue attachment
   e. periodontal ligament fibers
   f. crestal alveolar bone
   g. cemetum

7. From the bone structures listed, select the correct location of the structure from the list provided.

Structure	Location of Structure
1. alveolar bone proper	a. between the roots of a multi-rooted tooth
2. interradicular bone	b. lines the tooth socket
3. interdental bone	c. between roots of different teeth
4. trabecular bone	d. cancellous porous bone surrounding marrow spaces lies subjacent to cortical bone
5. radicular bone	e. covers the root of the tooth

8. From the following list, select the items associated with the junctional epithelium
   a. vascular
   b. lymph supply
   c. few cells thick
   d. contains a lamina propria
   e. surrounds the tooth
   f. continuous with the free gingiva
   g. contributes to attachment of the gingiva to the tooth

9. All of the following structures are avascular except one. Which one is the exception?
   a. enamel
   b. cementum
   c. junctional epithelium
   d. lamina propria

10. Arteries that supply blood and lymphatics to the free gingiva originate from all of the following parts of the periodontium except one. Which one is the exception?
    a. supraperiosteal
    b. periodontal ligament
    c. alveolar bone
    d. cementum

Case Study

A 55-year-old female patient complains that her gingiva between some teeth is "moving away" from the tooth. Medical history reveals she has diabetes (fasting blood glucose is 95; glycosylated hemoglobin is 6%). She has smoked one pack of cigarettes per day for the last 25 years. She does not brush or floss regularly. She was previously seen by a periodontist but did not go for regular recare appointments. Periodontal examination reveals generalized bleeding on probing with probing depths ranging from 4–6 mm. There is some tooth mobility. There is generalized heavy supra and subgingival calculus. The dentist diagnosed the case as generalized chronic moderate periodontitis.

1. What is the cause of the chief complaint?
   a. Smoking
   b. Uncontrolled diabetes
   c. Destruction of gingival fibers
   d. Resorption of alveolar bone

Answer: C. The gingiva is held in close proximity to the tooth by the presence of gingival fiber or connective gingival attachment. The gingival fibers include circular, dentogingival, and transeptal fibers. The free gingiva is "pulled up" against the tooth surface via the circular fibers. The gingiva becomes retracted from the tooth surface when there is lateral movement of the free gingival margin away from the tooth surface. In this case, gingival retraction has occurred because of the destruction of the circular fibers that encircle the tooth keeping the free gingiva in close proximity to the tooth. Destruction of the fibers occurs due to periodontal disease whereby the collagen fibers that make up the gingival fibers are destroyed by the enzyme collagenase. Usually there are also heavy calculus deposits on the tooth. Healing occurs after debridment.

2. Which of the following tissues makes up the margin and lateral borders of the interdental papillae?
   a. Junctional epithelium
   b. Connective tissue
   c. Free gingiva
   d. Col area

Answer C. The margin and lateral borders of the interdental gingival are an extension of the free gingiva, whereas the remaining parts are attached gingival.

3. What other structure, besides the gingival fibers, is responsible for holding the gingiva against the tooth?
   a. Epithelial attachment
   b. Connective tissue papillae
   c. Alveolar mucosa
   d. Sulcular epithelium

Answer A: The junctional epithelium, through the epithelial attachment, contributes to the attachment of the gingiva to the tooth surface, and thus serves a significant role in periodontal health and disease, when this attachment is lost.

References

Alfano, M. 1974. The origin of gingival fluid. *J. Theor. Biol.* 47:127–136.

Bartold, P. M. 2006. Periodontal tissues in health and disease. Introduction. *Periodontology 2000* 40(1):7–0.

Bartold, P. M., and A. S. Narayana. 2006. Molecular and cell biology of health and diseased periodontal tissues. *Periodontology 2000* 40(1):29–49.

Beertsen, W., C. A. G. McCulloch, and J. Sodek. 1997. The periodontal ligament: A unique, multifunctional connective tissue. *Periodontology 2000* 13:20–40.

Gargiulo, A., F. Wentz, and B. Orban. 1961. Dimensions and relations of the dento-gingival junction in humans. *J. Periodontol.* 32:261–267.

Goldman, H. M. 1951. The topography and role of the gingival fibers. *J. Dent. Res.* 30:331–336.

Gordon, J. M., C. B. Walker, J. C. Murphy, J. M. Goodson, and S. S. Socransky. 1981. Tetracycline: Levels achievable in gingival crevice fluid and in vitro effect on subgingival organisms. Part 1. Concentrations in crevicular fluid after repeated doses. *J. Periodontol.* 52:609–612.

Hassell, T. M. 1993. Tissues and cells of the periodontium. *Periodontology 2000* 3:9–38.

Kornman, K., R. Page, and M. Tonetti. 1997. The host response to the microbial challenge in periodontitis: Assembling the players. *Periodontology 2000* 14:33–53.

Moss-Salentijn, L., and M. Hendricks-Klyvert. 1990. Oral mucosa-epithelium. In eds. L. Moss-Salentijn & M. Hendricks-Klyvert, *Dental and oral tissues*, 27–44. Philadelphia: Lea & Febiger.

Mukherjee, S. 1985. The significance of crevicular fluid. *Compendium Cont. Educ. Dent.* 6:611–616.

Nakib, N., N. M. Bissada, J. W. Simmelink, and S. N. Goldstine. 1982. Endotoxin penetration into root cementum of periodontally healthy and diseased human teeth. *J. Periodontol.* 53:368–378.

Nanci, A., and D. D. Bosshardt. 2006. Structure of periodontal tissues in health and disease. *Periodontology 2000* 40(1):11–28.

Ritchey, B., and B. Orban. 1953. The crests of the interdental alveolar septa. *J. Periodontol.* 24:75–87.

Schroeder, H. E. 1991. Oral mucosa. In ed. H. E. Schroeder, *Oral structural biology*, 350–391. Stuttgart and New York: Georg Thieme Verlag.

Schroeder, H. E., and M. A. Listgarten. 1997. The gingival tissues: The architecture of periodontal protection. *Periodontology 2000* 13:91–120.

Squier, C. A., and M. W. Hill. 1998. Oral mucosa. In ed. A. R. Ten Cate, *Oral histology*. St. Louis, MO: Mosby.

Stern, I. B. 1965. Electron microscopic observations of oral epithelium I. Basal cells and the basement membrane. *Periodontics* 3:224–238.

Tonetti, M. S., M. Imboden, I. L. Gerber, and N. P. Lang. 1995. Compartmentalization of inflammatory cell phenotypes in normal gingiva and peri-implant keratinized mucosa. *J. Clin. Periodontol.* 22:735–742.

Visit www.pearsonhighered.com/healthprofessionsresources to access the student resources that accompany this book. Simply select Dental Hygiene from the choice of disciplines. Find this book and you will find the complimentary study tools created for this specific title.

Epidemiology of Periodontal Diseases

Mary Elizabeth and Aichelmann-Reidy

OUTLINE

Introduction and Definitions
Indices
Accuracy of Methodology
Prevalence of Periodontal Diseases
Incidence and Disease Progression
Epidemiologic Variables
Treatment Needs
Future Trends
Dental Hygiene Application
Key Points
Self-Quiz
Case Study
References

EDUCATIONAL OBJECTIVES

Upon completion of this chapter, the reader should be able to:

- Describe epidemiology and its descriptive terms: prevalence, incidence, extent, and severity.
- Explain the significance of epidemiologic data to future treatment.
- Describe the role of indices in private practice and population surveys.
- Describe the prevalence and incidence of periodontal diseases.
- Identify risk factors and risk indicators for periodontal diseases.
- Discuss future periodontal treatment needs and future trends that may have an impact on dental hygiene practice.

GOAL: To provide an understanding of the prevalence, extent, and severity of periodontal diseases in the population.

KEY WORDS

Introduction and Definitions

Epidemiology is the study of health and disease in the human population. The rationale for the study of epidemiology is to identify events and **risk factors** in populations that lead to disease so that future health problems can be anticipated, prevented, and controlled. A risk factor is an event or characteristic associated with a given disease. It is important to identify risk factors so that healthcare measures can target people at risk for a particular disease, perhaps altering the future course of the disease (Raul & Dietrich 2012; American Academy of Periodontology, 2005a). It is important to note that risk is not causative.

Epidemiologic studies focus on populations rather than individuals. Much of what we know about **periodontal diseases** comes from national or **population surveys**. Population surveys evaluate representative samples of individuals within a study population to assess the true risk for disease and quantify how many individuals are or will be affected by disease. This quantification of disease is referred to as disease **prevalence** and **incidence**. Prevalence is the proportion or number of individuals in a population having the disease (both old and new cases) at a given time. Incidence is defined as the rate of new cases occurring within a certain period of time. Disease prevalence and incidence can only be understood by looking at a large number of individuals within a population. Population surveys also provide insight into the severity and extent of a particular disease, say, periodontal disease, in populations. **Severity** is defined as the degree or amount of periodontal disease involvement and quantifies the amount of attachment loss, bone loss, or probing depth (Oliver, Brown, & Löe, 1998). The **extent** of periodontal disease refers to the number or percentage of diseased teeth or sites per individual.

Epidemiologic research is used to detect the underlying patterns of a disease and its associated factors to help find the cause of the disease. Trends are detectable when data collected from large numbers of individuals within a study population are combined. For a survey to be useful, the clinical assessments must be standardized so that population means (averages) can be determined.

Epidemiologic data are collected through the use of a specific methodology that differs from patient evaluations in private practice. Complete, full-mouth periodontal examinations, which are necessary to establish an individual's diagnosis and to determine treatment needs, are too time-consuming for use on a large scale in an epidemiologic survey. The survey methods used to evaluate periodontal diseases in a population usually involve screening tools designed to quantify and simplify the disease assessment. These tools are referred to as **indices** (singular: index). An index is a numerical expression of values, with upper and lower limits, that is used to describe a specific condition. Indices are used in both clinical practice and research as the system of measurement for collecting data. They provide the private practitioner with information for patient treatment planning and the researcher with information about the prevalence and incidence of disease.

Indices

Significance of Indices

Epidemiology is used to identify disease patterns, and indices are the measurement systems used for collecting the necessary data. For the study of periodontal diseases, assessments of plaque, calculus, gingival inflammation, periodontal attachment level, bleeding, and mobility are necessary to determine individual disease status. An index is a tool for standardized data collection and can measure the presence, absence, or severity of a disease condition on a specific tooth, area, or whole mouth and then can be extrapolated to the population. Unlike subjective clinician assessments of parameters of disease, an index is a numerical expression given to conditions that can then be quantified, tabulated, and used in comparisons to predict disease patterns, progression, and trends in study populations.

If a dental hygienist examines a patient and subjectively describes the condition of oral cleanliness in the mouth as "a fair amount of plaque and calculus on the teeth," this description could be interpreted differently by another clinician and might be interpreted as light or moderate plaque levels. Terms such as fair, light, moderate, and heavy have different meaning for different practitioners and therefore need to be standardized. The use of indices can help to standardize and reproduce findings for the purpose of assessment and monitoring patients' progression in private practice.

Dentists and dental hygienists formulate treatment plans based on full-mouth data collection. Becoming aware of the periodontal problem, assessing its severity, and presenting the findings to the patient require the practitioner to record and chart data in formats that can be compared over time. Periodontal charting forms and indices tabulate the measurements to be interpreted for treatment plans.

Criteria for Indices

There are many types of indices a practitioner can select from, depending on the specific method of data collection and the meaning to be given to the data collected. When selecting an index or set of indices, the following properties should be considered.

- Simplicity or ease of use is critical to provide a fast and reproducible method to collect the data. Reproducibility creates a reliable instrument that can be used by different examiners or the same examiner over time to produce the same results.
- The index should be quick to perform and practical. Whether in the field for research purposes or in a dental practice, the method of data collection must not be time consuming, be costly, or involve many instruments.
- Sensitivity requires the index to detect small changes. Sensitivity determines if the disease is really present and can be seen. A true-positive result (e.g., the

Rapid Dental Hint

Indices are important for patient assessment because indices are intended to be reproducible by other clinicians. Therefore, other clinicians that perform the same index that you do will obtain the same results.

Did You Know?

Oral biofilm deposits are closely correlated with gingivitis, a relationship long considered one of cause and effect.

patient has the condition and tests positive for the condition) would indicate that the disease or condition exists. A true-negative result is when the individual does not have the disease and the test results are negative for the disease. A false-positive is when the individual does not have the condition but the test results are positive for that condition.

- Validity provides the correlation of the disease with the measure employed. If bleeding on probing is to be measured, then the index can be confounded by other variables such as probing pressure, spontaneous bleeding, or instrumentation differences. A valid index must measure what it is intended to measure.
- Reliability describes the consistency of a set of measurements. It is the extent to which the indices remain constant over repeated testing of the same subject.
- Risks that are involved in participation should be acceptable to subjects.
- Indices should be amenable to statistical analysis that allows the results of the index to be interpreted through statistics.
- Indices should be clinically significant and meaningful to researchers.

There is no perfect index or one that assesses all categories of inquiry. There are numerous indices, and the practitioner must select the best ones to represent the disease under examination or the health of the patient. There are over 40 types of indices in periodontics. They fall into four general categories: oral hygiene indices (plaque, debris, and calculus), gingival indices, periodontal (destruction) indices, and treatment needs indices. An overview of historically important and commonly used indices is presented in Table 2–1 ■ and is reviewed briefly.

Plaque (Biofilm) and Debris Indices

Oral cleanliness is quantified by indices that measure plaque and debris and indices that measure calculus. Because bacterial plaque is considered a risk factor of periodontal diseases, methods of measuring plaque (or debris) are important epidemiologically and are useful to practitioners treating the disease. Many plaque indices are used today. Some are meant simply as screening tools in clinical practice to assess home-care practices, whereas others are designed to quantify and locate plaque as needed for the evaluation of plaque-control devices or products before and after use.

One of the simplest methods of monitoring patient plaque levels is the use of the O'Leary Plaque Index (O'Leary, Drake, & Naylor, 1972), also called the plaque control record. This index merely indicates the presence of plaque and is most suited for patient education and motivation in private practice rather than epidemiologic surveys.

A visual record of plaque control is made using a disclosing agent. A diagram is made of plaque-covered surfaces that can be shared with patients to visually help them identify problem areas and focus their efforts at home. O'Leary and colleagues (1972) recommended reduction of plaque levels to 10% of the available tooth surfaces as the patient's goal for home-care mastery.

Other common plaque indices are the Plaque Index (PlI; Silness & Löe, 1964), the Debris Index (DI-S) of the Simplified Oral Hygiene Index (Greene, 1967), and the modified Quigley-Hein Plaque Index (Turesky, Gilmore, & Glickman, 1970). These plaque indices provide numerical values that quantify the amount of plaque present, unlike the O'Leary Index.

The Plaque Index (PlI; Silness & Löe, 1964) scores the plaque thickness along the gingival margin of the tooth, whereas the Debris Index (DI-S) measures plaque surface area. The Debris Index is a component of the Simplified Oral Hygiene Index (OHI-S) developed by Greene and Vermillion (1964). The other component of the OHI-S is a Calculus Index (CI-S). The OHI-S is used primarily for epidemiologic and longitudinal dental studies.

Another plaque index used more specifically for clinical trials is the Turesky Modification of the Quigley-Hein Index (Turesky et al., 1970). Plaque is assessed on all facial and lingual tooth surfaces (excluding third molars) after a disclosing agent is applied. The additional scoring categories of this index allow researchers to quantify improvement or change in plaque levels after the use of a plaque-control device or topical antimicrobial. Both the modified Quigley-Hein Index and the Plaque Index (PlI) are suitable for the evaluation of topical antimicrobials and plaque-removal devices (Fischman, 1986).

In summary, a number of plaque indices are used today. Four plaque indices were presented, and each serves different purposes. The plaque control record (O'Leary et al., 1972) is used most commonly in periodontal practice, whereas the others are used more frequently in clinical trials and population surveys.

Table 2–1 Indices Used for Periodontal Disease Assessments

Index	Type of Evaluation	Teeth Measured	Method of Measurement	Scale of Measurement	Purpose	Advantages	Disadvantages	Uses
O'Leary (O'Leary, Drake, & Naylor, 1972)	Plaque	All teeth are scored at the cervical third of the tooth. Four surfaces of each tooth (M,B,D,L,) are measured.	A plaque record is made by marking a tooth diagram with the surface location of plaque. Mark each tooth surface with plaque as positive (disclosing agent used).	Calculation: Surfaces with plaque divided by the total number of surfaces. Multiply by 100 to get the percent of surfaces with plaque. Patient goal of 10% or less of plaque is ideal.	Visual record of plaque distribution; shows patients where they are insufficient in plaque removal; patient motivation.	Complete assessment of all tooth surfaces to determine areas of cleaning deficiency.	Will not pick up changes in plaque quantity at each tooth surface; time consuming.	Private practice.
Plaque Index (PI; Silness & Löe, 1964)	Plaque	All teeth (distal, facial, mesial, lingual) or selected teeth.	Sweep a probe along the tooth surface at the gingival margin. (No disclosing agent is used.) The score (0, 1, 2, or 3) per tooth is obtained by summing the four different surface scores and dividing by four. Adding each tooth score and dividing by the number of teeth evaluated generates a patient score. Excellent: 0 Poor: 2.0–3.0	0: No plaque. 1: A thinly adherent layer of plaque visible only when a probe is run across the tooth. 2: A visible layer of plaque, which is thin to moderately thick. 3: Heavy plaque accumulation in the crevice and the gingival margin.	Measures the thickness or amount of plaque along the gingival margin.	Good for research purposes because qualitative changes can be measured; not as time consuming if selected teeth are used.	Limited to the cervical portion of the tooth; not for patient motivation.	Clinical studies, epidemiologic surveys.

Table 2–1 Indices Used for Periodontal Disease Assessments (continued)

Index	Type of Evaluation	Teeth Measured	Method of Measurement	Scale of Measurement	Purpose	Advantages	Disadvantages	Uses
Simplified Debris Index (DI-S) of the Simplified Oral Hygiene Index (OHI-S; Greene & Vermillion, 1964)	Soft debris	Six tooth surfaces per mouth are scored: facial surfaces of teeth nos. 3, 8, 14, and 24 and lingual surfaces of teeth nos. 19 and 30. If the first molars are missing, choose the first fully erupted tooth distal to the second premolar.	Each tooth is divided into gingival, middle, and incisal thirds. Scoring is done by moving a no. 23 explorer from the incisal third toward the gingival third of the tooth. No disclosing agent is used. Score as 0, 1, 2, or 3. Calculation: Total of surface scores divided by the number of surfaces scored. Good score: 0.0–0.6 Poor score: 1.9–3.0	0: No stain or debris. 1: Soft deposit covering ≤ 1/3 of the surface or the presence of extrinsic stain. 2: Soft deposit covering more than 1/3 but less than 2/3 of the tooth surface. 3: Soft deposit covering > 2/3 of the tooth surface.	Measures plaque surface area.	Measures the quantity of debris rather than the presence or absence; not as time-consuming.	Cannot be used subgingivally.	Epidemiologic and research projects.
Turesky Modification of the Quigley-Hein Index (Turesky, Gilmore, & Glickman, 1970)	Plaque	Facial and lingual surfaces of all teeth excluding the third molars.	Score as 0, 1, 2, 3, 4, or 5. Disclosing agent is used. Calculation: Total of all scores divided by the number of surfaces examined.	0: No plaque. 1: Flecks of plaque at the cervical margin. 2: Thin, continuous band of plaque (≤ 1 mm) at the cervical margin. 3: Band of plaque wider than 1 mm but covering less than 1/3 of crown.	Measures surface area of plaque.	The additional scoring categories allow the researcher to quantify improvement or change in plaque levels after the use of a plaque-control device or topical antimicrobial.	Well-defined criteria	Index of choice in clinical trials.

(continued)

Table 2–1 Indices Used for Periodontal Disease Assessments (continued)

Index	Type of Evaluation	Teeth Measured	Method of Measurement	Scale of Measurement	Purpose	Advantages	Disadvantages	Uses
				4: Plaque covering at least 1/3 but less than 2/3 of the crown. 5: Plaque covering more than 2/3 of the crown.				
Simplified Calculus Index (CI-S); part of the OHI-S (Greene, 1967)	Calculus	Six teeth surfaces per mouth are scored: facial surfaces of teeth nos. 3, 8, 14, and 24 and lingual surfaces of teeth nos. 19 and 30. If the first molars are missing, choose the first fully erupted tooth distal to the second premolar.	Score as 0, 1, 2, or 3. Calculation: Total calculus scores divided by the number of surfaces scored. To tabulate the total OHI-S, add the DI-S + CI-S. Combined OHI-S: Good: 0.0–1.2 Poor: 3.1–6.0	0: No calculus present. 1: Supragingival calculus covering ≤ 1/3 of the exposed tooth. 2: Supragingival calculus covering more than 1/3 but 2/3 or less of exposed tooth or separate flecks of subgingival calculus in the cervical region. 3: Supragingival calculus covering more than 2/3 of exposed tooth or a continuous heavy band of subgingival calculus.	Quantifies calculus.	Well-defined criteria, allows for interexaminer reproducibility.	Combines location and quantity.	Epidemiologic and longitudinal studies.

Table 2–1 Indices Used for Periodontal Disease Assessments (continued)

Index	Type of Evaluation	Teeth Measured	Method of Measurement	Scale of Measurement	Purpose	Advantages	Disadvantages	Uses
Volpe Manhold Calculus Assessment (Volpe, Manhold, & Hazen, 1965)	Calculus	Mandibular incisors and cuspids (lingual surfaces).	With a probe, the coronal extension of supragingival calculus is measured in millimeters. Three readings are made bisecting the dimension of calculus at the direct lingual and mesial and distal line angles. These readings are averaged to generate a tooth score, and the individual tooth scores are averaged to provide the total patient score.	Readings are scored in millimeter markings from the probe.	Measures the height or dimension of calculus.	Ability to measure the rate of calculus formation.	Difficult to master.	Clinical studies and epidemiologic studies.
Calculus Index of the National Institute of Dental Research (Miller et al., 1987)	Calculus	Mesiobuccal and midbuccal surfaces of all fully erupted permanent teeth present in two randomly selected quadrants (one mandibular and the other maxillary).	Detected by explorer or probe.	0: No calculus. 1: Supragingival calculus only (calculus on the crown and root not extending more than 1 mm below the gingival margin). 2: Subgingival calculus is detected with or without supragingival calculus.	Presence or absence and location supra- or subgingival.	Simple.	Unable to quantify amount of calculus.	Used in the National Health and Nutrition and Examination Survey (NHANES III).

(continued)

Table 2–1 Indices Used for Periodontal Disease Assessments (continued)

Index	Type of Evaluation	Teeth Measured	Method of Measurement	Scale of Measurement	Purpose	Advantages	Disadvantages	Uses
Gingival index (GI; Löe, 1967)	Gingival inflammation	Four gingival areas (buccal, mesial, distal, and lingual) for all teeth or select teeth.	Probe is inserted into the gingival crevice and moved with a sweeping along the pocket wall. Probe is also pressed lightly against the gingiva to determine its firmness. Calculation: Each of the four gingival areas per tooth is given a GI score of 0 to 3. Total the scores for each area, and divide by the number of teeth scored. Good: 0.0–1.0 Fair: 1.1–2.0 Poor: 2.1–3.0	0: Normal gingiva. 1: Mild inflammation with slight changes in color and edema (swelling); no bleeding on probing. 2: Moderate inflammation with redness, edema, and glazing; bleeding on probing. 3: Severe inflammation with marked redness and edema; tendency to spontaneously bleed.	Measures severity of gingivitis.	Can detect change in degree of inflammation.	Time consuming.	Patient education and motivation; monitors progress of disease; Epidemiologic and clinical studies.
Sulcus Bleeding Index (Mühlemann & Son, 1971)	Gingival inflammation	Four gingival areas (facial and lingual marginal gingival and mesial and distal interdental papillae) for all teeth.	Insert probe in the sulcus and withdraw it. Wait 30 seconds to score the area. Calculation: Total the scores for each tooth, and divide by the number of teeth.	0: Healthy appearance with no bleeding on probing. 1: Healthy but with bleeding on probing. 2: Bleeding on probing and color change but no swelling.	Presence or absence and severity of gingival inflammation.	More gradations of severe inflammation.	Criticized for scores beyond clinical gingivitis.	Clinical and epidemiologic studies.

Table 2–1 Indices Used for Periodontal Disease Assessments (continued)

Index	Type of Evaluation	Teeth Measured	Method of Measurement	Scale of Measurement	Purpose	Advantages	Disadvantages	Uses
				3: Bleeding on probing, color change, and slight edema. 4: Bleeding on probing and obvious swelling with or without color change. 5: Bleeding on probing and spontaneous bleeding and color change, marked swelling with or without ulceration.				
Mühlemann Papillary Bleeding Index (Saxer & Muhleman, 1975)	Bleeding, inflammation	Mesial and distal aspects of the papillae.	The maxillary right and mandibular left quadrants are probed lingually and the maxillary left and mandibular right quadrants are probed bucally	0: no bleeding after probing 1: single bleeding point 2: several bleeding points or one fine line of blood 3: interdental triangle filled with blood 4: blood flows into the sulus scores are totaled and divided by the number of paillae examined	Quantify bleeding	More sensitive than an all or nothing index; good for patient motivation	More time consuming	Clinical practice and research

(continued)

Table 2-1 Indices Used for Periodontal Disease Assessments (continued)

Index	Type of Evaluation	Teeth Measured	Method of Measurement	Scale of Measurement	Purpose	Advantages	Disadvantages	Uses
Periodontal Index (PI) (Russell, 1967)	Inflammation, pocket depth, tooth mobility (visual assessment, without periodontal probing)	All teeth.	Each tooth is given a score from 0 (no disease) to 8 (advanced disease) Calculation: Add up the scores for all teeth, and divide by the number of teeth scored. 0.0–0.2: Normal periodontal condition. 0.3–0.9: Simple gingivitis. 1.0–1.9: Early destructive periodontitis. 1.6–5.0: Established periodontitis. 3.8–8.0: Terminal disease.	0: Tooth with healthy periodontium. 1: Mild gingivitis, localized and does not involve the entire tooth. 2: Gingivitis encircling the entire tooth. 6: Gingivitis with pocket formation with no loss of function or mobility. 8: Advanced destruction with tooth mobility.	Measures the severity of the periodontal condition.	Objective measures.	Visual assessment that often underestimates disease; evaluates both gingivitis and periodontitis in the same index.	National epidemiologic surveys including the National Health and Nutrition Examination Survey (1971–1974).
Community Periodontal Index of Treatment Needs (Ainamo et al., 1982)	Periodontal pockets, calculus, gingival bleeding	Ten teeth: 2, 3, 8, 14, 15, 18, 19, 24, 30, 31.	A 0.5 mm ball-tip probe with demarcations for shallow (3.5 mm) and deep (5.5 mm) pockets (CPITN probe) is used to detect and record the presence of bleeding, calculus, and periodontal pockets.	Code 0: No pocketing or inflammation. Code 1: Bleeding on probing. Code 2: Calculus present. Code 3: Pocketing extending in to the black area of the probe (4–5 mm).	Measures severity of the periodontal condition and treatment needs.	Simple.	Only selective teeth are measured, which may underestimate the disease.	Epidemiologic surveys (specifically designed by the WHO to compare population surveys internationally).

32

Table 2–1 Indices Used for Periodontal Disease Assessments (continued)

Index	Type of Evaluation	Teeth Measured	Method of Measurement	Scale of Measurement	Purpose	Advantages	Disadvantages	Uses
			The individual is scored by sextant assigning the worst tooth score per sextant as the overall sextant score. Treatment needs are assigned based on the highest code received by each sextant. 0: No further therapy needed. 1: Patient only requires oral home-care instruction. 2: Patient requires oral hygiene improvement and professional debridement. 3: Patient requires oral hygiene improvement and professional debridement. 4: Patient requires complex treatment (scaling and root planning with dental anesthesia and may require periodontal surgery).	Code 4: Pocketing extending beyond the black area of the probe (≤ 6 mm).				

(continued)

Table 2–1 Indices Used for Periodontal Disease Assessments (continued)

Index	Type of Evaluation	Teeth Measured	Method of Measurement	Scale of Measurement	Purpose	Advantages	Disadvantages	Uses
Periodontal Screening and Recording (PSR)	Periodontal pockets, calculus, bleeding, and defective restorations	Mouth is divided into sextants. All teeth are measured.	Each tooth in the sextant is probed, and the tooth with the worst score determines the sextant score. The highest-scoring sextant determines the individual's overall management. If two or more sextants have a score of 3 or any one sextant has a score of 4, then a complete periodontal charting is advised. Scores of 0 or 1 require preventive measures inclusive of home-care instructions. Scores of 2 or greater require the patient to have additional professional cleaning and correction of defective restorations.	Code 0: No calculus, defective margins, or bleeding, and the black band of the probe is completely visible (probing depth less than 3.5 mm). Code 1: No calculus or defective margins, but there is bleeding, and the black band of the probe is completely visible. Code 2: Supragingival or subgingival calculus or defective markings are present, but the black band is still visible. Code 3: Calculus, defective restorations, and bleeding may or may not be present, and the black band is partly visible (probing depth more than 3.5 mm but less than 5.5 mm).	Screening of periodontal disease in private practice.	Simplifies the charting of an individual's periodontal condition when extensive treatment is not required.	Cannot be substituted for a complete periodontal charting necessary for the treatment of periodontitis patients.	Private practice.

Table 2-1 Indices Used for Periodontal Disease Assessments (continued)

Index	Type of Evaluation	Teeth Measured	Method of Measurement	Scale of Measurement	Purpose	Advantages	Disadvantages	Uses
				Code 4: The black band of the probe is not visible (probing depth more than 5.5 mm). An asterisk (*) is added if any additional pathology is present, such as furcations.				Private practice.
Miller Index of Tooth Mobility (Miller, 1950)	Pathologic tooth mobility	All teeth in dentition.	Take blunt end of two instruments (e.g., probe and mirror). Using finger rests apply ends of instruments to the labial and lingual surfaces of teeth. Move tooth in facial-lingual direction.	0 = No pathologic movement. I = First distinguishable sign of tooth movement in a facial/lingual direction. II = Movement of the crown in a facial/lingual direction up to 1 mm. III = Movement of the crown in a facial/lingual direction more than 1 mm and/ or depressed in a vertical direction.	Determine the amount of movement of a tooth.	Results are reproducible.	This index is actually the only referenced index for tooth mobility. There are no disadvantages	Private practice.

CALCULUS INDICES In clinical practice, calculus is not monitored by a numeric index, but it is in epidemiologic surveys. Numerous methods have been devised to quantify this deposit, and three commonly used calculus indices will be presented here (see Table 2–1).

The simplified Calculus Index (CS-1), which is part of the OHI-S mentioned previously (Greene, 1967), is valuable for epidemiologic surveys and longitudinal studies. It quantifies calculus by location and surface area. Another common calculus evaluation is the Volpe Manhold Calculus Assessment (Volpe, Kupczak, & King, 1967; Volpe, Manhold, & Hazen, 1965), which measures the height and dimension of the calculus present. It was designed originally for use on the lingual surfaces of the mandibular incisors but can be used throughout the mouth.

National epidemiologic studies, conducted through the National Institute of Dental Research (NIDR), have developed and used their own calculus index (Miller, Brunelle, Carlos, Brown, & Löe, 1987). The NIDR Index merely indicates the presence or absence of calculus supragingivally or subgingivally. This index was used for the third National Health and Nutrition Examination Survey (NHANES III), conducted by the National Center for the Health Statistics in collaboration with the National Institute for Dental Research from 1988 to 1991.

Gingival Indices

The epidemiologic tool used to quickly assess gingival inflammation is the gingival index. A gingival index is designed to measure the degree of visible inflammation of the gingival tissues. Visible signs of gingival inflammation are bleeding, redness, and swelling. These are accepted clinical signs of inflammation and also have been incorporated into indices for evaluation of the periodontal status of individuals and populations.

The Gingival Index (GI) of Löe and Silness (Löe, 1967) is based on the assessment of the visual indicators of gingival inflammation. The degree of inflammation is subdivided into three categories, with moderate inflammation determined by the presence of bleeding and severe inflammation determined by spontaneous bleeding. The GI historically has been used for epidemiologic studies. Lobene, Weatherford, Ross, Lam, and Menaker (1986) modified this index for use in clinical trials evaluating plaque-control products. The Modified Gingival Index (Lobene et al., 1986) assesses gingival health by looking only at qualitative changes in the gingiva. Unlike the GI, which uses bleeding as an indicator of increasing severity of gingival inflammation, this index does not use bleeding on probing and has more gradations. The Modified Gingival Index is scored to pick up subtle changes earlier with four different scores for gingival inflammation.

Other gingival indices based primarily on bleeding include the Sulcus Bleeding Index (Mühlemann & Son, 1971) and the Eastman Interdental Bleeding Index (Caton & Polson, 1985). Gingival bleeding as a measure of gingival inflammation is considered a more objective measure, whereas gingival color and consistency are more subjective. For this index, gingival bleeding is determined by gently inserting a probe in the sulcus and withdrawing it. Mühlemann and Son (1971) based the Sulcus Bleeding Index on bleeding being the earliest symptom of gingivitis, but it has been criticized because distinctions are not made beyond the clinical point of gingivitis.

A novel approach to determining bleeding is the use of a triangular toothpick (e.g., Stimudent) rather than a periodontal probe. The Interdental Bleeding Index (Caton & Polson, 1985) uses interdental cleaners to evaluate bleeding in the midproximal gingival tissues where periodontal changes are most likely to be found. The interdental cleaner is inserted between teeth and removed, depressing the interdental papilla 1 to 2 mm. Fifteen seconds after insertion and removal, bleeding is recorded.

In an attempt to achieve a more objective measure, gingival bleeding is being used increasingly for the determination of gingival changes in epidemiologic studies. The presence or absence of bleeding has been used in current demographic studies, in the NIDR Adult Survey (1985–1986; Brown, Oliver, & Löe, 1989), and in NHANES III (1988–1991; Brown, Brunelle, & Kingman, 1996). Gingival bleeding also has been used to monitor patient home oral hygiene practices. The percentage of bleeding sites is considered a more accurate representation of the patient's true level of daily home care. Bleeding and gingival indices also have been monitored along with individual attachment levels and pocket bacteria to find markers or predictors of disease activity.

Indices of Periodontal Destruction

Another essential measure eused in epidemiologic studies is evaluation of periodontal destruction. Indices of periodontal destruction are designed to measure disease severity and extent by observing the outcomes of periodontal destruction. This is done by measuring clinical attachment loss and probing depth and recording bone loss and loss of function. Current national studies use direct measures of these disease outcomes. These measures are taken at the midbuccal and mesiobuccal levels of all fully erupted teeth (Brown et al., 1996). Even though current national surveys do not use periodontal indices or directly measure the outcome of destruction, much of the historical data pertinent to periodontal diseases in the United States have been compiled using periodontal indices.

The Periodontal Index (PI; Russell, 1967) has been a standard measure for the large national surveys that are responsible for early views of periodontal disease prevalence and incidence in the United States. The PI is a visual index and does not use a periodontal probe. The presence

---

Did You Know?

In a national survey of employed adults conducted in 1985–1986, 47% of males and 39% of females aged 18 to 64 exhibited at least one site that bled on probing.

of inflammation, pocket formation, and loss of function is assessed visually as criteria for numeric scoring of teeth.

Two additional indices of epidemiologic importance evaluate periodontal destruction and designate treatment needs. The Community Periodontal Index of Treatment Needs (CPITN; Ainamo, Barmes, Beargie, Cutress, & Martin, 1982) was developed by an initiative of the World Health Organization (WHO) expressly for population studies. Its primary focus is to assess treatment needs.

The CPITN was modified to the Periodontal Screening and Recording (PSR) system for general-practice use. The PSR system was developed to evaluate individual treatment needs and to be used as a quick screening tool to document new patient periodontal findings in lieu of a complete periodontal charting. It has been endorsed by the American Academy of Periodontology and the American Dental Association as a quick and easy method to record the periodontal status of a patient in the private-practice setting. This screening tool reduces the number of patients who need a complete periodontal charting simply by identifying those with periodontal treatment needs and therefore the need for a complete periodontal charting.

The CPITN probe is used in the PSR system, and the same parameters employed by the CPITN are evaluated— bleeding, calculus, and probing depth. The CPITN probe has a ball tip to aid in calculus detection and a black band that demarcates probing depth from 3.5 to 5.5 mm. It was developed to increase the recognition and treatment of periodontal disease in the general dental practice.

Accuracy of Methodology

Thus far the tools used for assessing the periodontal condition in epidemiologic studies have been described. These tools define or identify individuals within a population with periodontal disease. The sampling methodology for population studies differs from that used in clinical periodontics and can influence the accuracy of the data obtained. Epidemiologic data-collection tools do not measure all the periodontal findings a clinician might use to establish a diagnosis and prognosis, such as furcation involvement or tooth mobility. Population studies, because of their large sample sizes, use indices as assessment tools, unlike diagnostic evaluations in clinical practice, and thus only score a portion of the mouth. To streamline the examination process, partial mouth scores are incorporated into indices. Partial mouth observations improve study efficiency but reduce the accuracy of overall reporting of periodontal disease prevalence and incidence.

For example, the CPITN measures only 10 teeth in the mouth. Baelum, Manji, Fejerskov, and Wanzala (1993) found that the prevalence of teeth with moderate to deep pockets was underreported in the partial mouth scores of the CPITN. This was especially true for advanced periodontal conditions. In another report, Baelum, Manji, Wanzala, and Fejerskov (1995) concluded that the CPITN scores tend to underestimate prevalence and severity in younger age groups and overestimate the same in the elderly.

The methodology used by the NIDR for the most recent survey, NHANES (1999–2000; Borrell, Burt, & Taylor, 2005), also involves a partial mouth evaluation. As described earlier, periodontal probing is performed in half the mouth. When half-mouth and full-mouth scores were compared (Hunt & Fann, 1991), the results were similar. Half-mouth examination was considered accurate in estimating the prevalence of periodontal disease but still underestimated the percentage of the population with more advanced disease (periodontal attachment loss). A review by Papapanou (1996) concluded that the current NIDR methodology is inadequate because it is a combination of partial scores (e.g., only two sites per tooth are measured in only one-half of the mouth). Papapanou contended that the location of the pocket and the number of probing measures could have a profound influence on the outcome of the study. Partly because previous studies comparing half-mouth scores with full-mouth scores had used partial scores for their comparison, not all probing sites encircling a tooth were measured. When combining partial mouth scores with measures at only the midbuccal and mesiobuccal sites, current methodology actually could produce a mean percentage underestimation of deep pockets of 40% and an underestimation of the prevalence of these deep pockets of 58%.

The validity of an index in describing a population also can be affected by tooth loss. Missing teeth may have been the ones most severely affected by periodontitis. Because they are no longer present to be measured, there is a built-in selection bias for the healthier teeth still present, potentially underestimating both severity and prevalence of the disease (periodontitis). Thus the overall reliability of an index is affected by the method of data collection. It is difficult to have one tool that will be representative, accurate, and efficient at the same time for all periodontal measures. Historical and modern data are based on methodologies that have been criticized, but some researchers contend that they still render an adequate estimation of disease.

Prevalence of Periodontal Diseases

National surveys have helped build our knowledge of the prevalence, severity, and extent of periodontal diseases in the United States. Based on the results of these surveys, the commonly accepted model for periodontal diseases has changed and evolved. Historically, periodontal disease was considered inevitable, and all individuals were susceptible to advanced periodontal disease, gingivitis being its precursor. In essence, periodontal disease was considered universal, and the susceptibility to periodontitis increased with age (Waerhaug, 1966).

Information gathered from more recent national surveys, however, suggests otherwise. More severe disease (advanced periodontitis) was found in only 5% to 20% of adults (U.S. Public Health Service, 1987), and moderate disease (periodontitis) was found in the majority of adults (U.S. Public Health Service, 1987). Thus only a few individuals will be susceptible to advanced disease. Today, periodontitis is not considered part of the aging process but occurs because of the interaction of bacteria and the immune response of the individual.

Prevalence of Gingivitis

Gingivitis is the most common form of periodontal disease found in individuals of all ages; it can even occur in early childhood (Ayers, Abrama, & Lausten, 1979). In the U.S. Health and Resources and Service Administration (HRSA) study of 1981 (Brown, Oliver, & Löe, 1989), 54% of adults over age 18 were affected with gingivitis involving at least six or more teeth. Another national study of employed adults between the ages of 18 and 64, the NIDR Adult Survey (1985–1986), reported less gingivitis, finding that 44% of the sample had gingivitis (defined by gingival bleeding; Miller et al., 1987). The average involvement was 2.7 sites per person, and the extent of gingivitis increased with age. In the NHANES III study (Brown et al., 1996), gingival bleeding was present in 63% of those examined, and 12% of all sites examined bled on probing. Gingivitis was slightly more prevalent in teenagers (13 to 17 years). The extent was similar among all age groups, ranging from 10% to 15% of the sites examined. Plaque and calculus deposits correlated with the prevalence of gingivitis, and subgingival calculus were found in 67% of the population and at 22% of the sites evaluated. Compared with the more recent NHANES (Borrell et al., 2005) there has been a decrease in bleeding compared to the NHANES III.

When compared with earlier national surveys, gingivitis has declined in the United States, most likely due to the current focus on oral hygiene as part of a daily personal hygiene routine (Burt, 1996). In the early 1960s, visual assessments revealed that 85% of men and 79% of women had gingivitis. Current surveys report that 63% of the population has gingival bleeding and that gingivitis is found in 44% to 54% of the population. This differs considerably from reports from Third World countries, where gingivitis in the presence of extensive plaque and calculus is considered normal among adults (Löe, Anerud, Boysen, & Smith, 1978).

Prevalence of Periodontitis

Chronic periodontitis is not commonly found among young individuals and is more prevalent with age. The NHANES III study (1988–1994; Brown et al., 1996; $n = 7,447$ surveyed) found that over 90% of individuals over age 13 had some attachment loss, with only 15% of the population having advanced disease (defined as 5 mm or more of attachment loss). If the definition of attachment loss were limited to 3 mm or more, the prevalence was 40%. One-quarter of the individuals surveyed showed moderate attachment loss (3–4 mm). With increasing age, the prevalence of moderate and severe attachment loss increased, but the prevalence of pockets 4 mm or greater and 6 mm or greater in size remained the same. Because the extent and prevalence of attachment loss were found to increase with age and the prevalence of 4 mm or greater pocket depths did not, increased gingival recession was deemed responsible for the increased attachment loss experienced with age (Oliver et al., 1998).

A recent study (Borrell et al., 2005) examined change in the prevalence of periodontitis between the NHANES III and the NHANES 1999–2000 and differences in the prevalence of periodontitis among racial/ethnic groups in the United States. Results showed that the prevalence of periodontitis has *decreased* between the NHANES III and the NHANES 1999–2000 for all racial/ethnic groups in the United States. This may be attributed to awareness and changes in health-risk behaviors such as smoking. The overall prevalence of periodontitis for the NHANES III was 7.3%, whereas for the NHANES 1999–2000 it was 4.2%.

In the HRSA survey (Brown et al., 1989), periodontitis (at least one tooth with a pocket 4 mm or deeper) was found in 36% of the 7,078 individuals examined. The prevalence of the disease increased with age. Twenty-nine percent of individuals in the 19- to 44-year-old age group were affected, whereas almost 50% of individuals 45 years of age or older were affected. The percentage of elderly individuals (age 65 and older) with pockets was similar to that of the 45- to 64-year-old age group, although the number of teeth present decreased. Periodontitis, when present, usually involved only a few teeth, and advanced periodontitis was relatively rare.

In the NIDR study of employed adults between the ages of 18 and 64 (Brown et al., 1990), almost all had some attachment loss, with 44% experiencing attachment loss of 3 mm or more. Moderate pocket depths (4 to 6 mm) were present in only 13.4% of those examined, generally affecting only one to two sites. More advanced disease again was considered rare and was found in only 0.6% of the study population. Males experienced more disease than females, and blacks were more affected than whites.

In the NHANES III study (Brown et al., 1996), racial and gender differences were reported as well. Females overall were in better periodontal health than their male counterparts, and non-Hispanic whites had less periodontal disease than non-Hispanic blacks or Mexican Americans.

Rapid Dental Hint

Attachment loss is defined as the loss of collagen fiber attachment to the tooth with subsequent apical migration of the junctional epithelium.

Did You Know?

For many years, periodontitis was primarily viewed as the outcome from infection. It is now seen as resulting from a complex interplay between bacterial infection and host response, often modified by behavioral factors.

Overall, the United States has a relatively low prevalence and severity of periodontal disease compared with the rest of the world, and the severity and extent of disease have declined in the past 30 years (Oliver et al., 1998).

Prevalence of Aggressive Periodontitis

The prevalence of aggressive periodontitis has been estimated to be less than 1% of the general population (Papapanou, 1996). It is considered a rare form of periodontal disease. A review of national population studies indicates that approximately 3.6% of individuals between the ages of 18 and 34 (NIDR Adult Survey, 1985–1986; Oliver et al., 1998) have moderate periodontal disease. Among 14- to 17-year-olds (Löe & Brown, 1991), the prevalence of all forms of aggressive periodontitis was 2.27%, 0.53% were affected by localized aggressive periodontitis, and 0.13% were estimated to be affected by generalized aggressive periodontitis.

Racial differences also have been reported. Blacks were affected more often than whites by all forms of aggressive periodontitis. In a national (NIDR) study of over 11,000 adolescents between the ages of 14 and 17, gender differences existed and were influenced by race. For example, black males were 2.9 times more likely to have localized aggressive periodontitis than black females, and white females were more frequently affected by localized aggressive periodontitis than white males by the same amount. Males, in general, were 4.3 times more likely to have generalized aggressive periodontitis than females. When these results were extrapolated to the racial mix of the U.S. population in general, about 87,000 cases of localized and generalized aggressive periodontitis were estimated among 13 million 14- to 17-year-olds (Oliver et al., 1998).

Traditionally, black females have been reported to be two to three times more likely to have aggressive periodontitis than white females. It has been suggested that clinical trials and case reports used to establish this racial and gender predilection may have been skewed by ascertainment bias because more females will seek dental treatment and participate in clinical trials than males (Oliver et al.,

---

Rapid Dental Hint

Gingivitis is defined as inflammation of the gingival tissue without loss of connective tissue attachment.
Periodontitis is defined as inflammation and loss of the connective tissue of the supporting or surrounding structure of teeth with loss of attachment.

Did You Know?

Cats and dogs can also develop periodontal disease!

1998). Thus, a national survey that does not start out with this selection bias may more accurately reflect the national population prevalence.

In summary, the national status of periodontal disease has been gleaned by three recent national surveys: the NIDR, NHANES, and HRSA surveys. About 50% of all U.S. adults have gingivitis involving three to four teeth. Periodontitis is experienced in over 90% of the population over 13 years of age, but only 15% have advanced disease. There is a specific small subset of the population that has more advanced disease. Aggressive periodontitis is considered a rare disease in the United States and affects only 0.53% to 3.6% of individuals under age 35. Overall, the national prevalence of gingivitis has declined over the past 30 years. However, the prevalence of periodontitis has remained the same, but the severity of disease has decreased (Capilouto & Douglass, 1988).

Incidence and Disease Progression

National surveys used to estimate disease prevalence are cross-sectional, which means that the study population is evaluated at only one point in time. To determine the natural progression of periodontal diseases, longitudinal studies are necessary, where individuals are examined at multiple intervals. Few longitudinal studies are available because of the difficulty of conducting them. In a 15-year longitudinal study by Löe and colleagues (1986), 480 Sri Lankan tea workers with untreated disease were evaluated. About 8% had rapid progression of their periodontitis, and most had a moderate rate of disease progression. A small portion of this population (11%) showed no progression beyond gingivitis despite the presence of heavy plaque and calculus.

A parallel study run in Norway (Löe et al., 1978) showed a different rate of disease progression. No cases of aggressive periodontitis were found, unlike the Sri Lankan study. The mean annual rate of attachment loss was 0.08 mm for interproximal and 0.1 mm for buccal surfaces as individuals approached 40 years of age. In patients with moderate periodontitis, progression occurred slowly at any given site. The rate of periodontal destruction did not increase with age, and therefore, the progression of periodontitis (extent and severity) appeared to be slow and continuous in this population.

In a report by Beck, Koch, and Offenbacher (1994), detailing a longitudinal study of adults between the ages of 65 and 80 in North Carolina identified with extensive attachment loss, additional evidence of slow disease progression also can be found. Only 12% of this population experienced 3 mm or more of attachment loss on one or more teeth during the 3-year study period. Again, it appears that subjects with a past history of periodontitis can be quite resistant to future disease (breakdown). Future attachment loss was associated with greater baseline probing depths, but the vast majority of sites that lost attachment had probing depths of 3 mm or less at baseline. Individuals who experienced attachment loss in the first 18 months of the study were more likely to experience attachment loss in the subsequent 18-month period.

Racial differences also were detected. Blacks tended to experience more attachment loss during both 18-month periods of the study. Only 45% of blacks had no attachment loss during the 3-year period, whereas 63% of whites were free of attachment loss. Despite having advanced attachment loss at the outset of the study, both blacks and whites had a high frequency of no further disease progression. Similarly, adult subjects with gingivitis monitored over a 3-year period had no detectable increase in probing depth (Listgarten, Schifter, & Laster, 1985). In a review by Stamm (1986), the incidence of gingivitis was greatest at puberty, declined through age 17, and then remained steady.

These studies imply that only select individuals or a small portion of the population will have new disease or disease progression. In another U.S. study by Löe and Brown (1991), only a small portion of the study population had the highest rate of disease progression, as noted by attachment loss; this subset of the population was identified with aggressive periodontitis. In the Beck and colleagues (1994) study of elderly adults, disease progression was more likely when extensive bone loss and tooth loss were experienced at a young age, again alluding to a specific subset of the population with a higher incidence of disease. In sum, only a small portion of the population will experience incidence and progression of severe attachment loss. This attachment loss will not progress at the same rate but may be episodic. The progression of periodontal disease appears to be influenced by education level, socioeconomic factors, gender, and race. These variables will be discussed in the next section of this chapter.

Epidemiologic Variables

Risk Indicators

Risk indicators are demographic, behavioral, and socioeconomic characteristics that are associated with disease but not considered causal for the disease. Aging is considered a risk indicator for periodontal disease, but does not cause periodontal disease. With increasing age, the prevalence of periodontal disease increases, but the aging process is not responsible for the disease. It is believed that there is more disease with age because there is more exposure to plaque-induced inflammation over time. Other characteristics associated with an increased frequency of disease are the level of education, gender, and race. Females have less periodontal disease than males (Sheiham & Striffler, 1970). It is hypothesized that these differences are due to the availability and use of dental services, oral home care, and preventive practices. For example, the higher levels of periodontal disease reported in males versus females are attributed to higher levels of plaque and less use of dental services. Where extensive plaque, calculus, and gingival inflammation are considered normal among adults in Third World countries, an association is found with less education

and low income, and generally, there is more attachment loss than in industrial nations of the Western world.

Risk Factors

Risk factors are characteristics that have been shown to possibly put an individual more at risk for developing periodontal disease. Risk factors are used to predict the occurrence of disease. The presence of even a strong risk factor does not necessarily mean that an individual is very likely to get the disease. Also, just because risk factors predict disease, it does not necessarily follow that they will cause disease. Risk factors may or may not be causal (Fletcher & Fletcher, 2005). A risk factor that does not cause a disease is called a *marker of disease* because it marks the increased probability of disease (Fletcher & Fletcher, 2005). Even though a risk factor may not cause the disease, it is important to identify potential causal relationships so that oral disease can be prevented if a risk factor is modifiable. *Note that when the term risk factor is used throughout this text, it is referring to factors that predispose an individual to periodontal disease.* For example, it is accepted that bacteria in bacterial biofilms causes gingivitis, and thus biofilms are considered a risk factor for gingivitis. Poor oral hygiene has been correlated strongly with periodontal disease. The NHANES I data showed an inverse relationship between tooth loss and good oral hygiene. The periodontal index (PI) and oral hygiene (OHI-S) index scores were significantly better in individuals with the least tooth loss (Burt, Ismail, & Eklund, 1985). However, the causal relationship is not clear-cut with periodontitis. Supragingival plaque and supragingival calculus are not as strongly correlated with periodontitis as with gingivitis (Bakdash, 1994; Löe et al., 1978). In a recent appraisal by Oliver and colleagues (1998), the presence of subgingival calculus appeared to be a better predictor of periodontitis but was not considered causal because there was an inconsistent relationship among the epidemiologic data regarding oral hygiene, plaque and calculus, and periodontitis. In the NHANES III survey (Brown et al., 1996), no bleeding was found 88% of the time when subgingival calculus was present. In addition, gingivitis does not always progress to periodontitis, which means that periodontitis will not always occur in the presence of plaque and calculus. One could infer from this inconsistency that poor oral hygiene is an important risk factor in individuals who are more susceptible based on their immune response to bacterial plaque. The NHANES study reported a decrease in bleeding for all ethnic/racial groups compared to the NHANES III (Borrell et al., 2005)

Other risk factors for periodontitis are diabetes and tobacco use. The prevalence and extent of periodontal pockets are greater in diabetics than in nondiabetics. This is especially true for poorly controlled diabetics, who experience more attachment and bone loss than well-controlled diabetics with similar plaque levels (Seppälä, Seppälä, & Ainamo, 1993). Oliver and Tervonen (1994) outlined diabetes as a risk factor for extensive, advanced periodontitis when the individual's diabetes is poorly controlled and the individual has extensive subgingival calculus from poor home care and lack of professional cleanings. In a recent report (Taylor et al., 1998), subjects with type 2 diabetes had more severe alveolar bone loss progression over a 2-year period than those without diabetes.

Smoking has been well documented as a risk factor for periodontitis. An early National Health and Nutrition Survey (NHANES I) in 1971–1974 first demonstrated the relationship between smoking and periodontitis (Ismail, Burt, & Eklund, 1983) in the United States. More recent longitudinal studies confirm this relationship. One longitudinal study showed that smokers lost proximal bone twice as fast as nonsmokers (Bolin, Eklund, Frithiof, & Lavstedt, 1993). Even when plaque accumulation is minimal, smokers have more teeth with deeper pockets and alveolar bone loss than nonsmokers (Bergström & Eliasson, 1987; Bergström & Floderus-Myrhed, 1983). In a 3-year study conducted by Beck, Koch, and Offenbacher (1995), disease was more likely to progress if the subject was a cigarette smoker, had the presence of gram-negative anaerobes in subgingival microbiota (especially *Porphyromonas gingivalis*), or had financial stress. All led to an increased risk for disease progression. Thus it is apparent that microbiota and stress could be considered risk factors for periodontitis.

Another longitudinal study running from 1959 to 1985 in Tecumseh, Michigan (Ismail, Morrison, Burt, Cafesse, & Kavanaugh, 1990), reported age, smoking, and the presence of tooth mobility as risk markers for future attachment loss (2 mm or more). It has been hypothesized (Papapanou, 1996) that periodontitis actually may have different factors associated with its initiation than those involved in its progression. Multiple factors may play a role in the induction and progression of periodontal disease. The commonly accepted risk factors are lack of oral cleanliness, smoking, and systemic disease (diabetes). Specific subgingival bacteria and socioeconomic stress also have been linked causally to periodontal disease through epidemiologic studies, but further evaluation is ongoing. Gender, race, and age may play a role in disease expression but are not causally linked to periodontal disease.

Treatment Needs

Information provided by epidemiologic surveys regarding gingival bleeding (gingival inflammation), subgingival calculus, and probing depths of 4 mm or greater is of great importance to the dental hygienist. These data represent clinical parameters used to decide when treatment of periodontal disease is necessary. Most individuals will need periodontal preventive care (Oliver et al., 1998), which is provided by the hygienist. Over 90% of people surveyed (NHANES III) have attachment loss, and only 15% of the population has advanced disease, suggesting that much of the treatment needs of the United States can be fulfilled by hygienists. More extensive, advanced disease is found among minorities and those with less income and education. However, these are the same individuals who are less likely to seek or perceive the need for dental services. Tooth loss due to periodontal disease remains high in the United States (Brown et al., 1989). This suggests that public awareness and education about the preventive services of dental hygienists are paramount if those individuals who are most affected are to be treated before tooth loss due to periodontitis occurs.

Future Trends

The hygienist plays an important role in the treatment of periodontal patients. Prevention and education are important responsibilities of the dental clinician. As epidemiologic studies elaborate and refine the interrelationship between periodontal infections and the systemic health of the patient, hygienists will need to include this information in patient education sessions. It has been documented that systemic conditions can contribute to the expression of periodontal disease. In recent years there is increasing evidence that supports the concepts that the relationship between systemic and oral health is bidirectional (Williams & Offenbacher, 2000). As patient awareness of periodontal disease and its systemic implications increases, more individuals will specifically seek the preventive and periodontal debridement services of the dental hygienist.

Healthy People (refer to www.healthypeople.gov) supports oral/dental and medical prevention efforts across the United States. It is part of the Department of Health and Human Services. Healthy People 2020 provides 10-year national objectives for improving the health of Americans. Healthy People 2010 started on December 2, 2010, has a mission to identify nationwide health improvement priorities; to increase public awareness and understanding of the determinants of health, disease, and disability; to provide measurable objective and goals; and to identify critical research, evaluation, and data collection needs. Healthy People 2020 strives to prevent and control oral

---

Did You Know?

A recent review reports that the risk of destructive periodontal disease is 5- to 20-fold higher for a smoker compared with a never-smoker.

Rapid Dental Hint

A *risk factor* is an environmental exposure, aspect of behavior, or inherent characteristic that is associated with a disease. Risk factors predispose an individual to a disease; they don't necessarily cause the disease.

A *risk indicator* describes plausible correlates of disease identified in cross-sectional studies.

Did You Know?

Periodontal diseases are possible risk factors for cardiovascular disease, diabetes, lung disease, and preterm low-birth-weight babies.

and craniofacial disease (e.g., dental caries, periodontal diseases, cleft lip and palate, oral and facial pain, and oral and pharyngeal cancers), conditions, and injuries and improve access to preventive services and dental care. The objectives are to increase awareness of the importance of oral health to overall health and well-being, to increase acceptance and adoption of effective preventive interventions, and to reduce disparities in access to effective preventive and dental treatment services.

Recent technological advances have revolutionized the ability to understand and apply genetic principles to the study of human diseases. These developments may soon alter the management of periodontal diseases (American Academy of Periodontology, 2005b).

Dental Hygiene Application

Epidemiology of the periodontal diseases is an important concept for the dental hygienist to know because it gives an overall assessment of the prevalence and incidence of periodontal disease in the general population. It is important to have healthcare programs for young adults for the early detection of periodontal diseases (Costa, Costa, Costa, & Pordeus, 2007).

Knowledge of epidemiology of periodontal diseases will help the dental hygienist understand risk factors and thus better prevent and treat periodontal diseases.

Key Points

- Healthy People 2020 is important for oral and dental health of all Americans.
- Epidemiologic measurements used to assess periodontal diseases include plaque, calculus, gingival, and periodontal indices.
- Periodontal indices may measure past disease activity rather than current disease activity or future periodontal breakdown.
- Gingivitis is the most common form of periodontal disease.
- Aggressive periodontitis is not common in the general population.
- Chronic periodontitis is prevalent in the general population.
- Risk factors are used to predict occurrence of disease; risk factors are not causal.
- Even though risk factors are not causal, they predict the probability of disease.

Self-Quiz

1. Which one of the following modalities would best determine disease prevalence?
   a. Comprehensive periodontal charting
   b. Epidemiologic population surveys
   c. Patient questionnaires
   d. National dental hygiene expenditures

2. Which one of the following terms describes the rate of new cases of periodontal disease occurring in a given time period?
   a. Prevalence
   b. Incidence
   c. Severity
   d. Extent
   e. Index

3. It is highly unlikely (infrequent) that an individual with advanced attachment loss at one point in time will again experience rapid attachment loss (> 3 mm) within the next 3 years. This patient will go into disease remission for the rest of his/her lifetime.
   a. The first statement is true, and the second statement is false.
   b. The first statement is false, and the second statement is true.
   c. Both statements are true.
   d. Both statements are false.

4. Which one of the following indices is best used to monitor a patient's plaque control (location of plaque) in private dental practice?
   a. Quigley-Hein Plaque Index
   b. Plaque Record (O'Leary)
   c. Periodontal Screening and Recording (PSR) system
   d. Sulcus Bleeding Index

5. Which one of the following best measures the severity of periodontal disease in a population?
   a. Radiographs
   b. Intraoral cameras
   c. Indices
   d. Surgical costs

6. All of the following are potential risk factors for periodontal disease except one. Which one is the exception?
   a. Age
   b. Smoking
   c. Diabetes
   d. Presence of plaque or debris

7. A risk indicator differs from a risk factor in that there is no causal relationship of the associated characteristic with the disease. Low income and less education are risk indicators for periodontal disease.
   a. The first statement is true, and the second statement is false.
   b. The first statement is false, and the second statement is true.
   c. Both statements are true.
   d. Both statements are false.

8. According to surveys, which of the following percentages of the U.S. adult population has advanced periodontal disease (advanced periodontitis)?
   a. 5–20
   b. 40–50
   c. 70–80
   d. 90–100

9. Which one of the following describes how the prevalence of gingivitis has changed over the past 30 years?
   a. Increased
   b. Decreased
   c. Remained the same
   d. Increased in the first 10 years and then decreased

10. Which one of the following describes the prevalence of aggressive periodontitis in the general population?
    a. Rare
    b. Frequent
    c. Universal
    d. Nonexistent

Case Study

A 50-year-old male patient has a chief complaint of "bad breath." The patient smokes (1ppd) and has no medical conditions. The clinical examination reveals heavy deposits of plaque and calculus and generalized bleeding on probing. There localized mild bone loss on the radiographs.

1. Which of the following factors are considered to be a risk indicator for this patient?
   a. Smoking
   b. Poor oral hygiene
   c. Bone loss
   d. Age of patient

Answer: D

2. In this patient, which of the following factors are considered to be risk factors for periodontal disease?

   a. Smoking and poor oral hygiene
   b. Localized mild bone loss
   c. Age of the patient
   d. Bleeding on probing

Answer: A

3. Which of the following indices is best for this patient to motivate him in his oral hygiene?
   a. Community Periodontal Index of Treatment Needs
   b. Periodontal Index (PI)
   c. Gingival Index (GI)
   d. O'Leary, Drake and Naylor

Answer: D

References

Ainamo, J., D. Barmes, G. Beargie, T. Cutress, and J. Martin. 1982. Development of the World Health Organization (WHO) Community Periodontal Index of Treatment Needs (CPITN). *Int. Dent. J.* 32:281–291.

American Academy of Periodontology. 2005a. Epidemiology of periodontal diseases. Position Paper.

American Academy of Periodontology. 2005b. Implications of genetic technology for the management of periodontal diseases. *J. Periodontol.* 76:850–857.

Ayers, C., A. Abrama, and L. Lausten. 1979. Oral health assessment of inner city preschoolers. *Dent. Hygiene* 53:465–468.

Baelum, V., F. Manji, O. Fejerskov, and P. Wanzala. 1993. Validity of CPITN's assumptions of hierarchical occurrence of periodontal conditions in a Kenyan population aged 15–65 years. *Commun. Dent. Oral Epidemiol.* 21:347–353.

Baelum, V., F. Manji, P. Wanzala, and O. Fejerskov. 1995. Relationship between CPITN and periodontal attachment loss findings in an adult population. *J. Clin. Periodontol.* 22:146–152.

Bakdash, B. 1994. Oral hygiene and compliance as risk factors in periodontitis. *J. Periodontol.* 65:539–544.

Beck, J., G. Koch, and S. Offenbacher. 1994. Attachment loss trend over 3 years in community-dwelling older adults. *J. Periodontol.* 65:737–743.

Beck, J., G. Koch, and S. Offenbacher. 1995. Incidence of attachment loss over 3 years in older adults: New and progressing lesions. *Commun. Dent. Oral Epidemiol.* 23:291–296.

Bergström, J., and S. Eliasson. 1987. Cigarette smoking and alveolar bone height in subjects with high standard oral hygiene. *J. Clin. Periodontol.* 14:466–469.

Bergström, J., and B. Floderus-Myrhed. 1983. Co-twin study of the relationship between smoking and some periodontal disease factors. *Commun. Dent. Oral Epidemiol.* 11:113–116.

Bolin, A., G. Eklund, L. Frithiof, and S. Lavstedt. 1993. The effect of changed smoking habits on marginal alveolar bone loss: A longitudinal study. *Swed. Dent. J.* 17:211–216.

Borrell, L. N., B. A. Burt, and G. W. Taylor. 2005. Prevalence and trends in periodontitis in the USA: From the NHANES III to the NHANES. *J. Dent. Res.* 84(10):924–930.

Brown, L., J. Brunelle, and A. Kingman. 1996. Periodontal status in the United States, 1988–91: Prevalence, extent, and demographic variation. *J. Dent. Res.* 75 (spec issue): 672–683.

Brown, L., R. Oliver, and H. Löe. 1989. Periodontal diseases in the U.S. in 1981: Prevalence, severity, extent and role in tooth mortality. *J. Periodontol.* 60:363–371.

Brown, L., R. Oliver, and H. Löe. 1990. Evaluating periodontal status of U.S. employed adults. *J. Am. Dent. Assoc.* 121:226–232.

Burt, B. 1996. Epidemiology of periodontal diseases. *J. Periodontol.* 67:935–945.

Burt, B., A. Ismail, and S. Eklund. 1985. Periodontal disease, tooth loss and oral hygiene among older Americans. *Commun. Dent. Oral Epidemiol.* 13(2):93–96.

Capilouto, M., and C. Douglass. 1988. Trends in the prevalence and severity of periodontal disease in the U.S.: A public health problem? *J. Public Health Dent.* 48:245–251.

Caton, J., and A. Polson. 1985. The Interdental Bleeding Index: A simplified procedure for monitoring gingival health. *Comp. Cont. Educ. Dent.* 6:88–92.

Costa, F. O., L. O. M. Costa, J. E. Costa, and I. A. Pordeus. 2007. Periodontal disease progression among young subjects with no preventive dental care: A 52-month follow-up study. *J. Periodontol.* 78:198–203.

Fischman, S. 1986. Current status of indices of plaque. *J. Clin. Periodontol.* 13:371–374.

Fletcher, R. W., and S. W. Fletcher. 2005. Risk: Looking forward. In: eds. R. W. Fletcher and S. W. Fletcher, *Clinical epidemiology. The essentials*, 4th ed., 75–90. Hagerstown, Maryland: Lippincott, Williams and Wilkins.

Greene, J. 1967. The Oral Hygiene Index. Development and uses. *J. Periodontol.* 38:625–637.

Greene, J., and J. Vermillion. 1964. The Simplified Oral Hygiene Index. *J. Am. Dent. Assoc.* 68:7–13.

Hunt, R., and S. Fann. 1991. Effect of examining half the teeth in a partial periodontal recording of older adults. *J. Dent. Res.* 70:1380–1385.

Ismail, A., B. Burt, and S. Eklund. 1983. Epidemiologic patterns of smoking and periodontal disease in the United States. *J. Am. Dent. Assoc.* 106:617–621.

Ismail, A., E. Morrison, B. Burt, R. Cafesse, and M. Kavanaugh. 1990. Natural history of periodontal disease in adults: Findings from the Tecumseh Periodontal Disease Study, 1959–1987. *J. Dent. Res.* 69(2):430–435.

Listgarten, M., C. Schifter, and L. Laster. 1985. Three-year longitudinal study of the periodontal status of an adult population with gingivitis. *J. Clin. Periodontol.* 12:225–238.

Lobene, R., T. Weatherford, N. Ross, R. Lam, and L. Menaker. 1986. A modified gingival index for use in clinical trials. *Clin. Prev. Dent.* 8(1):3–6.

Löe, H. 1967. The gingival index, the plaque index, and the retention index. Systems (Part II). *J. Periodontol.* 38:610–616.

Löe, H., A. Anerud, H. Boysen, and E. Morrison. 1986. Natural history of periodontal disease in man: Rapid, moderate and no loss of attachment in Sri Lankan laborers 14–46 years of age. *J. Clin. Periodontol.* 13:431–446.

Löe, H., A. Anerud, H. Boysen, and M. Smith. 1978. The natural history of periodontal disease in man: The rate of periodontal destruction before 40 years of age. *J. Periodontol.* 49(12):607–620.

Löe, H., and L. Brown. 1991. Early-onset periodontitis in the United States of America. *J. Periodontol.* 62: 608–616.

Miller S. C. 1950. *Textbook of periodontia*, 3rd ed., 125. Philadelphia: Blakiston.

Miller, A., J. Brunelle, J. Carlos, L. J. Brown, and H. Löe. 1987. *Oral health of United States adults. National findings 1985–1986.* Bethesda, MD: U.S. Public Health Service, U.S. Dept. of Health and Human Services.

Mühlemann, H. R., and S. Son. 1971. Gingival sulcus bleeding: A leading symptom in initial gingivitis. *Helv. Odont. Acta* 15:107–113.

O'Leary, T. J., R. Drake, and J. Naylor. 1972. The Plaque Control Record. *J. Periodontol.* 43(1):38.

Oliver, R., L. Brown, and H. Löe. 1998. Periodontal disease in the United States population. *J. Periodontol.* 69:269–278.

Oliver, R., and T. Tervonen. 1994. Diabetes: A risk factor for periodontitis in adults. *J. Periodontol.* 65:530–538.

Papapanou, P. 1996. *Annals of periodontology, section 1A: Periodontal diseases: Epidemiology.* 1996 World Workshop in Periodontics, Lansdowne, VA.

Raul, G., and T. Dietrich. 2012. Introduction to periodontal epidemiology. *Periodontology 2000.* 58:7–9.

Russell, A. L. 1967. The Periodontal Index. *J. Periodontol.* 38:585–591.

Saxer, U. P. & H. R. Miihlemann. 1975. Motivation und Aufklärung. *Schweiz* Monatscchr Zahnheilkd. 85:905–915.

Seppälä, B., M. Seppälä, and J. Ainamo. 1993. A longitudinal study on insulin-dependent diabetes mellitus and periodontal disease. *J. Clin. Periodontol.* 20:161–165.

Sheiham, A., and D. Striffler. 1970. A comparison of four epidemiological methods of assessing periodontal disease: I. Population findings. *J. Periodont. Res.* 5:148–154.

Silness, J., and H. Löe. 1964. Periodontal disease in pregnancy: II. Correlation between oral hygiene and periodontal condition. *Acta Odontol. Scand.* 22:121–135.

Stamm, J. 1986. Epidemiology of gingivitis. *J. Clin. Periodontol.* 13:360–366.

Taylor, G. W., B. A. Burt, M. P. Becker, R. J. Genco, M. Schlossman, et al. 1998. Non-insulin-dependent diabetes and the progression of bone loss over a two-year period. *J. Periodontol.* 68:76–83.

Turesky, S., N. Gilmore, and I. Glickman. 1970. Reduced plaque formation by the chloromethyl analogue of vitamine C. *J. Periodontol.* 41:41–43.

U.S. Public Health Service, NIDR. 1987. *Oral health in United States adults: National findings* (NIH Publication No. 87-2868), pp. 1–168. Bethesda, MD: National Institute of Health, NIDR.

Volpe, A., L. Kupczak, and W. King. 1967. In vivo calculus assessment: III. Scoring techniques, rate of calculus formation, partial mouth exams versus full mouth exams, and intra-examiner reproducibility. *Periodontics* 5:184–193.

Volpe, A., J. H. Manhold, and S. P. Hazen. 1965. In vivo calculus assessment: I. A method and its examiner reproducibility. *J. Periodontol.* 36:292–298.

Waerhaug, J. 1966. Epidemiology of periodontal disease: A review of literature. In *World workshop in periodontics*, 179–212. Ann Arbor: University of Michigan.

Williams, R. C., and S. Offenbacher. 2000. Periodontal medicine: The emergence of a new branch of periodontology. *Periodontol. 2000.* 23(1): 9–12.

Visit www.pearsonhighered.com/healthprofessionsresources to access the student resources that accompany this book. Simply select Dental Hygiene from the choice of disciplines. Find this book and you will find the complimentary study tools created for this specific title.

3

Dental Biofilm: The Microbiology of the Periodontium in Health and Disease

Charles A. Powell, Sangeetha Chandrasekaran, and Raymond A. Yukna

OUTLINE

EDUCATIONAL OBJECTIVES

Upon completion of this chapter, the reader should be able to:

- Describe biofilm development.
- Describe the differences in bacterial species present in periodontal health and disease.
- Describe the bacterial species present in peri-implant disease.
- Discuss the use of systemic antibiotics in the nonsurgical treatment of periodontal disease.

GOAL: To describe dental biofilm development and review its role in periodontal disease.

KEY WORDS

acquired pellicle 47
dysbiosis 48
peri-implant mucositis 52
peri-implantitis 52
red complexes 51

Introduction

The oral environment provides a rich medium for the development of biofilm. Because of the presence of non-shedding oral surfaces such as teeth and restorative materials, a surface for attachment is present. The term *biofilm* was first proposed in 1978 by Costerton and colleagues to describe the diverse microbial community that is attached to a surface (Schaudinn, Gorur, Keller, Sedghizadeh, & Costerton, 2009). Over time this term was applied to all attached communities in which sessile bacterial cells are enclosed in matrices composed primarily of polymers of their own production (Schaudinn et al., 2009). As a dental biofilm develops, the host mounts an inflammatory response as a result of the bacterial challenge from the dental biofilm at the tooth/gingival interface, resulting in inflammatory periodontal disease (Figure 3–1 ■). In this chapter we will explore the unique role dental biofilm serve, their development and composition in health and disease, and methods to combat their presence within the oral environment.

Biofilm Formation

The dental biofilm can be characterized as a microbial community that develops on a tooth or root surface that is embedded in a matrix of polymers derived from bacteria and saliva (Marsh & Martin, 2009). Bacterial cells represent 15% to 20% of the biofilm volume, with the glycocalyx, composed predominately of water and aqueous solutes, representing the remaining 75% to 80% of the volume. Exopolysaccharides (EPS) produced by the bacteria in the biofilm make up 50% to 95% of the dry weight (Lindhe, Lang, & Karring, 2008). The development of the biofilm occurs in a series of stages.

The first event in dental biofilm development is the adsorption of molecules to the tooth surface. These molecules are derived mainly from saliva, but in the subgingival environment they originate from the gingival crevicular

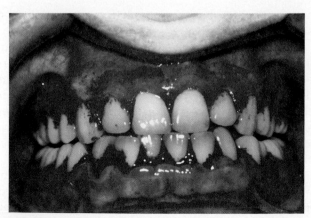

FIGURE 3–1 Clinical picture of supragingival plaque on teeth made more evident with disclosant.

> ### Did You Know?
>
> A biofilm is a complex aggregation of microorganisms marked by the excretion of a protective and adhesive matrix. Biofilm are found everywhere, not only in the mouth. Biofilm are also found on solid material submerged in or exposed to an aqueous solution. For example, biofilm grow in hot, acidic pools in Yellowstone National Park and on glaciers in Antartica.

fluid (Marsh, Moter, & Devine, 2011). The tooth surface therefore is altered by the formation of a conditioning film to allow interaction with bacteria.

Soon after development of the conditioning film, reversible adhesions occur between the charge on the microbial cell surface and the charge present on the conditioning film (Busscher, Norde, & van der Mei, 2008). Microbes collect on the conditioning film either passively through salivary or gingival crevicular flow or, in the case of a few motile species, by their own transport (Marsh et al., 2011). Irreversible adhesion then develops through the interaction of adhesions on the microbial cell surface and receptors present in the conditioning film (Marsh et al., 2011). These adhesions provide a strong bond for the biofilm. During this time both secondary and late colonizers adhere to receptors on bacteria that are already attached to the **acquired pellicle** (Society for General Microbiology, 2000). This leads to microbial diversity within the developing dental biofilm.

As these colonizers multiply there is an increase in biomass and synthesis of exopolymers to form a biofilm matrix (Marsh et al., 2011). These changes contribute to the structural integrity and resistance of biofilm to environmental factors and antimicrobial agents (Marsh et al., 2011). The matrix can be biologically active and retain water, nutrients, and enzymes, as well as exclude or restrict the penetration of other molecules (Marsh et al., 2011). The metabolism of the microorganisms produces gradients within the biofilm for nutrients, fermentation products, pH, and redox potential (Marsh et al., 2011). In response to these gradient changes, the microorganisms alter their pattern of gene expression (Forng, Champagne, Simpson, & Genco, 2000). The result is a heterogenous environment, which explains how microorganisms with apparent contradictory growth requirements can coexist within the

> ### Did You Know?
>
> Bacteria are used to make cheese, milk, sourdough bread, and yogurt.

Table 3–1 Properties of Biofilm and Microbial Communities (Marsh et al., 2011)

General Property	Dental Plaque
Open architecture	Presence of channels and voids
Microbial protection	Production of extracellular polymers to form a functional matrix; physical protection from phagocytosis
Host protection	Colonization; resistance
Enhanced tolerance to antimicrobials	Reduced sensitivity to chlorhexidine and antibiotics; gene transfer
Neutralization of inhibitors	Beta-lactamase production by neighboring cells to protect sensitive organisms
Coordinated gene responses	Production of bacterial cell-to-cell signaling molecules
Spatial and environmental heterogeneity	pH and oxygen gradients; coadhesion
Broader habitat range	Obligate anaerobes in an overly aerobic environment
More efficient metabolism	Complete catabolism of complex host macromolecules by microbial food chains and food webs
Enhanced virulence	Pathogenic synergism in periodontal diseases
Novel gene expression	Synthesis of novel proteins on attachment or on binding to host molecules
Communication with host	Downregulation of pro-inflammatory responses by resident oral bacteria; remodeling of the cytoskeleton of epithelial cells

dental biofilm (Marsh et al., 2011). (See Table 3–1 ■ and Figure 3–2 ■.)

Biofilm in Periodontal Health and Disease

It is estimated that over 700 bacterial species reside within the oral cavity, over half of which have never been cultivated (Aas, Paster, Stokes, Olsen, & Dewhirst, 2005). Periodontal diseases, like many other chronic diseases, appear to follow the microbial shift hypothesis. This shift, more commonly known as **dysbiosis**, refers to the concept that some diseases are due to a decrease in the number of beneficial symbionts and/or an increase in the number of pathogens (Berezow & Darveau, 2011). Within the mouth in the transition from periodontal health to disease, there is an oral microbiota shift from a population that is predominately

Rapid Dental Hint

Aggregatibacter actinomycetemomitans is an oral bacterium that causes localized aggressive periodontitis.

gram-positive aerobes to a population predominated by gram-negative anerobes.

The biofilm present when the gingiva is healthy and noninflamed consists mainly of gram-positive, saccharolytic, and facultative anaerobic bacteria (Marsh & Devine, 2011) that contain *Streptococcus* and additional species including *Actinomyces, Veillonella, Bacteroides,* and *Capnocytophaga. Streptococci* and *Actinomyces* may comprise over 85% of the microbial flora in health (Slots, 1979; Box 3–1).

Gingivitis has been characterized by a shift from a *Streptococcus*-dominated plaque to an *Actinomyces*-dominated plaque. Developing gingivitis has been associated with increased numbers of *Actinomyces israelii* and *Bacteroides,* especially *Porphyromonas gingivalis.* Gingivitis has also been associated with an increase in motile bacteria

Did You Know?

Scientists estimate that bacteria produce nearly half the oxygen found in the atmosphere.

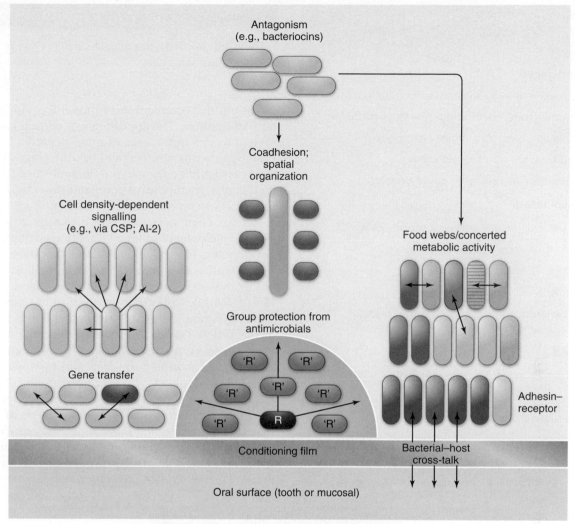

FIGURE 3–2 Schematic representation of the types of interaction (interbacterial and bacterial–host) that occur in a microbial community, such as dental plaque, growing as a biofilm. Bacteria adhere via adhesin–receptor interactions either to the conditioning film (derived either from saliva or gingival crevicular fluid) or to already attached cells (coadhesion). Bacteria interact synergistically to metabolize complex endogenous molecules (e.g., glycoproteins), and food webs can develop. Bacteria communicate with each other in a cell density-dependent manner via diffusible signaling molecules and with host cells. Cells are more tolerant of antimicrobial agents either because of the physical attributes of the biofilm, via gene transfer of resistance genes, or through protection by neighboring cells that produce neutralizing enzymes. Cells may also gain advantage by production of inhibitory molecules.

and spirochetes (Listgarten & Hellden, 1978). Moore and colleagues (Moore et al., 1982) described a great deal of individual variation in the development of gingivitis flora and reported a progression of species colonizing in a sequential manner in gingivitis. He associated gingivitis with specific *Actinomyces, Streptoccocus*, *Fusobacterium, Veillonella*, and

Treponema. Prevotella intermedia has been associated with pregnancy gingivitis (Kornman & Loesche, 1980).

In the classic experimental gingivitis study by Löe and his colleagues (Löe, Theilade, & Jensen, 1965), 12 subjects ceased all oral hygiene efforts and were monitored clinically and microbiologically. It was discovered that gingivitis began in 10 to 21 days and resolved within 1 week of renewed oral hygiene efforts. Three phases were described. On days 1 and 2, there was a transition from a sparse flora to a dense mat of gram-positive cocci and short rods. From this point until day 4, filamentous forms and rods increased, with cocci still present in large numbers. From days 6 to 10 there was a gradual shift to vibrios and spirochetes.

Did You Know?

There are more microbes on your body than there are humans on the entire planet.

Box 3–1: Types of Subgingival Dental Biofilm

Tooth Associated

- Densely packed strongly adherent to tooth surface (biofilm)
- Gram-positive rods, cocci, and filamentous bacteria
- Facultative aerobic or facultative anaerobes
- Removed by scaling and root planing
- Less virulent (limited ability to cause disease)

Tissue Associated

- Loosely packed, loosely adherent to soft tissue wall
- Gram-negative, motile, anaerobic
- Spirochetes, "bottle-brush" types
- More virulent (able to cause disease)
- Cannot be removed by scaling and root planing; needs to be surgically removed

Unattached

- Free swimming in pocket (not a biofilm)
- Gram-negative, motile, anaerobic
- Spirochetes and others
- More virulent (able to cause disease)
- Removed by flushing

Did You Know?

There are over 700 types of bacteria in the mouth!

Gram-positive cocci and short rods still comprised 45% to 60% of the flora. The appearance of clinical gingivitis was related to the appearance of gram-negative forms. When oral hygiene was resumed and healthy gingival conditions were reestablished, the gingival flora returned to one of predominantly gram-positive cocci and short rods. No vibrios or spirochetes were observed in health.

It has been suggested that a change in habitat such as the development of gingivitis can contribute to plaque development (Daly & Highfield, 1996; Ramberg, Furuichi, Volpe, Gaffar, & Lindhe, 1996). Thus the host plays a role in this dysbiosis. Socransky, Haffajee, Cugini, Smith, and Kent (1998) described this succession in terms of a color scheme (Figure 3–3 ■). Initial colonization is by members of the yellow (genus *Streptococcus*), green (*Capnocytophaga* species, *Aggregatibacter actinomycetemcomitans* serotype a, *Eikenella corrodens*, and *Campylobacter concisus*), and purple (*Veillonella parvula* and *Actinomyces odontolyticus*) complexes along with *Actinomyces* species. As this progression develops, members of the orange (*Campylobacter gracilis*, *C. rectus*, *C. showae*, *Eubacterium nodatum*, *Fusobacterium nucleatum* subspecies, *Fusobacterium periodonticum*, *Peptostreptococcus micros*, *Prevotella intermedia*, *Prevotella nigresens*, and *Streptococcus*

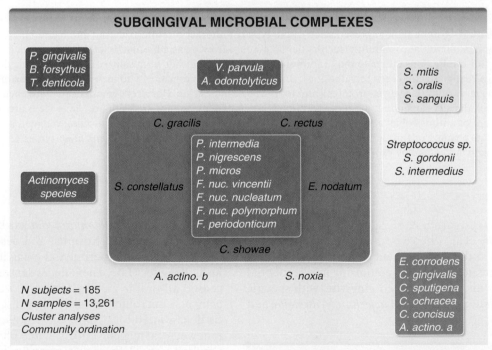

FIGURE 3–3 Diagram of the association among subgingival species. The complexes to the left are comprised of species thought to colonize the tooth surface and proliferate at an early stage. The orange complex becomes numerically more dominant later and is thought to bridge the early colonizers and the red complex species, which become numerically more dominant at late stages in plaque development.

constellatus) and red complexes (*Porphyromonas gingivalis, Treponema denticola*, and *Tannerella forsythia*) become more dominant (Socransky et al., 1998). The orange and the **red complexes** are comprised of species thought to be the major etiologic agents of periodontal disease. Haffajee, Teles, and Socransky (2006) in a study comparing patients with periodontal health and periodontal disease showed that the major differences between these patients was the increased counts, proportions, and prevalence of the red complex bacteria in patients with periodontal disease (Haffajee et al., 2006).

Oral Biofilm Formation

When a tooth begins to erupt, it is exposed to saliva, which contains all the acquired bacteria. At this point, the formation of dental plaque begins (Newman & Listgarten, 1999). The initial plaque formation is characterized by the numbers and kinds of bacteria that colonize the pellicle. Phase I, or initiation, begins in 1 to 2 days of plaque accumulation with no removal techniques. The microorganisms form as individual clones that extend both laterally and perpendicularly from the tooth surface to form parallel, palisading layers of bacteria (Fine, 1995; Figure 3–4 ■). The first colonies of bacteria are gram-positive cocci and short rods, including *Streptococcus mutans* and *Streptococcus sanguis*.

In the oral cavity, streptococci and *Actinomyces* form an essential component of the indigenous microbiota, as they are among initial colonizers in polymicrobial biofilms. The significance of *Actinomyces* is based on its ability to adhere to surfaces such as on teeth and to coaggregate with other bacteria.

Phase II begins in 2 to 4 days after abstaining from daily toothbrushing or leaving individual areas undisturbed. The early plaque masses provide the base for the next phase of colonies to infiltrate. The next bacteria to form are gram-positive rods and gram-negative cocci. The space between the layers of the first plaque provides an anaerobic environment for the arrival of anaerobic and facultative anaerobic (living with or without oxygen) bacteria. The cocci still dominate the plaque; however, filamentous forms and slender rods compete for the space (Fine, 1995; see Figure 3–4).

The matrix begins to form around the bacterial colonies derived mainly from salivary material, exudates (e.g., gingival crevicular fluid), and intermicrobial substances. Bacteria can form extracellular polysaccharides (carbohydrates) from sucrose. These glucans, levans, and fructans are significant to the adhesion process, and their insolubility

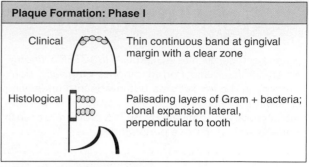

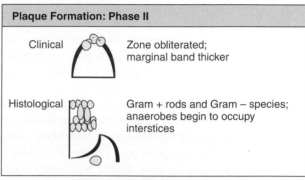

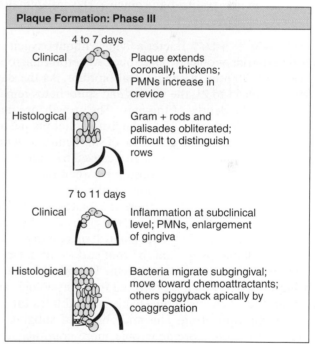

FIGURE 3–4 Illustration of different phases of oral biofilm formation.

increases the plaque resistance to removal. The levans and soluble glucans are an energy source for bacteria.

Days 4 to 7 mark Phase III of plaque formation with an increase in the filamentous bacteria. The rods, filaments, and fusobacteria commingle and interact with each other as nonmotile bacteria move with motile bacteria around the gingival margins. As the plaque matures, vibrios and spirochetes can colonize. New plaque may lie on the surface of mature plaque or spread coronally at the margin. This new plaque is characterized by cocci as before. The filaments at

---

Rapid Dental Hint

Remember that the names of two bacteria have been changed. *Aggregatibacter actinomycetemcomitans* and *Bacteriodes forsythus* are now *Tannerella forsythensis*.

Rapid Dental Hint

Some bacteria, such as *AGGREGATIBACTER* actinomycetemcomitans and *Porphyromonas gingivalis*, don't just stay in the pocket area but invade into underlying gingival connective tissue. Thus, systemic antibiotics are necessary to eliminate them. This problem is seen in patients with aggressive periodontitis.

the edge of the plaque serve as binding sites for these cocci, and a corncob formation appears. Gram-positive facultative filaments such as *Actinomyces* species bind with cocci such as *Streptococcus sanguis*.

Phase III continues as the plaque continues to mature over days 7 to 11. Due to a change in the environment at the tooth surface, spirochetes continue to multiply, and new species such as vibrios appear (see Figure 3–4). The host response to the plaque masses begins with early signs of inflammation observable in the gingiva. This inflammatory response is easily reversed by plaque removal.

SUBGINGIVAL BIOFILMS Bacteria living without oxygen are considered strict or obligate anaerobes. Anaerobic microbes thrive in the depths of subgingival biofilms. As the days progress from 14 to 21, the vibrios and spirochetes remain prevalent in the depths of the mass. The growth, accumulation, and pathogenicity of subgingival dental plaque are strongly influenced by the presence of supragingival dental plaque. Inflammation of the gingiva caused by supragingival plaque changes the relationship between the gingival margin and the tooth. In addition, swelling (edema) causes gingival enlargement, which alters the anatomic relationship between the tooth surface and the gingival margin and allows bacteria to invade the subgingival space and to form subgingival dental plaque on the root surface or adjacent to the epithelial tissue in the sulcus. This newly created subgingival space, which is protected from physiologic and mechanical oral cleansing mechanisms, facilitates further bacterial multiplication. The microbiota of subgingival plaque is generally more anaerobic, more gram-negative, more motile, and more asaccharolytic. There are also many motile organisms that are completely unattached to the plaque matrix. These microbes produce toxins, enzymes, and metabolic products that cause direct injury to the periodontium. More important, they act as antigens, and as the host responds to the irritant present, some destruction of the periodontal tissues occurs. Thus, elimination of subgingival plaque is critical to the prevention of periodontal diseases.

Biofilm in Peri-Implant Disease

Peri-implant disease has typically been characterized in two forms, peri-implant mucositis and peri-implantitis. **Peri-implant mucositis** describes an inflammatory lesion that resides in the mucosa, whereas **peri-implantitis** also affects the supporting bone (Lindhe & Meyle, 2008). Both of these conditions begin with biofilm formation. Using the experimental gingivitis model of Löe and others (1965), a cause-and-effect relationship between biofilm formation and implants and peri-implant mucositis has been demonstrated in humans (Pontoriero et al., 1994; Zitzmann, Berglundh, Marinello, & Lindhe, 2001).

Because the ecological environment with teeth and dental implants is the same, the formation of a biofilm is similar as well. One of the challenges in describing any biofilm relates to sampling methods. In dentistry, past methods for sampling a biofilm associated with an implant have been by insertion of a paper point into the peri-implant sulcus or removing a plaque sample by means of a curette. Due to these sampling methods, the three-dimensional architecture of the biofilm is destroyed. Therefore all data reported pertain to samples representing a largely uncontrolled mixture of bacteria from unspecified areas of biofilm associated with peri-implant diseases (Mombelli & Decaillet, 2011). In addition, the effectiveness of culture and sensitivity procedures has been questioned. In a study by Salkin et al. (2003), four different private periodontal practices participated in the collection of plaque samples, which were sent to two independent laboratories. Twenty individual subjects with generalized aggressive periodontitis or chronic periodontitis had microbiologic culture samples taken from their three deepest periodontal probing depth sites. Two paper points were inserted simultaneously at each site, with one point placed in each of the anaerobic culture transport tubes supplied by the laboratory. The two pooled sample tubes were sent to the same laboratory under identical conditions of carrier and time, and the laboratory results were collected and compared for similar findings of bacteria, similar threshold levels of those bacteria, similar antibiotic resistance or susceptibility of those bacteria, and the times both specimens revealed the same antibiotic for 100% kill for all pathogens. Results showed that the two labs very rarely agreed in their analysis, and even within the same lab there was often disagreement regarding two samples attained from the same pocket in a single patient. In only two samples (10% of samples) was there 100% agreement on the bacterial species, whereas antibiotic susceptibility agreed 80% of the time (Salkin et al., 2003).

The microbiota that has been described to be associated with peri-implant disease is mixed, rather variable, and in most cases dominated by diverse gram-negative anaerobic bacteria (Salkin et al., 2003). Ubiquitous organisms usually found in chronic periodontitis, such as *Fusobacterium* spp. and *Prevotella intermedia*, are regularly detected in specimens from peri-implantitis (Mombelli & Decaillet, 2011). Members of Socransky's "red complex" have also been detected. Checkerboard DNA–DNA hybridization for 40 bacterial species was used to analyze samples from 13 subjects with peri-implantitis and 12 subjects with mucositis (Maximo et al., 2009). *Porphyromonas gingivalis* and *Tannerella forsythia* were found at elevated levels in peri-implantitis cases, along with *Prevotella intermedia, Fusobacterium* ssp., *Streptococcus sanguinis, Streptococcus gordonii, Veillonella parvula*, and actinomyces. Maximo et al. (2009) also reported with regard to peri-implant mucositis cases elevated levels of *Capnocytophaga ochracea, Neisseria mucosa, Porphyromonas gingivalis, Prevotella nigresens, Fusobacterium* spp., and actinomyces.

There has been no reported evidence for the existence of one or a group of specific bacteria responsible for peri-implant disease. The possibility does exist that peri-implant disease may be linked to a microbiota substantially different than the microbiota associated with chronic periodontitis. Sporadic high numbers of the commensal organism peptostreptococci that has been associated with abscesses and necrotizing soft tissue infections, as well as staphylococci, which have been implicated in infections of implanted medical devices, have been reported with peri-implant disease (Mombelli & Decaillet, 2011). Therefore, any therapy to treat peri-implant disease must include disruption of the biofilm.

Disruption of Oral Biofilm: Treatment Modalities

The clinician is faced with many decisions when deciding on appropriate therapy for the periodontal patient or the patient with peri-implant disease. Scaling and root planing is considered the "gold standard" for treating periodontitis; however, the desired treatment outcome of resolution of inflammation and a decrease in probing depths may not occur. Because periodontitis is a microbial-based disease, the clinician may consider the use of antimicrobials as an adjunct to scaling and root planing. The host inflammatory response and its role in disease progression also must be taken into account, so consideration of treatment aimed at modulating the host response to suppress inflammation could be used.

Traditionally antibiotics can be given systemically or applied locally within the periodontal pocket. Administered as an adjunct to scaling and root planing, numerous studies that have utilized systemic antibiotics in conjunction with scaling and root planing (Ramberg et al., 2001; Rooney, Wade, Sprague, Newcombe, & Addy, 2002; Guerrero et al., 2005; Lopez, Socransky, Da Silva, Japlit, & Haffajee, 2006) have demonstrated clinical attachment gains superior to scaling and root planing alone in chronic and aggressive periodontitis patients. However, no study has proven systemic antimicrobials to be efficacious if the biofilm is not disrupted. This is due to several mechanisms. The biofilm itself offers protection of drug-sensitive microorganisms by neighboring commensal bacteria that can produce a neutralizing or drug-degrading enzyme, such as the production of beta-lactamase, which inactivates penicillin-based antibiotics. Phenotypic differences are also expressed by the micoorganisms within the biofilm when compared to their planktonic counterparts. Also, bacteria within the depths of the biofilm generally divide slower, which allows these slower-growing bacterial cells to be less sensitive to an antimicrobial agent (Marsh et al., 2011). In many instances these biofilm bacteria are up to 1,000 times more resistant to antimicrobial agents than planktonic bacteria (Jakubovics & Kolenbrander, 2010). There is no direct evidence demonstrating greater efficacy of a specific protocol when using systemic antibiotics with scaling and root planing. Indirect evidence does suggest that antimicrobial therapy should begin on the day of scaling and root planing completion and that scaling and root planing should be completed in less than 1 week (Herrera, Alonso, Leon, Roldan, & Sanz, 2008).

Dental Hygiene Application

Periodontal diseases have multiple risk factors. Therefore, it should not be expected that one risk factor will consistently be associated with the development of this kind of disease, and it should not be expected that control of one risk factor will completely eliminate the risk of developing the disease.

Dental biofilm are the primary etiologic factor in periodontal diseases. However, other local and systemic factors play an important role. By taking a thorough health and social history and correlating known local and systemic risk factors with periodontal clinical findings, clinicians can make patients who are at increased risk aware of the impact of these factors and the influence the factors have on their periodontal condition. Especially when treatment is unsuccessful, reevaluation of primary and secondary risk factors might improve future treatment results.

Metabolic interactions among different bacterial cell types probably play a dominant role in the changes in community composition during plaque maturation. Communication among different bacterial communities may help with nutrient availability and oxygen removal, favoring the proliferation of specific bacterial species (Kolenbrander et al., 2006)

The *Parameters of Care*, published by the American Academy of Periodontology (2000), suggests that the initial therapy for patients with periodontal inflammation should include the elimination, alteration, or control of risk factors that may contribute to chronic periodontitis. This represents significant progress because it is clear that periodontal diseases are infections initiated by bacteria and may have several associated risk factors. Management of these risk factors is likely to be the most successful approach to preventing periodontitis in the future. Physical removal of subgingival biofilm results in only a brief reduction in the numbers of colonizing bacteria. Within 2 to 7 days the bacterial mass of dental biofilm starts to be recolonized. Some bacteria such as *Streptococcus* recolonize very rapidly, whereas *T. forsythensis*, *P. gingivalis*, and *T. denticola* return slowly after mechanical debridement (Haffajee et al., 2006).

Also, because the presence of periodontitis is recognized as a risk factor for future and more severe periodontal disease (past attachment loss is a risk factor for future attachment loss), proper diagnosis and therapy of an existing condition is very important in helping prevent future occurrences.

Key Points

- The primary etiologic agent in periodontal disease is bacteria within a biofilm.
- There is a shift in bacteria from periodontal health to disease from a gram-positive, saccharolytic, facultative anaerobic bacteria to bacteria dominated by gram-negative anaerobes.
- The bacteria within the biofilm in peri-implant disease are similar to that found in periodontal disease.
- Systemic antibiotics should never be used as a stand-alone treatment in the nonsurgical management of periodontal disease.

Self-Quiz

1. From the following list, select the items associated with the term "biofilm."
   a. Diverse microbial community that is attached to a surface.
   b. Hard calcified bacteria by-products.
   c. Oral biofilm are bacterial populations adherent to each other.
   d. Biofilm are found only in the mouth.
   e. Microorganisms in biofilm are resistant to antibiotics.

2. All of the following are members of the "red complex" of bacteria except one. Which one is the exception?
   a. *Treponema denticola*.
   b. *Porphyromonas gingivalis*.
   c. *Tannerella forsythia*.
   d. *Aggregatibacter actinomycetemcomitans*.

3. From the following list, select the items associated with the features of oral biofilm.
   a. The majority of the biofilm volume is made up of bacterial cells.
   b. Bacteria adhere to the pellicle.
   c. Primarily composed of gram-negative obligate anaerobes.
   d. Live independently.

4. The microbiota that has been described to be associated with peri-implant disease is mixed, rather variable, and in most cases dominated by:
   a. gram-positive aerobes.
   b. gram-positive anaerobes.
   c. gram-negative aerobes.
   d. gram-negative anaerobes.

5. In the classic experimental gingivitis study by Löe and colleagues, a shift in microbial flora from a gram-positive cocci to a _____ flora was seen.
   a. gram-positive rod
   b. gram-negative anaerobe
   c. gram-positive anaerobe
   d. gram-positive cocci

6. Bacteria present within the biofilm are less resistant to antimicrobial agents than bacteria living in a planktonic state.
   a. True
   b. False

7. All of the following are examples of how the biofilm protects bacteria from antimicrobial agents except one. Which one is the exception?
   a. protection by neighboring commensal bacteria that can produce a neutralizing or drug-degrading enzyme.
   b. phenotype changes by the bacteria within the biofilm.
   c. slower growth of bacteria within the biofilm.
   d. genotype changes by bacteria within the biofilm.

8. All of the following were shown to be different in patients with periodontal health and disease except one. Which one is the exception?
   a. increased bacterial counts.
   b. increase in bacterial proportions.
   c. presence of yellow complex bacteria.
   d. presence of red complex bacteria.

9. Bacteria populate the biofilm either passively through salivary or gingival crevicular flow, or in the case of a few motile species, by their own transport.
   a. True
   b. False

10. *Aggregatibacter actinomycetemcomitans* is a member of which bacterial complex according to Socransky?
    a. Red
    b. Yellow
    c. Green
    d. Purple

Case Study

A 25-year-old female patient shows up in the dental office after disappointing many times. Her medical history is non-contributory. The periodontal examination reveals generalized edematous and erythematous gingiva with 1-4 mm probing depths. There is no radiographic bone destruction.

1. What is the most important part of therapy for this patient?
   a. To understand the importance of host response
   b. Have the patient make plans for periodontal surgical intervention
   c. Instruct the patient to brush for at least 2 minutes
   d. Refer the patient to a periodontist

Answer: A

2. What type of bacterial population is most likely present in this patient?
   a. *Bacteriodes*
   b. *Fusobacterium nucleatum*
   c. *Streptococcus-Actinomyces*
   d. *Porphyromonas gingivalis/Prevotella intermedia*

Answer: C

3. After this patient commences oral hygiene habits, about how long will it take for the gingivitis is resolve?
   a. 1 week
   b. 2 weeks
   c. 1 month
   d. 2 months

Answer: A

References

Aas, J. A., B. J. Paster, L. N. Stokes, I. Olsen, and F. E. Dewhirst. 2005. Defining the normal bacterial flora of the oral cavity. *J. Clin. Microbiol.* 43(11):5721–5732. Epub 2005/11/08.

American Academy of Periodontology. 2000. Parameters of Care. *J. Periodontol.* 71(5):847–883.

Berezow, A. B., and R. P. Darveau. 2011. Microbial shift and periodontitis. *Periodontol. 2000.* 55(1):36–47. Epub 2010/12/08.

Busscher, H. J., W. Norde, and H. C. van der Mei. 2008. Specific molecular recognition and nonspecific contributions to bacterial interaction forces. *Appl. Environ. Microbiol.* 74(9): 2559–2564. Epub 2008/03/18.

Daly, C. G., and J. E. Highfield. 1996. Effect of localized experimental gingivitis on early supragingival plaque accumulation. *J. Clin. Periodontol.* 23(3 Pt 1):160–164. Epub 1996/03/01.

Fine, D. 1995. Chemical agents to prevent and regulate plaque development. *Periodontology* 8:87–107.

Forng, R. Y., C. Champagne, W. Simpson, and C. A. Genco. 2000. Environmental cues and gene expression in *Porphyromonas gingivalis* and *Aggregatibacter actinomycetemcomitans*. *Oral Dis.* 6(6):351–365. Epub 2001/05/18.

Guerrero, A., G. S. Griffiths, L. Nibali, J. Suvan, D. R. Moles, L. Laurell, et al. 2005. Adjunctive benefits of systemic amoxicillin and metronidazole in non-surgical treatment of generalized aggressive periodontitis: A randomized placebo-controlled clinical trial. *J. Clin. Periodontol.* 32(10):1096–1107. Epub 2005/09/22.

Haffajee, A. D., R. P. Teles, and S. S. Socransky. 2006. Association of *Eubacterium nodatum* and *Treponema denticola* with human periodontitis lesions. *Oral Microbiol. Immunol.* 21(5):269–282. Epub 2006/08/23.

Herrera, D., B. Alonso, R. Leon, S. Roldan, and M. Sanz. 2008. Antimicrobial therapy in periodontitis: The use of systemic antimicrobials against the subgingival biofilm. *J. Clin. Periodontol.* 35(8 Suppl):45–66. Epub 2008/09/09.

Jakubovics, N. S., and P. E. Kolenbrander. 2010. The road to ruin: The formation of disease-associated oral biofilm. *Oral Dis.* 16(8):729–739. Epub 2010/07/22.

Kolenbrander, P. E., R. J. Palmer, A. H. Rickard, N. S. Jakubovics, et al. 2006. Bacterial interactions and successions during plaque development. *Periodontology 2000.* 42(1):47–79.

Kornman, K. S., and W. J. Loesche. 1980. The subgingival microbial flora during pregnancy. *J. Periodontal Res.* 15(2):111–122. Epub 1980/03/01.

Lindhe, J., N. P. Lang, and T. Karring. 2008. *Clinical periodontology and implant dentistry*, 5th ed. Oxford, UK; Ames, Iowa: Blackwell Munksgaard.

Lindhe, J., and J. Meyle. 2008. Peri-implant diseases: Consensus Report of the Sixth European Workshop on Periodontology. *J. Clin. Periodontol.* 35(8 Suppl):282–285. Epub 2008/09/09.

Listgarten, M. A., and L. Hellden. 1978. Relative distribution of bacteria at clinically healthy and periodontally diseased sites in humans. *J. Clin. Periodontol.* 5(2):115–132. Epub 1978/05/01.

Löe, H., E. Theilade, and S. B. Jensen. 1965. Experimental gingivitis in man. *J. Periodontol.* 36:177–187. Epub 1965/05/01.

Lopez, N. J., S. S. Socransky, I. Da Silva, M. R. Japlit, and A. D. Haffajee. 2006. Effects of metronidazole plus amoxicillin as the only therapy on the microbiological and clinical parameters of untreated chronic periodontitis. *J. Clin. Periodontol.* 33(9):648–660. Epub 2006/07/22.

Marsh, P. D., and D. A. Devine. 2011. How is the development of dental biofilm influenced by the host? *J. Clin. Periodontol.* 38(Suppl 11):28–35. Epub 2011/02/26.

Marsh, P., and M. Martin. 2009. *Oral microbiology*, 5th ed. Edinburgh; New York: Elsevier.

Marsh, P. D., A. Moter, and D. A. Devine. 2011. Dental plaque biofilm: Communities, conflict and control. *Periodontol. 2000.* 55(1):16–35. Epub 2010/12/08.

Maximo, M. B., A. C. de Mendonca, V. Renata Santos, L. C. Figueiredo, M. Feres, and P. M. Duarte. 2009. Short-term clinical and microbiological evaluations of peri-implant diseases before and after mechanical anti-infective therapies. *Clin. Oral Implants Res.* 20(1):99–108. Epub 2009/01/08.

Mombelli, A., and F. Decaillet. 2011. The characteristics of biofilm in peri-implant disease. *J. Clin. Periodontol.* 38(Suppl 11):203–213. Epub 2011/02/26.

Moore, W. E., L. V. Holdeman, R. M. Smibert, I. J. Good, J. A. Burmeister, K. G. Palcanis, et al. 1982. Bacteriology of experimental gingivitis in young adult humans. *Infection and Immunity*. 38(2):651–667. Epub 1982/11/01.

Newman, H. N., and M. A. Listgarten. 1999. The development of dental plaque: From preeruptive primary cuticle to acquired pellicle to dental plaque to calculus formation. In eds. N. O. Harris and F. Garcia-Godoy, *Primary preventive dentistry*, 5th ed., 21–39. Stamford, CT: Appleton and Lange.

Pontoriero, R., M. P. Tonelli, G. Carnevale, A. Mombelli, S. R. Nyman, and N. P. Lang. 1994. Experimentally induced peri-implant mucositis. A clinical study in humans. *Clin. Oral Implants Res*. 5(4):254–259. Epub 1994/12/01.

Ramberg, P., B. Rosling, G. Serino, M. K. Hellstrom, S. S. Socransky, and J. Lindhe. 2001. The long-term effect of systemic tetracycline used as an adjunct to non-surgical treatment of advanced periodontitis. *J. Clin. Periodontol*. 28(5):446–452. Epub 2001/05/15.

Ramberg, P., Y. Furuichi, A. R. Volpe, A. Gaffar, and J. Lindhe. 1996. The effects of antimicrobial mouthrinses on de novo plaque formation at sites with healthy and inflamed gingivae. *J. Clin. Periodontol*. 23(1):7–11. Epub 1996/01/01.

Rooney, J., W. G. Wade, S. V. Sprague, R. G. Newcombe, and M. Addy. 2002. Adjunctive effects to non-surgical periodontal therapy of systemic metronidazole and amoxycillin alone and combined. A placebo controlled study. *J. Clin. Periodontol*. 29(4):342–350. Epub 2002/04/23.

Salkin, L. M., A. L. Freedman, J. R. Mellado, M. D. Stein, D. B. Schneider, and L. Butler. 2003. The clinical relevance of microbiologic testing. Part 2: A comparative analysis of microbiologic samples secured simultaneously from the same sites and cultured in the same laboratory. *Int. J. Periodontics Restorative Dent*. 23(2):121–127. Epub 2003/04/25.

Schaudinn, C., A. Gorur, D. Keller, P. P. Sedghizadeh, and J. W. Costerton. 2009. Periodontitis: An archetypical biofilm disease. *J. Am. Dent. Assoc*. 140(8):978–986. Epub 2009/08/06.

Slots, J. 1979. Subgingival microflora and periodontal disease. *Journal of Clinical Periodontology*. 6(5):351–382. Epub 1979/10/01.

Society for General Microbiology. Symposium (59th: 2000: Exeter England), Allison, D. G. Society for General Microbiology. *Community structure and co-operation in biofilm*. Cambridge, UK; New York: Cambridge University Press; 2000.

Socransky, S. S., A. D. Haffajee, M. A. Cugini, C. Smith, and R. L. Kent, Jr. 1998. Microbial complexes in subgingival plaque. *J. Clin. Periodontol*. 25(2):134–144. Epub 1998/03/12.

Zitzmann, N. U., T. Berglundh, C. P. Marinello, and J. Lindhe. 2001. Experimental peri-implant mucositis in man. *J. Clin. Periodontol*. 28(6):517–523. Epub 2001/05/15.

4

Bacteria and the Host Response: Inflammatory and Immunology Fundamentals

Mea A. Weinberg

OUTLINE

EDUCATIONAL OBJECTIVES

Upon completion of this chapter, the reader should be able to:

- List three theories of periodontal disease activity.
- Describe the progression of gingivitis into periodontitis.
- Discuss bacterial components that stimulate the initiation of the inflammatory and immune systems.
- Describe the different levels of oral defense mechanisms.
- Describe the process of phagocytosis.
- Compare and contrast humoral immunity and cellular immunity.

GOAL: To provide an understanding of host response to the bacteria present in dental biofilms (biofilm).

KEY WORDS

Introduction

Gingivitis is defined as inflammation confined to the gingiva without clinical connective tissue attachment loss and bone loss. Gingivitis is a direct response of the host (body) to the accumulation of supragingival dental biofilms at the gingival margin. **Periodontitis** is defined as the loss of clinical connective tissue attachment (also referred to as clinical attachment loss) and alveolar bone loss with the formation of a periodontal pocket. **Connective tissue attachment loss** refers to the pathological detachment of collagen fibers from the cemental surfaces with the concomitant apical migration of the apical part of the junctional epithelium onto the root surface (Armitage, 1995). The events leading to clinical connective tissue attachment loss also result in the destruction of alveolar and supporting bone. The destruction that occurs in gingivitis and periodontitis is influenced by the *inflammatory and immune process* of the individual.

Periodontal Disease Activity

The development of chronic inflammatory periodontal diseases involves a series of host responses or reactions of the body to bacteria present in the dental biofilm (plaque), which is considered the invader or irritant. Host cells or cells normally found in the body are needed to fight this infection. Examples of host cells include blood cells present in the body, such as macrophages, lymphocytes, and polymorphonuclear leukocytes (PMNs) or, as sometimes called, neutrophils. PMNs are a type of white blood cell involved in the host defense system. The host defense is constantly being called on to ward off attacks of the microorganisms that are colonizing the oral cavity at any given time. This balance of host defense mechanisms against the microbial attack is kept in check until the microorganisms overtake the defense system, at which time infection and tissue damage develop (Bascones-Martinez et al., 2009). It is assumed that host cells mediate the destruction of soft and hard connective tissue because of the reaction to bacteria in the biofilm.

Periodontal disease activity (PDA) is defined as the *ongoing* loss of clinical connective tissue attachment and alveolar and supporting bone (Greenstein & Caton, 1990) at a certain point in time (e.g., at the clinical examination appointment). Detection of areas in the mouth that are in the active stage of destruction may be important in the implementation of treatment. However, it is extremely difficult to determine at a given time if a site is actively breaking down or will break down in the future.

Models of Disease Activity

Currently, three theories of periodontal disease activity have been described:

1. The continuous model theory
2. The random burst theory
3. The asynchronous multiple burst theory

Rapid Dental Hint

It is very difficult to determine or predict that a specific periodontal site in the mouth is "breaking down" and losing attachment and bone. It has been suggested that a 2 to 3 mm change in attachment level (level of the junctional epithelium, which is your probing depths measured from the CEJ) is required for a site to be disease active.

Rapid Dental Hint

Loss of connective tissue attachment (or loss of attachment, as it is sometimes referred to) is defined as the destruction of gingival connective tissue attachment (e.g., gingival fibers) due to disease, followed by apical migration of the junctional epithelium along the root surface.

The continuous model theory is based on the concept that periodontal destruction is slow and constant until tooth loss, and the severity of the disease increases with age (Löe, Anerud, Boysen, & Morrison, 1986). However, epidemiologic studies have not demonstrated whether destruction is continuous or new diseased sites actually develop (Greenstein & Caton, 1990).

The next theory is the random burst theory (Socransky, Haffajee, Goodson, & Lindhe, 1984). This theory states that periodontal diseases progress in short bursts of exacerbation (actively losing attachment), followed by a period of remission or quiescence, where there is no progressive attachment loss (Goodson, 1992; Socransky et al., 1984). Another proposed name for this theory is the episodic burst theory, which reflects the fact that periodontal diseases are site specific, and not all sites in the mouth are equally susceptible (Zimmerman, 1986).

The third concept, the asynchronous multiple burst hypothesis, states that periodontal disease activity occurs during a limited time period (e.g., acne during childhood may resolve during adulthood) followed by remission (Greenstein & Caton, 1990; Socransky et al., 1984).

In reality, all of the preceding theories may be interacting to explain periodontal disease progression. No one theory alone can explain the disease progression. It cannot be assumed that all sites will continuously get worse. Also, treatment should not wait until a burst of bone destruction has occurred. Periodontal destruction is cumulative over time. Because it is difficult to actually determine if a site is disease active, it is prudent to treat all inflamed sites (Greenstein & Caton, 1990).

Progression of Gingivitis into Periodontitis

Gingivitis must precede periodontitis. That is, periodontitis does not develop unless gingivitis existed previously. However, gingivitis may, but does not always, progress to periodontitis.

Why does periodontitis develop in some individuals whereas in others gingivitis does not progress into periodontitis? Currently, the *exact* cause for the progression of gingivitis into periodontitis is relatively unclear. Approximately 80% of the population is susceptible to periodontal diseases (Brown & Löe, 1993). Susceptibility to periodontal diseases involves changes in bacteria–host equilibrium. A failure of this equilibrium results in the initiation of periodontal disease. However, although bacteria are essential to this process, their presence alone is not enough to cause destructive periodontal disease. There must be a decrease in the number of beneficial (good) bacteria such as *Streptococcus* sp., a critical mass of pathogenic (disease-producing) bacteria, a conducive or favorable environment to cause disease, and a susceptible host that reacts to the pathogen. Gingivitis may progress into periodontitis if the host resistance decreases and if bacteria overwhelm the defense system and penetrate soft tissue. Some reasons for a decrease in host resistance include stress, chemotherapy, local tissue trauma, uncontrolled diabetes, leukemia, steroids, and fully developed acquired immunodeficiency syndrome (AIDS).

Rapid Dental Hint

Periodontitis does not develop unless gingivitis existed previously. Gingivitis may, but does not always, progress to periodontitis.

Rapid Dental Hint

Local etiologic factors and host response factors both contribute to the pathogenesis of inflammatory periodontal diseases.

The **host response** is in nature a defense mechanism (Kinane & Bartold, 2007; Shikawa, 2007; Weinberg, 2011). It is a natural response of the body to protect and defend the individual after the person's body has been challenged by an injurious agent such as a bacterium or virus. This same host response that provides protection to host tissues frequently also causes host tissue destruction (Figure 4–1 ■). When the repair of tissue is greater than its destruction, the tissue starts healing. Fortunately, host tissue destruction usually is not permanent because tissues have a great capacity for healing.

The Bacteria–Host Challenge

It is both the local etiologic factors, bacteria and the host factors, that contribute to the development of periodontal diseases (Hujoel, Zina, Cunha-Cruz, & Lopez, 2012). Both the microbiology and host response will be reviewed.

Microbiology

Bacteria that colonize early on the tooth surface at the gingival margin are predominately supragingival gram-positive facultative (i.e., can live with or without oxygen) *Streptococci* and *Actinomyces* species. If biofilm is not disrupted by toothbrushing and flossing, a more established and varied microbial colony develops. With increasing time and poor biofilm control, periodontitis-associated microbiota populate the subgingival pocket area, including gram-negative

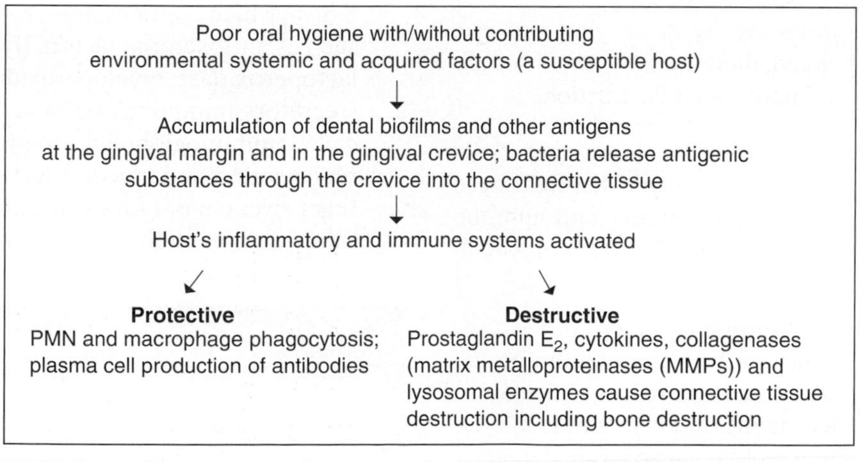

Poor oral hygiene with/without contributing environmental systemic and acquired factors (a susceptible host)

↓

Accumulation of dental biofilms and other antigens at the gingival margin and in the gingival crevice; bacteria release antigenic substances through the crevice into the connective tissue

↓

Host's inflammatory and immune systems activated

↙   ↘

Protective
PMN and macrophage phagocytosis; plasma cell production of antibodies

Destructive
Prostaglandin E_2, cytokines, collagenases (matrix metalloproteinases (MMPs)) and lysosomal enzymes cause connective tissue destruction including bone destruction

FIGURE 4–1 Pathway of pathogenesis showing the sequence of events leading to periodontal destruction.

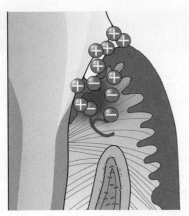

FIGURE 4–2 Gram-negative microorganisms live in the subgingival pocket environment and are no longer subjected to normal oral hygiene procedures.

anaerobes (oxygen intolerant) such as *Fusobacterium nucleatum, Porphyromonas gingivalis, Eikenella corrodens, Aggregatibacter actinomycetemcomitans*, and *Prevotella intermedia* (Listgarten, 1994; Figure 4–2 ■). In addition to the subgingival anaerobic bacteria found in the deeper subgingival biofilm, the bacteria found in direct contact with the junctional epithelium may be or has the potential to become pathogenic and cause disease. Anaerobic bacteria become established as the bacteria multiply and become thicker with less oxygen available to the bacteria. The rate of subgingival biofilm recolonization may depend on supragingival biofilm accumulation.

Bacteria, their metabolic wastes or by-products, and toxins that synthesize and release into the subgingival environment are foreign to the body and are termed **antigens**. Long-standing, chronic bacterial accumulation causes an excessive and persistent antigenic stimulus to the host response mechanisms. Thus, although bacteria initiate the disease process, it is enzymes and by-products produced by the host that are actually responsible for most of the breakdown of periodontal tissues. As a side effect, the reactions activated by the host response result in tissue inflammation in which surrounding cells, connective tissue, and bone are destroyed. Thus, host responses are basically protective by destroying antigens, but if the body is overwhelmed, then the host responses are destructive, causing soft- and hard-tissue destruction.

BACTERIAL COMPONENTS Bacteria release metabolic substances proven to be toxic to cells and tissues. These stimulate the initiation of the inflammatory and immune systems. The following substances are released from bacteria that affect the host:

- Endotoxin, a lipopolysaccharide (also termed lipooligosaccharide), is part of the outer membrane of all gram-negative bacteria. Endotoxins, which are released when the bacteria die and lyse (break apart), stimulate biologic activities that cause tissue damage and bone destruction.
- Leukotoxin, an exotoxin produced by *Aggregatibacter actinomycetemcomitans*, can kill PMNs.

- Bacteria synthesize and release various waste products (by-products) such as ammonia, which is toxic to many host cells, and hydrogen sulfide, which increases the permeability of the epithelium so that antigenic substances can more easily enter the lamina propria.
- Bacteria synthesize and secrete enzymes, which can break down tissue. Hyaluronidase, an enzyme found in periodontal pockets, may break down or degrade the "cementing substance" between epithelial cells, causing widening of the intercellular spaces and increased permeability.

Matrix metalloproteinases (MMPs) are a family of enzymes that cleave or break down the components of the extracellular matrix. This family of enzymes includes more than 25 members that are divided into collagenases (MMP 1,8,13), gelatinases (MMP 2,9), stromelysins (MMP 3, 10), matrilysins (MMP 7, 26), and membrane-type MMPs (MMP 14–17, 24; Birkedal-Hansen et al., 1993). Collagenase may break down collagen, and proteases degrade proteins, including the connective tissue ground substance and collagen fibers. Host cells such as PMNs and fibroblasts also secrete collagenase. Thus, these enzymes that bacteria and host cells synthesize and release prepare the tissues for absorption of toxic and otherwise harmful bacterial products.

Oral Defense Mechanisms

The host interacts with microorganisms at three different areas in the periodontium:

1. The supragingival environment
2. The gingival crevice
3. The gingival connective tissue

The first attempt at self-protection comes from the supragingival environment and involves nonspecific defenses. These responses are important in the prevention of the extension of supragingival biofilm into the subgingival area (the gingival crevice). Defense mechanisms include the following:

- Saliva, which contains numerous defensive substances such as antibacterial factors (lysozyme, lactoferrin, lactoperoxidase, myeloperoxidase) and antibodies (secretory immunoglobulin A [sIgA]). Antibodies called immunoglobulins are proteins present in the blood serum and mucosal secrections (e.g., saliva, tears, sweat, nasal fluids) produced following interaction with an antigen.

Rapid Dental Hint

Host responses are basically protective by destroying antigens. If the body is overwhelmed, then the host responses are destructive, causing soft- and hard-tissue destruction.

Rapid Dental Hint

Gingival crevicular fluid (fluid found in small amounts in gingival crevice) is important in cleansing substances from crevice and has antimicrobial properties

- Gingival crevicular fluid (GCF) functions as an outward flow cleansing the sulcus. The increased volume of GCF produced during the **inflammatory process** also serves to deliver more antimicrobial products from the deeper tissue toward the main site of supragingival bacterial colonization (e.g., tooth surface). These are the first substances to interact with the antigenic challenge (bacteria) to try to neutralize, isolate, or kill it.
- Oral epithelium also serves to prevent bacteria and their by-products from entering the underlying tissues. This is attained by the surface keratin and the close attachment of the epithelial cells.
- Shedding of epithelial cells from the oral mucosa into the oral cavity.

The Inflammatory Response and the Immune Response: Host Response to the Periodontal Diseases

If the body is unsuccessful in eliminating the pathogenic bacteria at the supragingival level, the inflammatory/immune response, working together, is further stimulated to eliminate the irritant and prevent the spread of infection. This system is activated when antigens (e.g., endotoxins, bacterial enzymes, and by-products) present in the biofilm mass in the gingival crevice pass through the protective wall of PMNs (leukocyte wall) interposed between the biofilm mass and the lining of the gingival crevice and junctional epithelium. After the antigens cross the junctional epithelial barrier, the deeper tissues are penetrated (Miyasaki, 1991; see Figure 4–3 ■). Only a few bacteria themselves actually enter the connective tissue. Usually, it is the products from the bacteria that enter the tissues while the bacteria remain in the crevice. However, it has been demonstrated that *Aggregatibacter actinomycetemcomitans*, *Porphyromonas* gingivalis, and spirochetes invade connective tissue (de Graaf, van Winkelhoff, & Goené, 1989; Renvert, Winström, Dahlén, Slots, & Egelberg, 1990; Saglie, Carranza, Newman, Cheng, & Lewin, 1982). Activation of the inflammatory/immune system results in the following:

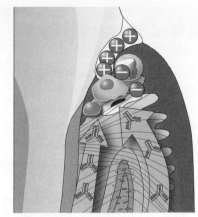

FIGURE 4–3 As the protective wall of neutrophils between the biofilm mass and the gingival crevice and junctional epithelium becomes compromised, the inflammatory response becomes magnified by the immune system. Once the antigens in the pocket pass through the wall of white blood cells and touch or penetrate the gingival connective tissue, a burst of immunological response results in gingival tissue damage and alveolar and supporting bone destruction.

(1) elimination or retardation of the invader (bacteria), (2) the limiting of further tissue destruction, and (3) the beginning of healing.

The Inflammatory Response

The inflammatory response to a bacterial challenge is a nonspecific reaction intended to prevent the spread of invading bacteria and, if possible, to destroy the damaging agent. This is accomplished through the process of inflammation.

When bacteria cause irritation to the gingival or periodontal tissues, a series of responses mediated by host defense cells is initiated. First, an acute inflammatory response occurs. Box 4–1 lists the cells involved in the inflammatory response (Van Dyke, 2007). If this is ineffective—the stimulus is not removed and healing does not occur—inflammation becomes chronic, and additional defense cells from the immune system become involved. After the events in the periodontal areas subside, the tissues

Rapid Dental Hint

Many substances or markers for periodontal disease are found in GCF, including collagenase, β-glucuronidase, and prostaglandin E_2.

Box 4–1: Key Elements in the Inflammatory Response

- Polymorphonuclear leukocytes (PMNs) or neutrophils (a white blood cell involved in phagocytosis or engulfing bacteria)

- Macrophages (phagocyte in connective tissue)

- Mast cells (cell found in connective tissue that contains granules and releases substances such as heparin and histamine)

- Serum complement (serum proteins that work with [*complement*] antibody activity to eliminate pathogens; stimulate inflammation)

are cleansed, repaired, and rebuilt. Unfortunately, sometimes the damage to some of these tissues is permanent and is present even after the infection is eliminated.

ELEMENTS OF THE INFLAMMATORY SYSTEM A clinically healthy gingiva that is relatively biofilm-free is characterized by a salmon pink color, firm consistency, no bleeding from the gingival crevice, and shallow sulci. In the healthy gingiva the junctional epithelium does not have long epithelial ridges and overlies the highly oriented collagen fiber bundles. Although clinically there may appear to be no inflammation, at a microscopic level there may be a mild inflammatory reaction. Thus, in the junctional epithelium of clinically healthy gingiva there are always inflammatory cells, primarily PMNs, which form a protective wall between the epithelium and the bacteria. PMNs constantly migrate from the junctional epithelium into the gingival crevice, where the older cells are shed into the oral cavity. With severe inflammation, a greater number of these cells are present.

THE INFLAMMATORY PROCESS Table 4–1 ■ describes three phases of the inflammatory process. If dental biofilm is allowed to accumulate at the gingival margin and is not disrupted, inflammation or gingivitis results. Biofilm removal every 48 hours can prevent gingivitis, but if it is allowed to accumulate for 72 hours, gingivitis will develop (Van Dyke, Offenbacher, Pihlstrom, Putt, & Trummel, 1999).

The gingiva reacts to the bacteria and its products by the first 3 days of biofilm accumulation at the gingival margin with signs of acute inflammation. The first inflammatory response to injury is vascular changes in the gingival connective tissue; the epithelium is avascular (no blood supply of its own) but depends on the connective tissue for its nutrition. Vasodilation of the blood vessels in the connective tissue results in the outflow of blood, fluids, proteins, and cells (PMNs) into the connective tissue (Figure 4–4 ■).

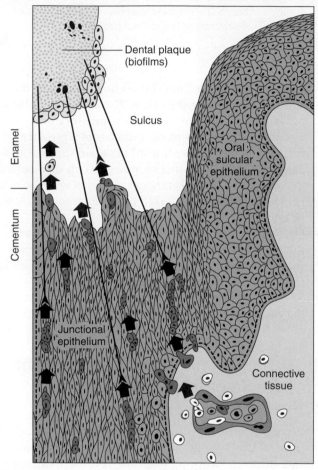

FIGURE 4–4 Schematic drawing of the relationship of the gingival sulcus to the epithelium and connective tissue in health. Note the dental biofilm on the tooth surface at the entrance to the gingival sulcus. Neutrophils are leaving blood vessels in the connective tissue and moving chemotactically through the semipermeable junctional epithelium but not through the oral sulcular epithelium of the lateral wall of the sulcus.

Table 4–1 Phases of the Inflammatory Process

Phase	Features
Phase 1: Acute transient phase	Local vasodilation and increased capillary permeability
Phase 2: Delayed subacute phase	Migration of PMNs and other phagocytic cells, including mast cells and macrophages into the tissue
Phase 3: Chronic phase	Tissue destruction

The primary substance responsible for the vasodilation and increased permeability of the blood vessel wall is histamine, which is released from mast cells found in the connective tissue. Another substance that is involved in the vasodilation is prostaglandin. **Prostaglandins** are fatty acids found in most cell membranes. Prostaglandins are synthesized in large amounts during gingivitis and periodontitis, and may be responsible for the pain and bone loss seen in periodontal diseases (Offenbacher, Heasman, & Collins, 1993; Figure 4–5a, b ■). Vasodilation clinically shows as gingival edema and erythema (redness). Thus, tissue edema or swelling is due to the increase of permeability of blood vessels, which causes the migration and accumulation of cells and fluid from the vessels to surrounding tissue. With the initiation of inflammation, the flow of gingival crevicular fluid increases from the connective tissue out through the junctional epithelium into the gingival crevice. Migration of PMNs through the junctional epithelium into the gingival sulcus and crevicular fluid flow both peak 6 to 12 days after the onset of clinically detectable gingivitis (Kowashi, Jaccard, & Cimasoni, 1980; Zappa, 1995). Table 4–2 ■ describes the differences between the acute and chronic inflammatory responses.

Gingival bleeding at the gingival crevice is an early and important sign of gingival inflammation. When the crevice is probed or stroked, it may bleed immediately because the sulcular epithelium (epithelium lining the sulcus) becomes ulcerated with tears in the epithelial lining. The bleeding on probing comes from the underlying vascular gingival connective tissue (lamina propria), which is engorged with blood because of the disease process (Rizzo, 1970).

The Neutrophil: The Phagocytic Cell. The neutrophil has been referred to as a "first line of defense" and the "hallmark of acute inflammation," meaning that it is one of the first defensive cells to be recruited to a site of inflammation

(Figure 4–6 ■). PMNs are the first cells to migrate from inside the blood vessels into the surrounding connective tissue and enter the gingival crevice and junctional epithelium in response to chemotactic substances such as toxins released by the bacteria and complement (proteins found in the serum; Miyasaki, 1991).

Neutrophils leave the bloodstream and get to the site of infection by first adhering to the endothelium of the blood vessel wall. This is called margination. Then, the neutrophil migrates between the endothelial cells and leaves through the capillary wall. This is called diapedesis.

Chemotaxis is the movement of cells in the direction of a chemical attractant. The PMNs create a wall between swimming, unattached bacteria and the junctional and sulcular epithelium. Once in the tissue, the neutrophil is ready to kill the foreign invader or bacteria. Once the PMN comes in contact with the bacteria, **phagocytosis** occurs. The PMN is the major phagocytic cell, whose fast arrival from the blood vessels in the connective tissue into the junctional epithelium and crevice plays an important part in removing bacteria and other foreign substances. Neutrophils live a very short time. Neutrophils come out of the bone marrow programmed to die in an average of about 5 days. Once at the site of injury, the bacteria are engulfed by the PMNs (endocytosis). Phagocytosis is a specific form of endocytosis involving the ingestion of solids such as bacteria versus fluids. The PMNs recognize the foreign material (bacteria, toxins, and by-products) and "eat and digest" it. Once inside

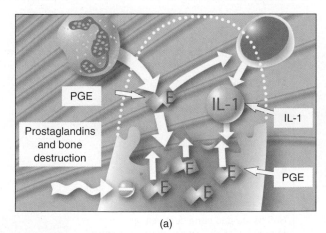

(a)

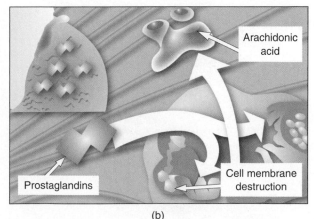

(b)

FIGURE 4–5 (a) Prostaglandins (PGs) are fatty acids produced in the body by the initiation of an inflammatory response involving the release of substances from the injured cell membrane of the tissue followed by production of PGs via arachidonic acid. (b) Prostaglandins are involved in the entire body process. Specifically, PGE_2 is involved in inflammatory periodontal disease, including destruction of alveolar bone.

Table 4–2 Acute versus Chronic Inflammatory Responses

	Acute Inflammation	Chronic Inflammation
What causes it?	Antigen such as bacteria in dental biofilm	Unresolved acute inflammation; continued presence of antigens
What cells are involved in the body's response to the causative agent?	PMNs, mononuclear cells (e.g., macrophages)	Monocytes, macrophages, lymphocytes, plasma cells
What substances (or mediators) are released from the cells that cause the signs and symptoms of inflammation?	Vasoactive amines (e.g., histamine, bradykinin)	Cytokines, growth factors, reactive oxygen species, hydrolytic enzymes
When does this inflammatory response first appear?	Immediate onset	Delayed onset
How long does this response last?	Several days	Long time (months to years)
After the response is over, what happens to the tissues?	Healing occurs if the inflammation is resolved	Tissue destruction

the PMN, the bacteria are degraded by enzymes called lysosomes. As the bacteria are engulfed, lysosomal enzymes "leak" out of the cell into the surrounding tissue causing destruction of host tissue. This process is called exocytosis, which refers to the movement of large amounts of material out of cells. Examples of lysosomal enzymes include collagenase, beta-glucuronidase, and alkaline phosphatase. High levels of these enzymes can be detected in the GCF during periodontitis.

Genetically, impaired PMN function is seen in patients with certain medical conditions. A depressed PMN chemotaxis and depressed phagocytic ability is seen in localized aggressive periodontitis and diabetes type 1. A depressed PMN chemotaxis is also seen in Chediak-Higashi syndrome and Papillon-Lefévre syndrome. A decreased number of circulating PMNs are seen in drug-induced agranulocytosis, cyclic neutropenia, and leukemia (Genco & Slots, 1984).

The Macrophage: The Other Phagocytic Cell. The other important phagocytic cell is the macrophage (Figure 4–7 ■). Monocytes (a type of white blood cell) in the blood differentiate or change into macrophages and migrate from the blood vessel into the inflamed connective tissues by chemotaxis, and a few continue into the gingival crevice. Similar to PMNs, macrophages kill bacteria by phagocytosis.

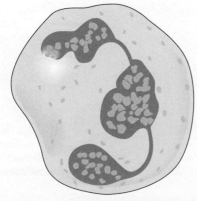

FIGURE 4–6 PMNs are the first cells to migrate to the infection site. Neutrophils comprise more than 90% of the circulating granulocytes, and move by chemotaxis.

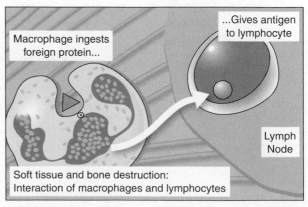

...Gives antigen to lymphocyte

Macrophage ingests foreign protein...

Lymph Node

Soft tissue and bone destruction: Interaction of macrophages and lymphocytes

FIGURE 4–7 A macrophage is a phagocyte that ingests foreign material such as periodontal bacteria.

Although neutrophils and macrophages arrive at the same time at the site of inflammation, neutrophils predominate initially because of their higher concentration in the circulation. The majority of macrophages remain in the inflamed connective tissue for months and function to clean up the body's damaged tissue and secrete prostaglandins and cytokines. **Cytokines** are proteins that are involved in regulating the activity of the cells that release them, as well as other cells (Kjeldsen, Holmstrup, & Bendtzen, 1993). The major cytokines released by macrophages as a result of phagocytosis are interleukin (IL-1) and tumor necrosis factor (TNF).

IL-1 worsens inflammation by stimulating mast cells to release histamine and attracts more PMNs and macrophages into the tissues (Offenbacher, 1996). As with PMNs, macrophages can also damage host tissue most likely a result of cytokines. IL-1 can increase the number of osteoclasts, which stimulate bone resorption seen in periodontitis (Ishikawa et al., 1997; Tatakis, 1993), and stimulates other cells to secrete prostaglandins, which are also involved in bone resorption. TNF is a less potent stimulator of bone resorption (Stashenko, Dewhirst, Peros, Kent, & Apo, 1987).

Phagocytosis: Opsonization. The process of phagocytosis is more effective if **opsonins** are present. Opsonins are antibodies or complement that bind to the surface of the bacteria, coating the bacteria and making it easier to be identified by PMNs and to be "swallowed."

The Complement System: A Group of Proteins. In addition to blood cells (e.g., PMNs) and fluids migrating from the blood vessels into the gingival tissues and crevicular area during inflammation, there is also a series of about 20 to 30 different plasma proteins called the **complement system**. The complement system works together with the rest of the immune system to destroy invaders and to signal to other immune system cells that the attack is occurring. The complement system plays an important role in the inflammatory and immune response by generating chemotactic factors, which attract PMNs, macrophages, and other leukocytes to the inflamed area. Also, it directly kills and lyses (breaks apart) bacteria.

Rapid Dental Hint

In addition to neutrophils and macrophages, monocytes and mast cells are phagocytes.

Did You Know?

Phagocyte means "eating cell" or "cell eater."

As with everything else in the immune system, the complement system must be activated before it can function. One way it is activated is when antibodies (proteins produced by plasma cells during the immune response) bind to the surface of bacteria (the antigen). This is called the "classical" pathway. The second way is called the "alternative" pathway, whereby endotoxins (lipooligosaccarides) activate the system. A third pathway involves the binding of specific proteins to proteins or carbohydrates on bacteria (Dennison & Van Dyke, 1997). Box 4-2 summarizes the important steps in acute inflammation.

The Immune Response

If, for any reason, inflammation does not subside within about 7 days, it will become a chronic reaction. Usually gingival inflammation progresses quickly into a chronic condition (Figure 4–8 ■). When the PMNs and macrophages are not strong enough to destroy the invaders, the immune system is further activated, although the inflammatory cells remain in the area.

Box 4–2: The Following Steps Review the Process of Inflammation

1st: The reaction of the tissue during acute inflammation following the presence of bacterial pathogens in the gingival crevice is increased blood flow due to dilation of the blood vessels. Increased capillary permeability allows fluid and blood proteins to move into the interstitial spaces (spaces in between the cells).

2nd: Now, the neutrophils, and a few macrophages, will prepare to migrate out of the capillaries into the interstitial spaces.

3rd: First, the neutrophils will undergo margination, which involves the formation of proteins on the surface of the neutrophil to allow them to attach to the blood vessel wall on its way out of the vessel.

4th: Then, the neutrophils bind to the endothelium of the blood vessels; this is referred to as adhesion.

5th: Once bound to the endothelium, the neutrophils begin to roll along the surface of the vessel and squeeze through gaps between adjacent endothelial cells into the interstitial fluid. This process is referred to as diapedesis.

6th: Once outside the blood vessel, the neutrophil is guided toward an infection by various chemotactic factors, such toxins released by the bacteria and complement, which are proteins found in the serum.

7th: Once the neutrophils have found the foreign bacteria, the bacteria are engulfed by the neutrophil (endocytosis), the lysosomal enzymes destroy the bacteria, and then the digestive enzymes and dead bacteria are dumped into the surrounding connective tissues (exocytosis), causing destruction and attracting more inflammatory cells.

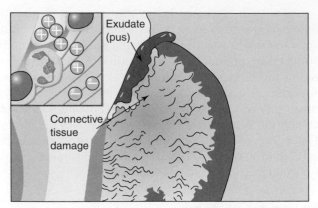

FIGURE 4–8 The inflammatory response triggers an immunologic response resulting in periodontal destruction.

Box 4–3: Key Elements in the Immune Response

- B lymphocytes
- Plasma cells
- Antibodies
- Macrophages
- Cytokines
- T lymphocytes
   T killer—directly involved
   T helper—"help" plasma cells

Activation of the "specific host response" or adaptive immune system is the next line of defense, with the purpose of the host developing immunity or resistance to specific antigens (e.g., bacteria and toxins; Figure 4–9 ■; American Academy of Periodontology, 2002; Ishikawa, 2006; Nagasawa et al., 2006). The objective of the immune response is to recognize the antigen and communicate with other defense cells to destroy or suppress the antigen. There is an interrelationship between the inflammatory and immune reactions. The same reactions and cells seen in the inflammatory level are also seen in the chronic state (e.g., PMNs and macrophages also belong to the immune system), but more cells are involved. There are two parts to the immune reaction: **humoral immunity** and **cellular immunity** (Mahanonda et al., 2011).

IMMUNE SYSTEM: CELLS The major cells in the immune system are white blood cells called lymphocytes (Box 4–3). The role of the immune system is to "patrol" the body, identifying foreign pathogens such as bacteria and viruses, cancer cells, or damaged tissue and eliminating them. Two kinds

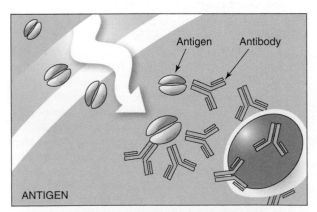

FIGURE 4–9 An antigen is any foreign material including bacteria. Antigens will eventually bind to antibodies with the intention of being eliminated from the body.

of lymphocytes originate in the bone marrow and travel to other areas of the body (Figure 4–10a ■). In fact, all cells in the inflammatory and immune systems, including blood cells, are made in the bone marrow from a stem cell. A stem cell is a cell from which all blood cells "stem" or originate. Lymphocytes predominate in the gingival connective tissue (Page & Schroeder, 1976). T lymphocytes, also referred to as *T cells*, are the mediators of cellular immunity. B lymphocytes, or *B cells*, are the mediators of humoral immunity (Figure 4–10b).

HUMORAL IMMUNITY Humoral immune mechanisms are most effective against bacteria such as those found in periodontitis. Although both the humoral and cellular immunity reactions occur almost at the same time, one or the other cells may predominate during a particular stage of periodontal diseases.

B lymphocytes or B cells are so named because much of the early research was done on chickens, in which the bursa (hence "B") of Fabricius is a center of B cell activation; there is no direct equivalent of this bursa in humans. B cells originate and mature in the bone marrow and then migrate and deposit in the blood and various lymphatic tissues (e.g., lymph nodes; Berglundh, Donati, & Zitzmann, 2007).

Humoral Immunity and Periodontal Disease. The following events depict the humoral response to biofilm accumulated at the gingival margin (Figure 4–11 ■):

1. In periodontal diseases, bacteria and their products, such as toxins and enzymes, accumulate in the gingival crevice. Then the toxins and enzymes penetrate through the protective wall of neutrophils and through the junctional epithelium, entering the lamina propria. Once this happens, an inflammatory/immune response is set off. As previously stated, if the inflammatory reaction cannot eliminate the antigens effectively, the immune response comes into play.

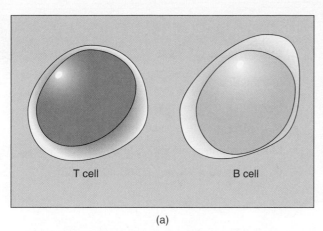

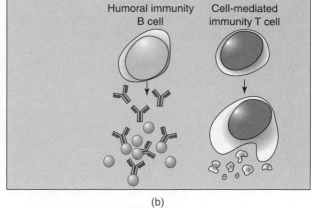

(a)

(b)

FIGURE 4–10 The antigen–antibody reaction involves the B lymphocytes and T lymphocytes.

2. From the tissues, these antigenic substances are carried to the local lymph nodes, probably by macrophages.

3. In the lymph nodes, the macrophages either present the antigens to B cells or the B cells by themselves recognize the antigens. The B cells then transform into plasma cells and memory cells.

4. Plasma cells make **antibodies** in the lymph nodes with assistance from T$_H$-cells and circulate in the blood to seek out and destroy the antigens.

5. The memory B cells remain inactivated, ready to respond should the same antigens appear again.

6. The plasma cells remain in the lymph nodes and secrete antibodies into the bloodstream. A local antibody response is also seen in the gingival tissues.

7. Antibodies belong to a family of large molecules known as **immunoglobulins** (Ig). Each immunoglobin has about a dozen parts and is designed for a specific invader (antigen). Antibodies float throughout the body and wait for invaders. Antibodies lock onto the antigen of the invader like a key fits into a lock. Antibodies will neutralize the enemy and tag it for attack. The primary antibody produced by the plasma cells is IgG (Note: "Ig" stands for immunoglobulin) with lesser amounts of IgM.

• There are five classes of immunoglobulins found in the serum, secretions, and tissues. IgG and IgM are primarily found in the periodontal tissues, and SIgA ("S" stands for secretory) is found in the saliva. IgE is found on mast cells and is responsible for the release of histamine causing vasodilation and allergy. In addition, there is IgD.

• Antibodies (e.g., IgG) are proteins that directly bind to and neutralize bacterial toxins (foreign antigens) forming an immune complex. This immune complex may activate the complement system or be phagocytosed by PMNs or macrophages for elimination.

8. Once the antigens and the surrounding tissue are destroyed, the tissue macrophages phagocytize and digest the debris and stimulate repair.

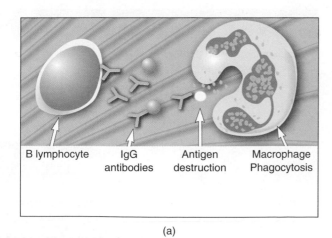

(a)

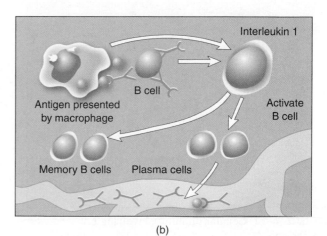

(b)

FIGURE 4–11 B lymphocytes function in periodontal disease (a) T cell and (b) B cell.

9. After the antigens have been eliminated, the short-lived plasma cells disappear into the gingival crevicular fluid and out through the gingival crevice, but the long-lived memory cells remain in circulation and are capable of maturing very rapidly into plasma cells if the antigens are encountered again.

Antibodies to various periodontal pathogens have been found in both serum and gingival crevicular fluids of patients with periodontal diseases (Ebersole & Taubman, 1994; Genco & Slots, 1984). Immune complex and complement will cause the release of prostaglandins from cell membranes of macrophages and PMNs. Prostaglandins of the E series (PGE$_2$) are potent stimulators of osteoclast activity responsible for bone resorption. B lymphocytes also release cytokines such as IL-1. Thus, it has been suggested that B cells may play a role in alveolar bone loss (Han, Kawai, Eastcott, & Taubman, 2006). Humoral immunity is activated in severe gingivitis and periodontitis. Thus, the proportion of B cells in connective tissue at sites with periodontitis can be as high as 90%.

CELLULAR IMMUNITY T cells undergo further maturation in the thymus gland located in the chest cavity. From the thymus gland, the T cells migrate into the bloodstream and lymph nodes. From the bloodstream, T cells enter the gingival tissues and "watch" the tissues (Figure 4–12 ■).

There are two major types of T cells: helper T cells (T$_H$) and cytotoxic T cells. Both types of T cells have protein receptors on the surface of their plasma membranes (Gemmell, Yamazaki, & Seymour, 2006). The helper T cells have a CD4 receptor, and the cytotoxic T cells have a CD8 receptor. There is a reduction in CD4 T$_H$-cells in AIDS patients. Once stimulated, helper T cells secrete cytokines that activate phagocytic cells to destroy target antigens (Box 4–4). T cells can directly cause alveolar bone

loss through stimulation of the synthesis of osteoclasts or indirectly through production of IL-1. T cells also activate other immune cells such as B cells. Cytotoxic T cells are sometimes called killer T cells and can directly kill virus-infected cells, cancer cells, parasites, and certain bacteria by making holes in them. Thus, cellular immunity is most effective against fungi, viruses, cancer, and foreign tissue such as transplanted organs and does not play an important role in periodontal diseases.

Cellular Immunity: Process. When a macrophage presents a foreign antigen to a T cell, it is stimulated to produce more T cells and cytokines. T cells are the target of the human immunodeficiency virus (HIV). AIDS is a manifestation of what happens when T cells are destroyed, showing the importance of T cells for a properly functioning body. Few lymphocytes are seen in healthy gingiva. Most T lymphocytes are evident in gingivitis. The T cells actually kill other cells on contact when the latter are recognized as foreign or have antigens attached. The main role of the cellular branch of the immune system in periodontal disease is the production of cytokines, such as interleukin, that can destroy bone.

Box 4–4: Cytokines Implicated in Periodontal Pathology

- IL-1 interleukin-1
- TNF tumor necrosis factor
- MAF macrophage activating factor
- MIF macrophage migration inhibitory factor
- CTX leukocyte-derived chemotatic factor

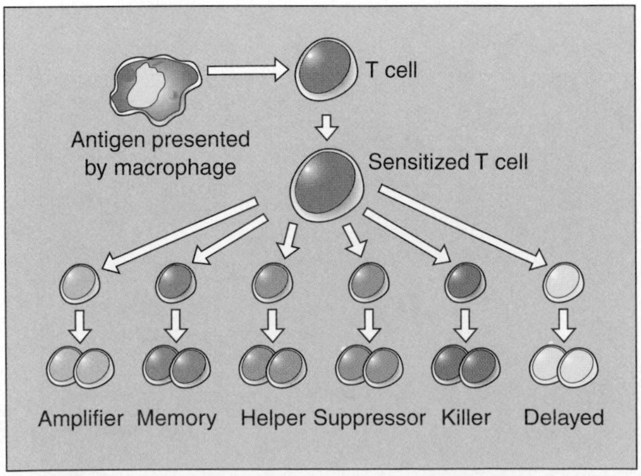

FIGURE 4–12 Cellular immunity involving T lymphocytes.

Did You Know?

B cells may play an active role in alveolar bone resorption; more research is needed.

Rapid Dental Hint

B cells produce antibodies (by way of plasma cells), and T cells produce cytokines.

Dental Hygiene Application

The pathway of destruction of inflammatory periodontal diseases is complicated, involving the host inflammatory and immune cells. Ideally, the overall outcome of these reactions is to eliminate harmful pathogens and prevent the spread of infection, while protecting the host tissues.

The basic concepts of biofilm control via periodontal debridement and patient oral home care both involve the inflammatory/immune pathways.

Key Points

- Overall, the host defenses are extremely successful in preventing infection around the teeth and in preventing destructive inflammatory periodontal diseases. However, a lot depends on the host or individual's response.
- There are two separate functions that lead to the damage seen in periodontal diseases: (1) direct effects of bacteria (e.g., enzymes, endotoxins) and (2) indirect effects of the body's own immune response.
- The host immune defense and inflammatory reactions are a double-edged sword; while being protective, the host can also suffer tissue damage.
- Bacterial products can enter the connective tissue and cause direct damage, but their effects are limited by the effectiveness of the host response.

- Weakened host defenses (e.g., because of a systemic disease) will not allow the host to ward off infection; the host will then develop signs and symptoms of destructive periodontal diseases.
- Neutrophils and macrophages are considered capable and efficient agents of phagocytosis.
- Clinical signs of gingival inflammation are first evident in the early lesion of gingivitis.
- B cells/plasma cells predominate in the body's response to periodontitis.
- Within the last decade, B cells have been found to also be involved in bone resorption.
- Elevated serum antibodies are seen in periodontitis.

Self-Quiz

1. Which one of the following types of cells is primarily recruited in high numbers to the site of acute inflammation?
   a. Mast
   b. Macrophage
   c. Neutrophil
   d. Lymphocyte

2. From the following list, select the cells that are phagocytic and involved in periodontal infections?
   a. Mast cells
   b. Lymphocytes
   c. Macrophages
   d. Melanocytes
   e. Neutrophils
   f. Monocytes

3. Which one of the following cells is mainly involved in the body's immune response to invading bacteria?
   a. Lymphocytes
   b. Mast
   c. Macrophages
   d. Neutrophils

4. Periodontal diseases are considered a group of infections characterized by destruction of the periodontium. The direct effects of the bacteria and indirect effects by the body's own immune response are responsible for the destruction.
   a. Both statements are true.
   b. Both statements are false.
   c. The first statement is true; the second is false.
   d. The first statement is false; the second is true.

5. The first attempt at self-protection from bacterial invasion comes from which one of the following areas in the oral cavity?
   a. Supragingival environment
   b. Subgingival environment
   c. Gingival connective tissue
   d. Tonsillar area

6. From the following list, select the items primarily associated with periodontal bone resorption.
   a. Cytokines
   b. Macrophages
   c. Prostaglandin E_2
   d. Neutrophils
   e. PMNs
   f. T lymphocytes

7. Which of the following cells remains in the bloodstream and does not function to phagocytize until it migrates into the tissues?
   a. PMN
   b. Macrophage
   c. Lymphocyte
   d. Neutrophil
   e. Monocyte

8. Which of the following cells/substances is involved in regulating the activity of other cells?
   a. Macrophages
   b. Cytokines
   c. Lymphocytes
   d. Neutrophils

9. Which of the following substances are associated with gram-negative bacteria and cause damage to the periodontium?
   a. Hyaluronidase
   b. Collagenase
   c. Leukotoxin
   d. Endotoxin

10. For each cell listed below, select the correct description from the list provided.

Cell	Description
1. plasma cell	a. makes histamine
2. mast cell	b. protein in serum that binds to bacteria
3. complement	c. makes antibodies
4. T lymphocytes	d. produces cytokines

Case Study

A 50-year-old female returns for a six month recall visit. A previous pocket depth on tooth #30 mesial lingual was 4 mm and did not bleed on the last visit. The new probing indicates a probing depth of 6 mm at mesial lingual and is currently bleeding upon probing. There is not recession at the site. The patient indicates regular brushing and flossing but has noticed the area bleeds upon flossing at times. She indicates she is under stress and is trying to stop smoking.

1. The increased pocket depth and current bleeding indicates
   a. Site is disease active
   b. Destruction of gingival connective tissue fibers
   c. Apical migration of the junctional epithelium
   d. B and C
   e. All of the above

Answer: E. all of the above. The increased probing depths and attachment loss, which is measured from the CEJ and bleeding, indicates that the site is disease active

2. This patient would have which host challenge to periodontal disease?
   a. Easily self-cleansed areas to maintain bacterial load
   b. Smoking increasing inflammatory response

   c. Gingivitis indicating progression to periodontitis
   d. Diabetes increasing inflammatory response

Answer: B. The patient smokes which increases her risk factor and decreases the patient host response. The patient does not indicate diabetes. Gingivitis does not always progress to periodontitis. A 6 mm pocket is not easily cleansed to maintain the bacterial load.

3. The bleeding at the 6 mm site on #30 indicates what event?
   a. Sulcular epithelium is ulcerated
   b. Lining muucosa is torn
   c. Brushing is too aggressive
   d. Blood vessels constricted

Answer: A. The sulcular epithelium is ulcerated as the vasodilation of the connective tissue blood vessels occurs and PMN invade the tissue. Histamines are released. Aggressive brushing would irritate the free gingiva; however, the bleeding in this case is *from the sulcus*.

References

American Academy of Periodontology. 2002. Modulation of the host response in periodontal therapy. *J. Periodontol*. 7:460–470.

Armitage, G. C. 1995. Clinical evaluation of periodontal diseases. *Periodontology 2000* 7:39–53.

Bascones-Martinez, A., M. Munoz-Corcuera, S. Noronha, et al. 2009. Host defense mechanisms against bacterial aggression in periodontal disease: basic mechanisms. *Med Oral Patol Oral Cir Buca*. 14:e680-e685.

Berglundh, T., M. Donati, and N. Zitzmann. 2007. B cells in periodontitis–friends or enemies? *Periodontology 2000* 45(1):51–66.

Birkedal-Hansen, H., W. G. Moore, M. K. Bodden, et al. 1993. Matrix Metallo proteinase: A review. *Crit. Rev. Oral Biol. Med.* 4:197–250.

Brown, L. J., and H. Löe. 1993. Prevalence, extent, severity and progression of periodontal disease. *Periodontology 2000* 2:57–71.

de Graaf, J., A. J. van Winkelhoff, and R. J. Goené. 1989. The role of *Aggregatibacter actinomycetemcomitans* in periodontal disease. *Infection* 17:269–271.

Dennison, D. K., and T. E. Van Dyke. 1997. The acute inflammatory response and the role of phagocytic cells in periodontal health and disease. *Periodontology 2000* 14:54–78.

Ebersole, J. L., and M. A. Taubman. 1994. The protective nature of host responses in periodontal diseases. *Periodontology 2000* 5:112–141.

Gemmell, E., K. Yamazaki, and G. J. Seymour. 2006. The role of T cells in periodontal disease: Homeostasis and autoimmunity. *Periodontology 2000* 43:14-40.

Genco, R. J., and J. Slots. 1984. Host response in periodontal diseases. *J. Dental Res*. 63:441–451.

Goodson, J. M. 1992. Diagnosis of periodontitis by physical measurement: Interpretation from episodic disease hypothesis. *J. Periodontol*. 63:373–382.

Greenstein, G., and J. Caton. 1990. Periodontal disease activity: A critical assessment. *J. Periodontol*. 61:543–552.

Han, X., T. Kawai, J. W. Eastcott, and M. A. Taubman. 2006. Bacterial-responsive B lymphocytes induce periodontal bone resorption. *The Journal of Immunology* 176:625–631.

Hujoel, P., L. G. Zina, J. Cunha-Cruz, and R. Lopez. 2012. Historical perspectives on theories of periodontal disease etiology. *Periodontology 2000* 58:153-160.

Ishikawa, I. K. 2006. Host responses in periodontal diseases: A preview. *Periodontology 2000* 43:9–13.

Ishikawa, I., K. Nakashima, T. Koseki, T. Nagasawa, H. Watanabe, et al. 1997. Induction of the immune response to periodontopathic bacteria and its role in the pathogenesis of periodontitis. *Periodontology 2000* 14:79–111.

Kinane, F., and P. M. Bartold. 2007. Clinical relevance of the host responses of periodontitis. *Periodontology 2000* 44(1):278–293.

Kjeldsen, M., P. Holmstrup, and K. Bendtzen. 1993. Marginal periodontitis and cytokines: A review of the literature. *J. Periodontol*. 64:1013–1022.

Kowashi, Y., F. Jaccard, and G. Cimasoni. 1980. Sulcular polymorphonuclear leukocytes and gingival exudate during experimental gingivitis in man. *J. Periodontol. Res*. 15:151–158.

Listgarten, M. A. 1994. The structure of dental biofilm. *Periodontology 2000* 5:52–65.

Löe, H., A. Anerud, H. Boysen, and E. Morrison. 1986. Natural history of periodontal disease in man. Rapid, moderate and no loss of attachment in Sri Lankan laborers 14 to 46 years of age. *J. Clin. Periodontol*. 13:431–440.

Mahanonda, R., N. Sa-Ard-Iam, P. Rerkyen, et al. 2011. Innate antiviral immunity of periodontal tissue. *Periodontology 2000* 56:143–153.

Miyasaki, K. T. 1991. The neutrophil: Mechanisms of controlling periodontal bacteria. *J. Periodontol*. 62:761–774.

Nagasawa, T. M. Kiji, R. Yashiro, et al. 2006. Roles of receptor activator of nuclear factor-κB ligand (RANKL) and osteoprotegerin in periodontal health and disease. *Periodontology 2000* 43:65–84.

Offenbacher, S. 1996. Periodontal diseases: Pathogenesis. *Ann. Periodontol*. 1:821–878.

Offenbacher, S., P. A. Heasman, and J. G. Collins. 1993. Modulation of host PGE_2 secretion as a determinant of periodontal disease expression. *J. Periodontol*. 64:432–444.

Page, R. C., and H. E. Schroeder. 1976. Pathogenesis of inflammatory periodontal disease. A summary of current work. *Lab Investigations* 33:235–249.

Renvert, S., M. Wikström, M. Dahlén, G. Slots, and J. Egelberg. 1990. On the inability of root debridement and periodontal surgery to eliminate *Aggregatibacter actinomycetemcomitans* from periodontal pockets. *J. Clin. Periodontol*. 17:351–355.

Rizzo, A. 1970. Histologic and immunologic evaluation of antigen penetration into oral tissues after topical application. *J. Periodontol*. 41:210–213.

Saglie, F. R., F. A. Carranza, Jr., M. G. Newman, L. Cheng, and K. J. Lewin. 1982. Identification of tissue-invading bacteria in human periodontal disease. *J. Periodontol. Res*. 17:452–455.

Shikawa, I. 2007. Host responses in periodontal disease: A preview. *Periodontology 2000* 44(1):9–13.

Socransky, S. S., A. D. Haffajee, J. M. Goodson, and J. Lindhe. 1984. New concepts of destructive periodontal diseases. *J. Clin. Periodontol*. 11:21–32.

Stashenko, P., F. E. Dewhirst, W. J. Peros, R. L. Kent, and J. Apo. 1987. Synergistic interactions between interleukin-1, tumor necrosis factor and lymphotoxin in bone resorption. *J. Immunol*. 138:1484–1468.

Tatakis, D. N. 1993. Interleukin-1 and bone metabolism: A review. *J. Periodontol*. 64:416–431.

Van Dyke, T. 2007. Control of inflammation and periodontitis. *Periodontology 2000* 45(1):158–166.

Van Dyke, T., S. Offenbacher, B. Pihlstrom, M. Putt, and C. Trummel. 1999. What is gingivitis? Current understanding of prevention, treatment, measurement, pathogenesis and relation to periodontitis. *J. International Acad. of Periodontol*. 1:3–10.

Weinberg, M. A. 2011. The fire within. *Dimensions of Dental Hygiene*. 9:21-24.

Zappa, U. 1995. Histology of the periodontal lesion: Implications for diagnosis. *Periodontology 2000* 7:22–38.

Zimmerman, S. O. 1986. Discussion: Attachment level changes in destructive periodontal diseases. *J. Clin. Periodontol*. 13:473–475.

Local Contributory Factors for Periodontal Diseases

Raymond A. Yukna and John D. Mason

OUTLINE

EDUCATIONAL OBJECTIVES

Upon completion of this chapter, the reader should be able to:

- List and explain contributing local factors.
- Describe the clinical significance of dental calculus.
- Discuss the specific role of dental calculus as a contributory factor for the periodontal diseases.

GOAL: To introduce the role of local contributory factors in the periodontal diseases.

KEY WORDS

Introduction

Many local factors can increase plaque deposition and retention, inhibit plaque control, and contribute to the development of gingivitis and periodontitis. These factors are termed **contributory** because they do not by themselves initiate gingival inflammation, but foster increased or long-standing plaque accumulation and make plaque removal more difficult. Awareness of these local factors can help the dental hygienist design more specific plaque-control activities, encourage patients to seek further corrective dental treatment, and contribute to the comprehensive care of periodontal patients.

Perhaps the most significant dentally related local factor strongly associated with an increased probability of developing periodontal diseases, but not directly involved in causing the disease, is the presence of established periodontal disease. Sites already or previously affected by periodontitis are at the greatest risk for future episodes (Douglass, 1998). More frequent professional care has been shown to reduce the risk.

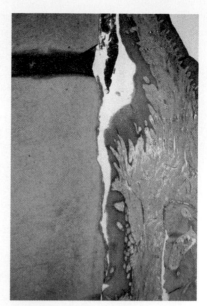

FIGURE 5–1 Histology of calculus with a plaque coating in a deep periodontal pocket.

Dental Calculus

Dental calculus is considered the most important *local* contributing factor. Calculus is not the cause of disease but rather the bacterial challenge. Calculus is essentially calcified dental plaque, but may form even in the absence of bacteria. Mineralization within plaque initially occurs supragingivally, but the rate of formation varies between individuals. Subgingival calculus forms more slowly in a thinner layer and, being firmly attached to the root, is usually more difficult to remove. Calculus is always covered by plaque and retains toxic bacterial products (Figure 5–1 ■).

Subgingival calculus is commonly deposited in rings or ledges on root surfaces, but may also appear in a veneer form and is associated with progressive periodontal disease (Figure 5–2 ■). It is porous and can provide a reservoir of bacteria and endotoxin. Long-term studies of periodontal patients support calculus removal to promote healing and prevent further loss of attachment (Pihlstrom, McHugh, Oliphant, & Ortiz-Campos, 1983).

"Tartar" is the common layperson's term for dental calculus and is often used by patients when referring to calculus. Tartar is used to describe the sediment or crust on the

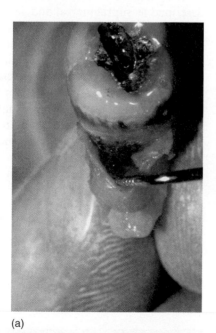

(a)

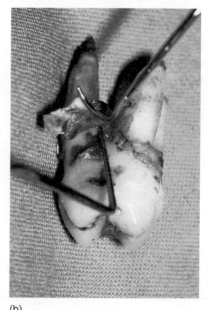

(b)

FIGURE 5–2 Clinical photographs of nodular calculus versus veneer-type calculus. (a) Nodular calculus is evident more coronally, whereas (b) veneer-type calculus is often found more apically.

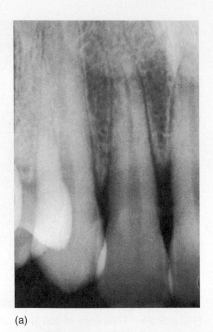
(a)

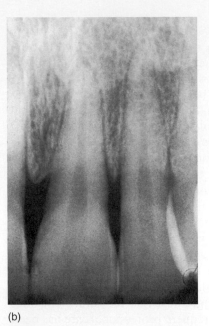
(b)

FIGURE 5–3 Radiographs of teeth in the same patient (a) with and (b) without calculus evident. Absence of calculus on radiographs does not mean that it is not present clinically (radiographs produce many false negatives).

side of a wine cask. The term was coined by a Swiss-German physician who identified all stony accretions in humans as tartars because they were similar in composition to the potassium bitartrate deposits on wine casks (Mandel, 1990). The term *calculus* is a Latin-rooted word meaning *pebble* or *stone*. Needless to say, the population has become more aware of the word *tartar* because of the advertising of "tartar-control" toothpaste and rinses, which reinforces the use of the common name.

Radiographic evaluation of calculus is not an effective diagnostic method. Only about 45% of surfaces with clinically visible calculus are detected radiographically (Figure 5–3 ■).

Clinical Significance of Calculus

The population is more aware of supragingival plaque and calculus and their relationship to gingivitis than it is of subgingival plaque and calculus and their relationship to periodontitis. Awareness is still lacking in the need to remove plaque to prevent periodontal disease and how to remove supragingival and subgingival plaque. The situation becomes increasingly confusing when descriptions are added of mineralized plaque becoming calculus or of loosely adherent plaque residing on top of mineralized calculus. Because calculus that forms above the gingival margin is both hard and visible, it

has become the focus of consumers for removal based on aesthetic reasons. Rather than being a mechanical irritant, as was once thought (Carranza, 1996), calculus contributes to the accumulation of plaque by having a porous surface. It is unknown if calculus covered with bacterial plaque is more damaging to tissues than plaque alone (Mandel, 1995).

Dental calculus can be defined as mineralized (calcified) plaque, although calculus has been shown to develop in germ-free animals. As with plaque, described according to its location in relationship to the gingival margin, calculus is also described as supragingival and subgingival. The mineralization process occurs separately for supragingival and subgingival plaque, and because of this, varying amounts of calculus can be found in the supragingival and subgingival areas.

Supragingival calculus can occur on any clinical crown, exposed root surface, prosthesis, or restoration. It is associated most frequently with sites that are adjacent to a salivary source, such as the parotid gland (maxillary molar area; Figure 5–4a ■) or floor of the mouth (Warton's duct) and salivary caruncle (lingual surfaces of mandibular anterior teeth; Figure 5–4b). Any retention site, such as a maligned tooth, a missed area of plaque removal, or an area where mastication does not remove all debris, is a primary site for supragingival calculus formation. The mineral components of supragingival calculus are derived from saliva.

The formation of supragingival calculus occurs in layers beginning closest to the tooth. The minerals are deposited within 24 to 72 hours of plaque formation. Minerals from

Rapid Dental Hint

Calculus is calcified plaque consisting of organic secretions and food particles deposited in various salts, such as calcium carbonate, between and within remnants of formerly live microorganisms.

Did You Know?

Cats and dogs also develop calculus buildup.

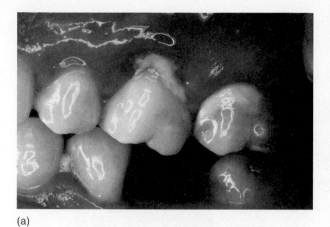

(a)

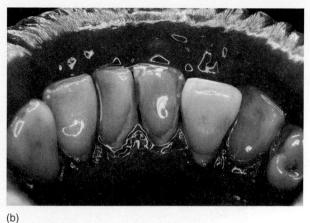

(b)

FIGURE 5–4 (a) Supragingival calculus on the maxillary first molar opposite Stensen's duct. (b) Supragingival calculus on the lingual surface of the mandibular anteriors in relation to the opening or orifice of the submandibular and sublingual salivary glands.

the saliva are deposited in the plaque matrix and around the filamentous bacteria. The process can take approximately 12 days or less for rapid formers. The actual mineralization process can occur in as few as 24 to 48 hours. Formation time varies according to the individual, the contents of the saliva, and the ability to remove plaque on all surfaces or various retention sites.

Subgingival calculus is derived from gingival crevicular fluid and any inflammatory exudates. More minerals become available as the inflammatory process continues, and the calculus contains more calcium, magnesium, and fluoride than supragingival calculus (Mandel, 1990). It most often forms in rings around the roots of the tooth or in ledges.

The mineralization process continues as crystals of hydroxyapatite, brushite, and whitlockite form. These crystals have different proportions of calcium and phosphate in combination with other ions, such as magnesium, zinc, fluoride, and other carbonates (Ellwood, Melling, & Rutter, 1979). The crystals form in the matrix and then on the surface of the bacteria; finally, they calcify the bacteria.

Other differences in subgingival calculus and supragingival calculus are the hardness of the calculus and the difficulty in removing it. Supragingival calculus is 30% mineralized, whereas subgingival calculus is 60% mineralized. Subgingival calculus is more difficult to remove because of this hardness. The color of the two calculus types varies from yellow-white for supragingival calculus to gray or black for subgingival calculus. Unless the subgingival calculus is minutely visible at the gingival margin, this coloration adds little to its removal. The gray or black color derives from the bacterial and blood pigments from the crevicular fluid.

The structure of calculus was described as layers in supragingival calculus. These layers build into incremental lines on the surfaces of a tooth. The surface of the calculus is irregular and rough. Plaque accumulates on the surface of the calculus. It can lodge in the pits and valleys of the calculus surface. In the subgingival calculus the outer surface may be less calcified. Again, subgingival plaque can accumulate. In either case, the plaque on the surface of the calculus contains living bacteria and is detrimental to the tissue. In this sense, calculus is a contributing factor for periodontal diseases. The calculus acts as an irritant to the gingival margin or the sulcular tissue. The overlying bacterial plaque continues to be the etiologic factor in periodontal disease.

There are many types of attachment of calculus to root surfaces. Calculus attaches to both tooth and implant surfaces. A classic article recognizes four modes of attachment of subgingival calculus to root surfaces (Zander, 1953):

1. Attachment by means of mechanical locking into irregularities in the cementum
2. Attachment into areas of cementum resorption
3. Attachment by means of an organic pellicle
4. Attachment by penetration into bacteria (not accepted by all researchers)

Both the bacterial plaque and the pellicle beneath the plaque calcify, making removal of the calculus via periodontal debridement very difficult. In addition, calculus binds to tooth surface irregularities, making mechanical calculus removal difficult. Calculus is not firmly attached to dental implants because the titanium surface is nonporous, which is just the opposite of natural teeth. Thus, calculus can actually be "chipped" off from dental implants (Lang, Mombelli, & Attström, 2003; Matarasso et al., 1996).

Anatomic Factors

Dental **anatomic factors** of importance to the accumulation of dental plaque include root morphology (size and shape) and position of teeth in the arch.

Rapid Dental Hint

Calculus is a *local* contributing factor for periodontal disease—it is *not* the cause of the disease. Plaque adheres to the surface of calculus.

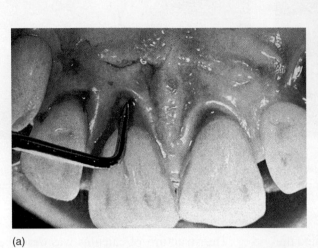

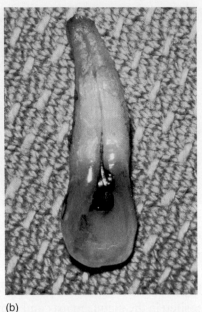

(a)

(b)

FIGURE 5–5 Clinical photographs of (a) a palatogingival groove with a deep pocket associated with it, and (b) an extracted lateral incisor exhibiting a deep palatal groove.

Root Morphology

Knowledge of dental morphology, supplemented by radiographs and the patient's dental history, is needed to identify dental anomalies. An anomaly is defined as a deviation from normal tooth development or function. Examples of dental anomalies include cervical enamel projections (CEPs), enamel pearls, and palatogingival grooves.

Several deviations in the shape or form of the tooth root can occur and often contribute to increased biofilm accumulation and more severe periodontal disease. Palatal grooves (also called **palatogingival grooves** or lingual grooves) are present on about 5% to 8% of maxillary incisors, tend to accumulate plaque, and can become the focus of a narrow, deep pocket (Hou & Tsai, 1993; see also Figure 5–5 ■). Likewise, biofilm may accumulate undisturbed in the deep mesial groove of the upper first premolars.

Enamel in the furcation area of the root surface may manifest as cervical enamel projections (CEPs; Figure 5–6a ■) or enamel pearls (Figure 5–6b). These ridges of enamel may allow increased plaque accumulation. Essentially, a CEP is an extension of enamel from the cementoenamel junction apically to the entrance of the

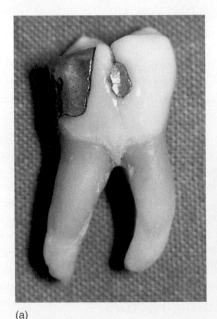

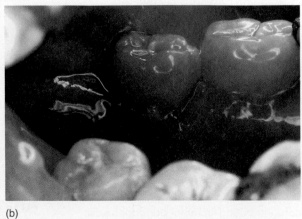

(a)

(b)

FIGURE 5–6 (a) Clinical photograph of a cervical enamel projection (CEP) at the furcation entrance. (b) Enamel pearl located at the lingual bifurcation on the mandibular first molar resembles a pearl. It is a potential plaque trap.

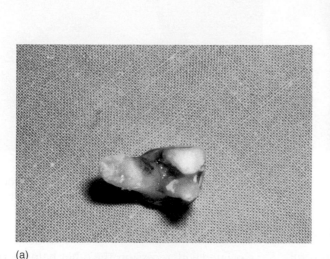

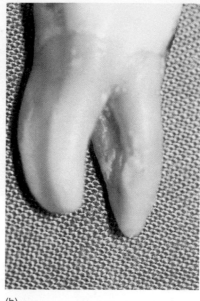

(a) (b)

FIGURE 5–7 Clinical photographs of calculus within furcations: (a) dark calculus evident on all internal surfaces of maxillary molar furcations; (b) more veneer like calculus in internal groove of mesial root of the mandibular molar.

furcation, which may predispose periodontal destruction within the furcation. It may be difficult to detect a CEP clinically because the area is covered by gingiva. The highest incidence of CEPs is on the buccal aspect of the mandibular second molars. An enamel pearl is similar to a CEP except that it consists of a clump of enamel most commonly located in the bifurcation of molar roots just apical to the cementoenamel junction. It is often mistaken for calculus.

Furcation involvements create a complication because they form a cul-de-sac that creates a plaque trap. Difficult access in this protected area fosters increased bacterial deposits and often leads to more severe periodontal disease. Proximal furcations on maxillary molars present particular problems because of even more limited access (Figure 5–7 ■).

Tooth Position

Tooth position may influence plaque accumulation and access for oral hygiene and therapy. Most studies that have evaluated the influence of crowding, tilting, rotations, and so on have found that such tooth position anomalies lead to increased plaque accumulation (and more tissue inflammation), especially in patients who do not have excellent oral hygiene practices (Figure 5–8 ■). Open contacts allow for food impaction, which may contribute to plaque-induced inflammation.

Iatrogenic Factors

A number of procedures, techniques, and materials used in dentistry indirectly, and on occasion directly, contribute to the initiation and/or progress of periodontal disease. These are termed **iatrogenic factors**.

Restorative Dentistry

Rough-surfaced and overcontoured amalgams, composites, crowns, bridges, and other types of restorations have been associated with increased gingival inflammation and periodontal disease. Plaque accumulation is enhanced by subgingival placement of restorations because of problems with greater surface roughness of the materials, fit of the margin to the remaining tooth structure, and contour of the restoration. Subgingival restorations that invade the biologic width and restorations with defective or overhanging margins may have a profound effect on periodontal health (Figure 5–9 ■).

Injuries to the gingiva can occur during restorative dentistry procedures. For example, a large portion of the interdental papilla can be destroyed by the careless use of a wedge during matrix stabilization. Also, retraction cord, impression material, and temporary restorations may result in irreversible damage to the periodontium.

Fixed crowns and bridges must be designed so that the patient can clean all surfaces of the restoration, including the pontic area. If removable partial dentures are designed so that they impinge on the soft tissue or they exert torque on the teeth, traumatic injury to the periodontium can occur.

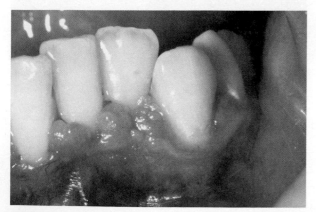

FIGURE 5–8 Crowded teeth with inflammation of the gingiva.

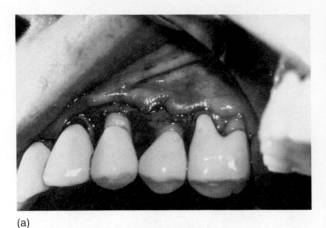

(a)

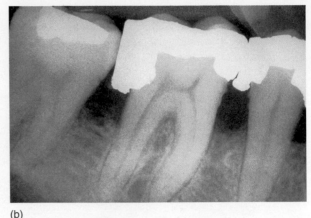

(b)

FIGURE 5–9 Overhanging restorations contributing to more advanced periodontitis: (a) clinical photograph of deficient crown margins exposed at surgery; and (b) radiograph of large overhang on mandibular molar resulting in more advanced bone loss on that tooth surface.

In the presence of dental plaque, these insults can result in more rapid, more severe destruction of periodontal structures.

Exodontics

Extractions can adversely affect adjacent teeth if their attachment apparatus is damaged. The soft tissue and bone supporting an adjacent tooth can be irreversibly destroyed. Failure to remove calculus from adjacent tooth surfaces during the extraction may negate the chance for proper healing on the adjacent teeth. An environment may be set up that actually fosters plaque accumulation. Frequently, patients stop eating on the side where teeth have been extracted. In addition to the decrease in masticatory (chewing) stimulation to the periodontium, plaque begins to form on those teeth, and patients avoid brushing the area.

Orthodontics

Orthodontic appliances have long been associated with increased plaque accumulation, gingivitis, and caries. Fixed appliances (bands, brackets, and wires) present excellent retentive areas for bacterial growth and can contribute significantly to inflammation. Special attention needs to be paid to these orthodontic plaque-retentive areas. More frequent recalls may be indicated for patients undergoing orthodontic therapy, especially adults (Figure 5–10 ■).

Traumatic Factors

Trauma to the periodontium from several sources can result in the loss of the attachment apparatus, changes in the local anatomy, and increased plaque accumulation and can contribute to the initiation and progression of periodontal diseases.

Toothbrush Trauma

Toothbrush trauma can completely destroy a narrow band of attached gingiva and result in extensive recession. In fact, toothbrush abrasion is one of the two most common factors

associated with recession, the other being permanent tooth position. Such abrasion also results in extensive grooving of the root surfaces, creating plaque traps and causing cleaning problems for the patient (Figure 5–11 ■).

Factitious Disease

Occasionally, patients may persistently gouge or "scratch" their gingiva with their fingernails or other devices (factitious disease). This action usually results in extensive exposure of the root surface and localized inflammation. Although relatively rare, whenever isolated areas of recession are noted and a thorough evaluation fails to identify the etiology of the condition, factitious disease should be

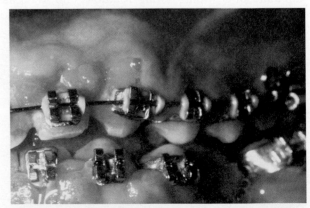

FIGURE 5–10 Clinical photograph of orthodontic bands and brackets with increased plaque and inflammation.

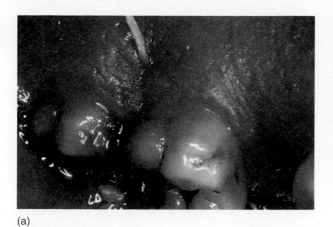

(a) (b)

FIGURE 5–11 Examples of trauma to tissues from home-care procedures due to overzealous use of devices: (a) dental floss lesions between maxillary molars; and (b) toothbrush abrasion in cervical area of teeth.

considered. The change in the local gingival anatomy often leads to greater plaque accumulation and inflammation (Figure 5–12 ■).

Food Impaction

Food impaction is one of the more common local factors that may contribute to the initiation and progression of inflammatory periodontal disease. Open contacts, uneven marginal ridges, irregular positions of teeth, and nonphysiologic contours of teeth and restorations can result in the impaction of food on the gingiva and into the gingival sulcus (Figure 5–13 ■). The cause of the initial breakdown in an area of food impaction or food retention is not clear. Forceful wedging of food beneath the gingival tissues may produce inflammation from physical trauma, and/or food retention leads to food degradation and chemical irritation that affords an excellent breeding ground for bacteria that can initiate and perpetuate the disease process.

Chemical Injury

Indiscriminate use of topically applied aspirin tablets, dental bleaching materials, strong mouthwashes, and various other topical drugs (including cocaine) may result in

ulceration or burning of the gingival tissue. Injuries of this nature are usually transient, but may temporarily interfere with plaque control and contribute to periodontal inflammation (Figure 5–14 ■).

In-office dental bleaching commonly uses a higher concentration of hydrogen/carbamide peroxide (up to 37%) than home bleaching systems (10% carbamide peroxide). Gingival irritation is a common adverse effect. Usually, these burns show up as a white lesion followed by a red rim. If patients feel burning or tingling of the gingiva during bleaching, the procedure should be stopped and the area rinsed with water. Gingival protection with rubber dams or soft tissue protectors should be used with high peroxide concentrations. Good-fitting bleaching trays will also minimize gingival problems.

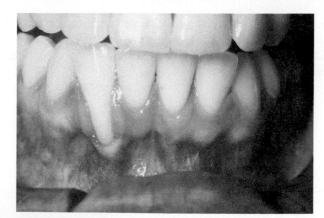

FIGURE 5–12 Clinical photograph of a factitious habit; recession area on the mandibular right central incisor.

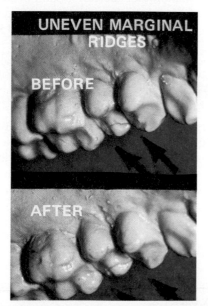

FIGURE 5–13 Example of uneven marginal ridges that can cause food impaction. Lower panel shows condition after reshaping of marginal ridges.

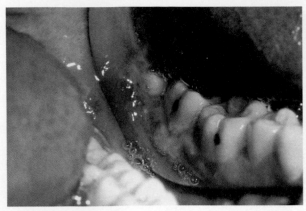

FIGURE 5–14 Clinical photograph of local cocaine application mimicking an aspirin burn.

Occlusion

In the past, occlusal trauma was considered to be a major factor in the initiation of periodontal diseases. It has been conclusively proven that occlusal trauma does not initiate gingival or periodontal inflammation or pocket formation. Heavy occlusal forces can, however, cause clinical tooth mobility and the radiographic appearance of bone loss. However, these changes involve the periodontal ligament and bone, not the marginal gingival surface tissues.

Occlusal trauma may increase the rate of progression of periodontitis if plaque-induced inflammation is also present. In this regard, trauma from occlusion acts as a contributing local factor in the presence of inflammation, but is not a primary etiologic factor by itself.

Oral Piercings

Oral piercing is frequently seen in patients today. Lip piercing may cause dental/periodontal injury on the facial aspect of the mandibular incisors (Chambrone & Chambrone, 2003), whereas tongue piercing affects the lingual aspect of the mandibular incisors (Figure 5–15 ■). Dental

> ### Rapid Dental Hint
>
> When your patient says that she takes aspirin for a toothache, make sure that she doesn't apply the tablet directly to the gingiva around the tooth—it is acidic and can "burn" the tissue.

complications from oral piercing include tooth chipping or fracture, gingival recession, bone loss, interference with speech and swallowing, and increased salivary flow with calculus formation (Choe, Almas, & Schoor, 2005). Insertion of jewelry into oral structures is usually done by individuals not familiar with oral anatomy.

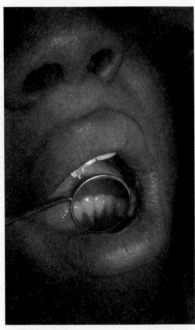

FIGURE 5–15 Example of tongue piercing causing gingival recession on the mandibular incisor. (Source: Ferhan Aziz)

Dental Hygiene Application

The dental hygienist must be able to recognize other factors that may contribute to a patient's periodontal condition. Oral biofilms are a primary risk factor for periodontal diseases. Other than the primary risk factors, contributory or secondary factors to periodontal diseases include calculus, which is "dead" bacteria with a porous surface that harbors biofilms, tooth aberrations, and occlusion. It is important to recognize these contributory factors. When possible, they should be eliminated.

Key Points

- Inflammatory periodontal diseases are infections caused by bacteria.
- Certain secondary local and systemic contributing factors influence the initiation and progression of the disease.

- Dental calculus is not a cause for the periodontal diseases, but a LOCAL contributing factor.

Self-Quiz

1. Which one of the following sources accounts for the mineralization of subgingival calculus?
   a. Salivary proteins
   b. Crevicular fluid
   c. Dental plaque
   d. Acquired pellicle

2. Which one of the following reasons explains the finding of supragingival calculus on the lingual surfaces of the mandibular incisors?
   a. Difficulty in cleaning the area with a toothbrush
   b. Inability of efficient salivary flow to that area
   c. Presence of the parotid duct
   d. Presence of Warton's duct

3. Which one of the following reasons makes calculus an important local etiologic factor for periodontal diseases?
   a. It is porous and can provide a reservoir for bacteria.
   b. It directly irritates the epithelial lining of the pocket.
   c. Minerals cause a breakdown in the epithelial attachment.
   d. The presence of lipooligosaccharides causes the tissues to erode.

4. All of the following anatomic factors may predispose a site to periodontal disease except one. Which one is the exception?
   a. Tooth position
   b. Furcation area
   c. Crown surface
   d. Root surface

5. On which of the following surfaces do palatogingival grooves usually appear?
   a. Lingual surface of mandibular lateral incisor
   b. Lingual surface of mandibular central incisor
   c. Palatal surface of maxillary lateral incisor
   d. Palatal surface of maxillary central incisor
   e. Palatal surface of maxillary canine

Case Study

A 60-year-old male is seen for the first time in the office as a new patient. The data is collected and first chart records of the dental and periodontal conditions are recorded. The dental records indicate gingival recession on the buccal of tooth #13, 14, and 15. There is a missing tooth for #19. There is mild interproximal subgingival calculus in the posterior regions and supragingival calculus on the lingual of #23, 24, 25, and 26.

1. Which factor is a contributory local factor for biofilm retention?
   a. Pocketing of 4 mm or more
   b. Restorations on #14 and #15
   c. Supra and subgingival calculus
   d. Age 60 years old

Answer: C. Dental calculus is considered the most important contributing factor. Dental bacterial biofilm is the main cause of the inflammatory response. Restorations alone are not contributory unless they are rough and biofilm retentive. Age is not a contributory factor unless there are difficulties in dexterity.

2. What impact does the missing #19 have as a contributory factor?
   a. Food impaction site to retain more plaque
   b. Possible occlusal trauma for rotated #18
   c. Open contact harder to cleanse
   d. All of the above

Answer: D. All of the responses can contribute to periodontal disease. Food impaction sites may also harbor more biofilm. Occlusal trauma on #18 can contribute to periodontal disease. Open contacts require additional maintenance and cleansing steps to completely remove biofilm.

3. Supra- and subgingival calculus removal has what effect on periodontal disease?
   a. Removes the causal factor
   b. Smooth tooth surface is less biofilm retentive
   c. Removal opens more areas for recession
   d. Periodontal fibers will regenerate

Answer: B. The smooth surface will be less retentive for more bacterial harboring biofilm. Response to the bacteria is the etiology. Although there may be recession exposed after removing the supragingival calculus the calculus did not create the recession. Periodontal fibers may or may not have been effected yet do not regenerate.

References

Carranza, F. A., Jr. 1996. Dental calculus. In eds. F. A. Carranza, Jr., and M. G. Newman, *Clinical Periodontology*, 9th ed., 150–160. Philadelphia: W. B. Saunders.

Chambrone, L., and L. A. Chambrone. 2003. Gingival recessions caused by lip piercing: Case report. *J. Can. Dent. Assoc.* 69(8):505–508.

Choe, J., K. Almas, and R. Schoor 2005. Tongue piercing risk factor to periodontal health. *NY Dental J.* 71(5):40–43.

Douglass, C. 1998. Risk assessment for periodontal disease in adults. *Oral Care Report* 8:1–11.

Ellwood, D., J. Melling, and P. Rutter. 1979. The accumulation of organisms on the teeth. In ed. Society for General Microbiology, *Adhesion of micro-organisms to surfaces*, 137–164. New York: Academic Press.

Hou, G. L., and C. C. Tsai. 1993. Relationship between palato-radicular grooves and localized periodontitis. *J. Clin. Periodontol.* 20:668–682.

Lang, N. P., A. Mombelli, and R. Attström. 2003. Dental plaque and calculus. In J. Linde, T. Karring, and N. P. Lang, *Clinical periodontology and implant dentistry*, 4th ed., 81–105. Oxford, UK: Blackwell Publishing.

Mandel, I. D. 1990. Dental calculus (calcified dental plaque). In eds. R. J. Genco, H. M. Goldman, and D. W. Cohen, *Contemporary periodontics*, 135–146. St. Louis, MO: Mosby.

Mandel, I. D. 1995. Calculus update: Prevalence, pathogenicity and prevention. *J. Am. Dent. Assoc.* 126:573–580.

Matarasso, S., G. Quaremba, F. Coraggio, E. Vaia, C. Cafiero, and N. P. Lang. 1996. Maintenance of implants: An *in vitro* study of titanium implant surface modifications subsequent to the application of different prophylaxis procedures. *Clinical Oral Implants Research* 7:64–72.

Pihlstrom, B. L., R. B. McHugh, T. H. Oliphant, and C. Ortiz-Campos. 1983. Comparison of surgical and nonsurgical treatment of periodontal disease. A review of current studies and additional results after 6 1/2 years. *J. Clin. Periodontol.* 10:524–541.

Zander, H. 1953. The attachment of calculus to root surfaces. *J. Periodontol.* 24:16–19.

The Oral–Systemic Disease Connection

Toula A. Palaiologou and John D. Mason

OUTLINE

EDUCATIONAL OBJECTIVES

Upon completion of this chapter, the reader should be able to:

- List and discuss possible systemic risk factors for periodontal diseases.
- Discuss periodontal diseases as a risk factor for specific disease entities such as diabetes mellitus, cardiovascular disease, obesity, vitamin D deficiency, and preterm low-birth-weight babies.
- Describe the role of diabetes mellitus as a risk factor for periodontal diseases.
- Discuss the importance of smoking as a risk factor for periodontal diseases.
- Discuss the association of hormones and periodontal diseases.
- Discuss the adverse effect of osteonecrosis of the jaws in dental patients taking bisphosphonates.

GOAL: To introduce the concept of risk factors for periodontal diseases and the relationship of periodontal diseases as a risk factor for other medical diseases.

KEY WORDS

bisphosphonates *87*
C-reactive protein *93*
osteonecrosis of the jaw (ONJ) *87*
risk factors *84*
systemic diseases *92*

Introduction

The oral–systemic disease connection is a rapidly advancing area of research. Many published research articles have found a potential link between periodontal disease and coronary heart disease, adverse pregnancy outcomes, diabetes, bacterial pneumonia, and Alzheimer's disease. More research is still needed to find a definitive connection.

Systemic Risk Factors for Periodontal Diseases

Although it must be assumed that general health affects a patient's resistance to the development of periodontal diseases, no specific systemic disease has been shown to produce periodontal diseases in the absence of local irritating factors. In fact, the presence of certain systemic conditions may actually enhance or intensify the response to the oral biofilms beyond what would occur if the systemic condition were not present.

Although it is not possible to include every systemic disorder that has an impact on periodontal disease progression, numerous conditions potentially modify biofilm accumulation and disease progression.

Periodontal diseases are no longer regarded as infections to which everyone is equally susceptible. Research is trying to determine why some patients are more at risk than others for destructive periodontal diseases. Although bacteria are essential for the development of periodontitis, they are insufficient by themselves. A susceptible host is also necessary, so host factors play a substantial role. Advances in the understanding of the pathogenesis of many chronic systemic diseases have increased awareness of the significant interactions and associations that can occur between oral diseases such as periodontal diseases and systemic diseases (Barnett, 2003). A rather large number of genetic and environmental or acquired factors place individuals at risk for periodontitis (Box 6–1).

Genetics

It is now known that host susceptibility factors play an important role in high-risk periodontal patients. Evidence for genetic control of **risk factors** for some forms of periodontal disease includes the following:

- A consistent association of periodontitis with certain genetically transmitted traits

Box 6–1: Social Factors Contributing to Periodontal Disease

- Tobacco
- Stress
- Alcohol
- Drugs
- Obesity

- Studies of separated twins with chronic onset forms of periodontitis
- Genetic studies of aggressive forms of periodontitis

Periodontal diseases can no longer be thought of as a prevalent condition for which all people are at equal risk if they fail to practice good oral hygiene. It appears that microbial and host factors are both important to disease susceptibility, but neither, independently, accounts for all degrees of periodontal disease. Because periodontal diseases are more than likely diverse in etiology, any thought of a universal host risk factor is probably also inappropriate. An association has been found between the susceptibility and severity of periodontitis and the presence of a substance called *interleukin-1* (IL-1). IL-1 is a cytokine that is released from inflammatory cells in the body for the purpose of altering either its own function or those of adjacent cells. An IL-1 gene-positive patient is about seven times more likely to develop or have advanced periodontal disease than a gene-negative patient, and this genotype occurs in approximately 30% of the population (Newman, 1998). In recent years, however, though a modest effect on disease risk is noted, one group determined that evidence is lacking to establish if a positive IL-1 genotype status adds to progression of periodontitis and/or treatment outcomes (Huynh-Ba et al., 2007). Recent studies provide evidence that cytokines appear to interact functionally in networks in the periodontium and integrate aspects of innate and adaptive immunity. However, our understanding is far from complete, particularly in how molecular and cellular pathways relate to disease pathogenesis (Preshaw & Taylor, 2011).

As with many other diseases, susceptibility to periodontal diseases may, to some extent, be genetically determined. Several congenital diseases with periodontal manifestations have been identified, such as hereditary gingival fibromatosis, cyclic neutropenia, Down syndrome, Papillon-Lefévre syndrome, Chediak-Higashi disease, and hypophosphatasia, among others.

It is now clear that genetic factors that act on and modify host responses to the microbial challenge are major determinants of susceptibility to periodontitis, as well as determinants of the rates and extent of disease progression and disease severity. Roughly 50% of the enhanced risk for severe periodontitis can be accounted for by heredity alone. Studies of families with aggressive periodontitis and groups of individuals with chronic periodontitis have shown that certain chromosomes, and in some cases specific gene loci, are linked to enhanced susceptibility for periodontitis (Newman, 1998).

Periodontal findings in twins who were reared together or apart have shown a significant genetic component for probing depth, attachment loss, and plaque that could not be explained by differences in family environment such as oral hygiene practices and frequency of dental visits (Michalowicz et al., 1991). A further twin study (Michalowicz et al., 2000) reemphasized the fact that about half of disease variance can be attributed to the genetic biologic variance in immunological host defenses.

Past conceptual models of the pathogenesis of periodontal disease did not capture the dynamic nature of the biochemical processes (i.e., *that innate differences among individuals* and changes in environmental factors may accelerate biochemical changes or dampen that shift). With emerging genomic, proteomic, and metabolomic data and systems biology tools for interpreting data, it is now possible to begin describing the basic elements of a new model of pathogenesis. Such a model incorporates gene, protein, and metabolite data into dynamic biologic networks that include disease-initiating and resolving mechanisms. New models in the next few years will be merely frameworks for integrating key knowledge as it becomes available from the "-omics" technologies (Kornman, 2008).

Our understanding of gene mapping and the human genome may allow for presymptomatic identification of individuals with elevated disease susceptibility, and this will lead to revolutionary changes in dental education and practice in the future (Johnson et al., 2008).

Age, Gender, and Race

Epidemiologic studies have shown that the incidence (rate of occurrence) of periodontal diseases increases with age (Abdellatif & Burt, 1987). This is likely the result of the cumulative effects of bacterial irritation of the tissues over many years, rather than a reduction in host resistance as a function of the aging process. Evidence strongly suggests that periodontal health can be maintained throughout life if local etiologic factors are controlled, and recent studies support that the level of education has a clear effect on the periodontal health status in the elderly (Siukosaari, Ajwani, Ainamo, Wolf, & Närhi, 2012).

The National Institute of Dental and Craniofacial Research Survey of Oral Health of Adults in the United States show that males have a greater incidence and severity of periodontal diseases.

No firm evidence documents that race is a significant risk factor in destructive forms of periodontitis other than as it may be related genetically within particular families.

Stress

Long-term physical and psychological stress seems to increase susceptibility to periodontal infection. Stress (along with depression, financial problems, social isolation, and other psychosocial factors) is another systemic risk factor for periodontitis because it may depress the immune response to periodontal pathogens, thereby increasing the severity of periodontal disease (Genco et al., 1998; Peruzzo et al., 2007; Semenoff-Segundo et al., 2012). Stressful life events such as divorce, joblessness, and lifestyle factors have been correlated with increased severity of periodontal disease (Kloostra, Eber, & Inglehart, 2007). Stress works in two ways. People under stress change their behavior and may pay less attention to oral hygiene. Also, their bodies increase the production of glucocorticosteroids (hormones made in the body that have anti-inflammatory actions and protect against stress) and cortisone, a type of glucocorticosteroid,

which results in immunosuppression and a reduced resistance to infection. Stress variables also seem to have an effect on healing (Broadbent, Petrie, Alley, & Booth, 2003).

Endocrine System

DIABETES   Diabetes mellitus is a group of diseases that results in hyperglycemia (high blood sugar or glucose). Diabetes mellitus is classified into type 1 and type 2 diabetes. Type 1 is caused by a severe insulin deficiency resulting from a destruction of beta-cells of the pancreas, which produce and secrete the hormone called insulin. Insulin is needed to control blood glucose levels because it helps bring blood glucose from the diet and that produced in the liver into the cells. The cells utilize glucose for energy. These patients are treated with insulin injections.

In type 2 diabetes, which is more common than type 1, insulin is being secreted from the pancreas, but not in sufficient amounts. Most probably, the insulin receptors on the cells surface of the tissues are not sensitive enough for the insulin to bind to the cell and allow for glucose uptake into the cell. This is referred to as insulin resistance.

Diabetes is associated with a reduced ability to cope with infections and with impaired wound healing. The balance of evidence suggests that both type 1 diabetes and type 2 diabetes carry an increased risk of severe gingivitis and periodontitis (Botero et al., 2012; Moritz & Mealey, 2006; Page & Beck, 1997). Diabetics may be more susceptible to developing periodontal disease. The relationship between diabetes and periodontal diseases is more likely to be observed in poorly controlled individuals (Nishimura, Takahashi, Kurihara, Takashiba, & Murayama, 1998; Ryan, Carnu, & Tenzler, 2006; Taylor et al., 1996). Patients with chronic, poorly controlled diabetes appear to have more attachment loss and bone loss than diabetics with good metabolic control (Safkan-Seppälä & Ainamo, 1992; Figure 6–1 ■). Poorly controlled diabetics had a 2.9-fold increased risk of having periodontitis compared to nondiabetics and well-controlled diabetics (Tsai, Hayes, & Taylor, 2002).

Epidemiologic studies on type 1 and type 2 diabetic patients indicate that although persons on optimal control

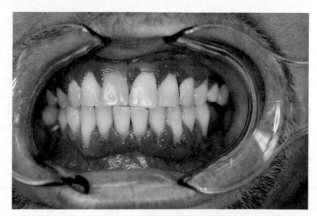

FIGURE 6–1 A 56-year-old patient with type 2 diabetes mellitus. Note the clinical appearance of the gingiva.

are at equal risk for developing periodontal disease, too few diabetics are optimally controlled, and maintaining strict control is difficult in the long term.

Elevated blood sugar levels (hyperglycemia) may suppress the host's immune response and lead to poor wound healing and recurrent infections such as multiple or recurrent periodontal abscesses. Impaired polymorphonuclear leukocyte chemotaxis (Manouchehr-Pour, Spagnuolo, Rodman, & Bissada, 1981; McMullen, Van Dyke, Horoszewicz, & Genco, 1981) and phagocytosis (Cutler, Eke, Arnold, & Van Dyke, 1991) have been implicated as factors in the predisposition of patients to severe periodontal destruction. The host's immuno-inflammatory response may also be altered by a hyperinflammatory production of cytokines by macrophages in response to bacteria antigens. These cytokines, like TNF-alpha, then appear in the gingival crevicular fluid and can result in increased periodontal inflammation and destruction of the supporting structures of the teeth (Mealey & Rose, 2008). Women with a family history of type 2 diabetes or diagnosed as prediabetic may be at higher risk for gestational diabetes. Close periodontal supervision would seem prudent and early intervention vital. Recent evidence indicates that *meticulous control* of the diabetic state is associated with periodontal health (Grossi & Genco, 1998).

It has been concluded that poor metabolic control of type 1 diabetes together with smoking is extremely detrimental for clinical attachment loss (Syrjala, Ylostalo, Niskanen, & Knuuttila, 2003).

HORMONES Gingivitis and periodontitis have been noticed clinically to be more severe in some patients during periods of change or imbalance in estrogen/progestin levels (Amar & Chung, 1994). In pregnant, pubertal, and postmenopausal patients, an exaggerated inflammatory response to local irritation may be evident. Hormonal status in general does have an influence on the inflammatory response.

Pregnancy. Although evidence suggests that pregnancy itself may not be associated with an increased risk of periodontitis, pregnant patients often exhibit exaggerated gingival inflammatory changes in the second and third trimesters, sometimes called pregnancy gingivitis (Figure 6–2 ■). Teeth often become more mobile during pregnancy due to changes in the periodontal ligament, but return to normal state after delivery.

Oral Contraceptives. Oral contraceptives act by elevating hormonal levels simulating pregnancy to prevent ovulation. Thus, it is expected that the same gingival changes seen during pregnancy will also be seen in women taking oral contraceptives. Gingival changes may include inflammation and enlargement with increased amount of fluid flow into the tissue. As with pregnancy-associated gingivitis, gingival inflammation in women on oral contraceptives occurs in the presence of very little plaque. The most profound gingival changes are seen in the first few months of initially taking the contraceptive. If the condition worsens, a different formulation may be tried. Maintenance of meticulous oral hygiene is important. Once the woman discontinues the contraceptive, the gingival condition usually reverses.

Since the inception of oral contraceptives, the newer formulations contain a lower concentration of hormones. Unfortunately, most of the clinical studies investigating oral contraceptive usage were done in the 1960s. One report suggests that because of the lower concentrations in the current oral contraceptive formulations, the inflammatory response of the gingiva to dental plaque was not affected, so no gingival changes were found (Preshaw, Knutsen, & Mariotti, 2001). A more recent study failed to validate the theory that earlier high- or current low-dose oral contraceptive use is associated with increased levels of gingivitis or periodontitis and suggests an important reexamination of the perceived association between OC use and periodontal diseases (Taichman, 2005).

Puberty. Hormonal imbalance is also felt to contribute to the increased severity of gingivitis seen at puberty, when there is an exaggerated response to plaque. The mechanisms are probably similar to those present in pregnancy. Gingival inflammation and enlargement can occur in both males and females, but it is more prevalent in females. Changes in hormonal levels (estrogen and progesterone) and gingival inflammatory changes are transitory and will revert to normal levels post–circumpubertal period.

Menopause/Osteoporosis. Osteoporosis as a result of estrogen depletion causes bone to become more porous, with less trabeculation and decreased thickness of the cortical plate (Jeffcoat, 1998). In fact, estrogen deficiency may play a role in the progression of periodontitis (Lerner, 2006). Under sufficient dental plaque stimulus, this can lead to more severe periodontal disease, including tooth loss. A correlation has been found between osteoporosis and both periodontal disease and tooth loss in postmenopausal women (Bando, Nitta, Matsubara, & Ishikawa, 1998; Jeffcoat, 1998; Oh, Bashutski, & Giannobile, 2007; Renvert, Berglund, Persson, & Persson, 2011), but it is not considered a definitive risk factor.

Certain risk factors associated with osteoporosis include age, calcium intake (e.g., through the consumption of milk, yogurt, cheese, fish, and calcium supplements), physical activity (e.g., walking, tennis), body build, and smoking status. A study by Bando and colleagues (1998)

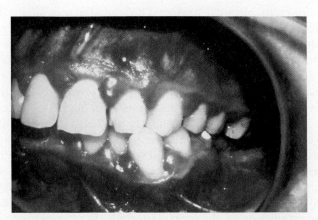

FIGURE 6–2 Example of pregnancy gingivitis exhibiting proximal puffiness and easy bleeding on probing, reflecting an exaggerated response to local irritants due to hormonal factors.

found that normal masticatory function in periodontally healthy postmenopausal women might inhibit or delay the progress of osteoporotic changes in skeletal bone.

Another study by Jeffcoat (1998) related systemic osteoporosis to oral bone loss, and Kribbs (1990) and Nitta (Nitta, Bando, Matsubara, & Ishikawa, 1997) discussed the impact of periodontal health on osteoporosis in postmenopausal women. In the latter study, 12 edentulous postmenopausal women were compared with 14 periodontally healthy postmenopausal women: "The edentulous patients had less bone mineral density of the lumbar spine and less occlusal force." Preliminary evidence suggests that supplementation with biphosphonates, such as alendrolate (Fosamax®, Merck & Co., West Point, PA), may be helpful in stabilizing dental supporting bone because it helps improve total bone mineralization. Calibrating dental radiographs (i.e., subtraction radiography) as a diagnostic tool for systemic osteoporosis may help in early detection of both oral and systemic bone loss (Jeffcoat, 1998). More recent information on **bisphosphonates** (Marx, 2010), however, has put a cloud over this treatment for *alveolar* bone loss. Overall, it can be concluded that current knowledge regarding the effects of osteoporosis/osteopenia on periodontal diseases and alveolar bone loss is inconclusive. Regarding implant placement, there are no convincing data that dental implant placement is contraindicated in the osteoporotic patient (Otomo-Corgel, 2012).

BISPHOSPHONATES Many dental patients with osteoporosis (reduction in bone mass due to loss of calcium), Paget's disease, or bone metastasis (with or without hypercalcemia) associated with multiple myeloma, breast, and prostate cancer are taking a bisphosphonate (Gross, 2008). Bisphosphonates are drugs that inhibit bone resorption and reduce increased levels of blood calcium caused by cancer. Bisphosphonates inhibit bone removal or resorption by osteoclasts (cells that resorb bone), thereby allowing the buildup of new bone. This will then help to prevent fractures of the hip and spine. Normally, equilibrium exists between osteoblasts (cells that lay down new bone) and osteoclasts. The problem arising in patients taking bisphosphonates is that there are no more osteoclasts to resorb or "eat" necrotic (dead) bone, so the new bone is laid down with the diseased bone. If necrotic bone cannot be resorbed by the osteoclasts using normal healing, then the necrotic bone will inhibit healing and affect blood supply to the area, resulting in **osteonecrosis of the jaw (ONJ)** (also referred to as bisphosphonate-related osteonecrosis of the jaw [BRONJ]; Ruggiero, 2008). Many invasive dental procedures may precipitate the development of ONJ.

Although first observed in 2004 in patients taking intravenous bisphosphonates, cases of ONJ are being seen in patients taking oral bisphosphonates. Patients are considered to be at risk for ONJ if they are currently taking or previously were taking a bisphosphonate. Bisphosphonates, once taken into the body, bind to bone and stay there for long periods of time, even if discontinued. This long half-life of about 10 years or more is of concern because even if the drug is discontinued before dental procedures, it is still in the body.

There are two subclasses of bisphosphonates: nonnitrogenous and nitrogenous bisphosphonates (Table 6–1 ▪). The nonnitrogenous or first-generation bisphosphonates are not as potent as the nitrogenous, second- and third-generation

Table 6–1 Bisphosphonates (AAOMS, 2009)

Subclass of Bisphosphonate	Trade Name	Generic Name	Route of Administration	Primary Indication	Potency
Nonnitrogenous	Didronel	etidronate	oral	Paget's disease	1
Nonnitrogenous (not avail. in U.S.)	Bonefos	clodronate	oral	Bone metastasis	10
Nitrogenous	Skelid	tiludronate	oral	Paget's disease	50
Nitrogenous	Aredia	pamidronate	IV	Bone metastasis	1000–5000
Nitrogenous	Fosamax	alendronate	oral	Osteoporosis	1,000
Nitrogenous	Boniva	ibandronate	oral, IV (quarterly)	Osteoporosis	1,000
Nitrogenous	Actonel	risedronate	oral	Osteoporosis	1,000
Nitrogenous	Zometa, Reclast	zoledronate	IV	Zometa for bone metastasis Reclast for osteoporosis (once a year injection)	10,000+

of bisphosphonates, which contain nitrogen and appear to be implicated in causing ONJ.

Clinically, patients are considered to have ONJ if they have (1) current or previous treatment with a bisphosphonate; (2) exposed, necrotic bone in the maxillofacial region (more common in the mandible than maxilla) that has persisted for more than 8 weeks; and (3) no history of radiation therapy (Figure 6–3 ■ and Figure 6–4 ■; Marx, 2010, American Association of Oral and Maxillofacial Surgeons [AAOMS], 2009). Osteonecrosis of the jaws can be triggered by precipitating causes such as extractions (highest incidence), implant placement, periodontal procedures, endodontic therapy, or orthodontic therapy and can even occur spontaneously without any treatment (Otomo-Corgel, 2007). The following factors are thought to be risk factors for ONJ: (1) corticosteroid therapy, (2) diabetes, (3) smoking, (4) alcohol use, (5) poor oral hygiene with clinical and radiographic evidence of periodontitis, and (6) chemotherapeutic drugs.

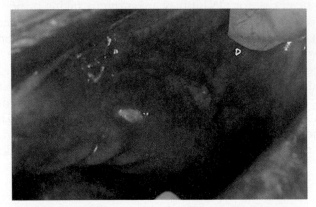

FIGURE 6–3 Edentulous patient had pieces of bone that became necrotic and continued to slough off after tooth extractions. (Courtesy of Jacqueline Plemons, DDS, Baylor College of Dentistry.)

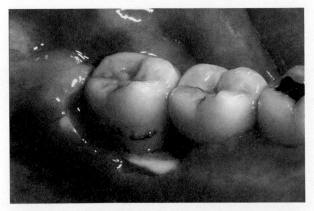

FIGURE 6–4 Case of ONJ that occurred spontaneously. Note the white area, which is exposed necrotic bone. (Courtesy of Jacqueline Plemons, DDS, Baylor College of Dentistry.)

Prior to treatment with bisphosphonates, the patient should have a thorough oral examination and all invasive dental procedures including extractions and restorative, endodontic, and periodontal therapies (AAOMS, 2009; Wade & Suzuki, 2007). Patients should be encouraged to practice good oral hygiene.

Once a patient has been taking an oral bisphosphonate for more than 3 years, the risk of developing ONJ increases (Zak, Spina, Spinazze, Perkinson, & Spinazze, 2007a, 2007b). *Although the risk of developing ONJ seems low in patients taking oral bisphosphonates* (Edwards, Hellstein, Jacobsen, 2008; Migliorati et al., 2005; AAOMS, 2009), dental treatment may need to be altered. There is currently no data from clinical trials evaluating dental management of patients on oral bisphosphonate therapy. In general, conservative treatment is recommended. Treatment regimens have been suggested based on staging (Table 6–2 ■; AAOMS, 2009; Marx 2010; Williamson 2010).

Preventive care is extremely important to reduce the incidence of ONJ. Recommendations focus on conservative surgical procedures, proper sterile technique, appropriate use of oral disinfectants, and the dentist's clinical and professional judgment (American Dental Association of Scientific Affairs, 2006). Consultation with the patient's physician is necessary.

Patients taking oral bisphosphonates for less than 3 years can have invasive dental treatment, but if the patient has been taking bisphosphonates for more than 3 years, the C-terminal cross-linked telopetide (CTx) blood test can be performed to determine the amount of bone resorption. The CTx test is performed by Quest Diagnostics and sent to its lab in California (http://www.questdiagnostic.com). If the results of the CTx blood test are greater than 150 pg/mL, then invasive dental procedures can usually be performed. Values less than 100 pg/mL are associated with a high risk of developing ONJ (Fugazzotto, Lightfoot, Jaffin, & Kumar, 2007; Grant, Amenedo, Freeman, & Kraut, 2008; Marx 2010). It is recommended to discontinue the drug for 3 months prior to the planned procedure and send for CTx testing. CTx values were noted to increase between 25.9 and 26.4 pg/mL for each month of a drug holiday. Once treatment is done, extend the "drug holiday" for an additional 3 months (Cartsos, Zhu, & Zavras, 2008; Marx, Cillo, & Ulloa, 2007; Marx, Sawatari, Fortin, & Broumand, 2005). Thus, patients on long-term oral bisphosphonates should be treated with caution (Wang, Weber, & McCauley, 2007).

On the other hand, while patients are taking IV bisphosphonates, any invasive dental procedures should be avoided. Dentists need to exercise their professional judgment, perhaps after consultation with the patient's physician, in deciding whether invasive treatment is needed under the particular clinical situations (American Dental Association Council on Scientific Affairs, 2006).

It is important to be aware that bisphosphonates are not all the same, and patient responses to treatment may vary depending on which bisphosphonates they are taking.

Table 6–2 Staging and Treatment Strategies

ONJ Staging	Treatment Strategies
At risk category No apparent necrotic bone in patients who have been treated with either oral or IV bisphosphonates	• No treatment indicated • Patient education
Stage 0 No clinical evidence of necrotic bone, but nonspecific clinical findings and symptoms	• Systemic management, including the use of pain medication and antibiotics
Stage 1 Exposed and necrotic bone in patients who are asymptomatic and have no evidence of infection	• Antibacterial mouth rinse • Clinical follow-up on a quarterly basis • Patient education and review of indications for continued bisphosphonate therapy
Stage 2 Exposed and necrotic bone associated with infection as evidenced by pain and erythema in the region of the exposed bone with or without purulent drainage	• Symptomatic treatment with oral antibiotics • Oral antibacterial mouth rinse • Pain control • Superficial debridement to relieve soft tissue irritation
Stage 3 Exposed and necrotic bone in patients with pain, infection, and one or more of the following: exposed and necrotic bone extending beyond the region of alveolar bone (i.e., inferior border and ramus in the mandible, maxillary sinus and zygoma in the maxilla) resulting in pathologic fracture, extra-oral fistula, oral antral/oral nasal communication, or osteolysis extending to the inferior border of the mandible of sinus floor	• Antibacterial mouth rinse • Antibiotic therapy and pain control • Surgical debridement/resection for longer-term palliation of infection and pain

Due to the risks of osteonecrosis (ONJ), dental clinicians should work closely with their medical colleagues prior to the physician prescribing oral bisphosphonates. Ideally, optimal periodontal and dental health should be established before the patient commences bisphosphonate therapy (Otomo-Corgel, 2012).

Hematologic System

Several blood dyscrasias have been associated with uncommon, unusual, extreme forms of periodontal diseases. Agranulocytosis and neutropenia (including cyclic neutropenia) are associated with an increased severity of gingivitis and periodontitis as well as necrotic ulcerations. Acute leukemia is characterized by purple-colored gingival enlargement, ulceration, inflammation, and spontaneous severe bleeding. These changes are attributable to infiltration of malignant cells, neutropenia, impaired phagocytosis, platelet deficiency, and decreased effectiveness of associated immune mechanisms. Patients with these medical problems require special attention.

HIV/AIDS

Human immunodeficiency virus (HIV) seropositive individuals appear to be vulnerable to aggressive necrotizing periodontal diseases, including necrotizing ulcerative gingivitis (NUG) and necrotizing ulcerative periodontitis (NUP; Murray, 1994). The development of severe forms of gingivitis and periodontitis is focused on an impairment of the host response (i.e., functional defects in the host's neutrophils) to combat infections. It appears that the degree of immunodeficiency influences the prevalence and severity of these periodontal diseases in the HIV-infected population and may also influence treatment expectations and prognosis (Figure 6–5 ▪).

The development of highly active antiretroviral therapy (HAART) has significantly modified the course of HIV disease into a manageable chronic disease with longer

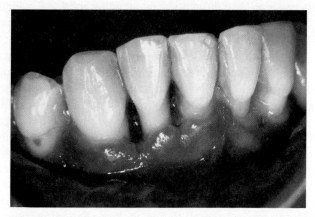

FIGURE 6–5 Periodontal lesions associated with HIV infection: more advanced lesions that resemble necrotizing ulcerative periodontitis (NUP) and that are nonresponsive to typical therapy.

survival and improved quality of life in HIV-infected subjects. It appears that HAART is also associated with a lower prevalence and modified course of HIV-associated periodontal disease in adults. Higher prevalence of opportunistic microorganisms has been frequently detected in the subgingival flora of HIV-infected individuals, probably due to the immune status of those patients, as colonization and overgrowth of atypical pathogenic species is facilitated by immunosuppression (Mataftsi, Skoura, & Sakellari, 2011).

Nutritional Status

Nutritional deficiencies have not been shown to cause periodontal diseases. Nutrition studies are commonly done by inducing a deprivation state of a single nutrient or a group of related nutrients in laboratory animals that result in decreased formation of the periodontal ligament, bone, and cementum. Very few patients have a diet that is totally lacking in a single nutrient or group of related nutrients; therefore, the information gained from these experimental laboratory studies in animals may not apply to the human clinical situation.

Vitamin deficiencies are probably given more significance in the etiology of periodontal diseases from a clinical standpoint than other nutritional substances. The vitamin most often studied is ascorbic acid (vitamin C), which plays an important role in the normal functions of fibroblasts, osteoblasts, and odontoblasts. When vitamin C levels are greatly reduced (i.e., scurvy), wound healing is impaired.

Another vitamin that has presented some interest in the periodontal literature is vitamin D. Vitamin D deficiency has been associated with periodontitis as well as a negative effect of the treatment outcome (Bashutski et al., 2011; Yao & Fine 2012).

Some other considerations concerning the diet may be important in the overall dental problems of some patients. Tough or coarse foods do not provide functional stimulation to the gingiva, nor do they help to remove plaque below the contact points or cervical bulge on the teeth.

Patients who regularly eat between meals present a problem in that they constantly provide a food source for the bacteria and may have difficulty in maintaining good oral hygiene.

Drug and Tobacco Use Status

TOBACCO PRODUCTS Cigarette smoking is a major (and maybe the most significant) risk factor for severe periodontal diseases. Fifty-three percent of periodontitis cases in the United States are attributable to smoking (Tomar & Asma, 2000). Smokers are about two to six times more likely to have periodontal destruction than nonsmokers, yet they can exhibit less gingival bleeding on probing (Heasman et al., 2006; Jansson & Lavstedt, 2002; Krall, Hayes, Garvey, & Garcia, 1997; Tonetti, 1998). Multiple studies report that smokers are at greater risk for loss of attachment, alveolar bone loss, and tooth loss compared to nonsmokers (Papantonopoulos, 2004). They also may respond less favorably to surgical and nonsurgical periodontal therapy (Fisher et al., 2008).

A study by Krall and colleagues (1997) found that current male cigarette smokers had significantly fewer teeth than those men who reported never smoking. The number of missing teeth was positively related to pack/years of cigarette use, age, and coffee consumption and inversely related to level of education. It is more accurate to use the term "pack/years" rather than "pack/day" because it describes the exposure to toxins in a cumulative way. The study also found that current smokers had higher levels of tooth mobility, calculus deposition, and probing depth than men who had never smoked. Former cigarette smokers and men who smoked pipes or cigars were similar to men who never smoked in regard to tooth loss.

Generally, the periodontal status of former smokers has been found to be intermediate between that of never smokers and current smokers (Haber & Kent, 1992; Haber et al., 1993). It has been suggested that the past effects of smoking on the periodontium cannot be reversed, but that smoking cessation is beneficial to periodontal health (American Academy of Periodontology, 1999). The effects may not be totally reversed, but a study of the data from the NHANES III survey showed an odds ratio of current smokers developing periodontitis declining from four times normal to almost equal to never-smokers or one (1.15), 11 years after quitting (Tomar & Asma, 2000). The inflammatory function in the periodontal tissues of smokers who quit reverts back to normal (Nair, Sutherland, Palmer, Wilson, & Scott, 2003).

Although smoking does not dramatically affect the oral microbiota, studies have shown that smoking and tobacco products directly modulate the subgingival microflora by favoring colonization with periodontal pathogens (Grossi et al., 1996). In addition, smoking may suppress the host-defense system, which may promote periodontal disease progression (Kibayashi et al., 2007). Thus, smoking increases the risk for periodontal diseases and interferes with the ability of the gingiva and bone to respond to treatment (Gunsolley et al., 1998; Tonetti, 1998). This mechanism is probably through an altered host response. Effects of smoking seem to be related not only to the local effects in the oral cavity (heat, dryness, and increased plaque and calculus deposits), but also to a suppression of the immune system altering the host response to periodontal pathogens. To adequately deal with bacterial infections, functioning neutrophils are necessary. It has been well documented that cigarette smoke can have harmful effects on various neutrophil functions (Kenny, Kraal, Saxe, & Jones, 1977). For example, tobacco smoke can impair the chemotaxis and phagocytosis of neutrophils (Lannan et al., 1992). Thus, the PMNs do not function properly in eliminating invasive, pathogenic bacteria. Individuals with alterations in their host-defense system would then be more susceptible to periodontal infections by preexisting pathogenic bacteria.

Another problem associated with smoking is that products of cigarette smoke remain on the root surfaces and in the gingival crevicular fluid, thereby providing a reservoir of irritants for the soft tissue and preventing tissue attachment. Recent studies have shown that exposure of periodontal ligament fibroblasts to cigarette smoke extract resulted in reduced survival of the cells and thus may inhibit tissue remodeling, an important step in the process of healing (Bulmanski, Brady, Stoute, & Lallier, 2012).

Research has found that the presence of a specific gene (interleukin-1 beta) has been associated with risk for periodontal disease severity. It has also been reported that in heavy cigarette smokers, carriage of interleukin-1 gene complex was associated with an increased risk for peri-implant (around the implant) bone loss (Feloutzis et al., 2003). A review of 35 studies found smoking to be a significant risk factor for implant treatment and any accompanying augmentations (Strietzel et al., 2007).

Smokeless tobacco for some may be an alternative to cigarette smoking. However, research has shown that smokeless tobacco may also contribute to periodontal diseases and may eventually lead to cancerous changes in the soft tissues (Figure 6–6 ■). A common finding is gingival recession adjacent to the site of tobacco placement. More research is needed to determine whether smokeless tobacco use is associated with an increased level of plaque-associated gingivitis. New studies have found that cigar and pipe smoking may be as harmful to periodontal tissues as cigarette smoking (Krall, Garvey, & Garcia, 1999).

Strict supragingival plaque control has been documented to reduce indicators of subgingival inflammation and destruction to a similar extent in smokers and never-smokers (Gomes et al., 2007).

Cannabis (marijuana) smoking may be a risk factor for periodontal disease that is independent of the use of tobacco. An article in *Journal of the American Medical Association* (*JAMA*) documented that although tobacco smoking was strongly associated with increased incidence of periodontal disease, there was no interaction between cannabis use and tobacco smoking in predicting the condition's occurrence (Thomson et al., 2008).

ALCOHOL Alcohol abuse may also contribute to periodontal diseases. Chronic alcohol intake presents an increased risk for periodontitis because of poor oral hygiene due to overall neglect and a tendency to malnutrition. Alcohol consumption is related to increased incidence (Drake, Hunt, & Koch, 1995) and prevalence of tooth loss, especially in men (Krall et al., 1997; Kranzler, Babor,

Goldstein, & Gold, 1990). It also adversely affects the host defense (PMNs), clotting mechanism, bone metabolism, and healing. Researchers have found a moderate but consistent dose-dependent relationship between alcohol consumption and periodontal disease (Tezal, Grossi, Ho, & Genco, 2004).

It has been proposed that ethanol consumption could represent a risk indicator for periodontal disease. More evidence of this was found in a recent study in rats, where alcohol was shown to augment the expression of inflammatory markers (Dantas et al., 2012).

XEROSTOMIA DUE TO DRUGS Several medications, such as diuretics (antihypertensive drugs) and psychotropic drugs (i.e., anti-anxiety drugs such as Valium; antidepressants such as Elavil; and antipsychotic drugs such as Clozaril and Risperdal) can cause xerostomia or dry mouth, which can be uncomfortable for the patient, interfere with plaque control, and thereby increase periodontal inflammation. The reduced salivary flow has also been associated with increased caries.

GINGIVAL OVERGROWTH DUE TO DRUGS Gingival enlargement or overgrowth in response to plaque accumulation can be exaggerated by medications such as phenytoin (used for seizures), calcium channel blockers such as nifedipine or diltiazem (for cardiovascular problems and hypertension), and cyclosporine (in transplant patients). The alveolar bone and attachment apparatus are not affected by these drugs (Ciancio, 1996; Figure 6–7 ■).

The areas of enlargement generally begin interproximally and slowly grow to form triangular tissue masses that eventually unite in a continuous curtain of firm gingival tissue across facial and lingual surfaces. The enlarged tissue interferes with oral hygiene and is often inflamed. Gingival overgrowth has been reported to occur in about 50% of patients receiving phenytoin (Ciancio, Yaffe, & Catz, 1972), 15% of patients receiving nifedipine (Barak, Engelberg, & Hiss, 1987), and 25% of patients receiving cyclosporine (Daley, Wysocki, & May, 1986).

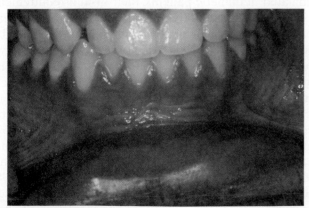

FIGURE 6–6 Clinical example of smokeless tobacco lesions damaging the periodontium. (Courtesy of Dr. Reid Lester)

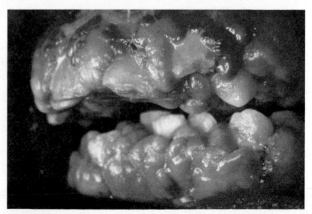

FIGURE 6–7 Example of drug-induced gingival overgrowth related to the use of cyclosporine.

Steroids. According to the American Academy of Periodontology, there is a lack of influence of steroids on periodontal disease (Kinane, 1999). Systemic steroids are used in the management of asthma and other inflammatory conditions including skin conditions and ear problems.

Obesity

The prevalence of obesity has increased substantially over the past decades in most industrialized countries (Pischon et al., 2007). Obesity is defined as body mass index (BMI) > 30 Kg/m^2 and predisposes to a variety of comorbidities and complications that affect overall health. It is generally accepted that obesity is associated with many other multiple-risk factor syndromes such as hypertension, hyperlipidemia, atherosclerosis, and type 2 diabetes mellitus and is associated with increased mortality (Nishimura et al., 2003). The growing prevalence of increased body weight and obesity in the United States has raised significant public health concerns. Cross-sectional studies suggest that obesity is also associated with oral diseases, particularly periodontal disease (Pischon et al., 2007).

Positive associations between periodontal disease and obesity were found in NHANES III based studies (Al-Zahrani, Bissada, & Borawskit, 2003; Genco, Grossi, Ho, Nishimura, & Murayama, 2005). Obesity was found to be positively correlated with increased periodontal disease prevalence as measured by probing depth and clinical attachment loss (Alabdulkarim, Bissada, Al-Zahrani, Ficara, & Siegel, 2005), and it significantly increased odds of having periodontitis (Khader, Bawadi, Haroun, Alomari, & Tayyem, 2009). The association between BMI and obesity may be modified by several factors (e.g., age, gender, and smoking). BMI, blood pressure, triglycerides, fasting blood glucose, and glycosylated hemoglobin A1c (HbA1c) were significantly elevated in patients with periodontal pockets of ≥ 4 mm (Morita et al., 2009).

Obesity is also associated with high plasma levels of TNF-α and its soluble receptors, which in turn may lead to a hyperinflammatory state increasing the risk for periodontal disease and also accounting in part for insulin resistance (Genco et al., 2005). Prevention and management of obesity may promote better systemic and periodontal health (Alabdulkarim et al., 2005). Promotion of healthy nutrition and adequate physical activity may be additional factors to prevent or halt the rate of progression of periodontal disease. Thus this connection between obesity and periodontal disease is complex and bidirectional, with obesity contributing to periodontal disease, and periodontal disease potentially contributing to obesity.

Periodontal Diseases as Risk Factors for Systemic Conditions

Although inflammatory periodontal diseases are local infections of the gingiva and bone, it has been shown that the presence of periodontitis may itself be a risk factor for other

Did You Know?

The U.S. Surgeon General stated that the oral cavity may be the initial site of disease that can serve as the portal of entry of microorganisms into the general circulation, which can have an adverse effect on your patient's general health status.

infections in the body, **systemic diseases**, and pregnancy-related problems (American Academy of Periodontology, 1998; Costerton & Keller, 2007; Kim & Amar, 2006). This means that although a relationship may have been found, it is not yet known that it is a cause-and-effect relationship; risk factors are not causative. Risk factors may predict disease, but it does not necessarily follow that they will cause disease. Examples of systemic conditions with such a relationship include cardiovascular disease and stroke (Gapski & Cobb, 2006), type 2 diabetes mellitus (Moritz & Mealey, 2006), respiratory conditions (Scannapieco & Ho, 2001), adverse pregnancy outcomes (Paquette, 2006), and possible Alzheimer's disease (Stein, Scheff, & Dawson, 2006). In addition, in 2007, pancreatic cancer may have been shown to be linked to periodontal disease (Michaud et al., 2007).

Diabetes

A conference on oral health and systemic health that was held in Switzerland in December 2002 (Barnett, 2003) concluded that evidence showed that untreated periodontitis can complicate glycemic control of patients with diabetes (Saremi et al., 2005). Diabetics may be *more susceptible* to developing periodontal disease, but diabetes does not cause it. Of all the systemic diseases, diabetes and periodontal diseases have been the most extensively studied. It has been shown that periodontal diseases may be responsible for higher levels of blood glucose in diabetics (Grossi & Genco, 1998). A study that evaluated periodontitis in diabetics with different interleukin (IL-1) genotypes concluded that the prevalence of severe attachment loss increased with decreasing diabetic control (Guzman, Karima, Wang, & Van Dyke, 2003). When these infections are controlled or eliminated in diabetic patients, their insulin requirements can often be reduced (Ryan et al., 2006). Effective treatment of periodontal diseases can result in a reduced need to gear up tissue metabolism to fight the infection and lower blood sugar levels, thereby reducing insulin requirements and helping in diabetic control with an additional benefit of reducing other complications (e.g., blindness, renal failure, neuropathy, and coronary artery disease) of diabetes. According to the American Academy of Periodontology, control of infections, including periodontal diseases, may be essential to the establishment of good metabolic control in diabetics (American Academy of Periodontology, 1998). Though the presence of periodontal disease may adversely affect glycemic control in diabetes, and there seems to be a trend toward improved glycemic control after periodontal treatment, it is really not conclusive. It cannot be predicted with certainty that the treatment of a patient's periodontal condition will have any effect on their blood sugar or glycemic control as measured by the HbA1c value (Jones et al., 2007; Mealey & Rose, 2008).

Cardiovascular Disease

In the late 1990s, researchers found a possible link between periodontal diseases and coronary heart disease (CHD) with an increased risk for atherosclerosis and thromboembolisms, independent of other risk factors for these cardiovascular diseases (Genco, Glurich, Haraszthy, Zambon, & DeNardin, 1998). This *association* between periodontal disease and atherosclerotic vascular disease (ASVD), independent of known confounders, is supported by the latest American Heart Association (AHA) statement and confirms that periodontal disease is a *risk factor* for ASVD (AHA, 2012). This link may have been explained by the systemic inflammatory burden caused by inflammatory periodontal diseases (Nakib et al., 2004). However, as with all the other systemic diseases mentioned in this chapter, *the studies are not conclusive of cause and effect*. Men with periodontitis, especially those under age 50, are 25% more likely to develop CHD (American Academy of Periodontology, 1998; Beck, 1996). Two different surveys have shown that heart disease is the most common condition shared by periodontitis patients (Umino & Nagao, 1993).

In the late 1990s, the connection between heart attacks and periodontal disease was felt to be so convincing that proper plaque control might actually be an exercise that saves a patient's life. Although it may seem unlikely that an infection in the mouth may result in heart disease, there are several possible links that might explain this association. For example, it is well known that if a person has periodontal disease, oral bacteria will enter the bloodstream even after chewing or toothbrushing. When bacteria from the inflamed gingival tissue enter the bloodstream, they trigger platelets to gather around them in a clump, possibly infecting and obstructing the blood vessels in the heart and the brain (Shanies & Hein, 2006). Forty percent of those bacteria, especially *Streptococcus sanguis* and *Porphyromonas gingivalis*, have been traced to the mouth (Genco, Glurich, et al., 1998). Patients have a 50% increased risk for heart disease (DeStefano, Andda, Kahn, Williamson, & Russell, 1993) and a 30% increased risk for stroke if they also have periodontitis.

Periodontitis and cardiovascular diseases are both associated with a systemic inflammatory response that contributes to elevated levels of serum **C-reactive protein**.

C-reactive protein (CRP) is an inflammatory serum marker or a predictor of increased risk for cardiovascular disease (Gapski & Cobb, 2006). A study by D'Aiuto, Ready, and Tonetti in 2004 found that periodontitis may result in an increased cardiovascular risk based on serum CRP levels and that successful periodontal therapy could decrease these serum inflammatory markers. In a review of studies, it appears that periodontitis elevated CRP levels and treatment lowered them (Paraskevas, Huizinga, & Loos, 2008).

In 2004 Nakib and colleagues reported on a study that was performed between 1996 and 1998 on 6,931 subjects. Results found that compared to subjects with no or mild periodontitis, subjects with moderate or severe periodontitis were more likely to have coronary artery calcification (CAC), but the difference was not statistically significant. Thus, these researchers suggested that periodontitis may not be strongly associated with CAC (Nakib et al., 2004). Future studies need to be conducted on this subject. Given that there has been no proven cause-and-effect relationship between periodontitis and CVD, recommending periodontal treatment for the prevention of artherosclerotic cardiovascular disease is not warranted based on present scientific evidence (Demmer & Desvarieux, 2006; AHA, 2012). Periodontal treatment is recommended because it will benefit the patient's oral health.

Adverse Pregnancy Outcomes

Women with periodontal disease may be seven to eight times more predisposed to deliver premature (< 37 weeks) infants with low birth weight (< 5.5 lb; Davenport et al., 1998). Periodontal disease in the mother may be responsible for many of the low-birth-weight, premature births (PLBW). Current data suggest a relationship between elevated prostaglandin E_2 (PGE_2) levels in the gingival crevicular fluid (GCF) as a marker of current periodontal disease activity and decreasing birth weight (Offenbacher et al., 1998). Also, the elevated levels of PGE_2 stimulate labor contractions (Doheny, O'Reilly, Sexton, & Morrison, 2007). The increased production of PGE_2 by the mother is due to a response to the anaerobic periodontal infection (e.g., *Porphyromonas gingivalis*, *Tannerella forsythia*, and *Camplytobacter rectus*). This twofold elevation in PGE_2, which is seen in the GCF and amniotic sac, was observed in PLBW compared with normal-birth-weight mothers (Hill, 1998). A study examined 124 pregnant or postpartum mothers for periodontitis at the University of North Carolina (Offenbacher et al., 1996). Mothers with a defined preterm low-birth-weight delivery demonstrated that periodontal disease was a "statistically significant risk factor for PLBW." PLBW status is defined as a birth weight of less than 2500 g (5.51 lbs) and/or a gestational age of less than 37 weeks at delivery or premature rupture of membranes. PLBW cases had significantly worse periodontal disease than respective normal-birth-weight (NBW) controls. PLBW is a major health problem because it occurs in 1 in 10 deliveries and results in infant mortality, long-term morbidity, and 5 million neonatal intensive care unit hospital stays per year. The emotional, social, and financial burdens on families are extraordinary (Dasanayake, 1998).

A clinical pilot study published in 2003 was conducted to determine whether treatment of periodontitis reduces the risk of spontaneous preterm birth. This study concluded that although this pilot study found that performing scaling and root planing in pregnant women with periodontitis might reduce spontaneous preterm birth, larger trials are needed (Jeffcoat et al., 2003) to confirm that periodontal therapy decreases the frequency of preterm delivery and neonatal complications. Though this seemed to be confirmed in a later study (Offenbacher et al., 2006), further intervention trials showed much less of an associated risk (Michalowicz et al., 2009).

Maternal periodontal disease, which is associated with systemic inflammation, has been associated with preterm birth. Intervention trials for treatment of periodontal disease during pregnancy, however, have not consistently shown a reduction in preterm birthrates. Despite, the lack of reduction in preterm birth, oral health maintenance is an important part of preventive care and should be supported during pregnancy (Horton & Boggess, 2012).

Effective maintenance should help the patient's health during pregnancy because it has been found that fetal exposures to periodontal pathogens also may increase the risk for maternal vaginal bleeding during pregnancy,

preeclampsia (hypertension occurring during pregnancy; can affect both mother and fetus), and intrauterine fetal growth restriction (Paquette, 2006).

Respiratory Diseases

Patients with periodontal disease may be at risk for respiratory diseases (Hayes, Sparrow, Cohen, Vokonas, & Garcia, 1998). Periodontal disease is added to the list of other risk factors for this problem, including the elderly, people who smoke, and individuals confined to nursing homes or hospitals. Examples of respiratory diseases include pneumonia (Azarpazhooh & Leake, 2006), bronchitis, and emphysema. Pneumonia may be the result of infection by anaerobic bacteria, which is a component of dental plaque (American Academy of Periodontology, 1998; Scannapieco & Mylotte, 1996).

Bacteria (oral biofilms) found in the oral cavity can be taken up into the lung to cause respiratory diseases. Many bacteria present in aspirated saliva are anaerobic, including *Porphyromonas gingivalis*, *Fusobacterium nucleatum*, and *Bacteroides oralis* (Terpenning, 2006). Recent hypotheses relate to the presence in saliva of enzymes and cytokines associated with oral pathogens, and that could alter the colonization of the respiratory tract or promote infection by respiratory pathogens (Mojon, 2003). Oral hygiene and frequent professional oral healthcare are useful in reducing the development of pneumonia in high-risk elderly people in nursing homes and hospitals (Azarpazhooh & Leake, 2006; Scannapieco, Wang, & Shiau, 2001). It is important to emphasize oral care in patients in hospital and nursing home environments.

Alzheimer's Disease

Early exposure to inflammatory diseases, including periodontal disease, may increase the risk for developing Alzheimer's disease later in life (Stein et al., 2006). Possible ways that oral bacteria are involved include spreading of gram-negative pathogens from the oral cavity to the brain, genetic predisposition, and injury to brain tissue due to the production of inflammatory mediators in response to periodontal bacteria (Stein et al., 2006). Studies seem to suggest that peripheral infections, such as periodontitis, contribute to the inflammatory state of the central nervous system (Kamer et al., 2008). Research is currently being conducted on this relationship.

Rapid Dental Hint

If your patient is pregnant, stress the importance of periodontal treatments to reduce the risk of adverse pregnancy outcomes.

Dental Hygiene Application

Oral conditions can significantly influence events elsewhere in the body. Periodontal disease is a risk factor for certain systemic conditions; certain systemic conditions are also a risk factor for periodontal disease. It is well known that medical conditions such as diabetes mellitus may modify the reaction to dental plaque, which may make the individual more susceptible to periodontal disease. In addition,

periodontal diseases have been documented to be risk factors for some medical conditions, including coronary heart disease, diabetes mellitus, low-birth-weight babies, respiratory diseases, and Alzheimer's. It then becomes apparent that periodontal clinicians are treating the "whole" patient and attempting to control both periodontal diseases and medical conditions.

Key Points

- Currently, evidence-based dentistry supports the use of risk assessment techniques to guide clinical decisions in the treatment of periodontal diseases.
- Although a relationship may have been found between certain medical conditions and periodontal disease, it is not yet known that it is a cause-and-effect relationship; risk factors are not causative.
- Other risk factors not strongly related but still associated with increased probability of periodontal diseases include aging, gender, genetic predisposition, stress, nutrition, and systemic diseases including immunosuppression.

- Not only do certain medical conditions predispose individuals to periodontal diseases, but also periodontal diseases predispose people to certain medical conditions.
- Patients taking oral bisphosphonates for osteoporosis must be assessed and monitored for osteonecrosis of the jaws (ONJ). Patients taking intravenous bisphosphonates should not have any elective, invasive dentistry performed on them.
- Attempts to manage risk factors are important in the prevention and treatment of periodontal diseases.

Self-Quiz

1. Which one of the following concerns should the dental hygienist be aware of in patients taking bisphosphonates?
   a. Diabetes
   b. Osteonecrosis of the jaw
   c. Stroke
   d. Hypertension
   e. Respiratory diseases

2. Which one of the following shows evidence exists to support the concept of a genetic predisposition to periodontal diseases?
   a. Presence of a specific type of bacteria
   b. Increased levels of bacterial enzymes in the blood
   c. Association of periodontitis with certain transmitted traits
   d. Transmission of bacteria through saliva from mother to child

3. Which one of the following mechanisms explains how increased stress adversely affects the periodontium?
   a. Increases in subgingival pathogenic bacteria
   b. Increases in estrogen levels results in gingivitis
   c. Less compliance with home care of teeth and gums
   d. Shifts in the concentration of available endotoxins

4. The hormonal changes associated with pregnancy cause an increased incidence of gingival disease because these changes are associated with an increase in sex hormone levels.
   a. Both the statement and the reason are correct and related.
   b. Both the statement and the reason are correct but not related.
   c. The statement is correct, but the reason is not.
   d. The statement is not correct, but the reason is correct.
   e. Neither the statement nor the reason is correct.

5. Smoking affects the periodontium by which one of the following mechanisms?
   a. Decreasing the number of melanocytes
   b. Suppressing of the immune system
   c. Altering the metabolism of fibroblasts
   d. Increasing the amount of fibrotic tissue
   e. Decreasing the number of periodontal pathogens

6. Which of the following cells are inhibited when a patient is taking a bisphosphonate for osteoporosis?
   a. Fibroblast
   b. Osteoblast
   c. Osteoclast
   d. Cementoblast
   e. Odontoblast

7. Which of the following statements about smoking and periodontal diseases is true?
   a. Smoking dramatically affects the oral microflora.
   b. Smoking cessation is beneficial to periodontal health.
   c. Past effects of smoking on the periodontium are usually reversible.
   d. Current smokers have a low level of tooth mobility.
   e. Smokeless tobacco does not increase the incidence of periodontal disease.

8. From the following list, select the items that have been a proven cause-and-effect relationship with periodontitis.
   a. Obesity
   b. Diabetes
   c. Preterm low-birth-weight babies
   d. Cardiovascular disease
   e. Chronic kidney disease
   f. Alcoholic liver cirrhosis

9. Which of the following bacterium in the mouth has been found to possibly infect and obstruct blood vessels in the heart and the brain?
   a. *Prevotella intermedia*
   b. *Fuscobacterium nucleatum*
   c. *Porphyromonas gingivalis*
   d. *Campylobacter rectus*
   e. *Tannerella forsythia*

10. Which of the following explains why patients with periodontal disease may be at risk for respiratory diseases, especially in hospitals and nursing homes?
    a. Neglected oral hygiene
    b. Decayed teeth
    c. Collapsed circulatory system
    d. Increased risk for heart failure
    e. Increased risk for other systemic diseases

Case Study

A 55-year-old woman returns for her dental recall visit. Since she was last seen she has gained 50 pounds. She describes herself as always tired, thirsty, and having trouble sleeping. She has moderate gingivitis and 4 mm pocketing on #30, #29, #18, and #15. There is no recession or bleeding upon probing.

1. What are the possible systemic disease for which she is at risk?
   a. Hypertension
   b. Diabetes
   c. Osteonecrosis
   d. Low-birth-weight babies
   e. All of the above

Answer: B. Given this patient with the increase in weight and thirst she is more likely to be at risk of Type 2 diabetes. There is no indication in the history of bisphosphonates, or high blood pressure. She is perhaps post-menopausal.

2. What dental hygiene referral for data would relate to this patient?
   a. Ctx
   b. HbA1C
   c. HAART
   d. All of the above

Answer: B. The HbA1c test of the glycosylated hemoglobin would be given as an indication of current or at risk status of diabetes. The Ctx is the blood test for bone resorption for bisphosphonate users. HAART is the highly active antiretroviral therapy for HIV.

3. If this patient were also a smoker what other systemic risks should the dental hygienist consider?
   a. More likely to have severe periodontal disease
   b. Increased risk for bone loss
   c. Increased host defense system
   d. A and B
   e. All of the above

Answer: D. The smoker is more likely to have severe periodontal risk than the non-smoker and increased risk for bone loss. The host immune system is more decreased or compromised from smoking and possible diabetes.

References

Abdellatif, H. M., and B. A. Burt. 1987. An epidemiological investigation into the relative importance of age and oral hygiene status as determinants of periodontitis. *J. Periodontol.* 66:16–33.

Alabdulkarim, M., N. Bissada, M. Al-Zahrani, A. Ficara, and B. Siegel. 2005. Alveolar bone loss in obese subjects. *J. Int. Acad. Periodontol.* 7(2):34–8.

Al-Zahrani, M. S., N. F. Bissada, and E. A. Borawskit. 2003. Obesity and periodontal disease in young, middle-aged, and older adults. *J. Periodontol.* 74(5):610–615.

Amar, S., and K. M. Chung. 1994. Influence of hormonal variation on the periodontium in women. *Periodontology* 6:79–87.

American Academy of Periodontology. 1998. Periodontal disease as a potential risk factor for systemic disease (position paper). *J. Periodontol.* 69:841–850.

American Academy of Periodontology. 1999. Tobacco use and the periodontal patient (position paper). *J. Periodontol.* 70:1419–1427.

American Association of Oral and Maxillofacial Surgeons (AAOMS): Position Paper on Bisphosphonate-related Osteonecrosis of the Jaw—2009 Update

American Dental Association Council on Scientific Affairs. 2006. Dental management of patients receiving oral bisphosphonate therapy. *JADA* 137(8):1144–1150.

American Heart Association: Scientific Statement. 2012. Periodontal disease and atherosclerotic vascular disease: Does the evidence support an independent association? *Circulation* 125:2520–2544.

Azarpazhooh, A., and J. L. Leake. 2006. Systematic review of the association between respiratory diseases and oral health. *J. Periodontol.* 77:1465–1482.

Bando, K., H. Nitta, M. Matsubara, and I. Ishikawa. 1998. Bone mineral density in periodontally healthy and edentulous postmenopausal women. *Ann. Periodontol.* 3:322–326.

Barak, S., I. S. Engelberg, and J. Hiss. 1987. Gingival hyperplasia caused by nifedipine—histopathologic findings. *J. Periodontol.* 58:639–642.

Barnett, M. L. 2003. Coordination Meeting on Oral Health and Systemic Health Periodontal Medicine: Health Policy Implications. Geneva, Switzerland. *J. Periodontol.* 74:1081–1086.

Bashutski, J., K. Eber, E. Benavides, S. Maitra, T. Braun, W. Giannobile, and L. McCauley. 2011. The impact of vitamin D status on periodontal surgery outcomes. *J. Dent. Res.* Aug; 90(*):1007–1012.

Beck, J. D. 1996. Periodontal implications: Older adults. *Ann. Periodontol.* 1:322–457.

Botero, J., F. Yepes, N. Roldan, C. Castrillon, J. Hincapie, J., Ochoa, et al. 2012. Tooth and periodontal clinical attachment loss are associated with hyperglycemia in diabetic patients. *J. Periodontol.* 83(10):1245–1250.

Broadbent, E., K. J. Petrie, P. G. Alley, and R. J. Booth. 2003. Psychological stress impairs early wound repair following surgery. *Psychosom. Med.* 65:865–869.

Bulmanski, Z., M. Brady, D. Stoute, and T. Lallier. 2012. Cigarette smoke extract induces select matrix metalloproteinases and integrin expression in periodontal ligament fibroblasts. *J. Periodontol.* 83(6):787–796.

Cartsos, V. M., S. Zhu, and A. I. Zavras. 2008. Bisphosphonate use and the risk of adverse jaw outcomes: A medical claims study of 714,217 people. *J. Am. Dent. Assoc.* 139:23–30.

Ciancio, S. G. 1996. Medications as risk factors for periodontal disease. *J. Periodontol.* 67:1055–1059.

Ciancio, S. G., S. J. Yaffe, and C. C. Catz. 1972. Gingival hyperplasia and diphenylhydantoin. *J. Periodontol.* 43:411–414.

Costerton, J., and D. Keller. 2007. Oral periopathogens and systemic effects. *Gen. Dent.* 55:210–215.

Cutler, C. W., P. Eke, R. R. Arnold, and T. E. Van Dyke. 1991. Defective neutrophil function in an insulin-dependent diabetic patient. A case report. *J. Periodontol.* 62:394–401.

D'Aiuto F., D. Ready, and M. S. Tonetti. 2004. Periodontal disease and C-reactive protein-associated cardiovascular risk. *J. Periodontol. Res.* 39:236–241.

Daley, T. D., G. P. Wysocki, and C. May. 1986. Clinical and pharmacological correlations in cyclosporin-induced gingival hyperplasia. *Oral Surg. Oral Med. Oral Patho.* 62:417–421.

Dantas, A. M., C. E. Mohn, B. Burdet, M. Zubilete, P. M. Mandalunis, J. C. Elverdin, and J. Fernandez-Solari. 2012. Ethanol consumption enhances periodontal inflammatory markers in rats. *J. Arch. Oral Biol.* 57(9):1211–1217.

Dasanayake, A. P. 1998. Periodontal disease as a risk factor in pregnancy. *Ann. Periodontol.* 3:206–212.

Davenport, E. S., C. E. Williams, J. A. Sterne, V. Sivapathasundram, J. M. Fearne, and M. A. Curtis. 1998. The East London study of maternal chronic periodontal disease and preterm low birth weight infants: Study design and prevalence data. *Ann. Periodontol.* 3:213–221.

Demmer, R. T., and M. Desvarieux. 2006. Periodontal infections and cardiovascular disease. *JADA* 137(10 supplement):14S–20S.

DeStefano, F., R. F. Andda, H. S. Kahn, D. F. Williamson, and C. M. Russell. 1993. Dental disease and risk of coronary heart disease and mortality. *Br. Med. J.* 306:688–691.

Doheny, H. C., M. J. O'Reilly, D. J. Sexton, and J. J. Morrison. 2007. THG113.31, a specific PGF2 alpha receptor antagonist, induces human myometrial relaxation and BKCa channel activation. *Reprod. Biol. Endocrinol.* 5:10. Published online 2007 March 16. doi: 10.1186/1477-7827-5-10.

Drake, C. W., R. J. Hunt, and G. G. Koch. 1995. Three-year tooth loss among black and white older adults in North Carolina. *J. Dent. Res.* 74:675–680.

Edwards, B. J., J. W. Hellstein, and P. L. Jacobsen. 2008. Updated recommendations for managing the care of patients receiving oral bisphosphonate therapy: An advisory statement from the American Dental Association Council on Scientific Affairs. *J. Am. Dent. Assoc.* 139:1674–1677.

Feloutzis A., N. P. Lang, M. S. Tonetti, W. Burgin, U. Bragger, et al. 2003. Il-1 gene polymorphism and smoking as risk factors for peri-implant bone loss in a well-maintained population. *Clin. Oral Implants Res.* 14:10–17.

Fisher, S., L. Kells, J. P. Picard, S. C. Gelskey, et al. 2008. Tobacco smoking and periodontal health in a Saudi Arabian population. *J. Periodontol.* 79(3):461–468.

Fugazzotto, P. A., W. S. Lightfoot, R. Jaffin, and A. Kumar. 2007. Implant placement with or without simultaneous tooth extraction in patients taking oral bisphosphonates: Postoperative healing, early follow up, and the incidence of complications in two private practices. *J. Periodontol.* 7819:1664–1669.

Gapski, R., and C. M. Cobb. 2006. Chronic inflammatory periodontal disease. A risk factor for cardiovascular disease and ischemic stroke? *Grand Rounds in Oral-Sys. Med.* 1:14–22.

Genco, R. J., A. W. Ho, J. Kopman, S. G. Grossi, R. G. Dunford, and L. A. Tedesco. 1998. Models to evaluate the role of stress in periodontal diseases. *Ann. Periodontol.* 3:288–302.

Genco, R. J., I. Glurich, V. Haraszthy, J. Zambon, and E. DeNardin. 1998. Overview of risk factors for periodontal disease and implications for diabetes and cardiovascular disease. *Compendium* (special issue) 19:40–45.

Genco, R. J., S. G. Grossi, A. Ho, F. Nishimura, and Y. Murayama. 2005. A proposed model linking inflammation to obesity, diabetes, and periodontal infections. *J. Periodontol.* 76(11 Suppl):2075–2084.

Gomes, S. C., I. B. Piccini, C. Susin, et al. 2007. Effect of supragingival plaque control in smokers and never-smokers: 6 month evaluation of patients with periodontitis. *J. Periodontol.* 78(8):1515–1521.

Grant, B. T., C. Amenedo, K. Freeman, and R. A. Kraut. 2008. Outcomes of placing dental implants in patients taking oral bisphosphonates: A review of its cases. *J. Oral Maxillofac. Surg.* 66:223–230.

Gross, H. B. 2008. Bisphosphonate-induced osteonecrosis: Dental considerations. *Compendium.* 29(2):112–113.

Grossi, S. G., and R. J. Genco. 1998. Periodontal disease and diabetes mellitus: A two-way relationship. *Ann. Periodontol.* 3:51–61.

Grossi, S. G., F. B. Skrepcinski, T. DeCaro, J. J. Zambon, D. Cummins, and R. J. Genco. 1996. Responses to periodontal therapy in diabetics and smokers. *J. Periodontol.* 67(Suppl.):1094–1102.

Gunsolley, J. C., S. M. Quinn, J. Tew, C. M. Gooss, C. N. Brooks, and H. A. Schenkein. 1998. The effect of smoking on individuals with minimal periodontal destruction. *J. Periodontol.* 69:165–170.

Guzman S., M. Karima, H. Y. Wang, and T. E. Van Dyke. 2003. Association between interleukin-1 genotype and periodontal disease in a diabetic population. *J. Periodontol.* 74:1183–1190.

Haber, J., and R. L. Kent. 1992. Cigarette smoking in periodontal practice. *J. Periodontol.* 63:100–106.

Haber, J., J. Wattles, M. Crowley, R. Mandell, K. Joshipura, and R. L. Kent. 1993. Evidence for cigarette smoking as a major risk factor for periodontitis. *J. Periodontol.* 64:16–23.

Hayes, C., D. Sparrow, M. Cohen, P. S. Vokonas, and R. I. Garcia. 1998. The association between alveolar bone loss and pulmonary function: The VA dental longitudinal study. *Ann. Periodontol.* 3:257–261.

Heasman, L., F. Stacey, P. M. Preshaw, G. I. McCracken, S. Hepburn, and P. A. Heasman. 2006. The effect of smoking on periodontal treatment response: A review of clinical evidence. *J. Clin. Periodontol.* 33:241–253.

Hill, G. B. 1998. Preterm birth: Associations with genital and oral microflora. *Ann. Periodontol.* 3:222–232.

Horton, A., and Boggess, K. 2012. Periodontal disease and preterm birth. *Obstet. Gynecol. Clin. North. Am.* 39(1):17–23.

Huynh-Ba, G., N. P. Lang, M. S. Tonetti, et al. 2007. The association of the composite IL-1 genotype with periodontitis progression and/or treatment outcomes: A systematic review. *J. Clin. Periodontol.* 34:305–317.

Jansson, L., and S. Lavstedt. 2002. Influence of smoking on marginal bone loss and tooth loss—A prospective study over 20 years. *J. Clin. Periodontol.* 29:750–756.

Jeffcoat, M. K. 1998. Osteoporosis: A possible modifying factor in oral bone loss. *Ann. Periodontol.* 3:312–321.

Jeffcoat, M. K., J. C. Hauth, N. C. Geurs, M. S. Reddy, S. P. Cliver, et al. 2003. Periodontal disease and preterm birth: Results of a pilot intervention study. *J. Periodontol.* 74:1214–1218.

Johnson, L., R. J. Genco, C. Damsky, et al. 2008. Genetics and its implications for clinical dental practice and education: Report of panel 3 of the Macy study. *J. Dent. Educ.* 72(Suppl):86–94.

Jones, J. A., D. R. Miller, C. J. Wehler, et al. 2007. Does periodontal care improve glycemic control? The Department of Veterans Affairs Dental Diabetes Study. *J. Clin. Periodontol.* 34:46–52.

Kamer, A. R., A. P. Dasanayake, R. G. Craig, et al. 2008. Alzheimer's disease and peripheral infections: The possible contribution from periodontal infections, model and hypothesis. *J. Alzheimers Dis.* 13(4):437–449.

Kenny, E. G., J. H. Kraal, S. R. Saxe, and J. Jones. 1977. The effect of cigarette smoke on human oral polymorphonuclear leukocytes. *J. Periodont. Res.* 12:227–234.

Khader, Y. S., H. A. Bawadi, T. F. Haroun, M. Alomari, and R. F. Tayyem. 2009. The association between periodontal disease and obesity among adults in Jordan. *J. Clin. Periodontol.* 36(1):18–24.

Kibayashi, M., M. Tanaka, N. Nishida, et al. 2007. Longitudinal study of the association between smoking as a periodontitis risk and salivary biomarkers related to periodontitis. *J. Periodontol.* 78:859–867.

Kim, J., and S. Amar. 2006. Periodontal disease and systemic conditions: A bidirectional relationship. *Odontology* 94:10–21.

Kinane, D. F. 1999. Periodontitis modified by systemic factors. *Ann. Periodontol.* 4:54–63.

Kloostra, P. W., R. M. Eber, and M. R. Inglehart. 2007. Anxiety, stress, depression and patient's responses to periodontal treatment: Periodontists' knowledge and professional behavior. *J. Periodontol.* 78:64–71.

Kornman, K. 2008. Mapping the pathogenesis of periodontitis: A new look. *J. Periodontol.* 79 (8 Suppl):1560–1568.

Krall, E., A. Garvey, and R. Garcia. 1999. Alveolar bone loss and tooth loss in male cigar and pipe smokers. *J. American Dent. Assoc.* 130:57–64.

Krall, E., C. Hayes, A. J. Garvey, and R. I. Garcia. 1997. Study finds a correlation between smoking and tooth loss. *J. Mass. Dent. Soc.* 46:20–23.

Kranzler, H. R., T. F. Babor, L. Goldstein, and J. Gold. 1990. Dental pathology and alcohol-related indicators in an outpatient clinic sample. *Community Dent. Oral Epidemiol.* 18:204–207.

Kribbs, P. J. 1990. Comparison of mandibular bone in normal and osteoporotic women. *J. Prosthet. Dent.* 63:218–222.

Lannan, S., A. McLean, E. Drost, M. Gillooly, K. Donaldson, et al. 1992. Changes in neutrophil morphology and morphometry following exposure to cigarette smoke. *Int. J. Exp. Pathol.* 73:183–191.

Lerner, U. H. 2006. Inflammation-induced bone remodeling in periodontal disease and the influence of post-menopausal osteoporosis. *J. Dent. Res.* 85:596–607.

Manouchehr-Pour, M., P. J. Spagnuolo, H. M. Rodman, and N. F. Bissada. 1981. Comparison of neutrophil chemotactic response in diabetic patients with mild and severe periodontal disease. *J. Periodontol.* 52:410–414.

Marx, R. E. 2010. *Oral and intravenous bisphosphonate-induced osteonecrosis of the jaws: History, etiology, prevention, and treatment.* 2nd ed. Chicago: Quintessence.

Marx, R. E., J. E. Cillo, and J. J. Ulloa. 2007. Oral bisphosphonate-induced osteonecrosis: Risk factors, prediction of risk using serum CTX testing, prevention, and treatment. *J Oral Maxillofac. Surg.* 65:2397–2410.

Marx, R. E., Y. Sawatari, M. Fortin, and V. Broumand. 2005. Bisphosphonate-induced exposed bone (osteonecrosis/osteopetrosis) of the jaws: Risk factors, recognition, prevention, and treatment. *J. Oral Maxillofae. Surg.* 63:1567–1575.

Mataftsi, M., L. Skoura, and D. Sakellari. 2011. HIV infection and periosontal diseases: An overview of the post-HAART era. *Oral Dis.* 17(1):13–25.

Mealey, B. L., and L. F. Rose. 2008. Diabetes mellitus and inflammatory periodontal diseases. *Curr. Opin. Endocrinol. Diabetes Obes.* 15:135–141.

Michalowicz, B. S., D. P. Aeppli, R. K. Kuba, J. E. Bereuter, J. P. Conry, et al. 1991. A twin study of genetic variation in proportional radiographic alveolar bone height. *J. Dent. Res.* 70:1431–1435.

Michalowicz, B. S., S. R. Diehl, J. C. Gunsolley, B. S. Sparks, et al. 2000. Evidence of a substantial genetic basis for risk of adult periodontitis. *J. Periodontol.* 71:1699–1707.

Michalowicz, G., J. Hodges, M. J. Novak, W. Buchanan, A. J. DiAngelis, P. N. Papapanou, . . . S. Matsesane. 2009. Change in periodontitis during pregnancy and the risk of pre-term and low birthweight. *J. Clin. Periodontol.* 36:308–314.

Michaud, D. S., K. Joshipura, E. Giovannucci, et al. 2007. A prospective study of periodontal disease and pancreatic cancer in U.S. male health professionals. *Journal of the National Cancer Institute* 99:171–175.

Migliorati, C. A., J. Casiglia, J. Epstein, P. L. Jacobsen, M. A. Siegel, and S.-B. Woo. 2005. Managing the care of patients with bisphosphonate-associated osteonecrosis: An American Academy of Oral Medicine position paper. *JADA* 136:1658–1668.

McMullen, J. A., T. E. Van Dyke, H. U. Horoszewicz, and R. J. Genco. 1981. Neutrophil chemotaxis in individuals with advanced periodontal disease and a genetic predisposition to diabetes mellitus. *J. Periodontol.* 52:167–173.

Mojon, P. 2003. Respiratory infection: How important is oral health? *Current Opinion in Pulmonary Medicine* 9(3):166–170.

Morita, T., Y. Ogawa, K. Takada, N. Nishinoue, Y. Sasaki, M. Motohashi, and M. Maeno. 2009. Association between periodontal disease and metabolic syndrome. *J. Public Health Dent.* 69(4):248–253.

Moritz, A. J., and B. L. Mealey. 2006. Periodontal disease, insulin resistance, and diabetic mellitus. *Grand Rounds Oral-Sys. Med.* 2:13–20.

Murray, P. 1994. Periodontal diseases in patients infected by human immunodeficiency virus. *Periodontology 2000.* 6:50–67.

Nair, P., G. Sutherland, R. M. Palmer, R. F. Wilson, and D. A. Scott. 2003. Gingival bleeding on probing increases after quitting smoking. *J. Clin. Periodontol.* 30:435–437.

Nakib, S. A., J. S. Pankow, J. D. Beck, S. Offenbacher, G. W. Evans, et al. 2004. Periodontitis and coronary artery calcification: The Atherosclerosis Risk in Communities (ARIC) study. *J. Periodontol.* 75(4):505–510.

Newman, M. 1998. Genetic, environmental, and behavioral influences on periodontal infections. *Compendium* (special issue) 19:25–31.

Nishimura, F., K. Takahashi, M. Kurihara, S. Takashiba, and Y. Murayama. 1998. Periodontal disease as a complication of diabetes mellitus. *Ann. Periodontol.* 3:20–29.

Nishimura, F., Y. Iwamoto, J. Mineshiba, A. Shimizu, Y. Soga, and Y. Murayama. 2003. Periodontal disease and diabetes mellitus: The role of tumor necrosis factor-alpha in a 2-way relationship. *J. Periodontol.* 74(1):97–102.

Nitta, H., K. Bando, M. Matsubara, and I. Ishikawa. 1997. *Impact of periodontal health on osteoporosis in postmenopausal women.* Periodontal Diseases and Human Health: New Directions in Periodontal Medicine. Sunstar–Chapel Hill, Chapel Hill, NC, March 24–25.

Offenbacher, S., B. Katz, G. Fertik, J. Collins, D. Boyd, et al. 1996. Periodontal infection as a possible risk factor for preterm low birth weight. *J. Periodontol.* 67:1103–1113.

Offenbacher, S., H. L. Jared, P. G. O'Reilly, S. R. Wells, G. E. Salvi, et al. 1998. Potential pathogenic mechanisms of periodontitis-associated pregnancy complication. *Ann. Periodontol.* 3(1):233–250.

Offenbacher, S., D. Lin, R. Strauss, et al. 2006. Effects of periodontal therapy during pregnancy on periodontal status, biologic parameters, and pregnancy outcomes: A pilot study. *J. Periodontol.* 77:2011–2024.

Oh, T. J., J. Bashutski, and W. V. Giannobile. 2007. The interrelationship between osteoporosis and oral bone loss. *Grand Rounds Oral-Sys. Med.* 2:10–21.

Otomo-Corgel, J. 2007. Implants and oral bisphosphonates: Risky business? *J. Periodontol.* 78:373–376.

Otomo-Corgrel, J. 2012. Osteoporosis and osteopenia: Implications for periodontal and implant therapy. *Periodontol 2000* 59(1):111–139.

Page, R. C., and J. D. Beck. 1997. Risk assessment for periodontal diseases. *Int. Dent. J.* 47:61–87.

Papantonopoulos, G. H. 2004. Effect of periodontal therapy in smokers and non-smokers with advanced periodontal disease: Results after maintenance therapy for a minimum of 5 years. *J. Periodontol.* 75:839–843.

Paquette, D. W. 2006. Periodontal disease and the risk for adverse pregnancy outcomes. *Grand Rounds in Oral-Sys. Med.* 4:14–25a.

Paraskevas, S., J. D. Huizinga, and B. G. Loos. 2008. A systematic review and meta-analysis on C-reactive protein in relation to periodontitis. *J. Clin. Periodontol.* 35:277–290.

Peruzzo, D. C., B. B. Benatti, G. M. D. Ambrosano, et al. 2007. A systematic review of stress and psychological factors as possible risk factors for periodontal disease. *J. Periodontol.* 78(8):1491–1504.

Pischon, N., N. Heng, J. P. Bernimoulin, B. M. Kleber, S. N. Willich, and T. Pischon. 2007. Obesity, inflammation, and periodontal disease. *J. Dent. Res.* 86(5):400–409.

Preshaw P., and J. Taylor. 2011. How has research into cytokine interactions and their role in driving immune responses impacted our understanding of periodontitis? *J. Clin. Periodontol.* 38(Suppl 11):60–84.

Preshaw P. M., M. A. Knutsen, and A. Mariotti. 2001. Experimental gingivitis in women using oral contraceptives. *J. Dent. Res.* 80:2011–2015.

Renvert, S., J. Berglund, R. Persson, and G. Persson. 2011. Osteoporosis and periodontitis in older subjects participating in the Swedish National Survey on Aging and Care (SNAC-BLEKINGE). *Acta. Odontol. Scand.* 69(4):201–207.

Ruggiero, S. L. 2008. Bisphosphonate-related osteonecrosis of the jaws. *Compendium.* 29(2):97–105.

Ryan, M. E., O. Carnu, and R. Tenzler. 2006. The impact of periodontitis on metabolic control and risk for diabetic complications. *Grand Rounds Oral-Sys. Med.* 2:24–34.

Safkan-Seppälä, B., and J. Ainamo. 1992. Periodontal conditions in insulin-dependent diabetes mellitus. *J. Clin. Periodontol.* 19:24–29.

Saremi, A., R. G. Nelson, M. Tulloch-Reid, et al. 2005. Periodontal disease and mortality in type 2 diabetes. *Diabetes Care* 28:27–32.

Scannapieco, F. A., and A. W. Ho. 2001. Potential associations between chronic respiratory disease and periodontal disease: Analysis of National Health and Nutrition Examination Survey III. *J. Periodontol.* 72:50–56.

Scannapieco, F. A., B. Wang, and H. J. Shiau. 2001. Oral bacteria and respiratory infection: Effects on respiratory pathogen adhesion and epithelial cell proinflammatory cytokine production. *Ann. Periodontol.* 6(1):78–86.

Scannapieco, F. A., and J. M. Mylotte. 1996. Relationships between periodontal disease and bacterial pneumonia. *J. Periodontol.* 67:1114–1122.

Semenoff-Segundo A, et al. (2012) Effects of two chronic stress models on ligature-induced periodontitis in Wistar rats. *Arch. Oral. Biol.* 57(1):66–72.

Shanies S., and C. Hein. 2006. The significance of periodontal infection in cardiology. *Grand Rounds Oral-Sys. Med.* 1:24–33.

Siukosaari, P., S. Ajwani, A. Ainamo, J. Wolf, and T. Närhi. 2012. Periodontal health status in the elderly with different levels of education: A 5-year follow-up study. *Gerodontology* 29(2):e170–e178.

Stein, P. S., S. Scheff, D. R. Dawson, III. 2006. Alzheimer's disease and periodontal disease; Mechanisms underlying a potential bidirectional relationship. *Grand Rounds Oral-Sys. Med.* 1:14–240.

Strietzel, F., P. Reichart, A. Kale, M. Kulkarni, B. Wegner, and I. Küchler 2007. Smoking interferes with the prognosis of dental implant treatment: A systematic review and meta analysis. *J. Clin. Periodontol.* 34:523–544.

Syrjala, A. M., P. Ylostalo, M. C. Niskanen, and M. L. Knuuttila. 2003. Role of smoking and HbA1c level in periodontitis among insulin-dependent diabetic patients. *J. Clin. Periodontol.* 30:871–875.

Taichman, S. L. 2005. Oral contraceptives and periodontal diseases: Rethinking the association based upon analysis of National Health and Nutrition Examination Survey Data. *Periodontol.* 76:1374–1385.

Taylor, G. W., B. A. Burt, M. P. Becker, R. J. Genco, M. Shlossman, et al. 1996. Severe periodontitis and risk for poor glycemic control in patients with noninsulin-dependent diabetes mellitus. *J. Periodontol.* 67:1085–1093.

Terpenning, M. S. 2006. The relationship between infections and chronic respiratory diseases: An overview. *J. Periodontol.* 6:66–70.

Tezal, M., S. G. Grossi, A. W. Ho, and R. J. Genco. 2004. Alcohol consumption and periodontal disease. The NHANES III Survey. *J. Clin. Periodontol.* 31(7):484–488.

Thomson, W. M., R. Poulton, J. M. Broadbent, et al. 2008. Cannabis smoking and periodontal disease among young adults. *JAMA* 299(5):525–531.

Tomar, S. L., and Asma, S. 2000. Smoking-attributable periodontitis in the United States: Findings from NHANES III. National Health and Nutrition Examination Survey. *J. Periodontol.* 71(5):743–751.

Tonetti, M. S. 1998. Cigarette smoking and periodontal diseases: Etiology and management of the disease. *Ann. Periodontol.* 3:88–101.

Tsai, C., C. Hayes, and G. W. Taylor. 2002. Glycemic control of type 2 diabetes and severe periodontal disease in the U.S. adult population. *Community Dent. Oral Epidimiol.* 30:182–192.

Umino, M., and M. Nagao. 1993. Systemic disease in elderly dental patients. *Int. Dent. J.* 43:213–218.

Wade, M. L., and J. B. Suzuki. 2007. Issues related to diagnosis and treatment of bisphosphonate-induced osteonecrosis of the jaws. *Grand Rounds Oral-Sys. Med.* 2:46–53b.

Wang, H. L., D. Weber, and L. K. McCauley. 2007. Effect of long-term oral bisphosphonates on implant wound healing: Literature review and a case report. *J. Periodontol.* 78:584–594.

Williamson, R. A., 2010. Surgical management of bisphosphonate induced osteonecrosis of the jaws. *Int. J. Oral. Maxillofac. Surg.* 39:251–255.

Yao, S. G., and J. B. Fine. 2012. A review of vitamin D as it relates to periodontal disease. *Compendium.* 33(3):166–171.

Zak, M., A. N. Spina, R. P. Spinazze, W. L. Perkinson, and D. J. Spinazze. 2007a. Bisphosphonates and the dental patient: Part 1. *Compendium.* 28(9):510–516.

Zak, M., A. N. Spina, R. P. Spinazze, W. L. Perkinson, and D. J. Spinazze. 2007b. Bisphosphonates and the dental patient: Part 1. *Compendium.* 28(9):510–516.

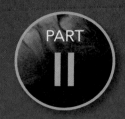

Periodontal Diseases: Classification

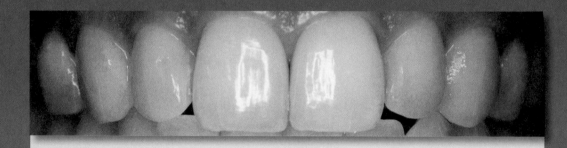

OUTLINE

Gingival Diseases

Surendra Singh

OUTLINE

Introduction
Gingival Diseases
Histopathogenesis of Gingivitis
Pathogenesis of Gingivitis
Classification of the Periodontal
    Diseases
Dental Hygiene Application
Key Points
Self-Quiz
Case Study
References

EDUCATIONAL OBJECTIVES

Upon completion of this chapter, the reader should be able to:

• Recognize and distinguish the two main forms of inflammatory periodontal diseases (1999 Classification of Periodontal Diseases).
• List and compare the plaque-induced gingival diseases and non-plaque-induced gingival diseases.
• List and describe the different stages in the histopathogenesis of gingivitis.
• Explain the host response to the presence of microorganisms within dental plaque.
• Explain the relationship of hormones and medications with periodontal diseases.
• Describe the clinical and histologic features of gingival inflammation.
• Discuss the clinical and histological relationship of the inflammatory and immune host responses to inflammatory periodontal diseases.

GOAL: To provide an understanding of the clinical features and histopathogenesis of gingival diseases.

KEY WORDS

Introduction

Periodontal diseases are not a single disease entity, but a group of lesions affecting the tissues that form the attachment apparatus of a tooth or teeth. Periodontal diseases, which consist of gingivitis and periodontitis, are microbial infections in which the microorganisms act in concert with a host's reduced capacity to resist disease. To successfully treat periodontal diseases, it is essential to be able to recognize different types of the diseases. When classifying inflammatory periodontal diseases, it is important to include not only diseases that have primary manifestation and etiology in the periodontium, but also periodontal manifestations of systemic diseases. In this chapter a comprehensive classification of the gingival diseases or conditions affecting gingival tissues is presented.

Gingival Diseases

Gingivitis is defined as an inflammatory lesion, mediated by host/microorganism interactions, which remains limited to the gingival tissues and does not involve the underlying periodontal ligament, cementum, or alveolar and supporting bone (American Academy of Periodontology, 2003). In this broad condition, the apical extent of the junctional epithelium and the coronal gingival connective tissue attachment remain at the cementoenamel junction; hence, there is no attachment loss. Gingivitis can affect children, adolescents, and adults.

Gingivitis has been further defined based on clinical manifestations, duration of the disease, and association with either dental plaque or systemic factors such as medical conditions or medications (Gurenlian, 2007; Page, 1986). Some professionals question whether gingivitis should be considered a periodontal disease because it does not cause loss of significant amounts of periodontal support or tooth

mortality (loss). However, most researchers have concluded otherwise (Page, 1986; Ranney, 1986, 1993).

Histopathogenesis of Gingivitis

Stages in the Histopathogenesis

As discussed in previous chapters, the reaction of the host to the presence of dental plaque (biofilm) is inflammatory in nature, initially developing into inflammation of the gingival unit. Inflammation confined to the gingiva (epithelium and lamina propria) results in gingivitis.

The **histopathogenesis**, or the events that occur in the periodontal tissues that lead to the development of gingivitis and periodontitis, is best explained by reviewing the different stages occurring in the initiation and progression of the periodontal disease as it relates to clinical signs. In a previous chapter, the role of the host immune system in the inflammatory process and periodontal disease progression was reviewed. In this section, the microscopic tissue changes seen as a result of periodontal diseases are discussed. It is important to remember that all these inflammatory and immunological events that occur during the time frame in the development of periodontal lesions are intermingled and must not be considered as separate entities.

Page and Schroeder (1976) described the development of periodontal diseases as a progression of inflammation through four different stages: initial lesion, early lesion, established lesion, and advanced lesion (Table 7–1 ■; Figure 7–1 ■). The initial and early lesions are representative of acute inflammation, whereas the established lesion is considered to be chronic gingivitis; the advanced lesion is periodontitis and will be discussed in the following chapter (Page & Schroeder, 1976). The information from the research by Page and Schroeder was obtained

Table 7–1 Page and Schroeder's Stages of Pathogenesis of Periodontal Disease

Stage	Onset Time After Plaque Accumulation	Histopathological Signs	Features
Initial	2 to 4 days	Acute inflammation; PMNs, machrophages; vasculitis	Subclinical; no signs of gingivitis; increased flow of GCF
Early	4 to 7 days	T cell lesion	Clinical signs of gingivitis first seen (redness, bleeding on probing, edema)
Established	2 to 3 weeks	B cell lesion; plasma cells	Chronic gingivitis (gingiva may appear bluish-red with increased probing depths)
Advanced	Undetermined	Alveolar bone loss, periodontal pocket formation; B cell lesion	Periodontitis

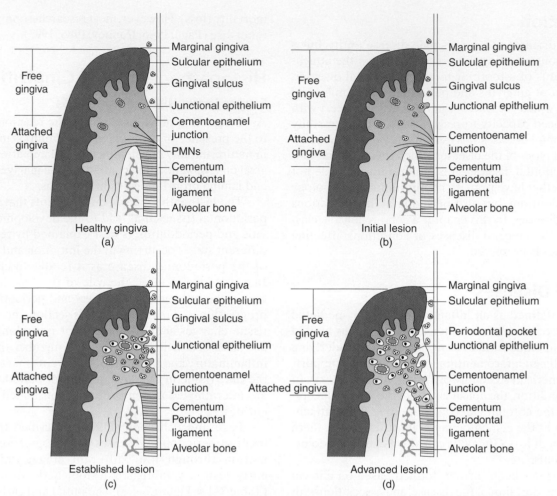

FIGURE 7–1 Page and Schroeder's histopathologic periodontal lesions. (a) Healthy gingiva: Little supragingival plaque accumulation; a few defense cells, primarily PMNs, migrate through the junctional epithelium into the gingival crevice and out into the oral cavity. (b) Initial lesion: This develops 2 to 4 days after plaque accumulation at the gingival margin. Vasodilation results in an increased emigration of PMNs from the blood vessels into the connective tissue and entering the gingival crevice. This is gingivitis but the lesion is not clinically visible. Early lesion: This lesion appears at the site of the initial lesion within 4 to 7 days following plaque accumulation. The same features seen in the initial lesion appear in the early lesion but they are accentuated with an increased number of PMNs and macrophages. T lymphocytes begin to migrate into the tissue and gingival crevice. A greater area of gingival connective tissue is affected. About 60% to 70% of collagen is destroyed. Acute inflammation features continue in the early lesion. This is still gingivitis. (c) Established lesion: This is characterized by the presence of PMNs, macrophages, and antibody-producing plasma cells (B lymphocytes), which comprise 10% to 30% of the infiltrate. More collagen has been destroyed. The bulk of plaque bacteria and cells in the gingival crevice cause the junctional epithelium to detach from the tooth. The pocket epithelium is mostly derived from junctional epithelium with the formation of epithelial ridges and microulcerations. This is chronic gingivitis and is still reversible if oral hygiene is reinstated. (d) Advanced lesion: This is periodontitis. Plasma cells (> 50%) are the primary cells involved in periodontitis. There is clinical attachment loss with loss of clinical connective tissue attachment to the tooth and apical migration of the junctional (pocket) epithelium, resulting in a periodontal pocket. In addition, the alveolar and supporting bone has been destroyed.

from animal specimens and a few human juvenile tissue samples. Also, because there are many factors involved in the initiation and progression of periodontal diseases, it is difficult to exactly pinpoint a clear delineation between the different stages, especially in humans. Also, it is unclear when and if an established lesion develops into an advanced lesion. Thus, even though this classic work by Page and Schroeder is primarily with nonhuman tissues, it is still the foundation from which the histopathogenesis of inflammatory periodontal diseases can be studied. The inflammatory and immune changes discussed earlier are involved in the histopathogenesis of periodontal diseases.

INITIAL LESION (PMN DOMINATED) The initial lesion develops after 2 to 4 days of plaque accumulation (Löe, Theilade, & Jensen, 1965; Page & Schroeder, 1976). Dental plaque accumulates on the tooth surface at the free gingival margin level (Figure 7–1b). The protective wall of PMNs (leukocyte wall) between the plaque mass and the junctional and sulcular epithelium becomes compromised (Miyasaki, 1991). Bacterial antigens cross the permeable junctional epithelium and enter the gingival connective tissue. The response of the tissue to the antigens is acute inflammation, developing within minutes of the insult. It is characterized by a dilation of blood vessels within the connective tissue subjacent to the junctional epithelium (Page & Schroeder, 1976). There is an increased flow of gingival crevicular fluid (GCF) into the crevice and migration of PMNs from the connective tissue into the junctional epithelium (Payne, Page, Ogilvie, & Hall, 1975) and gingival crevice in response to chemotactic factors released by bacteria and inflammatory cells. There is some loss of collagen in the lamina propria because of the action of collagenase that is replaced with inflammatory cells such as PMNs. This lesion is not clinically seen and is reversible with appropriate oral hygiene (Löe et al., 1965).

EARLY LESION (T-CELL DOMINATED) The early lesion evolves from the initial lesion after approximately 7 days of plaque accumulation and can continue for up to 14 days. Clinically, this lesion is observable as gingivitis. The presence and accentuation of the features in the initial lesion characterize the early lesion (see Figure 7–1b). PMNs continually migrate from the blood vessels through the junctional epithelium into the gingival crevice, and there is increased gingival crevicular flow. T lymphocytes accumulate immediately subjacent to the junctional epithelium. There is no apparent dividing line between the initial and early lesions. Approximately 60% to 70% of collagen is lost in the connective tissue. Changes start to occur in the junctional epithelium. As a result of the downgrowth of accumulating plaque, the gingival sulcus begins to deepen. This is still an acute gingivitis without clinical connective tissue attachment loss and no bone loss as yet. This lesion is reversible with adequate oral hygiene, healing without adverse consequences.

Bleeding on probing occurs when there are ulcerations in the epithelium lining the soft tissue wall of the pocket, and the engorged blood vessels from the underlying connective tissue protrude through the epithelium.

ESTABLISHED LESION (FEW B CELLS/PLASMA CELLS) As adverse clinical conditions progress, the early lesion develops into the chronic or established gingivitis lesion (Page & Schroeder, 1976). The gingiva responds to massive accumulations of plaque, which affects a greater area of tissue (see Figure 7–1c). The time period for the initiation of the established lesion has not actually been determined, but it can start within 2 to 3 weeks after plaque accumulation (Page & Schroeder, 1976). The manifestations of acute inflammation still persist. Established lesions may persist for months or years without progressing into periodontitis (Page, 1986;

Zappa, 1995). As gingivitis becomes clinically more severe, the proportion of T cells decreases, and B cells and plasma cells increase within the lamina propria (Zappa, 1995). More collagen is lost and replaced by an inflammatory cell infiltrate. The gingival fibers are still attached to the root surface; there is no clinical connective tissue attachment loss at this stage. Because of the massive amounts of subgingival plaque that advance in an apical direction, the junctional epithelium detaches laterally from the tooth surface to become pocket epithelium with elongation of epithelial ridges deeper into the connective tissue in an attempt to maintain epithelial integrity (Kinane & Lindhe, 1998); this leads to the formation of microulcerations, which may increase the permeability of the epithelium to bacteria and their by-products.

The gingival margin becomes swollen and enlarged, and the gingival margin can be separated easily from the tooth surface, forming a gingival pocket or pseudopocket. No alveolar bone loss occurs at this stage. Clinical signs are present and more severe than in the early lesion. Most of the changes that occur in the established lesion are still reversible. The advanced lesion (Figure 7–1d) is periodontitis and is discussed in the following chapter.

Pathogenesis of Gingivitis

The Gingival Pocket

In early periodontal lesions a **gingival pocket** (Figure 7–2 ■) is formed by gingival enlargement and coronal migration of the gingival margin. There is no loss of clinical connective tissue attachment (the gingival fibers remain attached to the root surface, and the junctional epithelium has not migrated apically onto the root surface). In addition, there is no alveolar and supporting bone loss. Gingival pockets are not true pockets; they are false or "pseudo," which means that the increased height of the gingiva creates an impression that a deep pocket has been formed when probing instruments are used around a tooth (Ranney, 1986). There is no attachment of gingival connective tissue above the cementoenamel junction, and because there is no loss of clinical connective tissue attachment to the root surface, it is not a true pocket. The pocket epithelium extends laterally and detaches from the tooth surface, permitting apical movement of the bacteria in plaque between the tooth and epithelium. A pseudopocket is often seen in drug-induced gingivitis (e.g., gingivitis produced by the use of phenytoin, cyclosporine, and certain calcium channel blockers), severe gingival inflammation, and hormone-induced gingivitis (e.g., during pregnancy or puberty).

Host Response to Gingival Inflammation

The gingiva reacts to the presence of microorganisms within dental plaque by alterations in the gingival vascular (blood) supply. The initial response from the gingival tissue is vasodilation of the blood vessels in the lamina propria (gingival connective tissue) in close proximity to the junctional epithelium. With this, there is an increased permeability

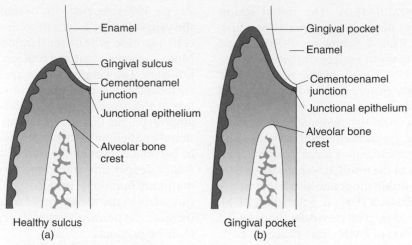

FIGURE 7–2 (a) Physiologic periodontium. (b) A gingival pocket. The gingival margin has migrated coronally, but there is no attachment loss or bone loss. There is a deepened pocket, but it is not a true pocket because the depth is due to the coronal position of the gingiva. This type of pocket is seen in gingivitis.

(increased opening) of the vessels allowing the exchange of fluid and cells between the blood and lamina propria. This allows for the increased migration of neutrophils (leukocytes) from the blood vessels into the lamina propria and junctional epithelium.

These changes in the underlying lamina propria and epithelium cause the clinical features of edema (fluid filled) and redness in the gingival tissues. Gingival redness occurs due to the increased vascularity at inflamed sites. Inflamed gingival is edematous because of the increased vascular permeability of blood vessels in the inflamed connective tissue. Fluid "leaks" out of blood vessels into the tissue, resulting in edema. The ulceration of the epithelium (due to the vascular changes) allows for a communication into the underlying lamina propria where there are an increased number of blood vessels. Thus, when a periodontal probe is placed in the gingival sulcus of inflamed gingiva, bleeding occurs. There is no loss of gingival connective tissue attachment (gingival fibers) and no alveolar and supporting bone loss. Gingivitis is reversible if the irritant is removed below the threshold of causing a host response.

Classification of the Periodontal Diseases

Over the years a number of classification systems have been developed to organize and name various disease entities or conditions affecting the periodontium. In 1989, the American Academy of Periodontology (AAP) recommended a classification based on the data from periodontal research that was used by the dental community to describe different forms of periodontal diseases. This was modified in 1992 (American Academy of Periodontology, 1992) in a position paper published by the Academy to include gingival diseases. In 1999 at the International Workshop for a Classification of Periodontal Diseases and Conditions the

American Academy of Periodontology proposed a new classification system (Armitage, 1999; Table 7–2 ■). This new classification system is not based on the age of the patient at the time of presentation but rather describes distinct forms of periodontal diseases based on clinical, radiographic, and historical data. Please note that the 1999 Classification lists both gingival diseases and periodontitis and other conditions relating to the periodontium. Box 7–1 lists the entire classification, not just gingival diseases (Holmstrup, 1999). Note that all periodontal diseases and conditions are listed, but only gingival diseases will be discussed in this chapter.

Dental Plaque-Induced Gingival Diseases

GINGIVITIS ASSOCIATED WITH DENTAL PLAQUE Gingivitis is a reaction of the host (body) to the bacteria present in the dental biofilm (plaque). Gingivitis, which exemplifies itself as inflammation of the gingiva, is the most common of the periodontal diseases (Page, 1985). Dental biofilms as the etiology or cause of gingivitis have been confirmed in Löe's classic "Experimental Gingivitis in Man" study (Löe et al., 1965). **Plaque-associated gingivitis** begins at the gingival margin and can spread throughout the remaining gingival unit. Plaque-induced gingivitis will not develop unless there are bacteria present (American Academy of Periodontology, 1992); however, the composition of the required oral microbiota is not specific (Moore, Moore, & Cato, 1987). Gingivitis is reversible following the removal of dental biofilms and maintenance of good oral hygiene self-care (Watt & Marinho, 2005). However, if oral hygiene procedures are discontinued and the level of oral hygiene is not adequate, allowing the accumulation of biofilms, clinical signs of acute gingivitis develop within 1 to 3 weeks. This classic model of gingivitis induction is used in clinical trials to test antigingivitis oral rinses.

Table 7–2 Common Gingival Diseases

Disease	Patient Population	Clinical Features	Causes of the Disease	Microbiologic Features	Figure
Gingivitis associated with dental plaque	Adolescents, adults	Gingival redness, bleeding, and enlargement Absence of clinical attachment loss and bone loss	Inadequate oral hygiene	No specific bacteria are demonstrated, although high levels of *Streptococcus sanguis, S. mitis, Fusobacterium nucleatum, Actinomyces viscosus,* and *Veillonella parvula* have been detected	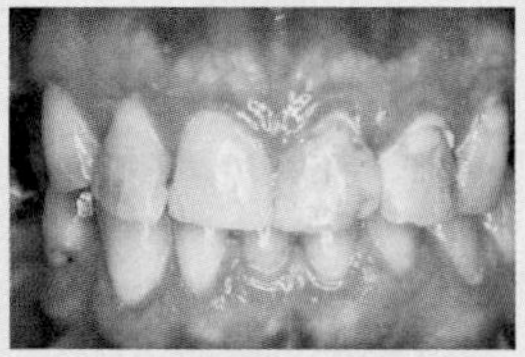 **FIGURE 7–3** Plaque-induced gingivitis.
Gingival diseases associated with the endocrine system	Pregnant patients, adolescents, diabetics	Intense gingival inflammation Absence of clinical attachment loss and bone loss	Changes in sex hormone level; exaggerated response to plaque	*Prevotella intermedia* (pregnancy gingivitis and puberty gingivitis)	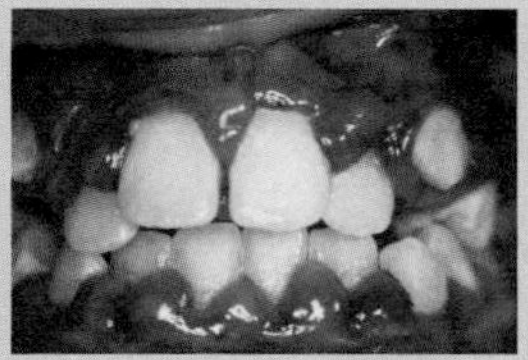 **FIGURE 7–4** Puberty gingivitis. 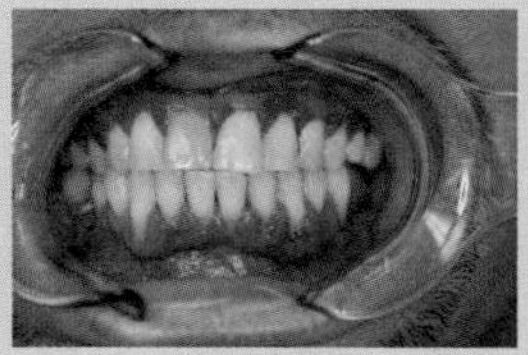 **FIGURE 7–5** Diabetes mellitus–associated gingivitis.
Gingival diseases associated with blood dyscrasias	Leukemia	Intense gingival inflammation, petechiae, mucosal ulcers, gingival bleeding	Abnormal proliferation and development of leukocyte	None	

(continued)

Table 7-2 Common Gingival Diseases (continued)

Disease	Patient Population	Clinical Features	Causes of the Disease	Microbiologic Features	Figure
Gingival diseases modified by medications	Patients taking phenytoin, calcium channel blockers, cyclosporine	Gingival enlargment or overgrowth Absence of clinical attachment loss and bone loss	Medications and dental plaque	No specific bacteria demonstrated	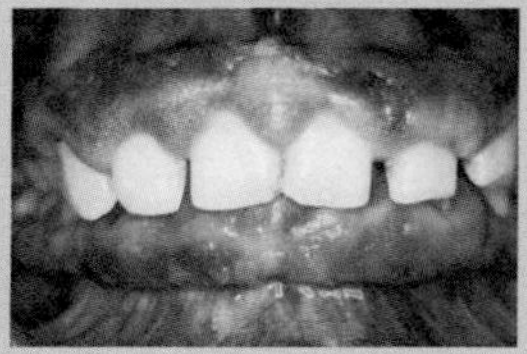 **FIGURE 7–6** Phenytoin-related gingivitis. 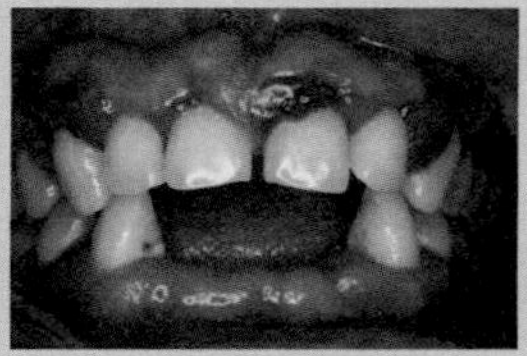 **FIGURE 7–7** Nifedipine-related gingivitis. 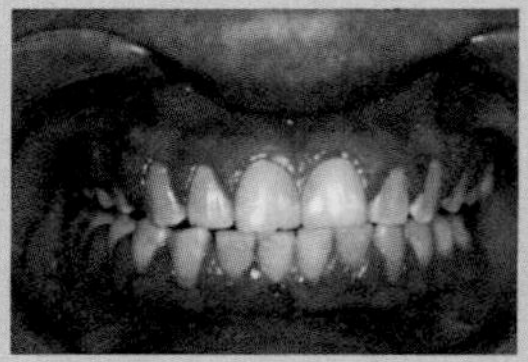 **FIGURE 7–8** Cyclosporine-related gingivitis.
Gingival diseases of viral origin	Herpes virus infections (primary herpetic gingivostomatitis, recurrent oral herpes, varicella-zoster infections)	Movable oral mucosa appears as vesicles that easily rupture to form painful ulcers affecting the gingiva	Herpes simplex viruses type 1 and 2, varicella-zoster virus	Viral, not bacterial	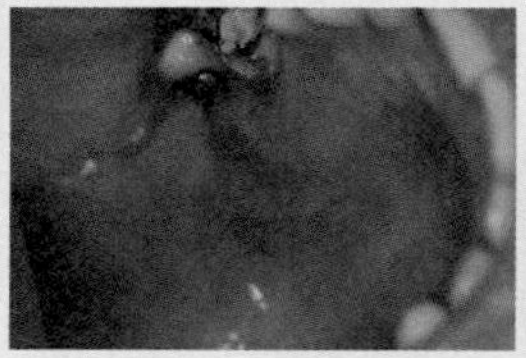 **FIGURE 7–9** Herpes simplex infection.

Table 7–2 Common Gingival Diseases (continued)

Disease	Patient Population	Clinical Features	Causes of the Disease	Microbiologic Features	Figure
Gingival diseases of fungal origin	Linear gingival erythema, antibiotic use, corticosteroid use	Denture sore mouth appears as red gingiva underlying a denture; may also show whitish patches that can be wiped off the mucosa leaving a slightly bleeding surface	Candida species (*Candida albicans*)	Fungal, not bacteria
(a)
(b)
FIGURE 7-10 (a) Chronic atrophic candidiasis (denture sore mouth). (b) Linear gingival erythema. |
| Gingival manifestations of systemic conditions, mucocutaneous disorders | These include skin diseases such as pemphigus, lichen planus, benign mucous membrane pemphigoid (BMMP), and others | Gingiva may appear blotchy red, have blisters or vesicles, or slough (peel) off from the underlying connective tissue | Abnormality in the immune system | None |
(a)
(b)
FIGURE 7-11 (a) Erosive lichen planus, and (b) pemphigus vulgaris. |

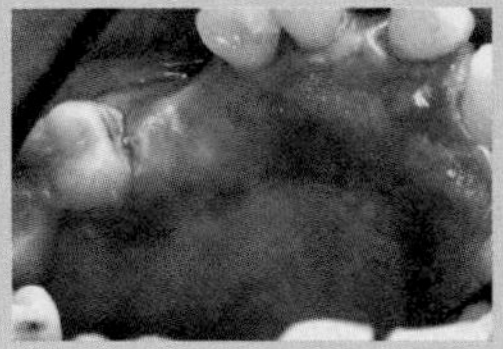

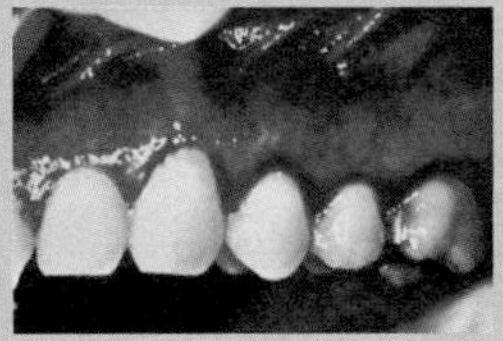

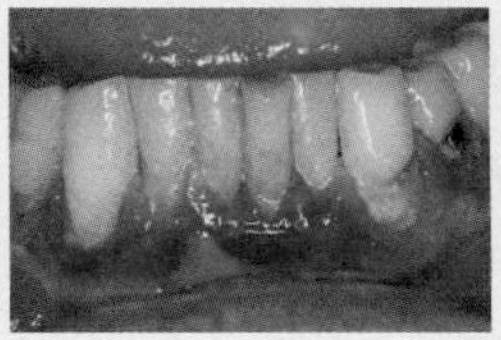

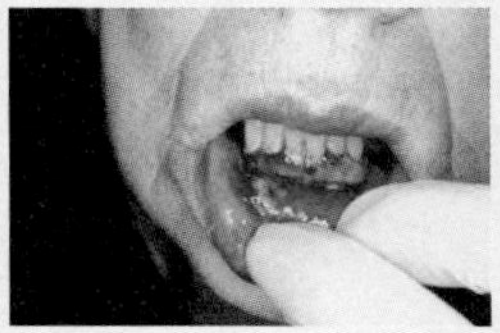

Box 7–1: Classification of Periodontal Diseases and Conditions

I. Gingival diseases
  A. Dental plaque–induced gingival diseases*
    1. Gingivitis associated with dental plaque only
      a. Without other local contributing factors
      b. With local contributing factors (see VIIIA)
    2. Gingival diseases modified by systemic factors
      a. Associated with the endocrine system
        (1) Puberty-associated gingivitis
        (2) Menstrual cycle–associated gingivitis
        (3) Pregnancy-associated
          (a) Gingivitis
          (b) Pyogenic granuloma
        (4) Diabetes mellitus–associated gingivitis
      b. Associated with blood dyscrasias
        (1) Leukemia-associated gingivitis
        (2) Other
    3. Gingival diseases modified by medications
      a. Drug-influenced gingival diseases
        (1) Drug-influenced gingival enlargements
        (2) Drug-influenced gingivitis
          (a) Oral contraceptive–associated gingivitis
          (b) Other
    4. Gingival diseases modified by malnutrition
      a. Ascorbic acid–deficiency gingivitis
      b. Other
  B. Non-plaque-induced gingival lesions
    1. Gingival diseases of specific bacterial origin
      a. Neisseria gonorrhea–associated lesions
      b. Treponema pallidum–associated lesions
      c. Streptococcal species–associated lesions
      d. Other
    2. Gingival diseases of viral origin
      a. Herpes virus infections
        (1) Primary herpetic gingivostomatitis
        (2) Recurrent oral herpes
        (3) Varicella-zoster infections
      b. Other
    3. Gingival diseases of fungal origin
      a. Candida species infections
        (1) Generalized gingival candidiasis

  b. Linear gingival erythema
  c. Histoplasmosis
  d. Other
    4. Gingival lesions of genetic origin
      a. Hereditary gingival fibromatosis
      b. Other
    5. Gingival manifestations of systemic conditions
      a. Mucocutaneous disorders
        (1) Lichen planus
        (2) Pemphigoid
        (3) Pemphigus vulgaris
        (4) Erythema multiforme
        (5) Lupus erythematosus
        (6) Drug-induced
        (7) Other
      b. Allergic reactions
        (1) Dental restorative materials
          (a) Mercury
          (b) Nickel
          (c) Acrylic
          (d) Other
        2. Reactions attributable to
          (a) Toothpastes/dentifrices
          (b) Mouth rinses/mouthwashes
          (c) Chewing gum additives
          (d) Foods and additives
        3. Other
    6. Traumatic lesions (factitious, iatrogenic, accidental)
      a. Chemical injury
      b. Physical injury
      c. Thermal injury
    7. Foreign-body reactions
    8. Not otherwise specified

*A section on gingival diseases (1A) was added to the current 1999 system. This includes plaque-induced gingivitis and **non-plaque-induced diseases** (1B). Also included in this classification system are gingival diseases that can be modified by systemic factors such as medications or diabetes mellitus.

Because the bacteria associated with chronic, long-standing, plaque-induced gingivitis are not very specific, recognition of gingivitis is primarily made clinically. However, the earliest changes may not be seen clinically and only histologically under the microscope. With the development of gingivitis, the healthy gingiva changes in color, contour, consistency, and surface texture. Plaque-associated gingivitis starts within the interdental papilla and is clinically characterized by gingival redness, gingival bleeding, swelling, and gingival sensitivity and tenderness (Löe et al., 1965; Suzuki, 1988). The features of dental plaque-induced gingivitis are summarized in Box 7–2 (Mariotti, 1999).

Treatment of gingivitis includes maintenance of adequate oral hygiene self-care and regular professional mechanical debridement.

Gingival Diseases Modified by Systemic Factors

GINGIVITIS ASSOCIATED WITH THE ENDOCRINE SYSTEM Altered hormonal balances elicit an apparent exaggerated response to dental plaque. Hormonal-influenced gingivitis manifests as puberty-associated gingivitis, menstrual cycle-associated gingivitis, and pregnancy-associated gingivitis. In addition, poorly controlled plasma glucose levels resulting in a diabetes-associated gingivitis may aggravate the inflammatory response of the gingiva to plaque.

Box 7–2: Clinical Features of Gingival Diseases

- Caused by nonspecific bacteria (although certain types of bacteria are associated with gingivitis, the condition is currently still considered of nonspecific bacterial origin)
- Dental plaque present at the marginal gingiva
- Clinical signs of inflammation are limited to the gingiva

- No clinical attachment loss
- It is reversible to health following the removal of the dental plaque causing it
- Even though bacteria are the primary risk factors, secondary factors apparently modify the clinical characteristics of the disease. This has resulted in many subclassifications.

Puberty Gingivitis. During puberty, the dramatic elevation in steroid hormones often can cause a gingival response that is similar to what has been described for pregnancy gingivitis. In addition to a rise in hormones (estrogen and progesterone), the incidence and severity of gingivitis in adolescents are influenced by a number of factors, including plaque levels, dental caries, mouth breathing, tooth crowding, and tooth eruption (Stamm, 1986). The distinguishing feature between plaque-induced gingivitis and puberty gingivitis is the development of gingival inflammation in the presence of a small amount of dental plaque. Meticulous oral hygiene is the recommended treatment.

Menstrual Cycle Gingivitis. During the menstrual cycle there are increased levels of estrogen and progesterone. These changes in hormone levels cause gingival inflammation characterized as enlarged, red interdental papilla. Connective tissue attachment loss and alveolar and supporting bone loss are not evident. All gingival changes are reversible after ovulation. It is important to note that gingival changes primarily are seen when plaque is present. Also, not every female patient will have this inflammatory response during menstruation.

Pregnancy Gingivitis. Pregnancy gingivitis is inflammation of the gingiva associated with pregnancy. The incidence of gingivitis during pregnancy ranges between 30% and 100%. The effects of pregnancy on preexisting gingivitis are seen by the second month of gestation and are most severe in the eighth month at the time of peak hormone levels (American Academy of Periodontology, 1992; Silness & Löe, 1963). Pregnant patients with healthy gingiva usually do not develop gingivitis, but if gingivitis or periodontitis is present, the course of the disease is aggravated by pregnancy.

Rapid Dental Hint

Gingivitis may develop without the patient even knowing. A patient may not recognize that he or she has periodontal disease. It is important for you to inform the patient of the signs and symptoms.

The degree of gingival inflammation is related to the state of oral hygiene of the patient. Accumulation of dental plaque parallels the gingival changes. The severity of the gingivitis is greater in pregnant than in nonpregnant women (Löe, 1965) but is not associated with more destructive periodontitis (Cohen, Shapiro, Friedman, Kyle, & Franklin, 1971). The condition regresses postpartum (Silness & Löe, 1963). However, gingivitis during pregnancy can be prevented or be resolved by adequate plaque control starting early in the pregnancy.

Dental plaque present at the gingival margin results in an exaggerated inflammatory response of the gingiva. Tissue inflammation and enlargement seen in pregnancy is not caused by the pregnancy itself but rather by the shifts in the hormonal levels, which aggravate the inflammation. Hormonal changes during pregnancy are due to elevated progesterone and estrogen levels, which in the final gestational month are 10 to 30 times greater than that seen during the normal menstrual cycle (Amar & Chung, 1994). Elevations in these steroids, especially progesterone, cause an increased permeability of the blood vessels (microvasculature; Lindhe & Bränemark, 1968) within the lamina propria, resulting in gingival redness, edema, and increased flow of gingival crevicular fluid (Amar & Chung, 1994; Lindhe, Lindhe, Attström, & Björn, 1968). Subgingival growth of *Prevotella intermedia* is enhanced because this bacterium can substitute progesterone, as well as testosterone and estradiol, as growth factors. Elevated levels of *Prevotella intermedia* are also seen in puberty gingivitis (Kornman & Loesche, 1980).

Pregnancy gingivitis is not synonymous with a pregnancy tumor. A pregnancy tumor is a non-neoplasm, pyogenic granuloma occurring in a pregnant patient. It arises from an analogue of a dormant (inactive) tumor and is stimulated during pregnancy. Clinically, it presents as a painless protuberant, mushroom-like exophytic mass that is attached to a base at the gingival margin. It will regress or completely disappear postpartum.

Treatment of pregnancy gingivitis consists of periodontal debridement and oral home care instruction. The gingiva may be erythematous and painful. Meticulous plaque control is important. The gingival condition will resolve postpartum.

Diabetes Mellitus–Associated Gingivitis. Diabetes mellitus is one of the important risk factors for periodontal diseases. Type 1 diabetes is not as common as type 2 diabetes, which is caused by the development of either resistance to insulin in muscle (insulin is not working to bring glucose into cells), impaired secretion of insulin from the pancreas, or increased glucose production by the liver. All causes result in an elevation of blood glucose levels or hyperglycemia, which causes complications related to accelerated artherosclerosis, retinopathy (blindness), renal (kidney) failure, neuropathy (diseases of the nervous system), altered wound healing, and periodontal conditions.

Diabetes mellitus–associated gingivitis is characterized by inflammation of the gingiva, especially where plaque is present without clinical attachment loss or bone loss. It is similar to plaque-induced gingivitis and is more commonly seen in children with poorly controlled type 1 diabetes.

Gingivitis Associated with Blood Dyscrasias

LEUKEMIA-ASSOCIATED GINGIVITIS Leukemia is a disease characterized by an abnormal proliferation of leukocytes (white blood cells) in the blood and bone marrow. Oral manifestations are seen as gingival bleeding and enlargement starting at the interdental papilla and spreading to the attached gingiva.

Treatment of patients with gingival diseases modified by systemic factors first involves getting the systemic disease under control followed by professional periodontal debridement and maintenance of oral home care.

Gingival Diseases Modified by Medications

DRUG-INFLUENCED ENLARGEMENTS Commonly used drugs can lead to the appearance of gingivitis (American Academy of Periodontology, 2004; Dongari, McDonnell, & Langlais, 1993). Many types of medications (Box 7–3) can cause gingival overgrowth or enlargement (Kanno et al., 2008).

No specific bacteria are associated with this type of gingivitis and no specific risk factors exist other than poor oral hygiene and use of the medication.

Based on current histological and ultrastructural findings, drug-influenced gingival changes are more accurately referred to as "gingival overgrowth" or "enlargement," rather than "gingival hypertrophy," which is defined as an increase in connective tissue volume, or gingival hyperplasia, which is defined as an abnormal increase in the number of fibroblasts (Hallmon & Rossmann, 1999).

The etiology of drug-induced gingival overgrowth is not exactly known. Either there is an excessive production of collagen by gingival fibroblasts, making the gingiva appear thickened or enlarged (Brown, Beaver, & Bottomley, 1991), or the action of collagenase, which breaks down collagen, is reduced (Hallmon & Rossmann, 1999). The highly active fibroblasts become sensitive to these medications in the presence of inflammation (Brown et al., 1991).

Box 7–3: Classification of Medications Associated with Gingival Enlargement

- Phenytoin (incidence 50%): Used to control convulsive or seizure disorders (Angelopoulos & Goaz, 1972; Dongari et al., 1993; Steinberg & Steinberg, 1982).

- Cyclosporine (incidence about 30%): Used for immunosuppressive or antirejection therapy when an individual receives an organ transplant (Greenberg, Armitage, & Shiboski, 2008; Seymour & Jacobs, 1992; Thomason et al., 1995).

- Calcium channel blockers (nifedipine, amlodipine, diltiazem): Used for the treatment of cardiovascular conditions such as hypertension, angina, and arrhythmias. Although nifedipine was the first calcium channel blocker (Barclay, Thomason, Idle, & Seymour, 1992) and is the one most frequently associated with gingival enlargement (incidence about 15%), the condition can occur with any drug in this class (Nishikawa et al., 1991).

- Sodium valproate: Used as an antidepressant and anticonvulsant (rare occurrence).

Enlargement often occurs within 1 to 3 months after the start of the medication (Nishikawa et al., 1991). Although the amount of the drug used daily and duration of use may be related to the severity of the overgrowth (Addy, McElnay, Eyre, Campbell, & D'Arcy, 1982), several studies have failed to see any relationship between these factors (Hassell & Hefti, 1991).

Although some clinical studies have shown the level of plaque accumulation affects the severity of the overgrowth, others have shown that, although plaque control and the removal of local irritants is of some benefit for gingival health, these measures alone do not prevent gingival overgrowth (Hefti, Eshenaur, Hassell, & Stone, 1994; Seymour & Smith, 1991). It is often difficult to determine whether the increased plaque accumulation preceded the gingival overgrowth or occurred because of ineffective oral hygiene in the presence of enlarged gingiva (Rees, 1998). Because hypertension is an adverse effect of cyclosporine, patients may also be taking a calcium channel blocker such as nifedipine, which may also induce gingival overgrowth. Other calcium channel blockers associated with gingival enlargement include diltiazem, verampamil, and amlodipine. Thus, it is difficult to assess the actual frequency of gingival overgrowth related to the use of cyclosporine (Lundergan, 1989).

If there is only gingival enlargement without bone loss, periodontal debridement with oral home care instruction is the mainstay. These procedures may be difficult because of the tissue contours. Surgical intervention (e.g., gingivectomy) may be necessary; however, as long as the patient is taking the medication, the gingiva will revert back to the original form. Thus, surgery may need to be done frequently.

Drug-Influenced Gingivitis

ORAL CONTRACEPTIVE–ASSOCIATED GINGIVITIS The etiology of oral contraceptive-induced gingival inflammation is similar to that seen in pregnancy (Pearlman, 1974) because the drugs used contain combinations of estrogen and progesterone that simulate pregnancy. Therefore, the same gingival changes observed during pregnancy are seen with oral contraceptive use (Mealey, 1996). However, much lower concentrations of hormones are used in today's oral contraceptive pills, thus reducing the incidence of gingival diseases (Preshaw, Knutsen, & Mariotti, 2001).

Non-Plaque-Induced Gingival Diseases

GINGIVAL DISEASES OF SPECIFIC BACTERIA ORIGIN This category includes gingival lesions caused by infections with *Neisseria gonorrhea*, *Treponema pallidum*, *Streptococci*, or other microorganisms. The gingival lesions appear as either erythematous (red), edematous (fluid-filled) ulcers, or inflamed, nonulcerated gingiva.

GINGIVAL DISEASES OF VIRAL ORIGIN This section is associated with gingivitis caused by viral infections such as herpes viruses (herpes simplex virus type 1 and 2, primary herpetic gingivostomatitis [Slots, 2005] and varicella-zoster virus). These viruses primarily affect babies and then become latent or dormant until adulthood at which time they appears as recurrent herpes labialis. Primary gingivostomatitis may also be seen during adolescence or adulthood.

GINGIVAL DISEASES OF FUNGAL ORIGIN This section is associated with gingivitis caused by fungal infections such as candidiasis, coccidioidomycosis, cryptococcosis, histoplasmosis, and others. Oral candidiasis (*C. albicans*) is usually seen in HIV-seropositive and other immunocompromised patients. The lesions appear as a band of erythema of the attached gingiva, which is termed linear gingival erythema (LGE). The prevalence of LGE in HIV-infected populations is relatively unknown because the stage of HIV

Rapid Dental Hint

Inflammation of a patient's gingival tissue can be due to many factors, including plaque, medications, or systemic diseases. Do a careful assessment of every patient.

disease varies among the population (Mealey, 1996), and more structured studies need to be conducted.

GINGIVAL LESIONS OF GENETIC ORIGIN Hereditary gingival fibromatosis clinically appears as a fibrotic gingival enlargement that is genetically derived and occurs rarely. The enlargement of the gingiva may cover the entire tooth surface.

GINGIVAL MANIFESTATIONS OF SYSTEMIC CONDITIONS Mucocutaneous diseases are lesions involving the mucous membranes, including the mouth and/or the skin. Oral manifestations of mucocutaneous diseases are seen in erosive lichen planus (Figure 7–11a; Endo et al., 2008), benign mucous membrane pemphigoid, bullous pemphigoid, and pemphigus vulgaris (Figure 7–11b). More adult women than men have been documented with the disease. Oral lesions may involve all or part of the gingiva and other mucous membranes of the oral cavity. Gingival involvement may manifest as desquamative gingivitis characterized by desquamation or sloughing (peeling) of the epithelium, leaving a red, painful underlying connective tissue surface. No specific bacteria have been identified. The cause of these mucocutaneous diseases is multifactoral, with some of the diseases being autoimmune in nature whereby the body attacks and destroys its own tissue (Weinberg, Insler, & Campen, 1997).

Allergic reactions due to ingredients or contents of dentifrices, mouth rinses, and chewing gum are relatively rare and are usually attributed to chemical additives.

TRAUMATIC LESIONS Physical injury to the gingival tissues may be due to thermal (e.g., burns from hot beverages), chemical (e.g., chemical products such as sloughing of tissues from oral rinses or dentifrices, aspirin burn), or physical (e.g., aggressive toothbrushing, incorrect use of dental floss, fingernails, or toothpicks) injury.

Dental Hygiene Application

Gingivitis is a type of inflammatory periodontal disease that is defined as a microbial infection that is confined to the gingival unit. Gingivitis is the result of the outcome of host–bacterial interactions and are modified by systemic factors including medical conditions and medications. Gingivitis is characterized by the presence of a gingival pocket in which there is neither loss of attachment nor bone loss.

The dental hygienist must be familiar with the clinical and histological features of gingivitis so that a distinction between the different gingival diseases can be made. This will allow for a more comprehensive treatment plan and definitive treatment for the patient.

Key Points

- Inflammatory periodontal diseases are broadly classified into gingivitis and periodontitis.
- Gingivitis is defined as inflammation confined to the gingiva.
- Gingivitis is reversible.
- Dental plaque (biofilm) is the major risk factor for gingivitis; other contributory risk factors include medications, hormones, and systemic diseases.

Self-Quiz

1. From the following list, select the items associated with gingivitis.
   a. Occurs primarily in children
   b. Extensive attachment loss
   c. Bone loss does not occur
   d. Primary risk factors include pathogenic bacteria and calculus
   e. Mild to moderate attachment loss
   f. Risk factors include poor oral hygiene and endocrine conditions

2. All of the following medications are contributing risk factors in causing gingival enlargement except one. Which one is the exception?
   a. Phenytoin
   b. Cyclosporine
   c. Ibuprofen
   d. Nifedipine
   e. Valproate

3. Which one of the following periodontal diseases is described by having inflammation of the gingiva without loss of clinical connective tissue attachment?
   a. Dental plaque-induced gingivitis
   b. Chronic periodontitis
   c. Aggressive periodontitis
   d. Refractory periodontitis
   e. Necrotizing ulcerative periodontitis

4. Which one of the following bacteria is found in high numbers in pregnancy gingivitis?
   a. *Porphyromonas gingivalis*
   b. *Prevotella intermedia*
   c. *Actinomyces viscosus*
   d. *Aggregatibacter actinomycetemcomitans*
   e. *Streptococcus sanguis*

5. Which periodontal lesion, according to the classification of Page and Schroeder (1976), is characterized by chronic gingival inflammation and the presence of plasma cells?
   a. Initial
   b. Early
   c. Established
   d. Advanced

6. Today most oral contraceptives do not cause gingival inflammation because of the lower levels of hormones used.
   a. Statement and reason are correct.
   b. Statement and reason are false.
   c. Statement is true but reason is false.
   d. Statement is false but reason is true.

7. Which periodontal lesion, according to the classification of Page and Schroeder (1976), is characterized by chronic gingival inflammation and the initial presence of PMNs?
   a. Initial
   b. Early
   c. Established
   d. Advanced

8. During the disease process, the junctional epithelium transforms into
   a. alveolar bone.
   b. periodontal ligament.
   c. pocket epithelium.
   d. sulcular epithelium.
   e. oral epithelium.

9. Which of the following lesions does clinical inflammation first appear?
   a. Initial
   b. Early
   c. Established
   d. Advanced

10. Which of the following features occurs first after 2 to 4 days of plaque accumulation?
    a. Dilation of blood vessels in the lamina propria
    b. Destruction of connective tissue by collagenase
    c. Influx of plasma cells
    d. Phagocytosis of bacteria by macrophages

Case Study

A 30-year-old pregnant female returns for her maintenance visit. She has had prior preventive visits with no pocketing, bone loss, or gingival inflammation. It is now six months later and she is returning for her recall. Her gingiva had been stippled, pink, narrow knife-like papillae with no edema. She states she is 3 months pregnant and her gums like red and swollen.

1. What would be her periodontal disease classification be from the previous preventive visit before she was pregnant?
   a. Gingival disease plaque induced
   b. Gingival disease modified by medications
   c. Gingival disease modified by system factors
   d. No gingival disease

Answer: D. As stated there was no gingival inflammation and therefore there was no gingival disease.

2. What is the patient's current periodontal disease classification?
   a. Gingival disease associated with dental plaque only
   b. Gingival disease modified by systemic factors
   c. Gingival disease modified by medications
   d. Not gingival disease but periodontal disease.

Answer: B. Pregnancy-associated gingivitis is a category of gingival disease which is modified by systemic factors. It is not a factor of medications and occurs as dental plaque induced and modified by pregnancy. It is not periodontal disease as there is no bone loss.

3. What is the rationale to classify gingival diseases in the classification of periodontal disease?
   a. Classification includes both gingival and periodontal condition
   b. Classification determines cost of dental therapy
   c. Classification determines Dental Hygiene treatment plan
   d. Classification determines ADA codes to use for billing

Answer: A. classification includes gingival and periodontal diseases. It does not determine cost or billing or therapy. Dental hygiene care plans are individualized and not necessarily related to the classification.

References

Addy, V., J. McElnay, D. Eyre, N. Campbell, and P. D'Arcy. 1982. Risk factors in phenytoin-induced gingival overgrowth. *J. Periodontol.* 54:373–377.

Amar, S., and K. M. Chung. 1994. Influence of hormonal variation on the periodontium in women. *Periodontology 2000* 6:79–87.

American Academy of Periodontology. 1992. The etiology and pathogenesis of periodontal diseases (Position Paper), 1–9. Chicago: Author.

American Academy of Periodontology. 2003. *Glossary of periodontal terms*, 4th ed. Chicago: Author.

American Academy of Periodontology. 2004. Drug-associated gingival enlargement. *J. Periodontol.* 75:1424–1431.

Angelopoulos, A. P., and P. W. Goaz. 1972. Incidence of diphenylhydantoin gingival hyperplasia. *Oral Surg. Oral Med. Oral Path.* 34:898–906.

Armitage, G. C. 1999. Development of a classification system for periodontal diseases and conditions. *Ann. Periodontol.* 84:1–6.

Barclay, S., J. M. Thomason, J. R. Idle, and R. A. Seymour. 1992. The incidence and severity of nifedipine-induced gingival overgrowth. *J. Clin. Periodontol.* 19:311–314.

Brown, R. S., W. T. Beaver, and W. K. Bottomley. 1991. On the mechanisms of drug-induced gingival hyperplasia. *J. Oral Pathol. Med.* 20:201–209.

Cohen, D. W., J. Shapiro, L. Friedman, G. C. Kyle, and S. Franklin. 1971. A longitudinal investigation of the periodontal changes during pregnancy and fifteen months post-partum. Part III. *J. Periodontol.* 42:653–657.

Dongari, A., H. T. McDonnell, and R. P. Langlais. 1993. Drug-induced gingival overgrowth. *Oral Surg. Oral Med. Oral Pathol.* 76:543–548.

Endo, H., T. D. Rees, W. W. Hallmon, et al. 2008. Disease progression from mucosal to mucocutaneous involvement in a patient with desquamative gingivitis associated with permphigus vulgaris. *J. Periodontol.* 79:369–375.

Greenberg, K. V., G. C. Armitage, and C. H. Shiboski. 2008. Gingival enlargement among renal transplant recipients in the era of new-generation immunosuppressants. *J. Periodontol.* 79(3):453–460.

Gurenlian, J. R. 2007. The role of dental plaque biofilm in oral health. *J. Dent. Hyg.* 81(5):116.

Hallmon, W. W., and J. A. Rossmann. 1999. The role of drugs in the pathogenesis of gingival overgrowth. *Periodontology 2000* 21:176–196.

Hassell, T., and A. F. Hefti. 1991. Drug-induced gingival overgrowth: Old problem, new problem. *Crit. Rev. Oral Pathol. Med.* 2:103–137.

Hefti, A. F., A. E. Eshenaur, T. M. Hassell, and C. Stone. 1994. Gingival overgrowth in cyclosporine A treated multiple sclerosis patients. *J. Periodontol.* 65:744–749.

Holmstrup, P. 1999. Non-plaque-induced gingival lesions. *Ann. Periodontol.* 4:20–29.

Kanno, C. M., J. A. Oliverira, J. F. Garcia, et al. 2008. Effects of cyclosporine, phenytoin, and nifedipine on the synthesis and degradation of gingival collagen in tufted capuchin monkey (Cebus paella): L Histochemical and MMP-q and -2 and collagen I gene expression analysis. *J. Periodontol.* 79(1):114–122.

Kinane, D. F., and J. Lindhe. 1998. Pathogenesis of periodontitis. In eds. J. Lindhe, T. Karring, and N. P. Lang, *Clinical periodontology and implant dentistry*, 189–225. Copenhagen: Munksgaard.

Kornman, K. S., and W. J. Loesche. 1980. The subgingival microflora during pregnancy. *J. Periodontol. Res.* 5:111–122.

Lindhe, J., and P. I. Bränemark. 1968. Experimental studies on the etiology of pregnancy gingivitis. *Perio. Abst.* 16:50–51.

Lindhe, J., J. Lindhe, R. Attström, and A. Björn. 1968. Influence of sex hormones on gingival exudation in dogs with chronic gingivitis. *J. Periodont. Res.* 3:279–283.

Löe, H. 1965. Periodontological changes in pregnancy. *J. Periodontol.* 36:209–217.

Löe, H., E. Theilade, and S. B. Jensen. 1965. Experimental gingivitis in man. *J. Periodontol.* 36:177–187.

Lundergan, W. P. 1989. Drug-induced gingival enlargements. Dilantin hyperplasia and beyond. *J. Calif. Dent. Assoc.* 17:48–52.

Mariotti, A. 1999. Dental plaque-induced gingival diseases. *Annals of Periodontology* 4:7–19.

Mealey, B. L. 1996. Periodontal implications: Medically compromised patients. *Ann. Periodontol.* 1:256–321.

Miyasaki, K. T. 1991. The neutrophil: Mechanisms of controlling periodontal bacteria. *J. Periodontol.* 62: 761–774.

Moore, L. V. H., W. E. C. Moore, and E. P. Cato. 1987. Bacteriology of gingivitis. *J. Dent. Res.* 66:989–995.

Nishikawa, S., H. Tada, A. Hamasaki, S. Kasahara, J. Kido, et al. 1991. Nifedipine-induced gingival hyperplasia: A clinical and in vitro study. *J. Periodontol.* 62:30–35.

Page, R. C. 1985. Oral health status in the United States. Prevalence of inflammatory periodontal diseases. *J. Dent. Educ.* 49:354–364.

Page, R. C. 1986. Gingivitis. *J. Clin. Periodontol.* 13:245–255.

Page, R. C., and H. E. Schroeder. 1976. Pathogenesis of inflammatory periodontal disease. A summary of current work. *Lab Investigations* 33:235–249.

Payne, W. A., R. C. Page, A. L. Ogilvie, and W. B. Hall. 1975. Histopathologic features of the initial and early stages of experimental gingivitis in man. *J. Periodont. Res.* 10:51–64.

Pearlman, B. A. 1974. An oral contraceptive drug and gingival enlargement: The relationship between local and systemic factors. *J. Clin. Periodontol.* 1:47–57.

Preshaw P. M., M. A. Knutsen, and A. Mariotti 2001. Experimental gingivitis in women using oral contraceptives. *J. Dent. Res.* 80:2011–2015.

Ranney, R. R. 1986. Discussion: Pathogenesis of gingivitis. *J. Clin. Periodontol.* 13:356–359.

Ranney, R. R. 1993. Classification of periodontal diseases. *Periodontology 2000* 2:13–25.

Rees, T. D. 1998. Drugs and oral disorders. *Periodontology 2000* 18:21–36.

Seymour, R. A., and D. J. Jacobs. 1992. Cyclosporin and the gingival tissues. *J. Clin. Periodontol.* 19:1–11.

Seymour, R. A., and D. G. Smith. 1991. The effect of a plaque control programme on the incidence and severity of cyclosporin-induced gingival changes. *J. Clin. Periodontol.* 18:107–110.

Silness, J., and H. Löe. 1963. Periodontal disease in pregnancy. *Acta. Odontol. Scand.* 21:533–551.

Slots, J. 2005. Herpes viruses in periodontal disease. *Periodontology 2000* 38(1):33–62.

Stamm, J. W. 1986. Epidemiology of gingivitis. *J. Clin. Periodontol.* 13:360–370.

Steinberg, S. C., and A. D. Steinberg. 1982. Phenytoin-induced gingival overgrowth in severely retarded children. *J. Periodontol.* 53:429–433.

Suzuki, J. B. 1988. Diagnosis and classification of periodontal diseases. *Dent. Clin. North America* 32:195–216.

Thomason, J. M., R. A. Seymour, J. S. Ellis, P. J. Kelly, G. Parry, et al. 1995. Iatrogenic gingival overgrowth in cardiac transplantation. *J. Periodontol.* 66:742–746.

Watt, R. G., and V. C. Marinho. 2005. Does oral health promotion improve oral hygiene and gingival health? *Periodontology 2000* 37(1):35–47.

Weinberg, M. A., M. S. Insler, and R. B. Campen. 1997. Mucocutaneous features of autoimmune blistering diseases. *Oral Surg. Oral Med. Oral Pathol. Oral Radiol. Endod.* 84:517–534.

Zappa, U. 1995. Histology of the periodontal lesion: Implications for diagnosis. *Periodontology 2000* 7:22–38.

Periodontitis and Other Periodontal Conditions

Surendra Singh

OUTLINE

EDUCATIONAL OBJECTIVES

Upon completion of this chapter, the reader should be able to:

- Define the course of the progression of periodontitis.
- Explain the pathogenesis of periodontitis.
- Explain changes in the 1999 Classification of Periodontal Diseases.
- Explain the different features of the various types of periodontitis.
- Discuss periodontitis as a risk factor for systemic diseases.

GOAL: To provide an understanding of the features of periodontitis.

KEY WORDS

aggressive periodontitis   *126*
bone loss   *121*
chronic periodontitis   *126*
connective tissue attachment
   loss   *118*
infrabony defects   *122*
peri-implant disease   *131*
periodontal pocket   *120*
periodontitis   *118*

Introduction

Periodontitis is widespread in the population, afflicting both children and adults. **Periodontitis** is defined as clinical attachment loss with subsequent bone loss. According to the 1999 Classification of the Periodontal Diseases, periodontitis is categorized into chronic and aggressive forms. Diagnosis of periodontitis is not based on the age of the patient but rather on clinical and radiographic findings. Dental biofilms are the primary risk factor for periodontitis. Modifying contributory factors such as systemic diseases are also involved in the development and progression of the periodontitis lesion.

Histopathogenesis of Periodontitis

INITIATION OF INFLAMMATORY PERIODONTAL DISEASES If gingivitis is not resolved, the inflammatory reaction may spread into the gingival connective tissue attachment, alveolar and supporting bone, and the principal fibers. At this stage, the disease is periodontitis.

This chapter deals primarily with the tissue changes that occur during the initiation and development of gingivitis and periodontitis. When these tissue changes occur within the periodontal tissues, the inflammatory and immune responses are also triggered. Thus, the features that are reviewed in this chapter occur as part of the entire inflammatory and immunological events.

The histological lesions presented in this chapter were initially classified and published in 1976 by Page and Schroeder. Page and Schroeder classified gingivitis and periodontitis according to histopathology from animal and some human adolescent specimens. This classification

> **Did You Know?**
>
> The periodontal ligament fibers are the most resistant to destruction and thus are the last structures to be lost during disease activity.

is still used in periodontic literature; however, it is not a realistic, up-to-date classification. The initial early and established lesions reflected the histopathology of clinically early and chronic gingivitis and were discussed in the previous chapter. The advanced lesion reflected the histopathology of the progression of gingivitis into periodontitis (Table 8–1 ■).

ADVANCED LESION (PLASMA CELL/ANTIBODY DOMINATED) The advanced lesion is characteristic of periodontitis. The inflammatory infiltrate extends into the alveolar and supporting bone and periodontal ligament (see Figure 8–1d ■). Periodontal pocket formation occurs with the clinical **connective tissue attachment loss** to the root surface and the apical migration of the apical aspect of the junctional epithelium along the root surface that was previously occupied by connective tissue; attachment loss occurs. Subsequently, there is alveolar and supporting bone loss. The apical and lateral migration of the junctional or pocket epithelium permits extension of subgingival plaque on the root surface. The lymphocytic infiltrate in the subjacent connective tissues is primarily B cells. The advanced lesion may become stable or progress continuously (Goodson, 1992).

Table 8–1 Page and Schroeder's Stages of Pathogenesis of Periodontal Disease

Stage	Onset Time after Plaque Accumulation	Histopathological Signs	Features
Initial	2 to 4 days	Acute inflammation; PMNs, machrophages; vasculitis	Subclinical; no signs of gingivitis; increased flow of GCF
Early	4 to 7 days	T cell lesion	Clinical signs of gingivitis first seen (redness, bleeding on probing, edema)
Established	2 to 3 weeks	B-cell lesion; plasma cells	Chronic gingivitis
Advanced	Undetermined	Alveolar bone loss, periodontal pocket formation; B-cell lesion	Periodontitis

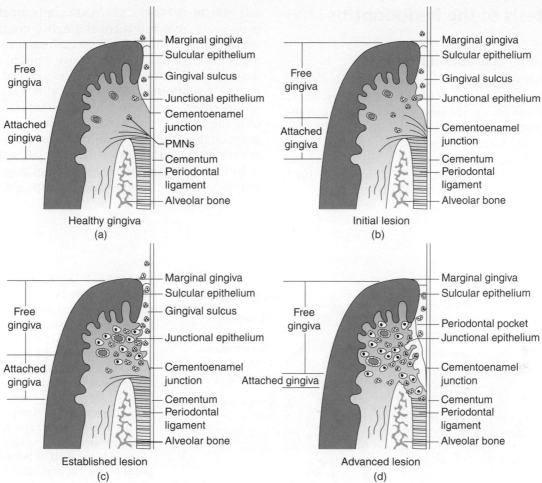

FIGURE 8–1 Page and Schroeder's histopathologic periodontal lesions. (a) Healthy gingiva: Little supragingival plaque accumulation; a few defense cells, primarily PMNs, migrate through the junctional epithelium into the gingival crevice and out into the oral cavity. (b) Initial lesion: This develops 2 to 4 days after plaque accumulation at the gingival margin. Vasodilation results in an increased emigration of PMNs from the blood vessels into the connective tissue and entering the gingival crevice. This is gingivitis, but the lesion is not clinically visible. Early lesion: This lesion appears at the site of the initial lesion within 4 to 7 days following plaque accumulation. The same features seen in the initial lesion appear in the early lesion, but they are accentuated with an increased number of PMNs and macrophages. T lymphocytes begin to migrate into the tissue and gingival crevice. A greater area of gingival connective tissue is affected. About 60% to 70% of collagen is destroyed. Acute inflammation features continue in the early lesion. This is still gingivitis. (c) Established lesion: This is characterized by the presence of PMNs, macrophages, and antibody-producing plasma cells (B lymphocytes), which comprise 10% to 30% of the infiltrate. More collagen has been destroyed. The bulk of plaque bacteria and cells in the gingival crevice cause the junctional epithelium to detach from the tooth. The pocket epithelium is mostly derived from junctional epithelium with the formation of epithelial ridges and microulcerations. This is chronic gingivitis and is still reversible if oral hygiene is reinstated. (d) Advanced lesion: This is periodontitis. Plasma cells (>50%) are the primary cells involved in periodontitis. There is clinical attachment loss with loss of clinical connective tissue attachment to the tooth and apical migration of the junctional (pocket) epithelium, resulting in a periodontal pocket. In addition, the alveolar and supporting bone has been destroyed.

Pathogenesis of the Periodontitis Lesion

Sequence of Events in Pocket Formation

A pocket is defined as a pathologically deepened gingival sulcus (American Academy of Periodontology, 2001). The development of a **periodontal pocket** between the root surface and the gingiva includes the transformation of a thin junctional epithelium into a pocket epithelium with the development of microulcerations and epithelial ridges (Müller-Glauser & Schroeder, 1982; Figure 8–2 ■).

THE PERIODONTAL POCKET As the inflammatory infiltrate progresses from the coronal gingival connective tissue subjacent to the junctional epithelium into the underlying connective tissue, an extensive amount of collagen is destroyed. The detachment of the gingival clinical connective tissue attachment (gingival fibers) to the tooth allows apical migration of the junctional epithelium onto the root surface. Apical and lateral migration of the junctional epithelium continues, and as this epithelium separates from the root surface, a periodontal pocket is formed. The junctional epithelium migrates apically only as a result of the destruction of the gingival collagen

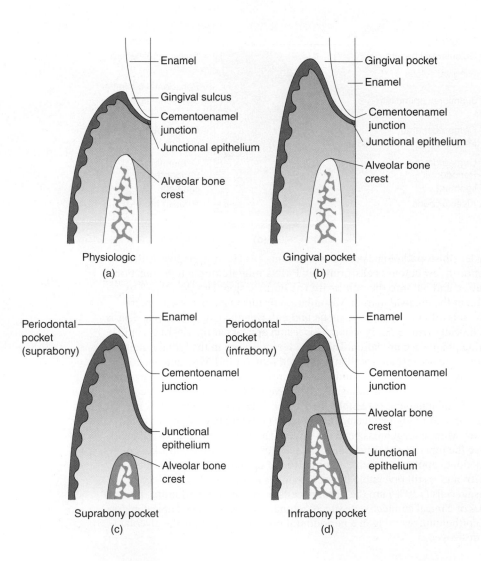

Physiologic
(a)

Enamel
Gingival sulcus
Cementoenamel junction
Junctional epithelium
Alveolar bone crest

Gingival pocket
(b)

Gingival pocket
Enamel
Cementoenamel junction
Junctional epithelium
Alveolar bone crest

Suprabony pocket
(c)

Periodontal pocket (suprabony)
Enamel
Cementoenamel junction
Junctional epithelium
Alveolar bone crest

Infrabony pocket
(d)

Periodontal pocket (infrabony)
Enamel
Cementoenamel junction
Alveolar bone crest
Junctional epithelium

FIGURE 8–2 (a) Healthy periodontium. (b) Gingivitis pocket seen in gingivitis. Note that the junctional epithelium is located at the CEJ. (c) A suprabony pocket is a type of periodontal pocket. The deepened pocket is caused by attachment loss. There is also bone loss. The base of the pocket is coronal to the crest of alveolar bone. This type of pocket is a result of the tissue destruction that occurs in periodontitis. (d) An infrabony pocket is another type of periodontal pocket. The base of the pocket is apical to the crest of bone. This type of pocket is seen in periodontitis.

fibers. With increasing periodontal pocket depths, it becomes an ideal environment for plaque accumulation, making it difficult to clean.

There are two types of periodontal pockets: suprabony and infrabony. The difference between the two kinds of pockets lies in the relationship of the base of the pocket or the coronal extent of the junctional epithelium to the alveolar crest and the type of bone destruction (Table 8–2 ■). Bone destruction occurs as the inflammatory infiltrate extends into the alveolar crest and then into the trabecular bone.

The base of a suprabony pocket (junctional epithelium) is coronal to the crest of bone (see Figure 8–2c), whereas the base of an infrabony pocket (junctional epithelium) is apical to the crest of bone (see Figure 8–2d). This is in contrast to the healthy periodontium (Figure 8–2a) and gingivitis (Figure 8–2b), where the junctional epithelium is at the CEJ. This can be identified on a radiograph when a dense object such as a periodontal probe is placed at the base of the pocket as the radiograph is taken.

ROOT SURFACE The areas of cementum that no longer have gingival or periodontal ligament fibers attached undergo changes. The surface of the cementum is rough because of the detachment of the previously inserting connective tissue. It was once thought that the surface of cementum becomes rough, easily absorbing endotoxins, bacteria, and their by-products onto and slightly into its surface. This cementum is referred to as necrotic cementum. However, current theory states that the influence of root surface roughness and endotoxin-contaminated cementum was overestimated. In 1987, it was documented that extensive root planing may not be warranted because the endotoxins were found to be very superficial and not embedded deeply into the cementum. They are weakly adherent to the cementum (Nakib, Bissada, Simmenlink, & Golstine, 1982). Excessive cementum removal to provide, a smooth, glass-like root surface is unnecessary (Greenstein, 1992; Hughes, Augr, & Smales, 1988).

Bone Resorbing Factors

The inflammatory process causes the resorption of alveolar and supporting bone. A consequence of pocket formation and loss of clinical connective tissue attachment is bone resorption. The process of **bone loss** involves the inflammatory cells including PMNs and macrophages. As the inflammatory infiltrate destroys more collagen in the connective tissue, the bone is approached.

Different substances involved in bone resorption include (1) prostaglandins, (2) endotoxins, (3) cytokines, and (4) B cells.

Numerous factors can act directly on osteoclasts to stimulate their activity to destroy bone. One of the main mechanisms of bone resorption is through the release of prostaglandins (PGE2) from macrophages or PMNs (Offenbacher, Heasman, & Collins, 1993). Prostaglandins activate resting osteoclasts, increase the number of osteoclasts, increase the number of macrophages, and inhibit bone collagen formation (Offenbacher et al., 1993). Prostaglandins are also produced in bone and have a direct resorptive effect on bone.

Bone resorption can also occur when bacteria release endotoxins, which activate inflammatory cells such as macrophages resulting in the production and release of cytokines such as IL-1 (Schwartz, Goultschin, Dean, & Boyan, 1997). IL-1 is most important in periodontal destruction (Ishikawa, Nakashima, Koseki, et al., 1997). IL-1 can also stimulate PGE2 production. Another theory of bone resorption is explained by the role of cytokines and prostaglandins

---

Did You Know?

In fact, on extracted teeth, endotoxins can be brushed away.

Table 8–2 Classification of Pockets

Type of Pocket	Pathogenesis	Relationship of Base of Pocket to Alveolar Crest	Pattern of Bone Loss
Gingival (pseudo-pocket) pocket	No clinical connective tissue attachment loss and no bone loss	At the cementoenamel junction	No bone loss
Periodontal pockets: Suprabony pocket	Connective tissue attachment loss and bone loss	Coronal to alveolar crest	Horizontal
Infrabony pocket	Connective tissue attachment loss and bone loss	Apical to alveolar crest	Vertical or angular

in stimulating collagenase production by PMNs (Reynolds & Meikle, 1997). Collagenase is an enzyme that destroys collagen, which is a component of bone.

Site Specificity

An important feature of inflammatory periodontal diseases is the site-specific localization of periodontal destruction. Pocket formation and bone loss do not occur in all areas of the dentition at the same time, but it could occur on a few teeth at a time or even on only some aspects of some teeth at any given time, while other teeth are healthy. The composition of subgingival plaque samples from different sites in the oral cavity of the same mouth has been shown to be different. These differences have presented a problem for research analysis and treatment response to therapy (Socransky & Haffajee, 1997).

Relationship of Bone Loss and Pocket Formation

Alveolar and supporting bone is destroyed as the pocket develops. Because the level of bone corresponds to previous periodontal destruction and changes in the soft tissue of the pocket wall reflect the present inflammatory condition, the degree of bone loss is not necessarily correlated with the depth of periodontal pockets. Radiographically, extensive bone loss can be associated with shallow pocket depths and vice versa. For example, a patient may have had severe periodontitis at one time but had periodontal treatment that stopped the progression of the disease. Clinically, the probing depths are shallow, but radiographically bone loss is evident.

Pattern of Bone Loss

The types of pockets that form and the pattern of bone loss depend on the route the inflammation takes from the gingiva to the underlying supporting structures. The route of extension of the inflammatory infiltrate from the gingiva into the interdental bone is by way of the blood vessels. The interdental bone is resorbed more rapidly than the bundle bone because it is more vascular and less resistant to resorption. Interproximally (between adjacent teeth), inflammation usually spreads along the interdental blood vessels from the gingiva through the crestal bone into the bone marrow spaces extending out to the periodontal ligament fibers (Figure 8–3a ■). On the facial and lingual surfaces of

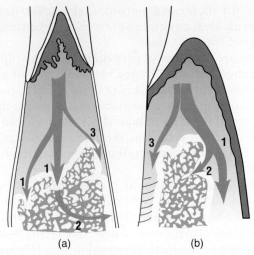

(a)   (b)

FIGURE 8–3 (a) The inflammatory infiltrate spreads from the gingiva through the lamina propria into the bone following the most vascular pathway, which is where most of the blood vessels are located. Sometimes the most vascular area (larger blood vessels) is on the side of the alveolar crest, allowing the inflammation to directly enter the periodontal ligament. (b) On the direct facial surface, inflammation extends along the supraperiosteal artery before entering bone.

teeth, the inflammatory infiltrate follows along the supraperiosteal blood vessels located in the periosteum on the outer surface of the bone (Figure 8–3b). Usually, the principal fibers are the most resistant to destruction and are the last to be resorbed.

The penetration of the inflammatory infiltrate into the marrow spaces and on the bone surfaces is associated with a loss of the equilibrium (balance) between bone formation and bone resorption, leading to loss of alveolar bone. The pattern of bone loss varies among individual teeth and on different surfaces of the same tooth. Bone destruction can occur on any surface of the tooth. The pattern of bone loss can occur in two different ways:

1. Horizontal bone loss when bone resorption occurs from its outer aspect buccal and lingual walls. Bone is lost equally on the surfaces of two adjacent teeth with the interproximal bone level remaining flat (Figure 8–4a ■), and the deepest portion of the pocket is located coronal to the alveolar crest.
2. Vertical or angular bone loss occurs when the inflammation travels directly from the gingiva into the periodontal ligament and then the bone. The interproximal bone level is not flat and even as in horizontal bone loss. Bone loss occurs at different rates around the tooth and is more rapid on one side of the tooth than the other. The base or the deepest portion of the bony defect is apical to the alveolar bone crest, creating an **infrabony defect**

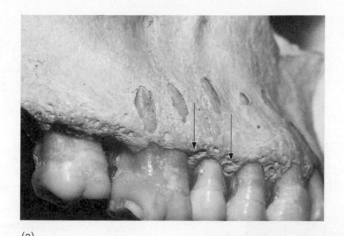

(a)

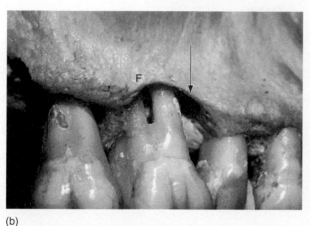

(b)

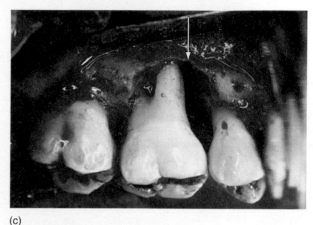

(c)

FIGURE 8–4 (a) Horizontal pattern of bone loss between the premolars and second premolar and first molar. Interproximal bone (arrows) is destroyed on both sides of adjacent teeth equally. (b) Left side: Dry skull specimen showing furcation involvement (F) and vertical pattern of bone loss on the mesial aspect of the first molar (arrow). Note that the interproximal bone is not flat as with horizontal bone loss. (c) Right side: After the gingiva has been reflected from the tooth and bone, a vertical defect is seen on the mesial aspect of the first molar.

(Figure 8–4b ■, c). If a sinus tract is present, a gutta percha point (it is radiopaque and will show up on an X-ray) is carefully inserted into the tract. In Figure 8–5 ■, a patient came in with an abscess. To determine the origin of this infection, a point was placed and then an X-ray taken.

The terms *infrabony* and *intrabony* have been used interchangeably to describe all vertical bony defects; however, these terms are frequently misused in the periodontal literature (Weinberg & Eskow, 2000). The term *intra-* translates to mean "within or inside the bone" and *infra-* to mean "below the crest of bone." An infrabony defect is a generic term to describe any periodontal vertical bony defect.

Periodontal infrabony defects are classified according to the number of osseous (bony) walls surrounding the pocket (Figures 8–6 ■ and 8–7 ■). There are four bony interproximal walls surrounding the tooth: the mesial, facial (buccal), distal, and lingual. Most vertical bone loss occurs interproximally, although vertical bone loss does occur on the direct facial and lingual walls. Types of defects include the following:

- Three-wall bony defect. The three-wall defect has three bony walls remaining interproximally or facially or lingually, with the tooth forming the fourth wall. An intrabony defect is a type of three-wall bony defect with specific characteristics (Prichard, 1979). As a result of the disease process, the bone lining the infrabony defect is usually composed of cortical bone. In an intrabony defect, the walls have cancellous bone behind them. The only way to determine if the defect is intrabony is during the surgical procedure when the bone is exposed. Thus, it is incorrect to refer to all infrabony defects as intrabony. A three-wall defect

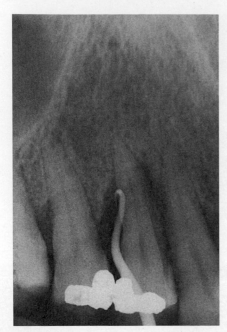

FIGURE 8–5 Note vertical bone loss on the distal of the premolar. A gutta percha point placed in the periodontal pocket before the radiograph was taken to show the origin of the abscess was the base of the pocket. This tooth had a hopeless prognosis, and treatment was planned for extraction.

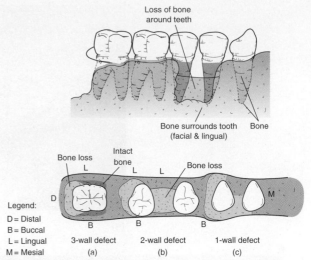

FIGURE 8–6 Vertical bone destruction is classified according to the number of bony walls surrounding the defect. In health there are four bony walls surrounding a tooth: mesial (M), buccal (B) or facial, distal (D), and lingual (L). In periodontitis one or more of the bony walls is destroyed. If three bony walls remain, it is called a three-wall defect (a). If the buccal and lingual bony walls remain, it is called a two-wall defect or crater (b). If one bony wall remains (e.g., buccal/lingual cortical plate or proximal [mesial, distal] wall of bone), it is called a one-wall defect or hemiseptum (c).

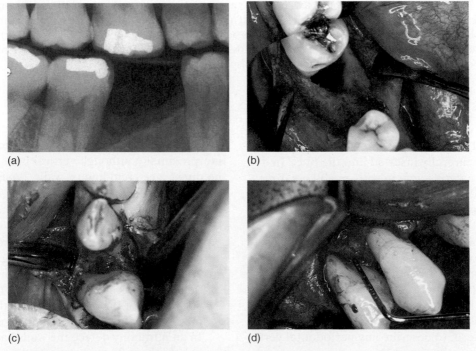

FIGURE 8–7 (a-b) X-ray of three-wall defect on the mesial of the mandibular molar; surgical entry exposes the three-wall defect. Note that the distal bony wall against the molar is resorbed. Thus, three walls remain: buccal, lingual, and mesial. (c) Surgical entry of a two-wall defect—the buccal and lingual walls remain. (d) Surgical entry of a one-wall defect—the buccal wall remains.

that wraps around the tooth and involves two or more adjacent root surfaces is referred to as a circumferential defect.

- Two-wall bony defect. The two-wall defect has two bony walls remaining. An interdental crater is the most common angular bony defect. It is a two-wall osseous defect with a buccal and lingual wall remaining.
- One-wall bony defect. The one-wall defect has one bony wall remaining and usually occurs interdentally. If the remaining wall is the proximal wall, the defect is referred to as a hemiseptum.

Factors Related to Pattern of Bone Loss

The bone destructive process radiates from the plaque mass, at the base of the periodontal pocket, 1.5 to 2.5 mm circumferentially (Tal, 1984; Figure 8–8 ■). Within this 2 mm "circle," bone destruction does not occur. Outside this 2 mm "circle," bone destruction occurs. Thus, the width and thickness of the interdental septum primarily determines if the pattern of bone destruction is horizontal or vertical. Bone destruction occurring where there is a wide interdental septum (>2 mm in width) will most likely not occur across the entire septum and results in a vertical pattern of bone loss. Bone destruction occurring where the interdental septum is narrow (< 2 mm) can be total and results in a horizontal pattern of bone loss.

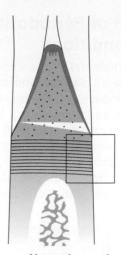

FIGURE 8–8 The range of bone destruction determines the pattern of bone loss. The area of bone destruction radiates from the plaque mass about 2 mm.

Teeth such as lower incisors, which have thin facial or lingual cortical plates of bone with little to no cancellous bone between the alveolar bone proper and the outer plate, will usually show a horizontal pattern of bone loss. Molars that have a thick facial cortical plate of bone will usually show a vertical pattern of bone loss. Figure 8–9 ■ is a panoramic radiograph showing different levels of bone loss.

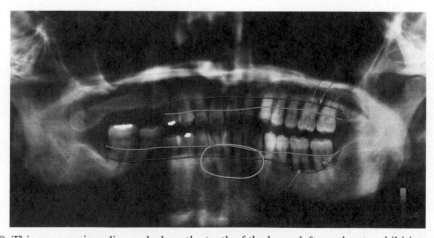

FIGURE 8–9 This panoramic radiograph show the teeth of the lower left quadrant, exhibiting generalized severe bone loss of 30% to 80%. The red line depicts the existing bone level, whereas the green line depicts where the bone was originally, prior to the patient developing periodontal disease. The orange arrows point to furcation involvement, or the loss of enough bone to reveal the location at which the individual roots of a molar begin to branch from the single root trunk; this is a sign of advanced periodontal disease. The blue arrow shows up to 80% bone loss on tooth #21, and clinically, this tooth exhibited gross mobility. Finally, the peach oval highlights the aggressive nature with which periodontal disease generally affects mandibular incisors. Because their roots are generally situated very close to each other, with minimal interproximal bone and because of their location in the mouth, where plaque and calculus accumulation is greatest because of the pooling of saliva, mandibular anteriors suffer excessively.

Classification of Periodontitis and other Conditions

Box 8–1 lists all periodontal diseases and conditions so that the student can see all diseases and conditions together. However, only periodontitis is discussed in this chapter.

Periodontitis is an inflammatory lesion mediated by host/microorganism interactions and results in clinical attachment loss and alveolar and supporting bone loss. Adolescents as well as adults can develop periodontitis. One of the changes that was made in the periodontitis classification was replacing the term "adult periodontitis" with "**chronic periodontitis**." Chronic periodontitis is subdivided as localized (≤ 30% of the sites affected) and generalized (>30% of the sites affected). Disease severity is divided into three groups, which are based on the amount of clinical attachment loss (CAL): slight = 1–2 mm CAL; moderate = 3–4 mm CAL; and severe = ≥ 5 mm CAL. The Academy decided that adults as well as adolescents could develop periodontitis and that "adult" was too restrictive. Thus, the age factor is eliminated from the criteria for periodontal diseases.

The term "early-onset periodontitis" was replaced with "**aggressive periodontitis**." Again, the age-dependent nature of the patient was a factor in changing the terms. The older

Box 8–1: Current Classification of Periodontal Diseases and Conditions

I. Gingival diseases (reviewed in Chapter 7)
  A. Dental plaque–induced gingival diseases*
  B. Non-plaque-induced gingival lesions
II. Chronic periodontitis†
  A. Localized
  B. Generalized
III. Aggressive periodontitis†
  A. Localized
  B. Generalized
IV. Periodontitis as a manifestation of systemic diseases
  A. Associated with hematologic disorders
    1. Acquired neutropenia
    2. Leukemias
    3. Other
  B. Associated with genetic disorders
    1. Familial and cyclic neutropenia
    2. Down syndrome
    3. Leukocyte adhesion deficiency syndromes
    4. Papillon-Lefèvre syndrome
    5. Chediak-Higashi syndromes
    6. Histiocytosis syndromes
    7. Glycogen storage disease
    8. Infantile genetic agranulocytosis
    9. Cohen syndrome
    10. Ehlers-Danlos syndrome (Types IV and VIIIAD)
    11. Hypophosphatasia
    12. Other
  C. Not otherwise specified (NOS)
V. Necrotizing periodontal diseases
  A. Necrotizing ulcerative gingivitis (NUG)
  B. Necrotizing ulcerative periodontitis (NUP)
VI. Abscesses of the periodontium
  A. Gingival abscess
  B. Periodontal abscess
  C. Pericoronal abscess

VII. Periodontitis associated with endodontic lesions
  A. Combined periodontal–endodontic lesions
VIII. Developmental or acquired deformities and conditions
  A. Localized tooth-related factors that modify or predispose to plaque-induced gingival diseases/periodontitis
    1. Tooth anatomic factors
    2. Dental restorations/appliances
    3. Root fractures
    4. Cervical root resorption and cemental tears
  B. Mucogingival deformities and conditions around teeth
    1. Gingival/soft tissue recession
      a. Facial or lingual surfaces
      b. Interproximal (papillary)
    2. Lack of keratinized gingiva
    3. Decreased vestibular depth
    4. Aberrant frenum/muscle position
    5. Gingival excess
      a. Pseudopocket
      b. Inconsistent gingival margin
      c. Excessive gingival display
      d. Gingival enlargement (see IA3 and IB4)
    6. Abnormal color
  C. Mucogingival deformities and conditions on edentulous ridges
    1. Vertical and/or horizontal ridge deficiency
    2. Lack of gingiva/keratinized tissue
    3. Gingival/soft tissue enlargement
    4. Aberrant frenum/muscle position
    5. Decreased vestibular depth
    6. Abnormal color
  D. Occlusal trauma
    1. Primary occlusal trauma
    2. Secondary occlusal trauma

*Can occur on a periodontium with no attachment loss or on a periodontium with attachment loss that is not progressing.
†Can be further classified on the basis of extent and severity. As a general guide, extent can be characterized as localized ≤ 30% of sites involved and generalized > 30% of sites involved. Severity can be characterized on the basis of the amount of clinical attachment loss (CAL) as follows: slight = 1–2 mm CAL; moderate = 3–4 mm CAL; and severe = ≥ 5 mm CAL.
Source: "Current Classification of Periodontal Diseases and Conditions" from Development of a classification system for periodontal diseases and conditions by from Armitage G. C. from *Ann Periodontal.* Copyright © 1999 by American Academy of Periodontology. Used by permission of American Academy of Periodontology.

Table 8–3 Definitions of the Extent and Severity of Chronic Periodontitis

Extent	
Localized	when ≤ 30% of the sites are affected
Generalized	when > 30% of the sites are affected
Severity	
Mild	1 to 2 mm clinical attachment loss (CAL)
Moderate	3 to 4 mm CAL
Severe	≥ 5 mm CAL

term "early-onset periodontitis" included prepubertal periodontitis, juvenile periodontitis (localized or LJP and generalized), and rapidly progressive periodontitis. Localized juvenile periodontitis is now termed localized aggressive periodontitis, and generalized juvenile periodontitis is now referred to as generalized aggressive periodontitis. Prepubertal periodontitis with complicating systemic involvement is now included under the heading of periodontitis as a manifestation of systemic diseases (IV).

Refractory periodontitis will no longer have a separate disease classification because any periodontal case can be considered refractory (e.g., localized aggressive periodontitis can be a refractory periodontitis case) or unresponsive to periodontal treatment (e.g., refractory chronic periodontitis).

Chronic Periodontitis

The current classification system of periodontitis (Table 8–1) does not rely on the age of the patient to make a diagnosis. Chronic periodontitis is the most common form of periodontal disease affecting both adults and adolescents and has a slow rate of progression (Löe, Anerud, Boysen, & Morrison, 1986). It is directly related to the presence of plaque. Recently, researchers have documented that genetics may play an important noncontrollable risk factor linked to periodontitis (Newman, 1998). Chronic periodontitis may be modified by and/or associated with systemic diseases (e.g., diabetes mellitus, HIV infection). Also, other nonsystemic factors such as smoking and stress may modify the progression of periodontitis. Table 8–2 reviews common features of different types of periodontitis.

For a person to develop periodontitis, gingivitis must have been present. Even though specific bacteria have been identified as related to the disease, it is still considered a nonspecific bacterial infection. Detection of *Porphyromonas gingivalis* indicates a high probability that periodontitis is present (Christersson, Zambon, Dunford, Grossi, & Genco, 1989). Other local risk factors include calculus, overhanging restorations, and other retentive conditions that favor microbial growth, smoking, systemic conditions, hormonal factors, and stress (American Academy of Periodontology, 1992).

Chronic periodontitis is classified according to the extent and severity of the disease. Extent is defined as the number of sites affected and is divided into localized and generalized (Table 8–3 ■): localized when ≤ 30% of the sites are affected and generalized if > 30% of the sites are affected. Severity is defined as how much disease has occurred and is based on the amount of attachment loss (measurement from the cementoenamel junction to wherever the base of the probe is. This is the clinical attachment level, which is used to determine the amount of attachment loss. Essentially, it is the amount of gingival recession plus the probing depth. If there is no gingival recession, then the attachment level is equal to the probing depth). Severity is classified into mild (or slight), moderate, and severe. Mild = 1 to 2 mm clinical attachment loss; moderate = 3 to 4 mm clinical attachment loss; and severe = ≥ 5 mm clinical attachment loss. When recognizing that the patient has chronic periodontitis, the extent and severity should also be noted. Figure 8–10 shows a case of generalized moderate to localized severe chronic periodontitis. Table 8–4 ■ lists common features of periodontitis.

Features of chronic periodontitis include pocket formation and alveolar and supporting bone destruction (see Figure 8–10). Tooth mobility may not necessarily be evident.

Established risk factors for chronic periodontitis include bacteria within dental plaque, smoking, and diabetes mellitus. Clinical features seen in smokers with periodontitis include deeper probing depths, enhanced gingival recession, more supragingival dental plaque, and more bone loss and attachment loss. There is little clinical gingival inflammation and bleeding because the tissues become less vascular and more fibrotic (thicker gingival tissue), which in a way masks the clinical appearance of inflammation. The nicotine present in tobacco appears to cause constriction of the blood vessels. Smokers also appear to have a decreased PMN migration into the oral cavity and depressed phagocytic function, resulting in a diminished immune host response to bacteria and impaired healing response.

Rapid Dental Hint

Latest news about the periodontitis-systemic connection is that deficiency in vitamin D may play a role in the development of periodontitis (Yao & Fine, 2012).

Table 8-4 Common Features of Periodontitis

Disease	Patient Population	Clinical Features	Causes of the Disease	Microbiologic Features	
Chronic periodontitis (Figure 8–10 ■)	Most prevalent in adults but can occur in children and adolescents	Pocket information; bone loss; inflammation	Primary etiologic factor is dental plaque (poor oral hygiene); many other risk factors (e.g., smoking, systemic diseases)	High numbers of *Porphyromonas gingivalis, Tannerella forsythensis, Prevotella intermedia,* and *Eikenella corrodens*	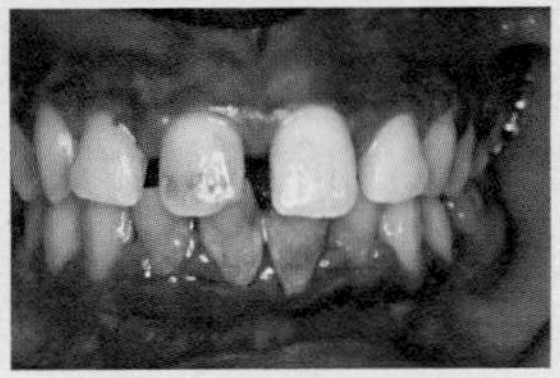 **FIGURE 8–10** Chronic periodontitis.
Generalized aggressive periodontitis (Figure 8–11 ■)	Usually affects persons under 30 years of age but patients may be older	Generalized: Severe gingival inflammation rapid bone destruction affecting at least three permanent teeth other than first molars and incisors	Defect in polymorphonuclear (PMN) and/or macrophage function	Some predominant bacteria include *Prevotella intermedia, Aggregatibacter actinomycetemcomitans*	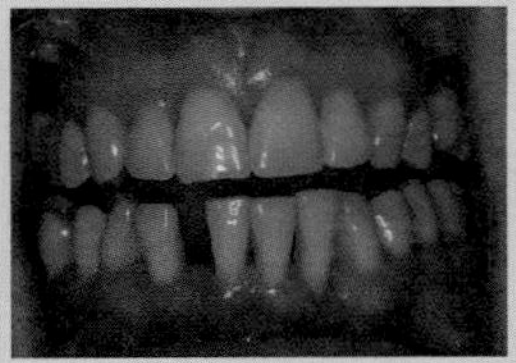 **FIGURE 8–11** Aggressive periodontitis in an adolescent.
Localized aggressive periodontitis (Figure 8–12 ■)	Except for the presence of periodontitis, patients are otherwise clinically healthy; puberty onset	Sparse amount of plaque and calculus; little inflammation Localized: Incisor and first molar sites	Defect in PMN chemotaxis	*Aggregatibacter actinomycetemcomitans, Capnocytophaga* species	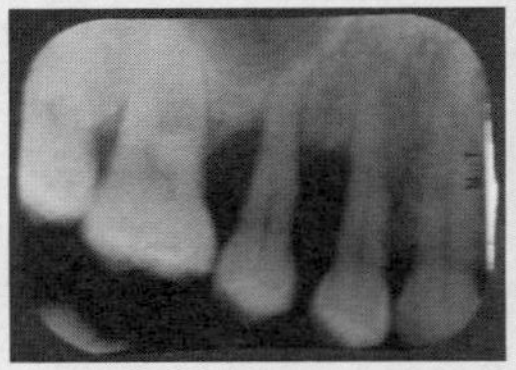 **FIGURE 8–12** Localized aggressive periodontitis.

Aggressive Periodontitis

At the 1999 International Workshop for a Classification of Periodontal Diseases and Conditions, the American Academy of Periodontology suggested to eliminate the old term "early-onset periodontitis" because it was too restrictive in terms of age. Early-onset periodontitis included prepubertal periodontitis, juvenile periodontitis, and rapidly progressive periodontitis. Aggressive periodontitis (AgP) can occur at any age, and the disease is not necessarily confined to individuals under age 35. The term "aggressive periodontitis" was chosen because it is a rapidly progressive form of periodontitis and is less dependent on the age of the individual than "early-onset periodontitis" (Tonetti & Mombelli, 1999; see Figures 8–12 ■, 8–13 ■).

Aggressive periodontitis (AgP) is divided into localized and generalized. *Localized aggressive periodontitis* (LAP) replaces the older term *localized juvenile periodontitis* (LJP), and *generalized aggressive periodontitis* (GAP) replaces the older term *generalized juvenile periodontitis* (GLP). Individuals with aggressive periodontitis have specific clinical and laboratory findings that make it distinctively different from chronic periodontitis. The common features of localized and generalized aggressive periodontitis are the following (Tonetti & Mombelli, 1999):

- Except for the presence of periodontitis, patients are otherwise clinically healthy.
- Rapid attachment loss and bone destruction.
- Familial disposition.
- Inflammatory infiltrate in the tissues is predominately plasma cells (Smith, Seymour, & Cullinan, 2010)

Secondary features that may be present include the following:

- Amounts of microbial deposits are inconsistent with the severity of the periodontal tissue destruction.

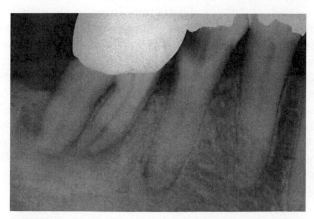

FIGURE 8–13 Radiograph of an endodontic-periodontic lesion. Mandibular first molar: The infection originated in the pulp and spread from the apex (periapical pathology) coronally into the periodontal ligament creating a probable pocket on the distal. Not only is there an endodontic infection but there is also deep probing depths with bone loss on the distal. The premolar has an endodontic lesion.

Rapid Dental Hint

Chronic and aggressive periodontitis are both plasma cell-dominated diseases.

- Elevated levels of *Aggregatibacter actinomycetem-comitans* and, in some populations, *Porphyromonas gingivalis*.
- Progression of attachment loss and bone loss may be self-arresting.
- Phagocyte abnormalities.

Features of localized aggressive periodontitis include the following:

- Circumpubertal onset.
- Serum antibody response to the bacteria.
- Localized first molar/incisor presentation with interproximal attachment loss on at least two permanent teeth, one of which is a first molar, and involving no more than two teeth other than first molars and incisors.

Features of generalized aggressive periodontitis include the following:

- Usually affecting individuals under 30 years of age, but can be older.
- Pronounced episodic nature of the destruction of attachment and bone.
- Poor antibody response to the bacteria.
- Generalized interproximal attachment loss and bone destruction affecting at least three permanent teeth other than first molars and incisors.

It should be noted that not all characteristics listed must be present to assign a diagnosis or classify the disease. The diagnosis may be based on clinical, radiographic, and historical data (Tonetti & Mombelli, 1999). Adjunctive lab testing may be used to help with the diagnosis.

To these primary classifications, secondary descriptors may be added. For example, risk factors that modify the disease progression include cigarette smoking, emotional stress, drugs, and sex hormones.

Rapid Dental Hint

How do you determine if an aggressive case is localized or generalized? Remember that generalized disease affects at least three permanent teeth other than first molars and incisors, and localized affects at least two permanent teeth, one a first molar, and involving no more than two teeth other than first molars and incisors.

Rapid Dental Hint

Remember, periodontitis can be linked to heart conditions and diabetes mellitus. That is why it is important to do appropriate patient assessments.

Etiology

A distinguishing feature found in AgP that is not seen in chronic periodontitis is the presence of polymorphonuclear (PMN) and macrophage defects (Page et al., 1983). These white blood cells do not function properly in eliminating the bacteria. Thus, there is a strong genetic or heredity component to this disease, which means that genetic factors may be important in the development of AgP. Children with GAgP are more prone to ear, skin, and upper respiratory tract infections (Suzuki, 1988).

Plaque accumulation is minimal in LAgP, there is slight gingival inflammation, and bone loss is not as rapid as in the generalized form. There is usually no accompanying infection. Patients may have either defective PMNs or macrophages, but not both. There is a defect in PMN chemotaxis and impaired phagocytosis in 70% to 80% of patients (Suzuki, Collison, Falkler, & Nauman, 1984). The PMNs are not working properly and arrive late to the diseased site (depressed chemotaxis), so they cannot properly devour the foreign material, including bacteria (impaired phagocytosis).

Predominant bacteria in LAP include *Aggregatibacter actinomycetemcomitans*, *Prevotella intermedia*, *Eikenella corrodens*, *Campylobacter rectus*, and *Capnocytophaga* species (American Academy of Periodontology, 1989). High numbers of *Aggregatibacter actinomycetemcomitans* in the subgingival pocket are associated with the localized form, and they may invade the soft tissue (epithelium and connective tissue) rather than just staying in the pocket (Saglie, Carranza, Newman, Cheng, & Lewin, 1982).

Refractory and Recurrent Periodontitis

Refractory periodontitis is a type of periodontitis wherein periodontitis patients previously treated conventionally (periodontal debridement, periodontal surgery, oral hygiene instructions) do not respond favorably to therapy and are

Rapid Dental Hint

Because about 90% of LAP have high counts of *Aggregatibacter actinomycetemcomitans*, these patients will require a systemic antibiotic because this periodontal pathogen does not stay in the pocket area and invades the soft tissues. Root debridement and surgery cannot reach the bacteria in the soft tissue.

considered resistant to treatment. Persistent periodontitis in patients with poor compliance with home care or heavy tobacco use precludes the use of the term *refractory*. These patients more likely have recurrent periodontitis. High numbers of *Prevotella intermedia*, *Tannerella forsythensis*, *Fusobacterium nucleatum*, and *Porphyromonas gingivalis* are found in subgingival refractory sites. Recurrent periodontitis is periodontitis that recurs.

Under the new classification system (Armitage, 1999), periodontitis associated with refractory and recurrent conditions has been eliminated as a separate disease category. It was concluded that only a small percentage of periodontitis cases are actually nonresponsive to treatment. Instead, the refractory designation could be applied to all forms of periodontitis (e.g., refractory chronic periodontitis, refractory aggressive periodontitis).

Periodontitis Associated with Endodontic Lesions

Lesions of the periodontal ligament and adjacent alveolar bone may originate from interactions of the periodontium or tissues of the dental pulp (Meng, 1999). Infections coming from the pulp can cause tissue destruction that proceeds from the apical region (apical foramen) of a tooth coronally toward the gingival margin. Thus, there may be communication between endodontic and periodontal lesions (Figure 8–13).

Periodontitis as a Manifestation of Systemic Diseases

Dental plaque initiates periodontal diseases but the form of disease and its progression is dependent on the host defenses to this challenge. Systemic conditions and environmental exposures may modify the normal defenses and influence the outcome of periodontal disease (Kinane, 1999). A reduction in the number of function of polymorphonuclear leukocytes (PMNs) usually results in increased rate and severity of periodontal tissue destruction. In addition, numerous drugs such as phenytoin, nifedipine, and cyclosporine predispose to gingival overgrowth in response to plaque and thus may be an effect in modifying preexisting periodontitis (Kinane, 1999). Several systemic diseases such as diabetes mellitus (Lalla, 2007; Mealey & Ocampo, 2007), Down syndrome, Papillon-Lefévre syndrome, hypophosphatasia, Chediak-Higashi syndrome, and HIV infection also appear to predispose individuals to periodontitis. These patients also have compromised host responses. Certain environmental conditions or exposures including cigarette smoking and emotional stress may modify periodontitis.

Periodontitis as a Risk Factor for Systemic Conditions

This topic is not included in the 1999 AAP Classification of Periodontal Diseases and is discussed thoroughly in Chapter 6. There is strong evidence relating periodontal disease and diabetes, cardiovascular disease, respiratory diseases, and adverse pregnancy outcomes.

Peri-Implant Diseases

Inflammatory conditions surrounding dental implants are becoming more common today, as more implants are being placed. Periodontal disease around implants is not listed in the original or new classification from the American Academy of Periodontology; however, inflammation and periodontal destruction around implants is clinically recognized. Loss of an implant after successful placement is often due to a bacterial infection. Gram-negative anaerobes, primarily the *Fusobacterium* species and *Prevotella intermedia*, are found in the subgingival pockets. **Peri-implant disease** is a collective term for soft-tissue inflammation surrounding an implant. Peri-implant mucositis is the term used to describe reversible inflammation in the gingiva around a functioning implant (Albrektsson & Isidor, 1994). Peri-implantitis is the term used for inflammatory changes in the soft tissues leading to loss of supporting bone around a functioning implant (Froum, Froum, & Rosen, 2012; Albrektsson & Isidor, 1994; Figure 8–14 ■). The primary risk factor for peri-implant diseases is the presence of certain bacteria (Mombelli & Lang, 1998).

Treatment of peri-implant diseases is based on proper clinical and radiographic assessment. It may include periodontal debridement, oral hygiene instruction, mouth rinses, systemic antibiotics, periodontal surgery, or removal of the implant.

Treatment of Periodontitis

The treatment for all types of periodontal diseases begins with oral hygiene care and nonsurgical therapy (scaling and root planing). Smoking cessation is also included in the treatment plan. Reevaluation of initial therapy at 4 to 8 weeks (Segelnick & Weinberg, 2006) will determine further treatment needs. Periodontal surgery may be required for pocket elimination or reduction. All patients will be placed on a maintenance schedule. Patients with chronic periodontitis do not require any systemic antibiotics. However, in selected cases, if the patient is having a difficult time with home care, a mouth rinse such as chlorhexidine may be recommended as an adjunct to periodontal debridement procedures. Patients with aggressive periodontitis will require a systemic antibiotic during scaling and root planing

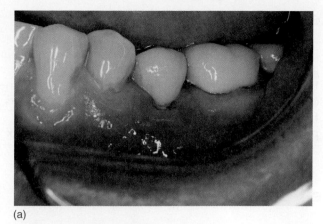

(a)

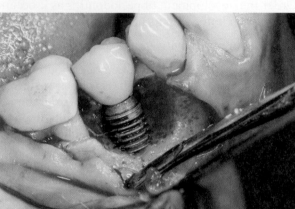

(b)

FIGURE 8–14 A case of peri-implantitis. (a) The gingiva was bleeding, was red, and had significant probing depth. (b) A gingival flap was reflected. Note bone loss is approximately to the sixth thread. Bone loss to the first thread is considered normal.

and periodontal surgery because *Aggregatibacter actinomycetemcomitans*, which is found in more than 90% of LAP, have invaded the epithelium and connective tissue, making root debridement and periodontal surgery ineffective in bacterial elimination (Renvert, Wikström, Dahlén, Slots, & Egelberg, 1990; Saglie et al., 1982).

Periodontal patients with diabetes who show poor oral health should be placed in a monitored oral health program that will take care of both the patient's dental and general health (Bakhshandeh, Murtomaa, Mofid, Vehkalahti, & Suomalainen, 2007).

Dental Hygiene Application

Periodontitis is classified based on clinical presentation rather than age, as was done in previous classification systems. Periodontitis is a microbial infection that is the result of host–bacteria interactions. Periodontitis is characterized by attachment loss with subsequent bone loss. Different patterns of bone loss are evident on radiographs. Periodontitis can be modified by systemic

factors wherein the host has a reduced capacity to resist infection.

The dental hygienist must differentiate between gingivitis and periodontitis because treatment options will differ. To treat a clinical case of periodontal disease, the dental hygienist must have an understanding of the the histogenesis and pathogenesis of the disease.

Key Points

- Periodontitis is inflammation that extends from the gingiva into the supporting periodontal structures.
- Periodontitis is most common in adults, although it does occur in a smaller number of children and adolescents.
- Dental plaque (biofilm) is the major risk factor for periodontal diseases; there are other contributory risk factors such as medications, hormones, and systemic diseases.
- Inflammatory periodontal disease is also seen around dental implants.
- Both chronic and aggressive periodontitis are plasma cell–dominated lesions.

Self-Quiz

1. Order the development of periodontitis as it occurs. Match each letter with its proper sequence number.

   Progression of gingivitis to periodontitis

   1. healthy gingiva
   2. initial lesion
   3. established lesion
   4. advanced lesion

   a. destruction of periodontal ligament fibers (principle fibers)
   b. apical and lateral migration of the junctional epithelium
   c. destruction of gingival fibers
   d. bone resorption
   e. formation of periodontal pocket
   f. PMNs present
   g. plasma cell predominate

2. The latest classification of periodontitis is based on all of the following factors except one. Which one is the exception?
   a. Age of patient
   b. Clinical presentation
   c. Radiographic survey
   d. Historical data
   e. Microbial profile

3. Which one of the following forms of periodontitis is associated with a chemotactic defect in the polymorphonuclear leukocytes or machrophages?
   a. Dental plaque–induced gingivitis
   b. Chronic periodontitis
   c. Puberty gingivitis
   d. Localized aggressive periodontitis
   e. Drug-influenced gingivitis

4. Which one of the following bacteria is found in high numbers in localized aggressive periodontitis?
   a. *Prophyromonas gingivalis*
   b. *Prevotella intermedia*
   c. *Actinomyces viscosus*
   d. *Aggregatibacter actinomycetemcomitans*
   e. *Streptococcus sanguis*

5. For each type of pocket listed, select the correct definition from the list provided.

   1. Gingival
   2. Suprabony
   3. Infrabony

   a. base of pocket located apical to the alveolar crest
   b. base of pocket located coronal to the alveolar crest
   c. marginal gingival enlargement with base of pocket at cementoenamel junction

6. For each type of severity and extent of periodontitis, select the correct definition or description from the list provided.

   Chronic periodontitis

   1. localized chronic periodontitis
   2. generalized chronic periodontitis
   3. mild chronic periodontitis
   4. moderate chronic periodontitis
   5. severe chronic periodontitis

   Description

   a. > 30% of sites are affected
   b. 1 to 2 mm of clinical attachment loss
   c. ≤ 30% of sites are affected
   d. 3 to 4 mm of clinical attachment loss
   e. > 5 mm of clinical attachment loss

7. Which periodontal lesion, according to Page and Schroeder (1976), is characterized by attachment loss and bone resorption?
   a. Initial
   b. Early
   c. Established
   d. Advanced

8. A periodontal pocket forms when
   a. the junctional epithelium migrates apically and laterally from the tooth surface.
   b. gingival fibers proliferate.
   c. bacteria multiply in the pocket.
   d. alveolar bone loss occurs.

9. All of the following factors are responsible for bone loss except one. Which one is the exception?
   a. Prostaglandins
   b. Endotoxins
   c. B cells
   d. Hyaluronidase

10. Order the stages of pathogenesis of periodontitis. Match each letter with its proper sequence number.

1.	a. Bone loss
2.	b. Destruction of periodontal ligament fibers
3.	c. Connective tissue attachment loss
4.	d. Apical and lateral migration of the junctional (pocket) epithelium

Case Study

A 50-year-old male has been a patient for several years. He has had periodontal pockets on several teeth with visible horizontal and vertical bone loss. He has received scaling and root planing in addition to maintenance visits every 4 months. He has no other systemic diseases, does not smoke, and his blood pressure is within normal limits. He asks why he continues to have bleeding points and some of his pockets have gotten deeper over the years. As a dental hygienist your role is to explain the following:

1. The major risk factor for periodontal disease is
   a. bone loss
   b. bacterial biofilm
   c. lose restorations
   d. high blood pressure

Answer: B. Bacterial biofilm is the major risk factor and then others aspects such as medications, hormones, or diseases can become contributory factors.

2. The pattern of his vertical bone loss would have been
   a. inflammation travels directly from gingival into periodontal ligament and then to bone
   b. bone resorption occurs form its outer aspect buccal and lingual walls
   c. inflammation travels to crestal bone and then to gingival fibers
   d. junctional epithelium destroyed and then bone

Answer: A. Inflammation extends from the gingival into the supporting periodontal structures, first to the periodontal ligament and then to the bone. The outer buccal and lingual aspects are resorbed in horizontal bone loss.

3. What other nonsurgical care therapies can be recommended to maintain the periodontal pocketing for this chronic periodontal patient?
   a. surgery pocket elimination
   b. systemic antibiotic
   c. chlorhexidine
   d. supragingival scaling

Answer: C. The major risk is biofilm and this does not require antibiotics. The request for nonsurgical care should first utilize modalities such as chlorhexidine to reach the subgingival bacterial biofilm.

References

Albrektsson, T., and F. Isidor. 1994. Consensus report of session IV. In eds. N. P. Lang and T. Karring, *Proceedings of the First European Workshop on Periodontology*, 365–369. London: Quintessence.

American Academy of Periodontology. 1989. *Proceedings of the World Workshop in Clinical Periodontics*, I-2–I-4. Chicago: Author.

American Academy of Periodontology. 1992. *The etiology and pathogenesis of periodontal diseases* (Position Paper), 1–9. Chicago: Author.

American Academy of Periodontology. 2001. *Glossary of periodontal terms*, 4th ed. Chicago: Author.

Armitage, G. C. 1999. Development of a classification system for periodontal diseases and conditions. *Ann. Periodontol.* 4:1–6.

Bakhshandeh, S., H. Murtomaa, R. Mofid, M. M. Vehkalahti, and K. Suomalainen. 2007. Periodontal treatment needs of diabetic adults. *J. Clin. Periodontol.* 34:53–57.

Christersson, L. A., J. J. Zambon, R. G. Dunford, S. G. Grossi, and R. J. Genco. 1989. Specific subgingival bacteria and diagnosis of gingivitis and periodontitis. *J. Dent. Res.* 68:1633–1639.

Froum, S. J., S. H. Froum, and P. S. Rosen. 2012. Successful management of peri-implantitis with a regenerative approach: A consecutive series of 51 treated implants with 3- to 7.5-year follow-up. *International Journal of Periodontics and Restorative Dentistry* 32:11–20.

Goodson, J. M. 1992. Diagnosis of periodontitis by physical measurement: Interpretation from episodic disease hypothesis. *J. Periodontol.* 63:373–382.

Greenstein, G. 1992. Periodontal response to mechanical nonsurgical therapy. *J. Periodontol.* 63:118–130.

Hughes, F. J., D. W. Augr, and F. C. Smales. 1988. Investigation of the distribution of cementum-associated lipopolysaccharides in periodontal disease by scanning electron microscope immunohistochemistry. *J. Periodont. Res.* 23:100–102.

Ishikawa, I., K. Nakashima, T. Koseki, et al. 1997. Induction of the immune response to periodontopathic bacteria and its role in the pathogenesis of periodontitis. *Periodontology 2000* 14:79–111.

Kinane, D. F. 1999. Periodontitis modified by systemic factors. *Ann. Periodontal.* 4:54–63.

Lalla, E. 2007. Periodontal infections and diabetes mellitus: When will the puzzle be complete? *J. Clin. Periodontol.* 34:913–916.

Löe, H., A. Anerud, H. Boysen, and E. Morrison. 1986. Natural history of periodontal disease in man. Rapid, moderate and no loss of attachment in Sri Lankan laborers 14 to 46 years of age. *J. Clin. Periodontol.* 13:431–440.

Mealey, B. L., and G. L. Ocampo. 2007. Diabetes and periodontal disease. *Periodontology 2000* 44(1):127–153.

Meng, H. X. 1999. Periodontic-endodontic lesions. *Ann. Periodontol.* 4:84–89.

Mombelli, A., and N. P. Lang. 1998. The diagnosis and treatment of periimplantitis. *Periodontology 2000* 17:63–76.

Müller-Glauser, W., and H. H. Schroeder. 1982. The pocket epithelium: A light- and electron-microscopic study. *J. Periodontol.* 53:133–144.

Nakib, N. M., N. F. Bissada, J. W. Simmenlink, and S. N. Golstine. 1982. Endotoxin penetration into root cementum of periodontally healthy and diseased human teeth. *J. Periodontol.* 53:638–678.

Newman, M. 1998. Genetic, environmental, and behavioral influences on periodontal infections. *Compendium* (special issue) 19:25–31.

Offenbacher, S., P. A. Heasman, and J. G. Collins. 1993. Modulation of host PGE2 secretion as a determinant of periodontal disease expression. *J. Periodontol.* 64:432–444.

Page, R. C., T. Bowen, L. Altman, E. Vandesteen, H. Ochs, et al. 1983. Prepubertal periodontitis I. Definition of a clinical disease entity. *J. Periodontol.* 54:257–271.

Page, R. C., and H. E. Schroeder. 1976. Pathogenesis of inflammatory periodontal disease. A summary of current work. *Lab Investigations* 33:235–249.

Prichard, J. F. 1979. Management of intrabony defects. In ed. J. F. Prichard, *The diagnosis and treatment of periodontal disease*, 358–361. Philadelphia: W. B. Saunders.

Renvert, S., M. Wikström, G. Dahlén, J. Slots, and J. Egelberg. 1990. On the inability of root debridement and periodontal surgery to eliminate *Aggregatibacter actinomycetemocomitans* from periodontal pockets. *J. Clin. Periodontol.* 17:351–355.

Reynolds, J. J., and M. C. Meikle. 1997. Mechanisms of connective tissue matrix destruction in periodontitis. *Periodontology 2000* 14:144–157.

Saglie, R. F., F. A. Carranza, Jr., M. G. Newman, L. Cheng, and K. J. Lewin. 1982. Identification of tissue-invading bacteria in human periodontal disease. *J. Periodontol. Res.* 17:452–455.

Schwartz, Z., J. Goultschin, D. D. Dean, and B. D. Boyan. 1997. Mechanisms of alveolar bone destruction in periodontitis. *Periodontology 2000* 14:158–172.

Segelnick, S. L., and M. A. Weinberg. 2006. Reevaluation of initial therapy: When is the appropriate time? *J. Periodontol.* 77:1598–1601.

Smith, M., G. J. Seymour, and M. P. Cullinan. 2010. Histopathological features of chronic and aggressive periodontitis. *Periodontology 2000* 53:45–54.

Socransky, S. S., and A. D. Haffajee. 1997. The nature of periodontal diseases. *Ann. Periodontol.* 2:3–10.

Suzuki, J. B. 1988. Diagnosis and classification of periodontal diseases. *Dent. Clin. North America* 32:195–216.

Suzuki, J. B., B. C. Collison, W. A. Falkler, and R. R. Nauman. 1984. Immunologic profile of juvenile periodontitis. II. Neutrophil chemotaxis, phagocytosis and spore germination. *J. Periodontol.* 55:461–467.

Tal, H. 1984. Relationship between the interproximal distance of roots and the prevalence of intrabony pockets. *J. Periodontol.* 55:604–607.

Tonetti, M. S., and A. Mombelli. 1999. Early-onset periodontitis. *Ann. Periodontol.* 4:39–52.

Weinberg, M. A., and R. N. Eskow. 2000. Osseous effects: Proper terminology revisited. *J. Periodontol.* 71:1928.

Yao, S. G., and J. B. Fine. 2012. A review of vitamin D as it relates to periodontal disease. *Compend. Contin. Educ. Dent.* 33:166–171.

9

Necrotizing Periodontal Diseases

Surendra Singh

OUTLINE

Introduction

Necrotizing Ulcerative Gingivitis (NUG)

Necrotizing Ulcerative Periodontitis (NUP)

Dental Hygiene Application

Key Points

Self-Quiz

Case Study

References

EDUCATIONAL OBJECTIVES

Upon completion of this chapter, the reader should be able to:

- Explain the current classification of ulcerative periodontal diseases.
- Describe the features of periodontal ulcerative gingivitis.
- Define the role of the dental hygienist in the treatment of necrotizing ulcerative gingivitis.
- Describe the features of periodontal ulcerative periodontitis.

GOAL: To provide an understanding of the etiology, clinical features, and treatment of necrotizing periodontal diseases.

KEY WORDS

necrotizing periodontal diseases *136*

necrotizing ulcerative gingivitis *136*

necrotizing ulcerative periodontitis *136*

Introduction

Necrotizing periodontal diseases are unique from other periodontal diseases. Necrotizing periodontal diseases include **necrotizing ulcerative gingivitis** (NUG) and **necrotizing ulcerative periodontitis** (NUP). The term *acute necrotizing ulcerative gingivitis* (ANUG) was changed to *necrotizing ulcerative gingivitis* (NUG). The American Academy of Periodontology decided that the term *acute* was a clinical descriptive term and should not be used as a diagnostic classification because there is no chronic form of NUG (Rowland, 1999).

Even though necrotizing periodontal diseases are classified as a separate entity, these conditions may actually be manifestations of underlying systemic problems (e.g., HIV infection). In addition, other risk factors include tobacco smoking, preexisting periodontal disease, and trauma.

Necrotizing Ulcerative Gingivitis (NUG)

Clinical features of necrotizing ulcerative gingivitis (NUG) are different from other periodontal diseases (e.g., biofilm-associated gingivitis). Necrotizing ulcerative gingivitis is a rapidly destructive, recurring, noncommunicable gingival infection. NUG is considered a type of necrotizing periodontal disease limited to the gingival tissues (Armitage, 1999). NUG is relatively uncommon (incidence 0.1% to 10%) and mostly affects young adults 18 to 30 years old (Škach, Zábrodský, & Mrklas, 1970). It has also been known as "trench mouth" or "Vincent's infection." During World War I, NUG reached very high levels of incidence and was called "trench mouth," referring to the trenches soldiers inhabited during the war. In addition to bacteria, other predisposing factors are emotional stress, cigarette smoking, or decreased nutritional intake. During stressful periods, oral hygiene measures may decrease, smoking may increase, and the immune function may be suppressed.

Clinical Features

NUG is clinically characterized by small, gray, ulcerative lesions that begin at the tips of the interdental papillae and spread to the gingival margin to form punched-out or cratered lesions. A grayish-white pseudomembrane covering the affected areas may be present. A prominent sign of NUG is punched-out, ulcerated (necrotic) interdental papillae, which are caused by ulcer formation on the tip of the papillae. Early on in the condition the lesions usually are confined to the top of a few interdental papillae and are often initially seen in the mandibular anterior region. The marginal gingiva is bright red, inflamed, and extremely painful. Patients complain of difficulty eating and a burning sensation in the mouth. There is spontaneous gingival bleeding (i.e., the gingiva bleeds when touched or during eating). There are usually heavy deposits of dental biofilm; oral hygiene is usually poor. These signs and symptoms are sudden in onset, localized, and recurrent. If left untreated, the infection may spread to the underlying periodontal structures. Lymphadenopathy (lymph nodes that are abnormal in size, consistency, or number), fever, and fetid oral odor (foul mouth odor) are variable findings and not always present. The signs and symptoms of NUG usually resolve a few days after adequate treatment, however (Table 9–1 ■ Figure 9–1 ■). *Three criteria must be present for a diagnosis, of NUG: (1) pain, (2) bleeding, and (3) interproximal necrosis.*

This condition is usually recognized on the basis of clinical signs and symptoms. It has a bacterial origin and is confirmed to be an infectious disease because reduction of dental biofilm either by mechanical debridement or the use of antibiotics will resolve clinical signs and symptoms.

Oral findings do not seem to correspond to supragingival dental biofilm accumulation (Mealey, 1996) because removal of dental biofilm does not improve the gingival condition as typically seen in chronic, biofilm-associated gingivitis. The lesion is confined to the gingiva and does not involve bone loss. Pain is the hallmark of NUG (Rowland, 1999). It is important for dental practitioners to recognize soft tissue lesions early because they may be the first signs of HIV infection (Mealey, 1996; Winkler, Grassi, & Murray, 1988; Winkler & Robertson, 1992).

A complete laboratory workup is indicated in the management of patients with NUG, especially if a systemic disease is suspected or if the patient does not respond to conventional therapy (Murayama, Kurihara, Nagai, Dompkowski, & Van Dyke, 1994).

Did You Know?

Necrotizing periodontal disease used to be called "trench mouth" because of its prevalence among soldiers who were stuck in the trenches during World War I without the means to properly take care of their teeth.

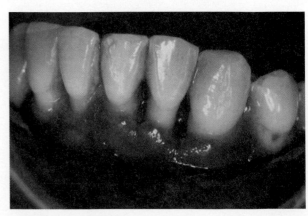

FIGURE 9–1 NUG.

Table 9–1 Common Features of Necrotizing Periodontal Diseases

Disease	Patient Population	Clinical Features	Causes of the Disease	Microbiologic Features	Figure
Necrotizing ulcerative gingivitis (NUG)	Usually young adults	Lesions develop quickly; punched-out interdental papillae, pain, and bleeding	Inadequate oral hygiene; emotional stress; cigarette smoking; immunosuppression	Specific bacteria: spirochetes, *Prevotella intermedia, Fusobacterium nucleatum*	See Figure 9–1
Necrotizing ulcerative periodontitis (NUP)	HIV-infected individuals	Periodontal involvement of deeper structures; rapid loss of attachment, bone loss	Immunodeficiency	Similar to chronic periodontitis; bacteria: *Porphyromonas gingivalis, P. intermedia, F. nucleatum.* Also *Candida albicans*	See Figure 9–2

Immunosuppression

Depressed PMN function (chemotactic, phagocytic) is suppressed in patients with NUG. NUG may also be the first sign of HIV infection. HIV-infected patients may present with severe forms of periodontal diseases. These patients are immunodeficient with a specific decrease in CD4+ lymphocytes. Conflicting reports concerning the classification system of HIV-associated periodontal lesions exist. New terminology was proposed in the early 1990s that is recognized by the United States and the rest of the world (EEC-Clearinghouse, 1993).

Necrotizing ulcerative gingivitis in HIV-infected patients is characterized by the destruction of one or more interdental papillae that became ulcerated, cratered, and necrotic (Murray, 1994), but there is no bone loss. NUG may represent an early form of NUP (Mealey, 1996).

Microbiological Features

Microbiological samples of the affected areas show specific bacteria. High numbers of *Prevotella intermedia*, spirochetes (*Treponema* sp.), and *Fusobacterium* sp. have been isolated (Loesche, Syed, Laughon, & Stoll, 1982). Spirochetes have been shown to penetrate deep into the connective tissue (Listgarten & Lewis, 1967). Normally, bacteria stay in the pocket and do not invade the underlying tissues. Thus, NUG is a manifestation of a mixed bacterial infection modified by particular systemic determinants.

The microorganisms present in the gingival lesions of HIV-positive patients are not similar to the microorganisms found in the gingival lesions of HIV-negative individuals but may be similar to those found in HIV-negative individuals who have chronic periodontitis (Mealey, 1996; Murray, Winkler, Peros, French, & Lippke, 1991). Implicating pathogens include *Porphyromonas gingivalis* (Pg), *Prevotella intermedia* (Pi), *Aggregatibacter actinomycetemcomitans* (Aa),

Fusobacterium nucleatum, spirochetes, and *Candida albicans* (fungus; American Academy of Periodontology, 1992).

Differential Diagnosis

Differential diagnosis of NUG includes primary herpetic gingivostomatitis, recurrent aphthous ulcer (canker sores), desquamatous gingivitis, acute leukemia, and infectious mononucleosis. Primary herpetic gingivostomatitis occurs in a much younger patient; an elevated temperature is more common, and the patient appears more ill and shows a general malaise. The oral lesions in primary herpes are vesicles that coalesce into ulcers, which occur on the attached gingival and oral mucosa. The papillae are not punched out as in NUG.

Thus, primary herpetic gingivostomatitis is a differential diagnosis of necrotizing ulcerative gingivitis. Actually, NUG can be easily recognized when interproximal papillae necrosis, bleeding, and pain are all seen. If these three features are not present, a diagnosis of NUG cannot be made.

Linear gingival erythema (LGE) is a condition with specific features. Originally LGE was directly linked with HIV-positive patients and hence called HIV-associated gingivitis (HIV-G). However, because research has shown that LGE can occur in HIV-negative patients, it is no longer named HIV-G. The clinical feature of LGE is a distinct red band about 2 to 3 mm in width around the free gingival margin. There is no specific treatment for LGE because it is not associated with the presence of biofilm.

Treatment

Severe pain is often the primary reason a patient seeks treatment. It is important to treat NUG immediately. If left untreated, extensive permanent papillae destruction can occur. Even with treatment, recurrent lesions are common. The patient is in a lot of pain, and even eating is a problem.

Because of this intense pain, it may be impossible to perform any type of periodontal debridement on the first office visit. If debridement is started, gentle ultrasonic or sonic instrumentation is the best choice. A systemic analgesic and antibiotic may be prescribed on the first office visit. After a few days, when the pain has reduced, the patient should return to the office for periodontal debridement.

Treatment of NUG is divided into two phases: acute and maintenance. The objective of the acute phase is to eliminate disease activity. Treatment on the first day consists of data collection (e.g., medical/dental history, chief complaint) and making the correct diagnosis. Initial supragingival debridement should be performed, if the patient can tolerate it. Usually, the patient is in too much pain, and the first step is to place the patient on a systemic analgesic (e.g., ibuprofen; make sure there are no drug/drug or drug/disease interactions) to eliminate the pain and a systemic antibiotic to eliminate the bacterial infection (Table 9-2 ■). Subgingival debridement is contraindicated during this initial visit because of possible spread of the infection to deeper tissues.

Because this is a bacterial infection with bacteria present within the gingival tissues, antibiotics may be indicated including metronidazole (250 mg three times a day), tetracycline, or penicillin. Although symptoms diminish within 24 hours, the antibiotic should still be taken for the prescribed time. Topical antibiotics (e.g., Arestin) are not indicated in the treatment of necrotizing ulcerative diseases.

Toothbrushing should be avoided, and instead patients are instructed to rinse twice daily with a mixture of 1 tablespoon of 3% hydrogen peroxide in 1/2 glass or one-half glass warm water, an oxygenating rinse such as GlyOxide (Wennström & Lindhe, 1979), or chlorhexidine; brushing is usually impossible due to extreme oral pain. The patient is advised to avoid alcohol and tobacco, eat a balanced diet, and rest. Within 1 day the patient should see much improvement, with alleviation of pain and the infection under control. The patient then returns to the office for supragingival debridement with ultrasonic or sonic scalers and hand instrumentation (anesthesia is given) and adequate water spray. Depending on the patient's tolerance, complete debridement may take a few visits. When debridement is finished, the patient will return in a few days so that a gingival examination can be done to evaluate the gingival architecture. When gingival tissues have healed, plaque control instructions are given and instruction on the elimination of other risk factors such as smoking cessation. The patient is instructed to use a soft toothbrush and interproximal devices (Box 9-1).

Box 9–1: Patient Education

- Good oral hygiene is critical.
- Resume daily brushing and flossing after the acute phase is treated.
- Use an ultrasoft bristled toothbrush.
- Drink fluids.
- Avoid smoking.
- Avoid spicy foods.
- Maintain proper nutrition.
- Get plenty of sleep/rest.
- Eliminate or reduce emotional stress.
- Frequent professional oral maintenance.
- Avoid eating or drinking for at least 30 minutes after rinsing with chlorhexidine.
- If metronidazole is prescribed, the patient must not intake any type of alcohol.

Table 9–2 Treatment Steps for Necrotizing Ulcerative Gingivitis

First appointment	Supragingival debridement, if the patient can tolerate it. If not, get the patient out of pain with an analgesic agent. Instead of brushing, instruct the patient to rinse twice daily with either chlorhexidine (twice a day), warm water/hydrogen peroxide, or an oxygenating agent.
Second appointment (day 1–2)	When patient is out of pain, supragingival debridement (power-driven scalers) is recommended to start.
Third appointment (successive days)	Continued periodontal debridement under topical/local anesthesia. Oral hygiene instructions given (ultrasoft toothbrush gently). Control of other risk factors (e.g., smoking cessation, emotional stress).
Fourth appointment	Maintenance phase: If necessary, referral to periodontist to surgically correct gingival architecture.
Fifth appointment	Two-month periodontal maintenance.

When the acute phase is completed, the maintenance phase begins. The patient is placed on a 2-month maintenance schedule. Once the necrotic gingiva has healed, the gingival craters may persist and act as plaque traps. Referral to a periodontist for surgical correction of gingival craters is recommended.

Necrotizing Ulcerative Periodontitis (NUP)

Necrotizing ulcerative periodontitis may also be the first clinical sign of underlying systemic disease, such as in human immunodeficiency virus (HIV) infection (Murayama et al., 1994).

Necrotizing ulcerative periodontitis is not limited to HIV infections and is often seen in patients who are immunosuppressed (Armitage, 1999). However, this form of periodontal disease in the HIV-positive patient may coexist with other forms of periodontitis such as aggressive or chronic periodontitis. NUP is characterized by the extensive necrosis of the gingiva with exposure, loss of attachment, and rapid destruction of the underlying bone extending past the mucogingival junction (Figure 9–2 ∎). If not successfully treated, NUP can spread into the adjacent maxilla and mandible (Mealey, 1996). Essentially, all NUP sites bleed on probing, and about 50% of sites show spontaneous bleeding (American Academy of Periodontology, 1992). Extensive clinical attachment loss is common, but deep periodontal pocket formation is not evident (American Academy of Periodontology, 1992).

The microbial population of subgingival sites with NUP is similar to that of chronic periodontitis, which is also similar to NUG. This may prove that NUG may be a precursor to the recession (attachment loss) and bone destruction seen in NUP (Murray, 1994).

Essentially, patients with necrotizing ulcerative periodontitis (NUP) have the same gingival features as seen in NUG except there is also loss of attachment and bone

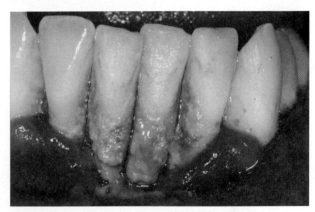

FIGURE 9–2 NUP.

destruction. Many NUP patients are immunosuppressed (low neutrophil levels; e.g., HIV). In NUP patients, treatment is aimed at periodontal debridement, improved oral hygiene self-care, and frequent use of an antiplaque rinse or irrigant such as chlorhexidine gluconate. Oral fungal infections are sometimes present due to the patient's immunosuppressed state, and these may require antifungal medication. Patients with HIV/AIDs are more prone to developing opportunistic infections because of a weakened immune system (e.g., CD4 count less than 500). Fungal infections are an example of an opportunistic infection. Antibiotic use is a common cause of the development of an opportunistic infection. Referral to a periodontist is recommended.

HIV-related oral lesions may not fully respond to therapy. Periodontal debridement may expose necrotic bone that should be removed. Local anesthesia, pain medication, and antibiotics may be necessary. Frequent periodontal maintenance visits are recommended. Oral care should be provided in collaboration with the patient's physician. Referral to a periodontist should be considered.

Dental Hygiene Application

The American Academy of Periodontology refers collectively to necrotizing ulcerative gingivitis (NUG) and necrotizing ulcerative periodontitis (NUP) as ulcerative periodontal diseases (Rowland, 1999). The reason for this is that both NUG and NUP may be considered the same disease but at different stages. Thus, they may not be separate diseases but named under the necrotizing ulcerative diseases. Both NUG and NUP are diseases related to a decreased systemic resistance, as seen in HIV-infected patients, to bacteria present in the periodontal tissues. NUG is confined to the gingival unit, and NUP involves gingiva and the attachment apparatus (bone, cementum, periodontal ligament). Three criteria (pain, bleeding, and papillae necrosis) must be present for a diagnosis of NUG.

Key Points

- NUG and NUP are ulcerative inflammatory periodontal diseases.
- Three criteria must be present for a diagnosis of NUG: pain, bleeding, and papillary necrosis.
- NUG involves the gingival unit only.
- NUP involves recession (attachment loss) and bone loss.

- *Prevotella intermedia* and spirochetes are associated with necrotizing gingivival lesions.
- Treatment of necrotizing ulcerative gingivitis first involves getting the patient out of pain before any debridement is started.

Self-Quiz

1. Which one of the following statements describes a patient with necrotizing periodontal disease?
   a. Higher prevalence in females than males.
   b. Higher incidence of skin lesions.
   c. Pain is a prominent feature.
   d. Geographic distribution shows a higher prevalence in the eastern United States.

2. Which of the following bacterium present in NUG patients may penetrate periodontal tissues?
   a. *Treponema denticola*
   b. *Prevotella intermedia*
   c. *Fusobacterium* species
   d. *Streptococcus sanguis*

3. Both necrotizing ulcerative gingivitis and necrotizing ulcerative periodontitis are currently categorized under the classification of
   a. acute necrotizing diseases.
   b. necrotizing ulcerative diseases.
   c. chronic periodontitis.
   d. aggressive periodontitis.

4. Necrotizing ulcerative gingivitis may be the first clinical sign of an underlying systemic disease such as
   a. human immunodeficiency virus infection.
   b. diabetes mellitus.
   c. osteoporosis.
   d. kidney failure.

5. Which of the following diseases must be differentiated from NUG?
   a. Herpes simplex type 2
   b. Primary herpetic gingivostomatitis
   c. Canker sores
   d. Acquired immunodeficiency syndrome

6. From the following list, select the items associated with NUG.
   a. Pain
   b. Bleeding
   c. Papillary necrosis
   d. Fever

   e. Emotional stress
   f. *Prevotella intermedia*
   g. *Porphyromonas gingivalis*
   h. Spirochetes

7. The distinguishing feature between NUP and NUG is
   a. amount of gingival bleeding.
   b. recession and alveolar bone loss.
   c. number of bacteria present in pocket.
   d. intensity of pain.

8. Which of the following conditions is a concern in immunosuppressed necrotizing ulcerative disease patients?
   a. Fungal infection
   b. Heart problems
   c. Stunting of growth
   d. Protozoa infection

9. A prominent sign of NUG is
   a. high fever.
   b. punched-out interdental papillae.
   c. gingival abscess formation.
   d. alveolar bone loss.

10. Order the treatment sequence as it occurs in necrotizing ulcerative gingivitis.

1.	a. Periodontal debridement with hand instrumentation
2.	b. Analgesics
3.	c. Resume regular toothbrushing and flossing
4.	d. Supragingival debridement with power-driven scaler
5.	e. Referral to periodontist

Case Study

A 20-year-old female comes to the dental hygiene visit in severe pain. The gingival tissue is ulcerated with the gingival margin in punched-out or crated lesions. There is a grayish-white pseudomembrane covering the tissue. The anterior mandibular gingival is bright red and inflamed. There is no apparent bone loss.

1. The most likely diagnosis of this condition is
   a. Aggressive periodontitiis
   b. Refractory periodontitis
   c. Necrotizing ulcerative gingivitis
   d. Necrotizing ulcerative periodontitis

Answer: C. Given the classic description of the gingival and lack of known bone loss the condition would most likely be NUG. The other three selections require bone loss

2. The dental hygienist would first begin to implement
   a. definitive scaling procedures
   b. chlorhexidine rinsing
   c. pain resolution
   d. brushing and antibiotics
   e. b and c
   f. all of the above

Answer: E. The patient is in too much pain to do definitive scaling and resolution of pain must come first. Then the patient can be instructed to use rinsing instead of brushing for the first appointment

3. Necrotizing ulcerative periodontitis may be a first sign for which systemic disease
   a. Acute gingivitis
   b. HIV
   c. Herpes simplex
   d. Chronic periodontitis

Answer: B. NUP may also be the first sign of underlying systemic disease such as HIV. There is no rapid destruction of bone with Herpes simplex or acute gingivitis. The gingiva is not punched out and very painful for chronic gingivitis.

References

American Academy of Periodontology. 1992. *The etiology and pathogenesis of periodontal diseases* (Position Paper), 1–9. Chicago: Author.

Armitage, G. C. 1999. Development of a classification system for periodontal diseases and conditions. *Ann. Periodontol.* 4:1–6.

EEC-Clearinghouse on Oral Problems Related to HIV Infections and WHO Collaborating Centre on Oral Manifestations for the Human Immunodeficiency Virus. 1993. Classification and diagnostic criteria for oral lesions in HIV infection. *J. Oral Pathol. Med.* 22: 289–291.

Listgarten, M. A., and D. W. Lewis. 1967. The distribution of spirochetes in the lesion of acute necrotizing ulcerative gingivitis: An electron microscopic and statistical survey. *J. Periodontol.* 38:379–386.

Loesche, W. J., S. A. Syed, B. E. Laughon, and J. Stoll. 1982. The bacteriology of acute necrotizing ulcerative gingivitis. *J. Periodontol.* 53:223–230.

Mealey, B. L. 1996. Periodontal implications: Medically compromised patients. *Ann. Periodontol.* 1:256–321.

Murayama, Y., H. Kurihara, A. Nagai, D. Dompkowski, and T. Van Dyke. 1994. Acute necrotizing ulcerative gingivitis: Risk factors involving host defense mechanisms. *Periodontology 2000* 6:116–124.

Murray, P. A. 1994. Periodontal diseases in patients infected by human immunodeficiency virus. *Periodontology 2000* 6:50–67.

Murray, P. A., J. R. Winkler, W. J. Peros, C. K. French, and J. A. Lippke. 1991. DNA probe detection of periodontal pathogens in HIV-associated periodontal lesions. *Oral Microbiol. Immunol.* 6:34–40.

Rowland, R. W. 1999. Necrotizing ulcerative gingivitis. *Ann Periodontol.* 4:65–73.

Škach, M., S. Zábrodský, L. Mrklas. 1970. A study of the effect of age and season on the incidence of ulcerative gingivitis. *J. Periodontal Res.* 5:187-190.

Wennström, J., and J. Lindhe. 1979. Effect of hydrogen peroxide on developing plaque and gingivitis in man. *J. Clin. Periodontol.* 6:115–130.

Winkler, J. R., M. Grassi, and P. A. Murray. 1988. Clinical description and etiology of HIV-associated periodontal diseases. In eds. P. B. Robertson and J. S. Greenspan, *Perspectives on oral manifestations of AIDS*, 49–70. Littleton, MA: PSG Publishing.

Winkler, J. R., and P. B. Robertson. 1992. Periodontal disease associated with HIV infection. *Oral Surg. Oral Med. Oral Pathol.* 73:145–150.

10

Occlusal Trauma

Mea A. Weinberg and Stuart J. Froum

OUTLINE

EDUCATIONAL OBJECTIVES

Upon completion of this chapter, the reader should be able to:

- List the classification of malocclusion.
- Identify and distinguish between the two types of occlusal trauma.
- Identify and describe the clinical and radiographic signs of occlusal trauma.
- Define the interrelationship between occlusal trauma and periodontitis.

GOAL: To provide information about the etiology, clinical manifestations, and therapy of occlusal trauma.

KEY WORDS

Introduction

Soon after the identification of microorganisms as a risk factor for periodontitis, the role of occlusion in periodontal diseases was considered. Although numerous studies using human and animal models have been published on this subject, it still remains a controversial issue.

Occlusion

Occlusion describes the contact relationship of teeth in function and dysfunction and is defined as any contact between the incisal or occlusal surfaces of the maxillary and mandibular teeth. It consists of all tooth contacts during swallowing and chewing. Centric occlusion (CO) is defined as maximal intercuspation or contact of the maxillary and mandibular teeth. The centric relation (CR) is the most retruded (posterior) position of the mandible in relation to the maxilla from which lateral movements of the jaw can be made.

An "ideal" or normal occlusion occurs where the arrangement of teeth is considered to be most correct. This is to say, on closing the mouth, all upper and lower teeth come together at the same time, and there are no crowded, malpositioned, or tipped teeth. Few patients have an ideal or normal occlusion. Usually, there are deviations from normal. Any deviation from the ideal or normal occlusion, for example, crowding, malpositioned, or tipped teeth, is referred to as **malocclusion**. However, malocclusion does not necessarily indicate occlusal disease. Classification of the various forms of malocclusion is done with Edward H. Angle's principles of defining occlusion. This classification is based on the interdigitation of the maxillary and mandibular teeth. Malpositioning is described in terms of crowding of individual teeth or groups of teeth. Figure 10–1 ■ describes the three classes of malocclusion. If the maxillary first molar is missing, the maxillary canine is used. The use

> ### Did You Know?
>
> Back in the 19th century there were strong overtones of religious belief in the concept of occlusion.

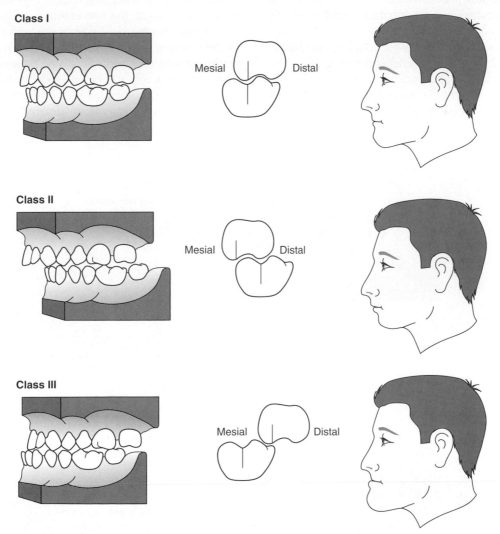

Class I

Mesial   Distal

Class II

Mesial   Distal

Class III

Mesial   Distal

FIGURE 10–1 Classification of malocclusion: Angle's classification.

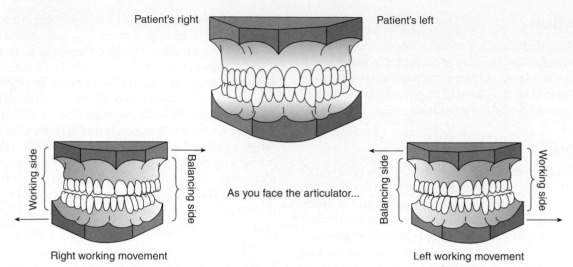

Patient's right   Patient's left

Working side   Balancing side   As you face the articulator...   Balancing side   Working side

Right working movement   Left working movement

FIGURE 10–2 Illustration of centric occlusion (*center*). Teeth close together with even pressure on both sides of the mouth. In right working movement (*left*), the mandible moves to the right. In left working movement (*right*), the mandible moves to the left.

of study casts to provide a better indication of occlusion is sometimes required. The main purpose for using this classification is for diagnostic consistency and treatment planning because malocclusion is a contributing risk factor for inflammatory periodontal diseases.

Functional occlusion consists of teeth that are in function when the mandible moves in lateral and protrusive excursions or movements. Lateral movements are defined by the direction in which the mandible is moving (Figure 10–2 ■). If the mandible moves to the left, the movement is called a left working movement, and the left side of the arch is known as the working side. In a left working movement, the right side is known as the nonworking (balancing) side. If the mandible moves to the right, the movement is called a right working movement, and the right side of the arch is then referred to as the working side. The left side is referred to as the nonworking (balancing) side. For some patients, a lateral movement results in contacts between the posterior teeth on the working side. This is called group function (Figure 10–3 ■). For other patients, a lateral movement results in contact only

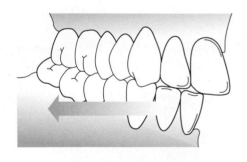

Right working movement
All posterior teeth are in
contact: group function

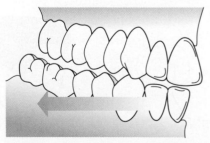

Right working movement
Only the canines are in
contact: canine protection

FIGURE 10–3 Group function: Lateral movement results in contact of all posterior teeth (*top*). Canine guidance: Lateral movement results in contact between the maxillary and mandibular canines (*bottom*).

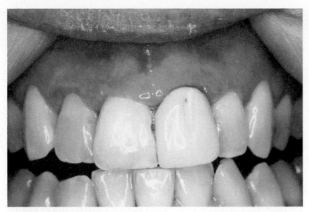

FIGURE 10–4 Protrusive occlusion (movement): Mandible moves forward from centric occlusion so that there is contact of the incisors.

Overbite (amount of vertical overlap of anterior teeth) and overjet (horizontal protrusion of upper teeth beyond the lower) are measured with a periodontal probe. Normally, the incisal edges of the lower incisors and the cingulum of the upper incisors establish the stops necessary to maintain tooth position. A deep overbite can occur as a result of skeletal relationship, extrusion or migration of teeth, or if posterior teeth are missing, causing the anterior teeth to handle the occlusal load. Overclosure of anterior teeth can cause trauma to the gingiva of the maxillary and/or mandibular anterior teeth (Figure 10–5 ■). This is referred to as a traumatic overbite. An open bite occurs when anterior and/or posterior maxillary and mandibular teeth do not occlude.

Terminology

Occlusal trauma (also termed trauma from occlusion, periodontal traumatism, or occlusal disease) is defined as injury to the attachment apparatus (bone, periodontal ligament, and cementum) as a consequence of normal or excessive occlusal force(s) applied to a tooth or teeth (American Academy of Periodontology, 2001). In addition to periodontal tissue damage, excessive occlusal force also can affect the temporomandibular joint, muscles of mastication, pulp tissue, and integrity of the restoration. Occlusal force is a force (or energy) transmitted to the teeth and their supporting structures by tooth-to-tooth contacts or through food substances or any other intervening material. When the magnitude (size), direction, frequency, and/or duration of these forces exceed the reparative capacity of the attachment apparatus, the result is occlusal disease. This

between the maxillary and mandibular canines on the working side. This is called canine protection or canine guidance (see Figure 10–3). It is generally believed that during lateral movements there should be no tooth contact on the nonworking side. However, balancing side contacts are probably prevalent in most patients. Denture wearers need tooth-to-tooth contacts on both the working and nonworking sides for the dentures to function effectively.

Protrusive occlusion is movement of the mandible in a direction anterior to centric occlusion (Figure 10–4 ■). Guidance for this movement should be on the anterior teeth, and edge-to-edge contact of the incisors should be possible. Any posterior contact during protrusive occlusion is considered undesirable. Posterior interference is seen frequently with an extruded or tipped tooth. A classic example of a prematurity occurs when an amalgam filling is too high (placed above the line of occlusion), and on biting down, the patient feels as though that particular area is touching first. Therefore, in this situation, one or more teeth are touching the occlusal surface rather than all the teeth touching simultaneously.

Cases where patients have occlusions that are not ideal but are symptom free and their dentition "survives" or "adapts" to a deviated occlusion are referred to as physiologic occlusion. Most people have some occlusal discrepancies, but in most cases, the dentition has "adapted" to the discrepancies and shows no signs of occlusal trauma. On the other hand, the dentition in a pathologic occlusion generally shows evidence of occlusal disease.

Pathologic occlusion occurs when patients show evidence or signs and have symptoms of occlusal disease (Goldman & Cohen, 1980).

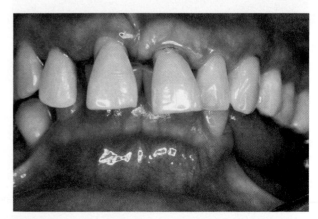

FIGURE 10–5 A deep overbite causes the mandibular incisors to touch the palatal gingiva of the maxillary anterior area.

is determined clinically by signs and symptoms. Traumatogenic occlusion is defined as any occlusion that produces forces that directly or indirectly cause injury to the attachment apparatus.

Premature occlusal contact (also called occlusal interference) occurs when there are interferences to closure of opposing teeth (Figure 10–6 ▪); that is, a tooth that occludes with an opposing tooth before full closure is achieved in centric occlusion. This premature contact prevents the other teeth in the arch from achieving contact simultaneously. Premature contacts also can occur during lateral movements when the mandible moves from one side to the other. In addition, an extruded (also termed supererupted) or a tipped tooth may cause posterior occlusal interferences. Premature contacts should be eliminated if there is evidence of damage to the attachment apparatus or increasing tooth mobility.

Parafunctional habits are activities of the masticatory (chewing) system that are beyond the normal range of function. Chewing and swallowing are normal, whereas grinding and clenching are abnormal or parafunctional activities. Parafunctional activities often occur during sleep or stressful situations. Premature contacts also may predispose to parafunctional habits. Occlusal therapy is designed to control the forces generated by tooth-to-tooth contact so they are tolerated by the attachment apparatus.

Parafunctional Habits

Bruxism, a type of parafunctional habit, is the unconscious grinding and/or clenching of the teeth when the patient is not swallowing or chewing. During sleep, it is called nocturnal bruxism and is often associated with stressful situations. Although most patients show signs of bruxism, only 5% to 20% are consciously aware of it (Hallmon, 1999). The early signs of bruxism may go undetected, but with increased duration, intensity, and direction of the habit, wear facets will be visible on tooth surfaces, and tooth mobility may be seen. Initially, this increase in functional demand will be accommodated by the periodontium. Other changes include

cusp fractures, increased thermal sensitivity, and increased tooth mobility, which can resolve when the parafunctional action is discontinued. Other examples of parafunctional habits include nail biting, tongue thrusting, and chewing of foreign objects between the teeth such as bobby pins, nails, pipes, and pencils.

Tongue thrusting or thumb sucking often creates a class II, division I malocclusion with an anterior and posterior open bite (Figure 10–7 ▪). During swallowing, the tongue is placed between the maxillary and mandibular anterior teeth and on the sides rather than on the hard palate near the rugae. The lips and chin muscles contract, visualized as a massive grimace. Tongue thrusting eventually can lead to a mouth-breathing habit, which may cause a localized gingival inflammation of the maxillary and mandibular incisor region that is unrelated to plaque accumulation. In addition, the lips will be dry and parted at rest. Parafunctional activity can produce symptoms from the musculature or TMJ. Palpation of the muscles of mastication can detect muscle spasms or pain. Parafunctional habits may lead to occlusal trauma. Occlusal trauma is defined as injury to the attachment apparatus as a result of excessive occlusal force.

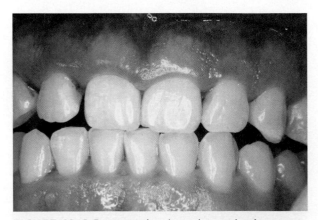

FIGURE 10–6 In protrusion (anterior teeth edge to edge), note that the initial interference is on the maxillary incisors, which prevents the right lateral incisor from occluding.

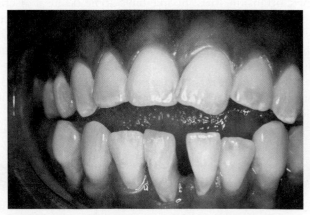

FIGURE 10–7 An anterior open bite caused by tongue thrusting.

Rapid Dental Hint

Do not forget to do an occlusal exam when performing a patient evaluation. Check for any occlusal interferences using articulating paper or floss.

The Role of Occlusal Trauma in the Initiation and Progression of Periodontal Diseases

Research has concluded that occlusal trauma alone does not cause gingivitis, periodontitis, pocket formation, or gingival recession (Harrel & Nunn, 2004; Ramfjord & Ash, 1981; Svanberg, King, & Gibbs, 1995). The gingival unit is independent, having its own blood supply, and is not affected by occlusal trauma (Keller & Cohen, 1955). In healthy conditions, the structure and adaptive nature of the attachment apparatus to occlusal forces permit a certain degree of physiologic mobility. Adaptation refers to alterations or adjustments that the body develops to accommodate to its environment. However, when occlusal forces are excessive, beyond the capability of the attachment apparatus to repair itself, tissue injury occurs, resulting in occlusal trauma.

A more complex and controversial issue is the interrelationship between periodontal inflammation and trauma from occlusion. Is the presence of inflammation **codestructive** and accelerated when occlusal trauma is also present? Numerous human and animal models were developed to determine the effects of occlusal forces on the progression of periodontitis. According to the codestructive theory, occlusal forces will accelerate the rate of periodontal destruction and result in connective tissue attachment loss, in the presence of preexisting inflammation. This concept is still controversial. It is also debatable whether these factors interfere with wound healing in the treatment of periodontal diseases. The conflicting results of different studies may be due to differences in animal species, the procedures used for producing occlusal trauma, and inherent measurement inaccuracies.

HUMAN STUDIES Glickman (1963) introduced the concept of codestruction, whereby inflammation and trauma from occlusion are synergistic factors in periodontal destruction. He suggested that although occlusion does not cause gingival inflammation or pocket formation, inflammation of the supporting tissues in the presence of occlusal trauma alters the pathway of inflammation. Subsequently, the inflammatory infiltrate will spread more rapidly through tissue damaged by excessive occlusal forces and move directly into the periodontal ligament space, causing the development of angular bone defects and infrabony pockets. Thus, according to Glickman, inflammation and occlusal trauma become codestructive, whereby the progression of periodontitis is accelerated by the presence of occlusal trauma.

However, other investigators (Shefter & McFall, 1984) reported no relationship between occlusal disharmonies and pathoses associated with inflammatory periodontal disease in patients with mild to moderate periodontitis.

ANIMAL STUDIES In an attempt to reproduce the kind of occlusal trauma that might occur in the human dentition, early studies placed high restorations on teeth to reproduce the jiggling forces caused by premature tooth contacts. Jiggling or reciprocating forces were applied in opposite directions on a tooth at the same time. This prevented the tooth from moving away from the force. Unilateral forces would have allowed the traumatized teeth to migrate away from the occlusal forces. In many studies, tissue inflammation was induced using silk ligatures placed around the teeth near the gingival margin to enhance plaque retention.

Primate Model. Meitner (1975) examined the effects of jiggling forces on marginal periodontitis in squirrel monkeys by forcing wedges into the embrasure between teeth. The wedges were moved every 48 hours, allowing the teeth to be subjected to reciprocating forces every other day. Although this type of trauma is quite different from that caused by premature contacts, there was no accelerated loss of connective tissue attachment.

Polson, Meitner, & Zander (1976) also found that there was no difference in loss of connective tissue attachment and bone destruction in periodontally involved teeth of squirrel monkeys subjected to a single episode of trauma.

Beagle Model. The results of several beagle dog studies (Ericsson & Lindhe, 1982; Lindhe & Svanberg, 1974) showed that when heavy occlusal forces were combined with plaque-induced periodontitis, the rate of clinical attachment loss was accelerated, but this model system also showed that trauma from occlusion does not aggravate gingival inflammation or cause loss of clinical attachment in chronic gingivitis (Ericsson & Lindhe, 1977). In the beagle, when jiggling forces were applied to a periodontally healthy tooth or a tooth with chronic gingivitis, the tooth became hypermobile.

Pathogenesis of Occlusal Trauma

The pathologic features of occlusal trauma are different from those of inflammation. With occlusal trauma, healing of traumatized tissue need not be considered an inflammatory process because no inflammatory/immune cells such as leukocytes, lymphocytes, or plasma cells are present. Thus repair is initiated after the trauma is removed, without the tissue exhibiting the classic signs of inflammation. The lesion of occlusal trauma in the normal, healthy periodontium usually develops following compression and tension of the periodontal ligament (PDL) fibers and resorption and deposition of bone. Compression of the PDL fibers results in obstruction of blood flow to the fibers, which in turn results in bone resorption. If the destructive process is greater than the repair potential of the periodontal tissue, injury may result. The alveolar bone undergoes osteoclastic resorption in areas of pressure, which results in the widening of the periodontal ligament space (Svanberg et al., 1995). Clinically, increased tooth mobility may result to accommodate for the widened PDL. Regardless of the status of the original attachment apparatus, there will be increasing tooth mobility until the PDL can adapt to the applied force. When adaptation is complete, new lamina dura may be seen radiographically, even though the increased PDL space of hypermobile teeth will remain. When the occlusal trauma is eliminated, bone repair will occur, and a functional width of the PDL will be reestablished. If, however, the trauma continues, excessive widening of the PDL results to accommodate the bone loss. This results in increasing tooth mobility.

The gingival connective tissue attachment is not affected, nor is there apical migration of the junctional epithelium. This same tissue reaction that occurs in a patient with a healthy periodontium also occurs in a patient with a reduced bony support who also has a healthy periodontium.

If the codestructive theory was correct, then the pathway of inflammation would be seen as proceeding not from the gingiva to the bone and finally to the PDL but rather from the gingiva directly into the PDL, inducing the formation of an infrabony pocket with associated vertical bone loss (Glickman & Smulow, 1965). Removal of the trauma but not the inflammation does not decrease tooth mobility, and the crestal bone does not repair (Polson, Meitner, & Zander, 1976). Kantor, Polson, and Zander (1976) removed both jiggling forces and inflammation, resulting in new bone formation without an increase in alveolar bone height. Collectively, these studies show that occlusal trauma does not initiate gingivitis or periodontitis. Although the importance of the role of dental plaque in inflammatory periodontal diseases is undisputed, the influence of occlusal trauma on the attachment level remains controversial (Hallmon, 1999).

Classification of Occlusal Trauma

Occusal trauma can be classified as either primary or secondary and either localized to a single tooth or generalized, affecting several teeth (Table 10–1 ■).

Primary occlusal trauma is defined as injury to the supporting structures (PDL, cementum, and bone) caused by excessive occlusal forces (forces greater than experienced during normal chewing function) placed on a tooth or teeth with normal periodontal tissue support (Figure 10–8 ■). Examples of causes of primary occlusal trauma include the following:

- A "high" restoration, where, on biting, the restored tooth creates a premature contact with the opposing tooth.
- Parafunctional habits involving tooth-to-tooth contact such as bruxism, clenching, or object-to-tooth contact such as biting on pencils or nail biting.
- A malpositioned or maligned tooth, including teeth that are extruded (moved occlusally) or tipped.
- A periapical (around the apex of the root) abscess or infection causing a tooth to be extruded.
- Physical "blow" to a tooth or teeth.
- A removable partial denture clasp around an abutment tooth.
- Orthodontic movement of teeth.

Parafunctional activity may result in primary occlusal trauma. This occurs when a tooth is subjected to greater

Table 10–1 Periodontal Occlusal Traumatic Lesions

Type of Occlusal Trauma	Etiology	Pocket Formation	Bone Height	Mobility	Treatment Options
Primary	Excessive occlusal force(s)	No	Normal height or slight bone loss	Adapted	Selective grinding, appliances, monitoring without treatment
Secondary	Normal or excessive occlusal force(s)	No/Yes. Periodontal pockets may be present, but due to periodontal destruction rather than the occlusal trauma	Reduced height (moderate/severe)	Progressive	Splinting if necessary, selective grinding, extraction, orthodontic movement, appliances, monitoring

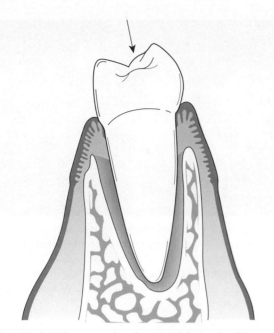

FIGURE 10–8 Primary occlusal trauma. A tooth with normal periodontal tissues is exposed to excessive occlusal load (arrow). As a result of bone resorption, the periodontal ligament space gradually increases in size on both sides of the teeth as well as in the periapical region.

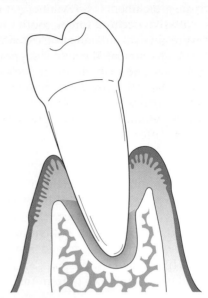

FIGURE 10–9 Secondary occlusal trauma. If a tooth with reduced periodontal tissue support has been exposed to excessive occlusal forces, a widened periodontal ligament space and increased mobility result.

forces over a longer period of time than what normally occurs in chewing and swallowing. Food chewing is not a cause of primary occlusal trauma because the forces are most likely not long-standing or severe enough to affect the attachment apparatus.

When the forces generated during bruxism exceed the adaptive capacity of the periodontium on a regular basis, occlusal trauma is initiated (Caffesse & Fleszar, 1992).

Secondary occlusal trauma occurs when normal (e.g., chewing) or excessive occlusal forces cause injury in a periodontium with reduced bone support (Figure 10–9 ■). Bone levels around the tooth are inadequate to support these forces, and the tooth is less resistant to occlusal loading. In other words, a tooth in secondary occlusal trauma has insufficient bone support, and normal chewing and swallowing forces are excessive, causing injury to the attachment apparatus. This can occur even when the periodontal tissues are healthy, but there is a reduced bone height. Therefore, the distinguishing feature between primary and secondary occlusal trauma is the amount of bony support surrounding the tooth.

Other parafunctional habits such as lip, nail, or cheek biting, tongue thrusting, or the placement of foreign objects between the teeth (e.g., pipe clenching and chewing, pencil biting, playing a wind musical instrument, and clenching fingernails or bobby pins) may affect the attachment apparatus. However, these do not appear to occur as frequently as tooth-to-tooth contact habits. A less common cause of primary occlusal trauma is occupational bruxism, which occurs in certain stressful occupations.

Clinical Findings in Occlusal Trauma

Tooth Mobility

The most common sign of occlusal trauma is increasing **tooth mobility** over a period of time. However, excessive occlusal forces may not always cause tooth hypermobility (Svanberg et al., 1995). Because mobility due to occlusal trauma is an adaptive function, it may not be considered pathologic (resulting in disease). A tooth with excessive occlusal load may adapt to the forces by exhibiting increased but not increasing mobility. However, if there is progressive tooth mobility over a period of several days or weeks, it may then be considered pathologic (Green & Levine, 1996). Consequently, for the proper recognition of occlusal disease, tooth mobility has to be assessed on two or more separate occasions (Svanberg et al., 1995).

A tooth in primary occlusal trauma may show mobility. In this case, the tooth becomes mobile so that it can adapt to the abnormal force placed on it. Thus the mobility of the tooth could be classified as an adapted mobility (Tarnow & Fletcher, 1986). For example, mobility of a tooth caused by a high restoration will come to a plateau and no longer increase; this is adapted mobility. Tooth mobility in absence of supporting alveolar bone may be characteristic of a parafunctional habit. However, tooth mobility does not occur in all patients who grind and clench their teeth. In some cases, tooth wear accommodates for the bruxing habit.

Tooth hypermobility, produced by excessive occlusal forces, does not cause gingival inflammation, worsen the severity of chronic gingivitis, or act as a primary cause for connective tissue attachment loss (Svanberg et al., 1995).

Besides excessive occlusal forces, tooth mobility may result from severe gingival inflammation extending into the connective tissue attachment, the loss of supporting alveolar bone, pregnancy, and orthodontic movement or may occur following surgical therapy. Tooth mobility will usually decrease by the fourth week after surgery. The cause and progression of the mobility must be determined because treatment options differ.

Fremitus

Fremitus is the vibrational movement of a tooth under occlusal function. Fremitus is detected by placing the index finger on the gingival-tooth interfaces (Figure 10–10 ■) of the maxillary teeth and asking the patient to tap the teeth up and down, grind from side to side, and move the jaw into an edge-to-edge (protrusive) occlusion. Centric prematurities are detected by the presence of fremitus.

Pain

Pain from percussion, pain on biting, and the pain of tooth hypersensitivity are symptoms of primary and secondary occlusal trauma. For example, after receiving a restoration, a patient may call to report tooth pain. An evaluation will reveal that the restoration is high, causing pain and mobility on biting or chewing. Once the restoration is reduced in height, the pain and mobility will disappear.

Tooth Migration

Pathologic tooth migration usually is indicative of moderate to severe periodontitis and secondary occlusal trauma (Towfighi et al., 1997). Pathologic migration is defined as a change in tooth position resulting from disruption of the forces that maintain teeth in a normal position (Chasens, 1979). Excessive occlusal forces, which include the normal forces of chewing or swallowing applied to teeth, and

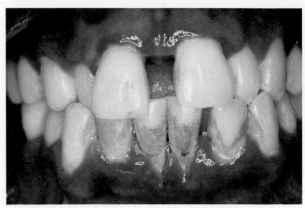

FIGURE 10–11 A 45-year-old patient with advanced periodontitis. Patient complaints of recently widened spaces, flaring of the maxillary incisors, and extrusion of the maxillary right central incisor are often an indication that the reduced attachment apparatus is reacting to occlusal forces.

extensive bone loss may cause teeth to migrate (Towfighi et al., 1997). Clinically, pathologic tooth migration results in widened spaces between teeth (diastemas), flaring or fanning of anterior teeth, and/or extrusion of teeth (Figure 10–11 ■). Although it is a common sign of secondary occlusal trauma, pathologic tooth migration may be caused by periodontal surgery or extensive inflammation extending into the PDL.

Attrition

Forces generated during bruxism frequently are greater than the adaptive capacity of the periodontium. Consequently, the contoured surface of a tooth may be ground flat, to the point where the dentin may be exposed (Figure 10–12 ■). Cracks and pits form on the worn edges and may become plaque traps. Clinical features of attrition include flattened occlusal or incisal surfaces of teeth. The canines and central and lateral incisors most commonly receive the heaviest and earliest lateral wear (Lytle, 1990). Exposed dentin may

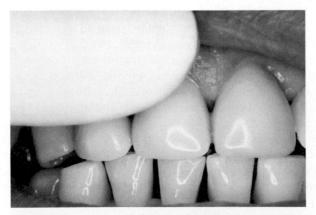

FIGURE 10–10 A technique for detecting fremitus. The index finger is placed partly on the facial tooth surfaces and the gingiva. Tooth movements can be detected when the patient taps the teeth together and grinds side to side.

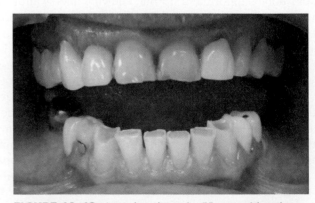

FIGURE 10–12 Anterior view of a 55-year-old patient who was unaware he was a bruxer. Note the generalized heavy wear such that all teeth appear flat and on the same plane. (Courtesy of Dr. Xiu Yan Li.)

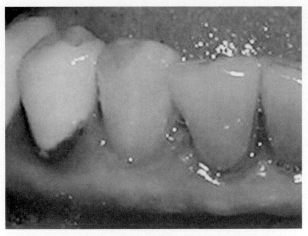

FIGURE 10–13 Showing a mandibular anterior teeth wear facet on the mandibular canine. (Courtesy of John Eum, DDS, New York University College of Dentistry.)

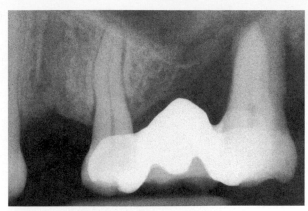

FIGURE 10–14 A radiograph showing a typical lesion of primary occlusal trauma. Widening of the periodontal ligament space has occurred due to a heavy occlusal force placed on the premolar. Note that there are no increased probing depths.

cause a tooth to become sensitive. Wear facets frequently are seen as a flat, shiny, worn spot on the side of a cusp of a tooth (Figure 10–13 ■). The presence of attrition and wear facets does not necessarily indicate occlusal habits. Wear on teeth also may be due to the patient's age or diet. Once a facet has developed, it remains. If a patient has wear facets for many years with no changes, it is probably not an active process.

Muscle/Temporomandibular Joint

Occlusal trauma may cause the muscles that work the jaw, the largest being the temporalis and the masseter, to become chronically sore, resulting in headaches and muscle pain. Pain usually occurs during chewing or on waking in the morning. This type of pain may be emanating from the temporomandibular joint (TMJ). The patient may report muscle spasms in the head, neck, and ear area. Pathology must be ruled out when a patient complains of any type of facial pain, including TMJ pain.

Tooth Structure

Tooth fractures and long-term chipping of enamel are additional signs of occlusal trauma related to the magnitude of forces that the teeth endure.

Radiographic Findings in Occlusal Trauma

Along with the clinical examination, radiographs are useful for recognizing the signs of occlusal trauma and/or the signs of adaptation to significant occlusal forces (Caffesse & Fleszar, 1992).

Widening of the PDL occurs as an adaptation response to accommodate excessive occlusal loading and also may result in the resorption of alveolar bone. Radiographically, when the PDL space is wider at the coronal third of the root, it is referred to as crestal funneling.

Radiographically, a tooth in primary occlusal trauma may or may not show vertical bone loss as a result of widening of the PDL space. However, this should not be confused with bone loss related to periodontitis (Ricchetti, 1998; Figures 10–14 ■ and 10–15 ■) because primary occlusal trauma does not show loss of connective tissue attachment, increased probing depth, and related infrabony pockets (Polson & Zander, 1983). The presence of angular bony defects is not necessarily a sign of occlusal trauma. If a widened PDL space is present but no tooth mobility exists, occlusal trauma is not necessarily present. The findings may be a functional adaptation to the occlusal forces. In addition, an increase in the density, referred to as osteoporosis, of the alveolar bone and the excessive deposition of cementum, referred to as hypercementosis, around the apical part of the root may be evident (Figure 10–16 ■).

Radiographically, a tooth in secondary occlusal trauma shows reduced bone levels that are inadequate to support

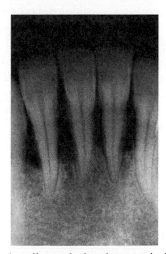

FIGURE 10–15 A radiograph showing a typical lesion of secondary occlusal trauma. The tooth has a reduced bony support and increasing tooth mobility. The tooth has an adverse crown-to-root ratio.

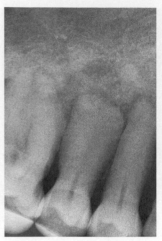

FIGURE 10–16 Hypercementosis (excessive deposition of cementum) seen on the root may be indicative of occlusal trauma.

the tooth under a normal load without increasing mobility, migration, or fremitus (Ricchetti, 1998). Vertical bone loss is accompanied by widening of the PDL. Occasionally, root resorption may occur.

Occlusal Overload in Implants

A dental implant responds differently than a natural tooth during occlusal trauma or biomechanical overload. As previously mentioned, when a natural tooth is subjected to occusal trauma, it can adapt to the forces. There will be bone loss in the socket, widening of the periodontal ligament space and subsequently tooth mobility. This is the tooth's way to avoid excessive force by "moving away" from the force. The tooth will become less mobile once the excessive force is removed. This is not the case with a dental implant where there is no periodontal ligament to adapt to the excessive force. Occlusal overloading is the primary cause of implant complications, including fracture or loosening of the implant fixture or prosthetic crown. In addition, the bond between the implant surface and bone (there is no periodontal ligament) is disrupted, resulting in bone loss around the implant and possible failure where the implant becomes mobile (Fu, Hsu, and Wang, 2012). At scheduled recare appointments, the dental hygienist must evaluate implants for occlusal overloading. A radiograph may be needed. Patient complaints of pain must be evaluated for occlusal trauma (Wingrove, 2011). Treatment of occlusal overload includes occlusal adjustment and repair of defective prosthetic components.

Outcomes of Treatment of Occlusal Trauma

The desired outcome of treatment of occlusal trauma is that the patient remains comfortable during chewing and is able to maintain the dentition in a state of health. The dental hygienist can determine if the reversal of signs and symptoms of occlusal trauma has achieved the following outcomes (American Academy of Periodontology, 1996). These include the following:

- Elimination or significant reduction of tooth mobility (the patient should be comfortable when in function)
- Elimination of occlusal prematurities and fremitus
- Elimination of parafunctional habits
- Prevention of further tooth migration
- Decrease or stability of radiographic changes
- Inadequate resolution of occlusal trauma is identified by increasing tooth mobility
- Progressive tooth migration
- Patient continuing to complain of discomfort with pain and tooth mobility
- Premature contacts remaining
- Radiographic signs remaining, including widening of the PDL space
- Parafunctional habits continuing
- TMJ problems remaining or worsening

Occlusal Therapy

The objective of **occlusal therapy** is to control the direction, duration, magnitude, and/or frequency of excessive occlusal forces. Practitioners have different views on whether occlusal therapy is necessary in the overall periodontal treatment plan.

Box 10–1 lists the most common approaches to treating trauma from occlusion. The key to treatment of occlusal trauma lies in the ability to determine if physiologic or pathologic occlusion exists. Physiologic occlusion does not need to be treated, whereas pathologic occlusion that shows signs and symptoms of occlusal problems requires treatment. Occlusal treatment has been shown to significantly reduce the progression of periodontal disease and be an important adjunct therapy in the comprehensive treatment of periodental disease (Harrel & Nunn, 2001).

Because primary occlusal trauma is caused by excessive occlusal forces, treatment is aimed at eliminating or reducing the forces. Treatment options include selective grinding, control of habits, orthodontic movement, or monitoring of the condition without treatment.

Box 10–1: Approaches to Treating Occlusal Trauma

- Selective grinding
- Control of habits
- Orthodontic tooth movement
- Splinting
- Restorative procedures
- Monitoring without treatment

In contrast to the primary occlusal traumatic lesion, the secondary occlusal traumatic lesion is not reversible because its cause is loss of bony support around a tooth or teeth. Treatment options for secondary occlusal trauma include splinting, selective grinding, orthodontic movement, extraction, or monitoring of the condition without treatment. Reductions in tooth mobility are limited because the mobility is due to a reduced periodontal support rather than to excessive occlusal force. Premature contacts on mobile teeth are detected and eliminated by selective grinding.

Selective Grinding

Selective grinding or occlusal equilibration is defined as the reshaping of the occlusal or incisal surfaces of teeth to create harmonious contacts between the upper and lower dentition. The goal of selective grinding is to eliminate premature contacts in primary or secondary occlusal trauma. Correction of prematurities should be done in centric occlusion, centric relation, and protrusive and lateral movements so that a traumatic contact of teeth occurs during movements of the mandible (Burgett, 1995). Prematurities are detected by the use of wax, articulating paper, or dental floss.

Selective grinding always should be completed after inflammation has been controlled. Once the inflammation is eliminated by periodontal debridement and oral hygiene self-care, the tooth mobility may decrease because the fibers of the connective tissue attachment repair and a tooth with an intact connective tissue attachment has additional rigidity. Once periodontal health is reestablished, the occlusal condition is reevaluated. A decision to perform selective grinding depends on the degree of patient discomfort and function rather than on the assumption that selective grinding is necessary to halt the progression of disease (Gher, 1996).

Primary occlusal trauma caused by a high restoration is treated by selective grinding. However, severe discrepancies may be resolved best by replacing the restoration. Selective grinding reshapes the occlusal surfaces of teeth to create harmonious contact relationships between the opposing teeth. This is accomplished with hand instruments or a high-speed handpiece and a bur. Tooth surfaces should be smooth so that patients do not develop secondary occlusal habits by "playing" with a rough surface. Selective grinding also can be performed on teeth in secondary occlusal trauma.

Control of Parafunctional Habits

APPLIANCES If the cause of the occlusal trauma is bruxism, selective grinding usually will not correct the problem; however, counseling the patient may alleviate the psychological component of clenching and grinding. Because such problems are difficult to resolve, a bite plane or Hawley appliance may be fabricated from an orthodontic resin material that disoccludes the posterior teeth. This does not permit the opposing arches to contact and permits the attachment apparatus to heal. The appliance also can be used as an adjunct to selective grinding to stabilize the occlusion and allow the attachment apparatus to rest.

During sleep, a night guard can be worn to control occlusal habits. A night guard serves to protect the teeth from abnormal occlusal wear due to bruxism. Occlusal contacts between the upper and lower teeth are eliminated, thus stabilizing the occlusion and negating the effects of grinding and clenching at night (Chasens, 1990). The night guard is made of either hard or soft acrylic, usually covering the occlusal surfaces of all teeth in the maxillary arch (Figure 10–17 ■). The night guard is adjusted so that all mandibular teeth make simultaneous contact in centric occlusion.

EXERCISE Besides using appliances to alter or control occlusal habits, exercise is important as well, especially if the patient clenches. An exercise to follow includes clenching for 5 seconds, then releasing, and repeating this five times in a row (for a total of 60 seconds). This should be done five times a day for 14 consecutive days. If one day is missed, the exercise must be started again.

Orthodontics

Orthodontic treatment may be indicated in periodontal patients exhibiting drifting, migration, extrusion, or flared anterior teeth. The goal is to move a tooth or teeth into a more functional, less-traumatic position.

Restorative Procedures

To establish a stable posterior occlusion, restorations may be placed if other treatment options, including orthodontics or selective grinding, are not possible. For example, if a patient has anterior teeth and some or all of the posterior teeth on both sides are missing, the anterior teeth may become overloaded. Thus, restorations (e.g., removable partial dentures [RPDs] or crowns) will restore the posterior occlusion and distribute the load to protect the anterior teeth.

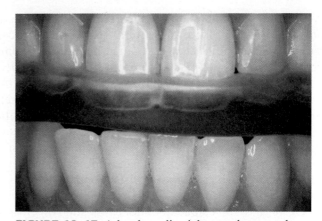

FIGURE 10–17 A hard acrylic night guard was made for this 35-year-old bruxer. It is used to protect the teeth during the night and help eliminate the habit. Night guards have full occlusal coverage and usually are made for the maxillary arch.

Splinting

Splinting of teeth is considered the treatment of choice for patients who complain of discomfort or if the examination reveals that the mobility interferes with chewing (mastication). Although tooth mobility that develops after periodontal surgery usually will subside within a few months, temporary splinting may be necessary to prevent secondary occlusal trauma. Splinting is also done on teeth in primary occlusal trauma if the mobility was caused by avulsion of the tooth or if the patient received a blow to the mouth resulting in loosening of a tooth or teeth.

Splinting permits healing of the attachment apparatus by holding a tooth in a totally fixed position. This allows the PDL to become narrower and the mobility to be reduced (Ricchetti, 1998). Instead of one tooth experiencing the brunt of forces, the forces are distributed and spread over several teeth, which are better able to absorb the trauma. If mobility is not increasing over time, it may not be necessary to splint. The attachment apparatus may have adapted to the excessive forces and is in a stage of repair (Chasens, 1990). Unfortunately, it is difficult to determine at any given point in time if a patient's attachment apparatus is in a state of repair. That is why monitoring mobility is so important.

Temporary splinting uses wires and composite material, acid-etching nylon mesh, or fixed bridges or crowns that are joined or soldered together (Figures 10–18 ■, 10–19 ■). A night guard is considered a type of occlusal splint.

Disadvantages of splinting include compromised aesthetics, reduced plaque-control efficacy, and a changed stable occlusion. Because of these disadvantages, splinting is not done routinely, and if it is selected, it should be considered with the preceding problems in mind.

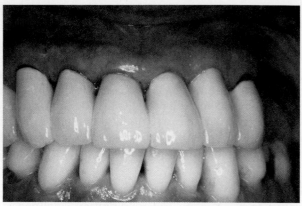

FIGURE 10–18 The fixed prosthesis consists of multiple crowns on the maxillary teeth that have been soldered. This represents a form of permanent splinting.

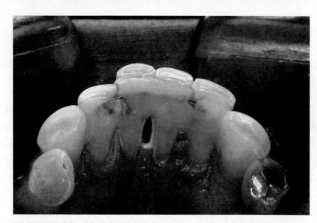

FIGURE 10–19 The incisors were splinted with wire and composite due to increasing mobility on these teeth that made the patient uncomfortable. This type of splinting is referred to as extracoronal because no channel was prepared in the tooth.

Dental Hygiene Application

Overall, the periodontal response to occlusal trauma can be considered a physiologic adaptation. This adaptation can result in permanently increased tooth mobility if the trauma continues. However, if plaque control is adequate, connective tissue attachment loss should not occur. Removal of the injurious occlusal forces allows the lesion to repair itself, but this may be compromised by the presence of dental plaque. Therefore, maintenance of adequate plaque control is of utmost importance in preventing and reversing the problem. The question of increased periodontal tissue destruction when periodontitis coexists with occlusal trauma remains unresolved.

Occlusal trauma alone does not cause gingivitis, loss of connective tissue attachment, or pocket formation. Unless there is compromised periodontal support, there is little or no damage to the teeth or the attachment apparatus from normal masticatory (chewing) forces. Normal forces are only traumatogenic in secondary occlusal trauma, when the periodontal support is reduced by disease.

The role of the dental hygienist in the identification of occlusal trauma on natural teeth as well as dental implants is important for the overall treatment of the patient. Treatment differs depending on the type of occlusal trauma and its etiology. To help distinguish between primary and secondary occlusal trauma, the dental hygienist can use radiographs and present and past dental history. The occlusal forces required to produce occlusal trauma generally are related to the remaining bony support for a given tooth.

Key Points

- Occlusal trauma does not initiate gingivitis or periodontitis, but in the presence of inflammation periodontal destruction may be accelerated.
- Parafunctional habits may cause occlusal trauma.
- The most common clinical sign of occlusal trauma is increasing tooth mobility.

- Pathologic tooth migration is usually indicative of moderate to severe periodontitis and secondary occlusal trauma.
- Dental implants respond differently than natural teeth when subjected to occlusal overload.
- Different treatments are available for occlusal trauma.

Self-Quiz

1. All the following parts of the periodontium are affected by occlusal trauma except one. Which one is the exception?
   a. Periodontal ligament
   b. Alveolar bone
   c. Gingiva
   d. Cementum

2. Which one of the following definitions pertains to primary occlusal trauma?

Type of Occlusal Force	Bone Support
a. Normal	Adequate
b. Excessive	Adequate
c. Normal	Reduced
d. Excessive	Reduced

3. From the following list, select the items associated with occlusal trauma.
   a. Tooth mobility
   b. Tooth migration
   c. Pain on chewing
   d. Occlusal erosion
   e. Periodontal pockets
   f. Attachment loss

4. From the following list, select the items associated with primary occlusal trauma.
   a. Radiographic widening of the periodontal ligament space
   b. Deposition of a cellular cementum
   c. Deposition of alveolar bone
   d. Receding pulp tissue
   e. Development of periodontal pockets
   f. Presence of wear facets
   g. Increasing mobility of teeth
   h. Occlusal restoration in hyperocclusion

5. Occlusal trauma in combination with chronic inflammatory periodontitis may result in greater tooth mobility and alveolar bone loss because occlusal trauma causes periodontal pocket formation.
   a. Both the statement and the reason are correct and related.
   b. Both the statement and the reason are correct but not related.
   c. The statement is correct, but the reason is not.
   d. The statement is not correct, but the reason is correct.
   e. Neither the statement nor the reason is correct.

6. Two days after a patient receives an amalgam restoration, he reports back to the office complaining of pain and looseness of the tooth. Which one of the following treatments would be most appropriate?
   a. Replace the amalgam with composite.
   b. Reduce the height of the restoration.
   c. Polish the restoration.
   d. Maintain the restoration as is.

7. From the following list, select the items associated with secondary occlusal trauma.
   a. Tooth with advanced bone loss
   b. Mastication
   c. Tongue thrusting
   d. Tooth with adequate periodontium
   e. Fremitus

8. A patient complains of soreness in the jaw on waking in the morning. She is having stressful problems at work. She complains that some of her lower teeth are "wearing down." Which one of the following conditions does this patient most likely have?
   a. Fractured jaw
   b. Parafunctional habit
   c. Severe periodontitis
   d. Necrotizing ulcerative gingivitis

9. A patient has returned for a 2-week follow-up visit after periodontal surgery complaining of tooth mobility. There was no mobility before the surgery was done. Which one of the following should be explained to the patient?
   a. Teeth must be splinted immediately.
   b. Mobility will decrease in time.
   c. Additional surgery will be needed.
   d. Systemic antibiotics are indicated.

10. Which one of the following conditions is best treated with a night guard?
    a. Tooth with severe bone loss
    b. Tongue-thrusting habit
    c. Teeth with severe abrasion
    d. Clenching and grinding

Case Study

A 50-year-old male has had a missing #14 for some years. Tooth #19 had been supererupted and torso. He recently had a new crown on #19 which now has slight mobility. The patient is having a preventive prophylaxis. The gingival assessment shows some slight gingivitis in the mandibular molar regions. The patient asks why his #19 feels loose and what can be done.

1. As a dental hygienist what would you discuss with the patient?
   a. improve homecare in mandibular molars region
   b. refer for selective grinding on crown of #19
   c. perform occlusal adjustment
   d. remove grinding habit
   e. all of the above

Answer: A. Occlusal trauma does not initiate gingivitis but in the presence of inflammation periodontal destruction may be accelerated. Dental consultation is necessary but not in the realm of the dental hygienist to determine whether the crown needs adjustment or other aspects to remove the occlusal trauma.

2. If the patient were to receive an implant to replace #14 what consideration would be necessary?
   a. Implants should never oppose natural teeth.
   b. Dental implants respond differently than natural teeth when subjected to occlusal overload.
   c. The mobility on #19 will get worse.
   d. Normal chewing forces will increase the mobility on #19.

Answer: B. There is no evidence that implants can not oppose natural teeth. Implants do respond differently as there is no periodontal ligament so the implant becomes loose with excessive force. Teeth do not become mobile with normal chewing forces if the periodontal support is normal.

3. What classification of occlusal trauma is represented by tooth #19?
   a. Parafunctional habits
   b. Primary occlusal trauma
   c. Secondary occlusal trauma
   d. Implant overload

Answer: B. Primary trauma example are injury to supporting structures caused by excessive occlusal forces on a tooth with normal periodontium. Parafunctional habits are activities of mastication beyond normal range. Secondary trauma occurs when there is already reduced bone support. Tooth #14 would be replaced by the implant.

References

American Academy of Periodontology. 1996. *Parameters of care.* Chicago: American Academy of Periodontology, Scientific and Educational Affairs Department.

American Academy of Periodontology. 2001. *Glossary of periodontal terms*, 4th ed. Chicago: Author.

Burgett, F. G. 1995. Trauma from occlusion. *Dent. Clin. North Am.* 39:301–311.

Caffesse, R. G., and T. J. Fleszar. 1992. Occlusal trauma. In eds. T. G. Wilson, K. S. Komman, and M. G. Newman, *Advances in periodontics*, 205–225. Chicago: Quintessence.

Chasens, A. I. 1979. Periodontal disease, pathologic tooth migration and adult orthodontics. *N.Y. J. Dent.* 49:40–43.

Chasens, A. I. 1990. Controversies in occlusion. *Dent. Clin. North Am.* 34:11–123.

Ericsson, I., and J. Lindhe. 1977. Lack of effect of trauma from occlusion on the recurrence of experimental periodontitis. *J. Clin. Periodontol.* 4:115–127.

Ericsson, I., and J. Lindhe. 1982. Effect of long-standing jiggling on experimental marginal periodontitis in the beagle dog. *J. Clin. Periodontol.* 9:497–503.

Fu, J. H., Y. T. Hsu, and H. L. Wang. 2012. Identifying occlusal overload and how to deal with it to avoid marginal bone loss around implants. *Eur. J. Oral. Implantol.* 5 Suppl:S91–103.

Gher, M. E. 1996. Nonsurgical pocket therapy: Dental occlusion. *Ann. Periodontol.* 1:567–580.

Glickman, I. 1963. Inflammation and trauma from occlusion: Codestructive factors in chronic periodontal disease. *J. Periodontol.* 34:5–10.

Glickman, I., and J. B. Smulow. 1965. Effect of excessive occlusal forces upon the pathway of gingival inflammation in humans. *J. Periodontol.* 36:141–147.

Goldman, H. M., and W. D. Cohen (eds.). 1980. Occlusal adjustment. In *Periodontal therapy*, 6th ed., 1065–1111. St. Louis, MO: Mosby.

Green, M. S., and D. F. Levine. 1996. Occlusion and the periodontium: A review and rationale for treatment. *J. Calif. Dent. Assoc.* 24:19–27.

Hallmon, W. W. 1999. Occlusal trauma: Effect and impact on the periodontium. *Ann. Periodontol.* 4:102–107.

Harrel, S. K., and M. E. Nunn. 2001. The effect of occlusal discrepancies on periodontitis. II. Relationship of occlusal treatment to the progression of periodontal disease. *J Periodontol.* 72(4): 495–505.

Harrel S. K., and M. E. Nunn. 2004. The effect of occlusal discrepancies on gingival width. *J Periodontol.* 75(1): 98–105.

Kantor, J., A. M. Polson, and H. A. Zander. 1976. Alveolar bone regeneration after removal of inflammatory and traumatic factors. *J. Periodontol.* 47:687–695.

Keller, G., and W. Cohen. 1955. India ink perfusions of the vascular plexus of oral tissues. *Oral Surg.* 8:539–542.

Lindhe, J., and G. Svanberg. 1974. Influence of trauma from occlusion on progression of experimental periodontitis in the beagle dog. *J. Clin. Periodontol.* 1:3–14.

Lytle, J. D. 1990. The clinician's index of occlusal disease: Definition, recognition, and management. *Int. J. Periodontic Restorative Dent.* 10:103–123.

Meitner, S. 1975. Codestructive factors of marginal periodontitis and repetitive mechanical injury. *J. Dent. Res.* 54:78–85.

Polson, A. M., S. W. Meitner, and H. A. Zander. 1976. Trauma and progression of marginal periodontitis in squirrel monkeys: IV. Reversibility of bone loss due to trauma alone and trauma superimposed upon periodontitis. *J. Periodontol. Res.* 11:290–298.

Polson, A. M., and H. A. Zander. 1983. Effect of periodontal trauma upon intrabony pockets. *J. Periodontol.* 54:586–591.

Ramfjord, S. P., and M. M. Ash. 1981. Significance of occlusion in the etiology and treatment of early, moderate and advanced periodontitis. *J. Periodontol.* 52:511–517.

Ricchetti, P. A. 1998. Treatment of the periodontium affected by occlusal traumatism. In eds. M. Nevins and J. T. Mellonig, *Periodontal therapy: Clinical approaches and evidence of success*, Vol. 1, 132–133. Chicago. Quintessence.

Shefter, G. J., and W. T. McFall. 1984. Occlusal relations and periodontal status in human adults. *J. Periodontol.* 55:368–374.

Svanberg, G. K., G. J. King, and C. H. Gibbs. 1995. Occlusal considerations in periodontology. *Periodontology 2000* 9:106–117.

Tarnow, D. P., and P. Fletcher. 1986. Splinting of periodontally involved teeth: Indications and contraindications. *N.Y. State Dent. J.* (May):24–25.

Towfighi, P. P., M. A. Brunsvold, A. T. Storey, B. M. Arnold, D. E. Willman, and C. A. McMahan. 1997. Pathologic migration of anterior teeth in patients with moderate to severe periodontitis. *J. Periodontol.* 68:967–972.

Wingrove, S. S. 2011. Dental implant maintenance: The role of the dental hygienist and therapist. *Dental Health* 50(5):8–13.

Visit www.pearsonhighered.com/healthprofessionsresources to access the student resources that accompany this book. Simply select Dental Hygiene from the choice of disciplines. Find this book and you will find the complimentary study tools created for this specific title.

11

Abscesses of the Periodontium

Surendra Singh

OUTLINE

EDUCATIONAL OBJECTIVES

Upon completion of this chapter, the reader should be able to:

- Identify and describe the clinical and radiographic findings of three types of abscesses of the periodontium.
- Define the role of the dental hygienist in the treatment of a gingival abscess.
- Define the role of the dental hygienist in the treatment of a periodontal abscess.
- Define the role of the dental hygienist in the treatment of an operculum.

GOAL: To educate about the etiology, clinical manifestations, and therapy of different types of acute periodontal conditions.

KEY WORDS

Introduction

An abscess is defined as an infection originating from the tooth or periodontium. Pain and swelling from an abscess usually brings the patient into the dental office as an emergency visit. Classification of abscesses is based on the location of the infection. For example, a gingival abscess is an infection located in the gingival unit, usually the free (marginal) gingiva; a periodontal abscess is an infection located within the tissues adjacent to the periodontal pocket; and a pericoronal abscess is an infection located within the tissue around the crown of a partially erupted tooth, usually the last tooth in the arch.

The 1999 American Academy of Periodontology Classification of Periodontal Diseases added abscesses of the periodontium. It was a consensus that gingival/periodontal abscesses are part of the clinical course of gingivitis and periodontitis, and thus specific diagnosis and treatment challenges are required (Armitage, 1999).

Gingival Abscess

Etiology and Clinical Features

A **gingival abscess** is an acute infection characterized by a localized, painful edema at the free gingival margin or interdental papilla. Usually, there are no signs of periodontitis in the patient's mouth. The etiology of a gingival abscess is usually foreign objects such as popcorn kernels, toothbrush bristles, fish bones, or seeds that become lodged in a previously healthy site. Calculus is usually not the cause (Corbet, 2004).

Because the abscess is sudden in onset, the patient often will know the cause. The infection usually rapidly expands from the gingival margin or interdental papilla. Within 24 to 48 hours, the lesion will appear fluctuant (soft and movable). Purulent exudate (pus) may be exuding from the surface. If treatment is not immediately given, the abscess will usually rupture on its own. Pus is a collection of white blood cells (neutrophils), dead (necrotic) tissue, and bacteria in tissue fluid. Before treatment is started, it is necessary to determine the origin of the abscess.

Differential Diagnosis

The differential diagnosis of a gingival abscess is a periodontal abscess or endodontic abscess. The gingival abscess is usually located more coronally than the periodontal or endodontic abscess. The gingival abscess is usually found just within the gingival sulcus, whereas the periodontal abscess is usually found at the lateral side (corresponding to a deep pocket), and the endodontic abscess is usually found at the apical area of the root.

Treatment

Treatment usually involves identity and removal of the etiologic agent by periodontal debridement. Because the gingiva may be friable, careful tissue manipulation is advised. It is best to place the finger of the nondominant hand on

Rapid Dental Hint

When a patient presents with an abscess, it is important to determine if the origin of the abscess is periodontal or endodontic.

the tissue to support it. Local anesthesia may be helpful, but the injection should never be directly into the infection, as the infection may spread. Scaling establishes drainage through the gingival crevice. The patient can be placed on a warm saline rinse (1/4 teaspoonful of salt to 8 oz of warm water; rinse every 1 to 2 hours for several days). Make sure the patient is not hypertensive (because of the salt). The patient should be instructed to use a soft-bristled toothbrush. Systemic antibiotics are not recommended, as there is no systemic infection. If treated adequately, the condition will resolve within 24 hours or so. A follow-up appointment is recommended after 24 to 48 hours.

Periodontal Abscess

Etiology and Clinical Features

A **periodontal abscess**, also called a lateral periodontal abscess, is the most common type of abscess involving the periodontium. It is a localized purulent nidus of acute inflammation as a result of invasion of bacteria into the periodontal tissues, specifically within the gingival wall of a periodontal pocket that may cause destruction of the periodontal ligament and alveolar and supporting bone (Meng, 1999; Figures 11–1 ■, 11–2 ■). A periodontal abscess contains bacteria, bacterial by-products, inflammatory cells, tissue breakdown products, and serum. In the gingival connective tissues an inflammatory reaction occurs due to the bacteria and bacterial by-products, resulting in the connective tissue becoming infiltrated with inflammatory cells (e.g., neutrophils, macrophages). As a result of the inflammatory infiltrate, there is destruction or breakdown of the gingival connective tissues (e.g., collagen). The bacterial mass becomes encapsulated with the resultant pus formation.

Factors associated with periodontal abscess formation include (1) preexisting, untreated advanced periodontitis (Jaramillo et al., 2005); (2) an endodontic infection where there are lateral canals; (3) furcation involvement; (4) inadequate or partial periodontal debridement, which may allow the calculus to remain in the deepest pocket area, whereas the resolution of the inflammation at the coronal pocket area will occlude the normal drainage, resulting in the formation of a periodontal abscess; and (5) patients with diabetes mellitus, who are also more susceptible to periodontal abscess formation.

A periodontal abscess usually occurs around teeth with deep periodontal pockets and in furcation sites because of anatomical limitations, which makes oral hygiene and professional instrumentation difficult.

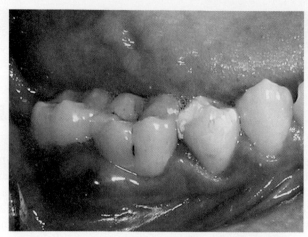

FIGURE 11–1 Periodontal abscess involving the mandibular molar. The buccal probed 10 mm. The pocket was occluded. Drainage was established after anesthesia was administered and the orifice of the pocket was opened with a curet. (Courtesy of John Eum, DDS, New York University College of Dentistry.)

Radiographically, the abscessed tooth, as well as other teeth, will most likely demonstrate advanced bone loss. The clinical probing depths should always be correlated with the radiographic findings.

Microorganisms found in the periodontal/gingival abscess resemble the microbiota of chronic periodontitic lesions. Microorganisms that colonize and are found in the exudate of the periodontal abscesses are primarily gram-negative anaerobic rods (Herrera, Roldán, & Sanz, 2000; Meng, 1999). Other bacteria associated with and found with high frequency in periodontal abscesses include *Porphyromonas gingivalis*, *Prevotella intermedia*, *Fusobacterium nucleatum*, *Campylobacter retus*, and *Capnocytophaga* sp. The eradication of *Porphyromonas gingivalis* from abscessed sites after treatment indicates that this bacterium is highly associated with abscess formation. *Aggregatibactor actinomycetemcomitans* is usually not found in the exudate.

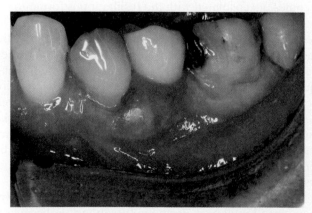

FIGURE 11–2 Periodontal abscess on the buccal surface of the mandibular premolar; 10 mm probing depths were recorded.

> ### Did You Know?
> Pus is generally a viscous, yellowish-white fluid formed in infected tissue, consisting of white blood cells, cellular debris, and necrotic tissue.

Acute versus Chronic

Periodontal abscesses can present as acute or chronic (long-standing). An abscess occurs if the acute abscess is not resolved or treated. A common chief complaint when a periodontal abscess is developing is that "I have pressure in my gums." The acute periodontal abscess presents as a shiny, swollen, discolored mass on the gingiva or mucosa at the lateral aspect of the root, but not at the free gingival margin as is the gingival abscess. It is usually located on the lateral aspect of the tooth surface where the periodontal pocket is. Finger pressure may produce purulent drainage. Clinically, the involved tooth may be tender to percussion (especially on chewing or mastication), mobile, with deep probing depths and edematous gingiva. Occasionally, patients may demonstrate localized lymphadenopathy (palpable lymph nodes) and fever. If the abscess is present on the lateral aspect of the tooth, there will be a radiolucent area, but if the abscess is formed on the facial or lingual part of the tooth, it will not show up on the radiograph so that probing the area is important. The patient does not usually display symptoms in an acute periodontal abscess, but some symptoms, such as a deep, dull pain or elevation of the tooth, may be present.

Differential Diagnosis

A differential diagnosis of a periodontal abscess is a periapical (endodontic) abscess (Figures 11–3 ■, 11–4 ■, 11–5 ■). By definition, an endodontic abscess usually occurs adjacent to the apex of a necrotic tooth and often heals following endodontic therapy. There may be a sinus tract draining the abscess, which originates from deep within the tissues and opens and drains onto the gingiva (Figure 11–3). Table 11–1 ■ shows the common features of periapical and periodontal abscesses. A sinus tract can be traced by taking a radiograph with a gutta percha point within the sinus tract. Often there is a combined endodontic/periodontic lesion where the tooth is nonvital, and a periodontal defect and deep pocket is present due to the periodontal tissue destruction from the lateral root canals. Clinicians often must be able to differentiate the origin of the infection, which is sometimes challenging.

> ### Did You Know?
> A gingival abscess occurs by the gingival margin. A periodontal abscess occurs where there is a deep pocket.

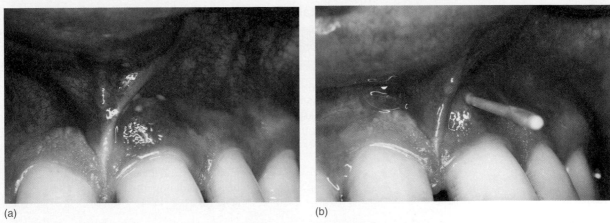

(a)   (b)

FIGURE 11–3 (a) A sinus tract is present on the maxillary central incisor. (b) To determine the origin of the infection, a gutta percha point is inserted into the fistula. Temperature testing revealed this tooth was nonvital, and an X-ray confirmed the gutta percha point ended at the apical region of the tooth.

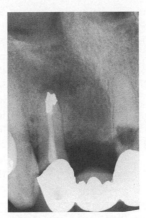

FIGURE 11–4 X-ray showing a previously endodontically treated tooth that still had a chronic infection. An apicoectomy was performed whereby the apical part of the root was excised, and a retrograde amalgam was placed.

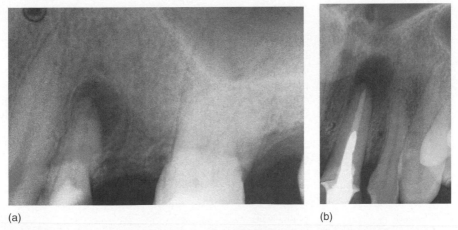

(a)   (b)

FIGURE 11–5 (a) Periapical pathology (PAP) on the premolar. The tooth tested nonvital. Endodontic therapy is indicated. (b) X-ray showing periapical pathology (PAP) on the central incisor. Root canal therapy was performed, and final post and crown were fabricated.

Table 11–1 Differences Between a Gingival, Periodontal, Periapical, and Pericoronal Abscess

	Gingival Abscess	Periodontal Abscess	Periapical Abscess	Periocoronitis (Pericoronal Abscess)
Symptoms	Swelling, warmth, redness, fluctuant mass near the gingival margin on the buccal aspect, pain	Swelling, warmth, redness, fluctuant mass on the lateral aspect of the tooth, may or may not have pain (Figures 11–1, 11–2)	Tender to percussion (tap the occlusal/incisal edge of tooth with a mirror handle); tender when chewing/biting; pressure tenderness; tooth is extruded; may be lymphadenopathy (Figures 11–3, 11–4, 11–5)	Trismus, difficulty in swallowing, facial swelling, lymphadenopathy (Figure 11–6)
Origin of infection	Gingiva	Periodontal ligament, bone	Pulp	Gingiva
Vital	Yes	Yes	No	Yes
Caries	No	No	Yes	No
Periodontal status	Previously health site	Deep pocket	No pocket—not probable except when the lesion extends into the periodontal ligament resulting in deep pocket. This lesion becomes an endodontic-periodontic lesion. Remember the lesion is pulpal in origin.	Good
Tooth mobility	No	Yes/no	Yes	No
Location of abscess	Abscess located by the gingival margin	Abscess usually located at lateral aspect of tooth	Sinus tract usually located in apical area	Partially erupted third molar
X-ray findings	No radiolucency	Lateral radiolucency	Apical radiolucency	Impacted third molar
Differentiation	Periodontal abscess	Endodontic abscess	Periodontal abscess	None
Treatment	Incision and drainage through pocket opening. Periodontal debridement.	Incision and drainage through pocket. Periodontal debridement. Definitive treatment may include extraction of the tooth or periodontal surgery. Antibiotics are not required if there is no systemic involvement (e.g., fever, lymphadenopathy)	Root canal. Antibiotics are not needed if the tooth is nonvital. Antibiotics are required if the tooth is vital and there is swelling and lymphadenopathy.	Antibiotics are usually needed if lymphadenopathy is present (penicillin drug of choice). Extraction of the third molar. Surgical removal of the operculum

Rapid Dental Hint

Always know the origin of the infection; is the infection coming from the pulp or from the periodontal tissues?

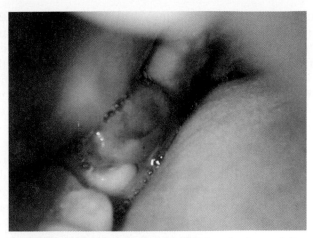

FIGURE 11–6 Pericoronitis. The third molar is partially covered by an operculum. (Courtesy of Dr. Michael Turner, New York University College of Dentistry.)

Treatment

Treatment of a periodontal abscess consists of two phases (Herrera et al., 2000). The first phase involves management of the acute signs and symptoms. Different therapies have been suggested for the acute lesion, including incision and drainage, scaling and root planing, administration of systemic antibiotics, periodontal surgery, and tooth extraction. Some clinicians prefer to wait until the acute lesion has subsided followed by periodontal debridement (López-Píriz, Aguilar, & Giménez, 2007), or periodontal surgery. The second phase involves more definitive treatment. Antibiotics should never be prescribed without subgingival debridement because antibiotics could not penetrate the biofilm without it being disrupted first with mechanical debridement.

If the decision is made to treat the acute lesion, then usually treatment involves incision and drainage. When giving infiltration anesthesia, injection into the abscess may cause spread of the infection. The opening of the periodontal pocket often is occluded because either there is healing at the coronal tissue area or there may be a foreign body (e.g., food), resulting in a buildup of pus. Because the pocket may be occluded, opening the pocket (incision) to drain the pus may be difficult. After obtaining profound anesthesia, the pocket should be carefully opened with a probe or curet to drain the pus. The tissue is very friable. Once the pocket is open, debridement of the pocket area and root under local anesthesia is performed. In the majority of cases, an antibiotic is not necessary. Only if there is systemic involvement (e.g., fever, lymphadenopathy) is an antibiotic necessary. After drainage is achieved, periodontal debridement is performed to remove the plaque and calculus from the root surface. The successfully treated patient will notice improvement within 24 hours of treatment. If symptoms fail to improve promptly, referral to a periodontist is recommended for surgery or extraction.

Pericoronal Abscess

Etiology and Features

Pericoronal abscess, also referred to as pericoronitis, is a localized infection involving the gingiva adjacent to a partially erupted tooth, usually the mandibular third molar region (Figure 11–6 ■). The **operculum** or gingival flap overlying the erupting tooth is usually red and edematous with food and debris collecting under the operculum. The operculum will disappear once the tooth fully erupts, but many of these teeth remain partially erupted indefinitely because of inadequate arch space for complete eruption or when the tooth is extracted.

Microbiology

The offending microorganisms are gram-negative anaerobes. The infection may spread posteriorly into the oropharyngeal area and medially to the base of the tongue and involve the regional lymph nodes (Meng, 1999). Patients may experience difficulty in swallowing, complain of a dull ache, and demonstrate limited jaw opening (trismus).

Treatment

Treatment initially is focused on controlling the infection. Irrigation with saline, iodine solution, or water is common therapy to flush out the food and debris found under the operculum. This area is very sensitive, so care must be taken when manipulating the tissues. If the infection is severe or systemic involvement (e.g., lymphadenopathy) is suspected, systemic antibiotics such as penicillin are indicated. Ultimately, extraction of the erupting tooth may be necessary but is better performed when the patient no longer has acute local infection or trismus.

Primary Herpetic Gingivostomatitis

Primary herpetic gingivostomatitis is a condition of the oral mucosa characterized by a *previous* infection with herpes virus (HSV 1), which is mainly a disease of infants and children and clinically detectable in about 90% of patients. After a brief prodromal period (1 to 2 days before development of blisters) of fever, headache, nausea, vomiting, and malaise, many small blisters (vesicles) form on the mucosa inside the lower lip. Vesicles also appear on the hard palate and tongue. These blisters quickly break and form painful, yellowish-gray ulcers, which form in groups surrounded by a red halo (inflammation). Rarely are the vesicles present at the time of the office visit because they quickly rupture. One of the most important distinguishing features, which is diagnostic for primary herpetic gingivostomatitis, is the presence of a generalized acute gingivitis. The gingival papillae are intact and not necrotic as in necrotizing ulcerative gingivitis (NUG). The gingiva is red (erythematous) and swollen (edematous). Submandibular lymphadenopathy is present. The patients do not have a past history of recurrent herpes labialis. When this disease is present in adults, it may be more difficult to diagnose because the typical signs and symptoms may not be present. Most patients develop the infection through direct contact with another person with active recurrent lesions (e.g., through kissing). Symptoms usually last for 1 to 2 weeks. However, a differential diagnosis (determination of which two or more diseases with similar symptoms is the one from which a patient is suffering) would be aphthous stomatitis (canker sores). Aphthous stomatitis occurs only on unattached mucosa, and there is a history of recurrence. Usually, there is no associated fever, whereas the ulcers in primary herpetic gingivostomatitis occur on both unattached and attached mucosa.

Treatment of primary herpetic gingivostomatitis in both children and adults is primarily palliative. The intense oral pain makes eating and drinking difficult. Dehydration must be prevented with frequent drinking of liquids. Rinsing with viscous xylocaine 2% before eating and drinking may be helpful to anesthetize the area. A palliative mouth rinse consisting of a mixture of Kaopectate and diphenhydramine may be helpful. Antipyretics such as acetaminophen are recommended to reduce the fever and pain. Antiviral drugs such as acyclovir (400 mg four times daily for 1 to 2 weeks is recommended) are used to reduce the duration of the infection.

Box 11–1: Treatment Steps for Gingival and Periodontal Abscesses

Gingival Abscess	Periodontal Abscess
First probe the site: relatively shallow or presence of pseudopocket (because of inflammation)	First probe the site: deep
Periodontal health	Periodontitis
Location is submarginal	Location is base of pocket
Incision and drainage: debridement and irrigate area	Incision and drainage: debridement and irrigate area
Rinse with warm water and salt	May require periodontal surgery for pocket elimination or extraction
No antibiotics required	Systemic antibiotics if lymphadenopathy is present

Dental Hygiene Application

An abscess is an infection originating from the tooth or periodontium. It is important to determine the point of origin so that proper treatment is given. The patient's chief complaint and a review of the dental history will help to determine the type of abscess. For instance, the patient should be asked if he or she recently had anything to eat that would cause a gingival abscess. The gingival abscess is confined to the marginal gingival or interdental papilla. If the patient has moderate to advanced periodontitis, then most likely it will be a periodontal abscess. Periodontal abscesses are part of the clinical course of the progression of periodontitis. Upon probing these sites, pus will usually come out of the pocket. The microbiota of a periodontal abscess is gram-negative anaerobic rods, which are similar to that found in deep periodontal pockets (Meng, 1999). This is a form of drainage that is necessary to eliminate the infection. A periapical abscess differs from a periodontal abscess in that the abscessed tooth is usually nonvital and will require endodontics therapy.

Oral examination of a patient complaining of pain and trouble opening his/her mouth will most likely reveal an operculum around a partially erupted mandibular third molar. The location of the infection will give a good indication on the type of abscess.

Box 11-1 summarizes the treatment sequence for a gingival and periodontal abscess.

Key Points

- Abscesses are bacterial infections.
- It is important to determine the origin of the abscess.
- Establish incision and drainage of the infection.
- Systemic antibiotics are only needed if there is systemic involvement.

- Five to 10% of patients initially infected with the herpes simplex virus develop primary herpetic gingivostomatitis.

Self-Quiz

1. A gingival abscess is localized to the
   a. periapical area.
   b. gingival margin.
   c. periodontal pocket.
   d. pericoronal area.

2. From the following list, select the items associated with patient management of an acute periodontal abscess without lymphadenopathy.
   a. Local delivered antibiotics (e.g., Arestin)
   b. Supragingival scaling
   c. Incision and drainage
   d. Leave alone until it becomes chronic
   e. Systemic antibiotics

3. From the following list, select the items associated with a gingival abscess.
   a. Popcorn kernel
   b. Deep periodontal pocket
   c. Partially erupted third molar
   d. Firm, pink gingiva
   e. Treat by debridement
   f. Treat with antibiotics

4. For each feature listed, select the correct condition from the list provided.

Feature	Condition
1. Apical radiolucency	a. Periodontal abscess
2. Trismus	b. Gingival abscess
3. Dental caries	c. Periapical abscess
4. Furcation defect	d. Pericoronitis
5. Operculum	
6. Deep pocket	
7. Fluctuant	

5. Which of the following is occurring when a pocket entrance is "opened" with a probe or curet on a tooth with an acute periodontal abscess?
   a. Transformation of the epithelium into connective tissue
   b. Conversion of the acute abscess into a gingival abscess
   c. Incision and drainage
   d. Laceration of the fistula tract

6. Which of the following treatments is used for a patient with a gingival abscess?
   a. Identify and remove the cause
   b. Use of systemic antibiotics
   c. Use of systemic analgesic
   d. Placement of controlled-drug antimicrobial such as Arestin.

7. From the following list, select the items associated with treatment of pericoronitis.
   a. Irrigation
   b. Extraction of third molar
   c. Removal of operculum
   d. Placement of Arestin
   e. Systemic antibiotics if lymphadenopathy is present

8. Which of the following conditions describes a localized purulent infection within the tissues surrounding the crown of a partically erupted tooth?
   a. Gingival abscess
   b. Periodontal abscess
   c. Pericoronal abscess
   d. Periapical abscess

9. From the following list, select the items associated with formation of a periodontal abscess.
   a. Preexisting, untreated advanced periodontitis
   b. From an endodontic infection where there are lateral canals
   c. Deep pocket associated with furcation involvement
   d. Inadequate or partial periodontal debridement
   e. Patients with diabetes mellitus

10. From the following list, select the bacteria associated with a periodontal abscess.
    a. *Porphyromonas gingivalis*
    b. *Prevotella intermedia*
    c. *Fusobacterium nucleatum*
    d. *Staphlococcus aureus*

Case Study

The dental hygienist upon gingival assessment and probing finds pus coming from the probing site on tooth #3. The dental hygienist has not yet exposed a radiograph of the area. In comparison to previous probing this tooth now has a 7 mm pocket when previous recordings were 4 mm.

1. What has caused the pus in the pocket?
   a. abscess at the apical end of the root
   b. infected operculum
   c. popcorn or other foreign object in gingival
   d. bacterial mass encapsulated

Answer: D. The inflammatory infiltrates cause the breakdown of the gingival connective tissue. The bacterial mass becomes encapsulated and pus forms. The operculum is related to pericoronitis. Foreign objects can infect the gingival for a gingival abscess. A periapical abscess occurs at the apex of the tooth.

2. Treatment of a periodontal abscess would include
   a. radiographs, incision, and drainage
   b. no radiographs, incision, and drainage
   c. radiographs and endodontic therapy
   d. irrigation, possible extraction

Answer: A. Radiographs are needed to determine bone loss. The area needs drainage. A gingival lesion does not have bone loss. A pericoronal abscess is a localized infection of the gingival adjacent to the partially erupted tooth. A periapical abscess occurs at the apex of a necrotic tooth.

3. How would the dental hygienist distinguish a periodontal abscess from primary herpetic gingivostomatitis?
   a. vesicles rupture quickly
   b. vesicles on lip mucosa and hard palate and tongue
   c. generalized acute gingivitis
   d. all of the above

Answer: D. All of the above are signs of primary herpetic gingivostomatitis. A periodontal abscess would be in one location on the attached gingiva adjacent to an infected tooth.

References

Armitage, G. C. 1999. Development of a classification system for periodontal diseases and conditions. *Ann. Periodontol.* 4:1–6.

Corbet, E. F. 2004. Diagnosis of acute periodontal lesions. *Periodontology 2000* 34:204–216.

Herrera, D., S. Roldán, and M. Sanz. 2000. The periodontal abscess: A review. *J. Clin. Periodontol.* 27:377–386.

Jaramillo, A., R. M. Arce, D. Herrera, M. Betancourth, J. E. Botero, and A. Contreras. 2005. Clinical and microbiological characterization of periodontal abscesses. *J. Clin. Periodontol.* 32(12):1213–1218.

López Píriz, R., L. Aguilar, and M. J. Giménez. 2007. Management of odontogenic infection of pupal and periodontal origin. *Med. Oral Patop. Oral Cir. Bucal.* 12(12):E154–159.

Meng, H. X. 1999. Periodontal abscess. *Ann. Periodontol.* 4:79–82.

Periodontal Diseases: The Assessment Phase

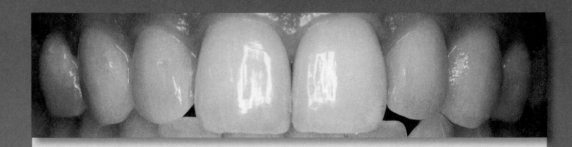

OUTLINE

12

Dental Hygiene Process of Care for the Patient with Periodontal Disease

Cheryl Westphal Theile

OUTLINE

Introduction
Assessment
Dental Hygiene Diagnosis
Planning
Implementation
Evaluation
Documentation
Dental Hygiene Application
Key Points
Self-Quiz
Case Study
References

EDUCATIONAL OBJECTIVES

Upon completion of this chapter, the reader should be able to:

- List and explain six phases of the dental hygiene process for periodontal patient care.
- Explain the importance of stating the goals for periodontal patient care.
- Understand the differences between a dental diagnosis and a dental hygiene diagnosis.

GOAL: To provide information on the procedures of patient care.

KEY WORDS

Introduction

The purpose of the dental hygiene process of care is to provide a framework within which the individualized needs of the patient can be met. The dental hygiene process of care is a whole process of care, and the assessment process is the first phase of the five phases (Mueller-Joseph & Petersen, 1995) of a search for clues leading up to the identification and classification of the nature of the disease and the steps in patient care needed to alleviate the problem (Bates, Bickley, & Hoekelman, 1995; DeGowin, 1994). Since this concept development in 1995, a sixth component has been added, documentation, to highlight the need to document each phase in the decision-making process. The American Dental Hygienists' Association (ADHA) states that the dental hygiene process of care encompasses all significant actions taken by the dental hygienist. The dental hygiene process of care provides a framework for the dental hygienist to provide care according to a critical thinking process, which first analyzes individual patient needs, identifies the causative or influencing factors, then prepares a care plan that includes modalities to eliminate, reduce, or prevent the factors and evaluates and documents the results (ADHA, 2008). The six components are

- Assessment
- Dental hygiene diagnosis
- Planning
- Implementation
- Evaluation
- Documentation

Assessment

Assessment is the systemic gathering of all relevant information concerning the patient, including medical/dental history, vital signs, extraoral and intraoral examination, periodontal and dental examination, radiographs, indices, and risk assessments (e.g., patient use of tobacco, presence of systemic disease). In the patient history assessment, clues are symptoms, which are abnormalities experienced by the patient. Information obtained by observations of and statements made by the patient are termed **subjective data**. In the clinical examination, on the other hand, clues are signs, which are abnormalities perceived by the practitioner. Information obtained from direct measurements and recorded data of the patient and statements made by the practitioner are termed **objective data**.

Data collection starts with recording the personal profile of the patient and then collecting the chief complaint and medical, dental, and social history, followed by the extra/intraoral examination, restorative charting, occlusal, gingival assessment, periodontal assessment, oral hygiene evaluation, radiographs, nutritional, risk assessment, and additional diagnostic laboratory tests if required. The data is assessed to determine factors that affect the periodontal patient such as autoimmune disorders, hormonal changes, cardiovascular disease, or medications that effect the oral environment. The data is also assessed to determine if any medical condition requires a modification in the planning or implementation of the care such as premedication, appointment timing, urgent needs, or medical complex status.

Social, Economic, and Cultural Considerations

From the moment the patient enters the care cycle within the practice, the whole person is assessed to understand aspects such as his or her health background, health beliefs, cultural background, social and economic background, educational background, oral health literacy, and work-related issues. These factors play an important role as a whole when determining a successful outcome for the dental hygiene care plan.

A review of the patient's dental and medical history from the viewpoint of social and economic concerns provides insight to the patient's ability to access dental care and afford subsequent dental follow-up home-care regimens. Often factors such as people's beliefs about the role they should play in their own healthcare and the part their home care habits play in causing periodontal disease will have an impact upon their desire to maintain their oral health after surgery or other extensive dental care. A cultural assessment should be obtained to determine if any health beliefs or practices will influence the patient's compliance. A complete discussion with the patient is crucial to elicit the information instead of a nonverbal form of the medical or social history questionnaire, often done without any review of these factors. Successful outcomes depend on the patient's and practitioner's agreement on the goals and interventions for the dental hygiene care plan.

Dental Hygiene Diagnosis

After the data are collected, the dental hygienist reviews and analyzes the information. A **dental hygiene diagnosis** is defined as the identification of an existing or potential oral health problem that the dental hygienist is educationally qualified and licensed to treat (ADHA, 2010). Many diagnostic models are used in planning dental hygiene care. The Dental Hygiene Process Model is based on identification of the patient's problem in terms of response and states the possible etiology of the response. The problems are classified into categories of general systems, soft tissue, periodontal, oral hygiene, and dental. A dental hygiene diagnosis differs from a dental diagnosis because a dental diagnosis gives a name to the disease, and the dental hygiene diagnosis identifies the patient's actual or potential response to the disease process (Mueller-Joseph & Petersen, 1995). The problem statement is written by stating the problem and a phrase "related to" for the etiologic factor. The purpose of a dental hygiene diagnosis is to keep the planning of patient care centered on problems or conditions that are responsive to dental hygiene intervention (Mueller-Joseph & Petersen, 1995). For example, a patient has inflamed gingiva, but no bone loss is shown on the radiographs. The dental hygienist should also understand the need to disrupt the pathogenic bacteria so that a more beneficial microflora will populate the tooth/soft tissue area.

After the etiology is determined, the practitioner determines a care plan that will eliminate or control the condition. The dental hygienist should know why the patient developed the condition for appropriate treatment to be rendered. For example, a patient complains of bleeding gums. The dental hygienist assesses the situation to determine the extent of gingivitis and periodontitis. The problem is stated as related to inadequate biofilm removal and possible faulty dental restorations leading to biofilm traps. The dental hygienist develops a plan to educate the patient in home care, removes the biofim, and adjusts or refers for the faulty restorations.

Planning

Planning is the establishment of realistic goals and treatment strategies to facilitate optimal oral health. A **dental hygiene care plan** involves the development of written interventions for the patient's individual needs based on data collection and assessment. Alternative options should be included in the plan that may be implemented instead of the ideal plan if the patient is in poor health, if the patient is not compliant or motivated to follow the ideal plan, if there are cultural barriers, or if the patient cannot afford the ideal treatment. The dental hygiene care plan must be presented to the patient and agreed on before any treatment is started. An appropriate sequence of treatments must be stated. Developing a plan involves knowledge from a variety of disciplines besides dental hygiene, including behavioral sciences, pharmacology, anatomy and physiology, chemistry, and microbiology. The dental hygiene care plan is part of the comprehensive dental treatment plan, and the care is sequenced with all phases of the master plan for initial, surgical, restorative, or maintenance phases or other supportive therapies such as nutritional counseling or tobacco cessation. Critical thinking and decision-making skills are necessary to provide effective and efficient dental hygiene services.

When developing a dental hygiene care plan, the goal or end result of treatment must be stated (Mueller-Joseph & Petersen, 1995). The goal is a statement that addresses and identifies the purpose for implementing the dental hygiene care. The individualized plan also identifies the interventions necessary to meet the healthcare goals of the patient. Interventions are procedures carried out by the dental hygienist to help the patient reach the desired goal. For example, let us say that a dental diagnosis is gingivitis modified by systemic factors for pregnancy-associated gingivitis. The dental hygiene diagnosis is gingival inflammation related to the elevated hormonal levels and inadequate home care of the teeth and gingiva by the patient. The aims of dental hygiene treatment are to reduce biofilm levels by oral hygiene instruction and educate the patient about the influence of biofilm and hormones on overall dental health. Dental hygiene intervention deals with the disruption of the biofilm by mechanical debridement or other modalities.

Implementation

Once the care plan is presented to the patient and an informed consent form is signed by the patient and dentist, treatment commences. This **implementation** phase includes (1) providing the patient with health education, preventive counseling, and nutritional counseling; (2) implementing pain management procedures; (3) carrying out periodontal debridement procedures; (4) providing and educating on use of antimicrobial therapies; (5) applying chemotherapeutic agents; (6) undertaking coronal polishing; (7) carrying out fluoride therapy or desensitizing therapies; (8) teaching the patient proper care of oral prostheses; (9) teaching the patient proper care and maintenance of restorations; (10) providing or referring for tobacco cessation; (11) providing any follow-up instructions; and (12) documenting the process properly. The order of the procedures is determined by the needs of the patient and assessment made after each visit to determine if the goals of each visit are accomplished.

The dentist may determine a dental diagnosis of gingivitis, whereas the dental hygiene diagnosis focuses on educating the patient on the need and benefit (Mueller-Joseph & Petersen, 1995) of proper biofilm control to reduce supragingival and subgingival microbial accumulation. Thus the dental hygiene implementation may be oral hygiene education (CDT D01330), full-mouth debridement (CDT D04355), prophylaxis (CDT D0110), and reevaluation to review outcomes and determine further treatments.

Evaluation

The **evaluation** phase of therapy addresses the feedback on the outcomes of the treatment and the patient's effectiveness or compliance. This phase occurs after treatment has been completed, when the patient returns for a follow-up visit a few weeks after the nonsurgical periodontal therapy (initial therapy or Phase I therapy) or surgical therapy has been completed, or for periodontal maintenance (recall/recare) procedures. Evaluation also occurs after each treatment visit in a series of appointments to determine if the goals of the previous visit were reached or if the clinician needs to return to previous treatment or consider additional modalities of care. For instance, if an area is still bleeding, the clinician needs to reassess the biofilm and calculus removal, patient home care compliance, or other factors preventing the improvement and healing of the site. Repeated scaling or additional modalities may be required, and this is then factored into the revised care plan. In addition, referrals may be necessary for further diagnostics or treatment.

Documentation

Because the process of care is an ongoing process, an appropriate method of written and visual **documentation** is required. The intraoral camera is an excellent technology to document various findings before and after the treatment procedure. The practitioner is able to view and record such conditions as biofilm retention sites, gingival conditions, faulty margins or caries, and stain or other deposits. The images can assist the practitioner to motivate the patient and secure agreement on treatment goals. The recordings help explain the condition and create a historical record that can be placed in the patient's file and used to show the patient any progress or degeneration of the periodontal condition being treated at subsequent appointments. Many dental practice management software systems and cameras are available for chair-side use. The intraoral camera can be employed during the charting, oral soft tissue exam, or oral hygiene evaluation to involve the patient in the process and discuss the findings. Fully integrated systems are available to network with electronic health or dental records and charting. Digital radiography and intraoral photography are combined to present a comprehensive documentation for the patient. Permanently saved images after case presentation are a valuable tool for patient education and increasing the likelihood that the recommended treatment procedures will be performed.

Computer technology is an essential component for the treatment record, appointment planning, recare visit booking, and patient documentation for running a dental practice. Oral hygiene evaluations as part of the computer record of the patient offer an array of visual presentations that can enhance treatment planning and patient compliance with the recommended procedures. Patients can be shown a pictorial display of their probing depths, caries, gingival recession, other gingival involvement, or potential treatment outcomes of surgery or prosthetic replacements.

Documentation of all aspects of the process of care is essential record keeping, even with computerized technology. Ongoing recorded progress notes include compliance with self-care, responses to treatment, and specific educational topics. Any specific notes related to the cultural variations, health beliefs, or practices should be noted. The documentation also includes a summary of the goals and outcomes of treatment in an ongoing process of care.

Dental Hygiene Application

The dental hygiene diagnosis provides the foundation for the development, implementation, and evaluation of the dental hygiene treatment plan (ADHA, 2008). It is a key element in identifying an existing or potential periodontal/oral problem.

Key Points

- Six components of the dental hygiene process enable the dental hygienist to identify the patient's periodontal problem, to determine the cause of the problem, and then to treat the problem.
- An intraoral camera can be useful to point out areas of recession, biofilm-retentive sites, bleeding points, and restorations.

- Documentation is an integral part of the dental hygiene process; written notes are an essential component of the treatment record.

Self-Quiz

1. All of the following are components of the dental hygiene process except one. Which one is the exception?
   a. Assessment
   b. Dental diagnosis
   c. Treatment planning
   d. Implementation
   e. Evaluation

2. Which one of the following reasons is important for determining the individual goals for periodontal patient care?
   a. Establishes a rapport with the patient
   b. Emphasizes the need for prevention in the care of the patient

   c. Identifies the purpose for treating the patient
   d. Evaluates for treatment needs after the first appointment

3. Which one of the following statements explains the purpose of a dental hygiene diagnosis?
   a. Keeps the planning of patient care centered on problems or conditions that are responsive to dental hygiene intervention
   b. Helps the dental hygienist determine the need for additional radiographs
   c. Identifies the type of periodontal disease
   d. Anticipates the effectiveness in achieving the desired outcome of therapy

4. Before undergoing any periodontal treatment, every patient should have his or her mouth and dentition photographed with an intraoral camera because the intraoral camera is an important part of documentation.

   a. Both the statement and the reason are correct and related.

   b. Both the statement and the reason are correct but not related.

   c. The statement is correct, but the reason is not.

   d. The statement is not correct, but the reason is correct.

   e. Neither the statement nor the reason is correct.

5. Which of the following reasons best explains the purpose of evaluation of periodontal therapy?

   a. Determines the need for additional periodontal intervention

   b. Deals with the feedback on the effectiveness of treatment

   c. Identifies the type of disease present

   d. Allows the dental hygienist to introduce oral hygiene care products for home use

Case Study

The dental hygienist is new to the dental practice and begins to review the charts to plan the care for each appointed patient of the day. Upon review of one patient the dental hygienist notices there is very little written in the progress notes and the periodontal charting was not updated at the last visit 6 months ago. It appears there was some pocketing then but no bleeding sites were recorded. The patient record does not indicate what home care was recommended or the goals for the dental hygiene treatment. There is a general dental treatment plan which indicates that the patient is to have 6 month "prophys".

1. What is the first step the dental hygienist should do for this patient?

   a. evaluate the bleeding to complete the periodontal charting.

   b. reassess all the data beginning with the chief concern and medical history.

   c. scale and polish while discussing the possible therapies.

   d. ask the dentist for the dental diagnosis.

Answer: B. A complete reassessment of all data needs to be done which may include collecting data that was previously not recorded. All data should be updated and reviewed for accuracy and completeness. It is the responsibility of the dental hygienist to create a dental hygiene care plan.

2. What data would be needed to formulate a dental hygiene diagnosis?

   a. existing or potential oral health problems

   b. dentist does treatment plan

   c. listing of the diseases such as caries or periodontal disease

   d. plan of interventions

Answer: A. The dental hygiene diagnosis differs from the dental diagnosis since the dental diagnosis gives a name to the disease and the dental hygiene diagnosis identifies the actual or potential response to the disease process. After the dental hygiene diagnosis is created the planned interventions are determined.

3. When does evaluation occur in the dental hygiene care planning process?

   a. after each visit in a series of visits

   b. at the beginning of the recall preventive visit

   c. after non-surgical care is complete

   d. B and C

   e. all of the above

Answer: E. All of the above. The evaluation phase is an ongoing phase to determine if the goals of the treatment are being met or if the clinician has to modify the treatment to meet the goals.

References

American Dental Hygienists' Association (ADHA). 2008. *Standards for clinical dental hygiene practice*, Available at http://www.adha.org/downloads/adha_standards08.pdf

American Dental Hygienists' Association (ADHA). 2010. *Dental hygiene diagnosis: An American Dental Hygienists' Association Position Paper*. Available at http://www.adha.org/downloads/ADHA_Policies.pdf

Bates, B., L. S. Bickley, and R. A. Hoekelman. 1995. *A pocket guide to physical examination and history taking*, 2nd ed. Philadelphia: Lippincott.

DeGowin, R. L. 1994. *DeGowin & DeGowin's diagnostic examination*, 3–4. New York: McGraw-Hill.

Mueller-Joseph, L., and M. Petersen. 1995. The dental hygiene process of care. In eds. L. Mueller-Joseph and M. Petersen, *Dental hygiene process: Diagnosis and care planning*, 1–19. Albany, NY: Delmar.

Visit www.pearsonhighered.com/healthprofessionsresources to access the student resources that accompany this book. Simply select Dental Hygiene from the choice of disciplines. Find this book and you will find the complimentary study tools created for this specific title.

13

Patient History

Rosemary DeRosa Hays

OUTLINE

EDUCATIONAL OBJECTIVES

Upon completion of this chapter, the reader should be able to:

- Explain the importance of data collection.
- Illustrate the importance of total health assessment in providing periodontal services.

GOAL: To provide information on the patient history-taking process.

KEY WORDS

Introduction

The patient's first visit is the time to collect subjective data. A complete **dental/medical history** is an essential aspect of the initial evaluation. It is here that the dental hygienist becomes an advantageous partner in the healthcare evaluation process. The hygienist interviews the patient for his or her history, which is divided into the personal profile, social history, chief complaint, history of the present illness, medical history, family history, and dental history. The collective diagnostic information developed through this interview provides a basis for future comparisons to evaluate the progress of disease, the efficacy of treatment, and the appearance of new findings. Therefore, taking the patient history is a mandatory first step in the treatment process.

Prevention survey systems can be designed on the computer to make data collection, results, and interpretation simpler.

The Interview

The **interview process**, so critical to the successful completion of the dental and medical history, demands a high level of communication between the patient and the dental hygienist. If done properly, an interview helps establish a rapport between the dental hygienist and the patient. Obtaining a proper history of the dental patient is important for accurate diagnosis and treatment (Rahman & Tasnim, 2007). History taking can be accomplished through a questionnaire, a patient interview, or a combination of both. The most practical and successful method for assessing the health status of a patient is a combination questionnaire and interview.

During the interview, open-ended questions such as "What changes in your health or medications have occurred since your last dental visit?" or "What in your mouth bothers you?" open doors to gaining more pertinent information. If good rapport develops, the patient will feel more comfortable, and as the interview progresses, he or she will volunteer more information. Open-ended questions put patients more at ease. Nevertheless, closed-ended questions also are necessary, such as, "When was your last dental visit?" These types of questions do not require much responding from the patient; rather, they can be answered usually in one sentence.

Personal Profile

The obvious place to begin the interview is by asking questions concerning the patient's identity. This personal profile consists of the patient's name, age, address, occupation, and telephone number. Some of this information is needed for identification purposes, whereas the patient's age and sex may be useful in the classification of the periodontal disease. Document the name, address, and telephone number of the patient's physician, which will be useful if consultation is necessary.

Social History

The social history includes the patient's occupation, lifestyle, marital status, diet, and use of alcohol and tobacco, both smoking and chewing tobacco. Habits such as cigarette smoking or use of smokeless tobacco should be noted because they are potential risk factors for periodontal diseases.

Cigarette smoking is reported in pack-years, which is determined by multiplying the number of packs of cigarettes smoked per day by the number of years the patient has smoked. Documenting the amount of smoking in pack-years gives a better understanding of the total exposure of nicotine during the lifetime of an individual. For example, if a person smoked one pack every day for 10 years, this is 10 pack-years.

The patient's lifestyle, including family and social structure, attitudes, and behaviors, is part of the social history. A patient's social perceptions, priorities, amount of stress, and ideas on aesthetics provide clues to compliance with dental care. A dental hygienist can work toward changing a patient's attitudes and behaviors by understanding the patient's cultural differences, motivation, patience, education, and expectations.

Chief Complaint

The next step is to ask the patient to identify his or her **chief complaint** (CC). The patient should state in his or her own words why he or she is seeking treatment. Determination of the CC assists in the identification of any ongoing disease process. Symptoms of periodontal problems include pressure in the gingiva or jaw or itchy gingiva. Signs of periodontal disease include bleeding, halitosis (bad breath), and/or tooth mobility. Given the insidious nature of periodontal diseases, many patients have no idea there is a problem. If the patient's CC involves something other than periodontal disease, such as pain of significant concern, this must be treated first before any other dental treatment is rendered.

History of Present Illness

The history of the CC expands on the patient's awareness of the problem and is also referred to as the history of present illness. The dental hygienist should inquire how long the

---

Did You Know?

Seventy-three percent of Americans would rather go grocery shopping than floss.

Rapid Dental Hint

The patient's chief complaint is very important. Ask him or her, "Why did you come to the dental office today?" You must address the chief complaint first before any other procedures are performed.

patient's problem has existed, any previous treatment(s), and if this problem has occurred before. For instance, if the patient's CC is "bleeding from the gums," the dental hygienist should ask about the onset, cause, location, and duration of the bleeding.

Medical History

The current and past status of the patient's general health, or medical history, should be the next area of investigation (Pickett & Gurenlian, 2005). A questionnaire, an interview, or a combination of questionnaire and interview can be used to accomplish this. Sometimes, however, a simple telephone call to the patient prior to the first appointment may screen for potential medical problems. A written questionnaire provides a baseline for treatment, whereas an interview provides both personal contact with the patient and supplementary information that may contribute to a more comprehensive evaluation. It is important to listen closely to the patient and have a genuine interest in what is said to provide insight, accuracy, and clarity in the history (McDaniel, Miller, Jones, & Davis, 1995). Allowing the patient to describe symptoms or complaints at length encourages trust and fosters a sympathetic professional relationship, but it is only necessary to record the relevant facts and details. Eliciting proper history from a patient is paramount in establishing an accurate diagnosis and management in medical practice (Rahman & Tasnim, 2007).

Questions concerning current medication use and drug allergies are crucial because the answers may have a direct effect on any treatment the dentist eventually prescribes. Both prescription and over-the-counter medications the patient is taking should be recorded. The name, dosage, and indications also should be written on the form. The hygienist should look especially for any potential drug–drug or drug–food interactions. Adverse side effects (undesirable effects of the drug on the body) of certain medications may be the source of dental problems. For example, antidepressant and antihypertensive medications may cause xerostomia, or dry mouth. Some medications for hypertension or epileptic seizures may cause enlargement of the gingiva, which can result in plaque-control problems. Absorption from the intestines of certain antibiotics such as tetracycline is delayed with food and calcium-containing products including milk and other dairy products. Consultation with the patient's physician may be necessary. If the patient does not know the names of the medications, ask him or her to bring the containers to the next office visit. If a patient is regularly taking medication for diabetes or hypertension, it is extremely important to ask if he or she took the medication as prescribed on that day; if so, the dosage and frequency of usage should be noted on the form. Sometimes a patient may forget to take high blood pressure (antihypertensive) medication and present with uncontrolled blood pressure. If this is the case, the hygienist should contact the patient's physician.

The medical history may uncover other conditions that can have an effect on periodontal health or treatment, such as diabetes mellitus, leukemia, or acquired immunodeficiency syndrome (AIDS; Neff, 1997). At this time a link between periodontal disease and certain discussed medical conditions that the patient has can be made. If the patient is suspected of being medically compromised, consultation with the patient's physician is indicated, and a written release should be obtained from the patient before treatment begins.

Infective endocarditis is of particular concern in dental care. Infective endocarditis is an infection of the tissue lining of the heart that can result in damage to the heart valves. Any dental procedure that causes bleeding could allow bacteria to enter the bloodstream, resulting in bacteremia. Before initiating any dental treatment that may cause bleeding in patients who are susceptible to developing infective endocarditis, proper antibiotic protection should be administered. The American Heart Association (AHA) recommends a prophylactic antibiotic regimen for such patients, and the 2007 guidelines of the AHA should be followed (Wilson et al., 2007; see Appendix C)

The medical history form is a legal document that provides a past and present profile of the patient's health (Robbins, 2002). After the medical history is complete, the document must be dated and signed by the patient and the dentist, and at each future visit, the form should be updated. The patient should review this information and sign the form again. A new form should be filled out yearly. Indelible ink, preferably black (because it will copy better than blue), should be used. If the patient is a minor, a parent or legal guardian should date and sign the form.

Family History

The family history consists of the present and past medical illnesses of family members. Such a record may help to identify disease trends in the family that are risk factors for dental/periodontal diseases such as diabetes and ischemic heart disease.

Dental History

The dental history includes past and present dental treatments, past dental problems, oral habits, nutritional profile, past response to treatment, and oral hygiene status. This information is collected by way of a written form and an interview with the patient.

The past dental history often provides insight into previous dental experiences, pleasant or unpleasant, in all areas of dentistry, including oral surgery, periodontics, restorative dentistry, endodontics, and orthodontics. Experiences with local anesthetics and nitrous oxide should be recorded. Questions especially pertinent to the dental hygiene visit

Rapid Dental Hint

If a patient does not know the name of drugs he or she is taking, ask him or her to bring in the pill containers.

include those regarding the patient's last dental visit, what was done, and how long since the last prophylaxis.

A nutritional or diet profile of the patient is helpful in assisting the dental hygienist in recognizing a caries-prone diet. During the interview, the dental hygienist can suggest ways in which the patient can alter his or her diet to promote better dental health.

Past dental history also provides information on the patient's dental health values. The periodontal history may be significant. For example, a patient should be asked if previous periodontal surgery was performed (make sure he or she understands what periodontal surgery is). The patient may respond that he or she has had periodontal surgery twice in the past year. On further questioning, it may become apparent that the patient returned to the dental office only once for a periodontal maintenance appointment. This information suggests that the patient is noncompliant with oral hygiene self-care and dental visits.

Other areas to explore include the patient's attitude toward dental care and the present surroundings and the level of desire for treatment. Question the patient on what specific oral hygiene regimen he or she follows, including the types of products used. Question the patient on what kind of toothbrush (e.g., soft, medium, or hard bristled), electric brushes, dental floss, and mouth rinse he or she uses. The frequency of product use should be documented, as well as compliance with recommended periodontal maintenance appointments.

Did You Know?

A survey shows that 83% of U.S. adults are very satisfied with the services they get from their dentists. This survey was done by Louis Harris and Associates in an effort to study U.S. attitude toward dentists.

Dental Hygiene Application

The initial step performed on a periodontal patient is to obtain a complete dental/medical, social, and family history. Determination and recording of medications the patient is taking are important because certain drugs affect the periodontium, and severe drug interactions can occur. Other factors, such as the number of cigarettes smoked, should also be recorded.

Key Points

- The interviewing process establishes rapport with the patient.
- Medical diseases and medications can affect conditions in the mouth.
- Update a patient's dental/medical history at every appointment.

Self-Quiz

1. Which one of the following pieces of information collected from the patient is subjective?
   a. Medical history
   b. Dental examination
   c. Periodontal examination
   d. Radiographic survey
   e. Oral hygiene evaluation

2. From the list provided, select the items associated with the importance of patient information collected during the interview.
   a. Anticipates patient's attitude about periodontal care
   b. Determines the number of visits for the patient
   c. Allows the patient to voice his or her opinions about treatment
   d. Provides a basis for future comparison
   e. Establishes a rapport between patient and hygienist

3. From the list provided, select the items that a dental hygienist should do before periodontal treatment is started if the patient cannot remember the names of the medications he or she is taking.
   a. Call the patient's pharmacist to confirm the medications.
   b. Call the patient's physician to confirm the medications.
   c. Tell the patient to bring the containers to the next appointment.
   d. Tell the patient to call home.

4. Which of the following parts of the interview determines the patient's smoking habits?
   a. Chief complaint
   b. Dietary profile
   c. Medical history
   d. Social history
   e. Dental history

5. All the following types of communications are most appropriate to determine the medical history of a patient except one. Which one is the exception?
   a. Telephone
   b. Questionnaire
   c. Interview
   d. Computer

Case Study

Age: 20   Blood Pressure: 140/90
Gender: female   Pulse Rate: 90
Height: 5'3"   Respiratory Rate: 19
Weight: 185

Medical History

Patient has a history of obesity. She has been on multiple fad diets since the age of 15. A year and a half ago the patient lost 70 pounds while taking fenfluramine (Fen-Phen) for a duration of six months. The patient has been diagnosed with clinical depression. She has noticed weight gain since she stopped taking the weight loss medication.

Medications

Oral contraceptives, Prozac (fluoxetine) 20 mg one tab in the morning and one in the afternoon

Family History

Father died of heart attack at the age of 61. Family history of hypertension and high cholesterol

Questions

1. The patient has extensive interproximal and surface caries. Which of the following may be contributing factors to her condition?
   a. Medication Prozac
   b. Diet
   c. High frequency consumption of sugary foods
   d. Improper home care
   e. All of the above

Answer: E.

2. After reviewing the patient's medical history what is the next appropriate action?
   a. Begin treatment.
   b. Conclude there are no significant medical findings that would contraindicate treatment.
   c. Consult a physician and obtain a written release before treatment.
   d. Wait 10 minutes and re-assess blood pressure.

Answer: C.

3. All of the following are appropriate dietary modification recommendations EXCEPT one. Which is the exception?
   a. Milk, cheese, and yogurt products after meals
   b. Chewing gum containing xylitol
   c. Drinking water after meals and snacks
   d. Eating dried fruit snacks throughout the day

Answer: D.

4. Which of the following would be the MOST appropriate referral for the patient?
   a. Psychiatrist
   b. Oral Surgeon
   c. Endodontist
   d. Nutritionist

Answer: D.

5. The patient is at high risk for all of the below:
   a. Heart problems
   b. Periodontal disease
   c. Morbid obesity
   d. Multiple chronic nutritional deficiencies

Answer: B

6. What is the clinical significance of the patient's previous use of fenfluramine (Fen-Phen)?
   a. At risk for infective endocarditis
   b. Pre-medication may be needed
   c. Valvular spasms
   d. All of the above

Answer: D

References

McDaniel, T. F., D. Miller, R. Jones, and M. Davis. 1995. Assessing patient willingness to reveal health history information. *J. Am. Dent. Assoc.* 126:375–379.

Neff, L. 1997. Oral health and systemic disease. *Access* 11(3):29–34.

Pickett, F. A., and J. Gurenlian. 2005. *The medical history: Clinical implications and emergency prevention in dental settings*. Philadelphia: Lippincott, Williams & Wilkins.

Rahman, A., and Tasnim.S. 2007. Twelve tips for better communication with patients during history-taking. *Scientific World Journal* 7(April 30): 519–524.

Robbins, K. S. 2002. Medicolegal considerations. In ed. S. F. Malamed, *Medical emergencies in the dental office*, 6th ed., 93–103. St Louis: Mosby.

Wilson W., K. A. Taubert, M. Gewitz, et al., 2007. Prevention of infective endocarditis: Guidelines from the American Heart Association: A guideline from the American Heart Association Rheumatic Fever, Endocarditis, and Kawasaki Disease Committee, Council on Cardiovascular Disease in the Young, and the Council on Clinical Cardiology, Council on Cardiovascular Surgery and Anesthesia, and the Quality Care and Outcomes Research Interdisciplinary Working Group. *Circulation* 116(15):1736–1754.

Visit www.pearsonhighered.com/healthprofessionsresources to access the student resources that accompany this book. Simply select Dental Hygiene from the choice of disciplines. Find this book and you will find the complimentary study tools created for this specific title.

14

Clinical Examination: Extraoral/Intraoral Examination and Dental Evaluation

Rosemary DeRosa Hays and Cheryl M. Westphal Theile

OUTLINE

Introduction
Extraoral/Intraoral Examination
Dental Evaluation
Tooth Stain Evaluation
Dentinal Hypersensitivity
Dental Hygiene Application
Key Points
Self-Quiz
Case Study
References

EDUCATIONAL OBJECTIVES

Upon completion of this chapter, the reader should be able to:

- Discuss the role of the dental hygienist in evaluating the dental and oral hygiene status of a patient.
- Describe the importance of performing an intraoral and extraoral examination.
- Describe the components of the dental examination.
- Explain how the findings of the dental evaluation relate to the recognition of periodontal diseases.
- Discuss the different types of tooth stains and their clinical significance.
- Discuss techniques for determining dentinal hypersensitivity.

GOAL: To explain the clinical components of a dental examination and how it relates to the periodontal condition.

KEY WORDS

caries *180*
dental charting *180*
dental implants *181*
dentinal hypersensitivity *186*
oral cancer *180*
tooth wear *183*

Introduction

After completing the patient history, the next aspect of patient assessment involves the collection of objective data by means of a physical examination of the patient. The dental hygienist's tools for this task include the extraoral/intraoral examination, the dental evaluation, the oral hygiene evaluation, the gingival assessment, and the periodontal examination. This section focuses on the extraoral/intraoral examination and the dental evaluation. The section concludes with a brief discussion of dental hypersensitivity.

Extraoral/Intraoral Examination

There are six steps to an extraoral and intraoral examination: (1) visual examination, (2) palpation, (3) instrumentation, (4) percussion, (5) electrical test, and (6) auscultation. Visual examination involves direct observation, radiographic examination, and transillumination to observe the patient. Palpation is the action of feeling by the sense of touch. Instrumentation uses examination instruments such as periodontal probe and an explorer for specific examination of the teeth and periodontal tissues. Percussion is the process of striking a part of the body (e.g., detection of the source of a painful tooth). Tapping the tooth with an instrument can give status of health or pain. An electrical pulp tester may be used to detect the presence or absence of vital pulp.

Auscultation is the act of listening to sounds from different parts of the body (e.g., using the stethoscope to hear temporomandibular joint [TMJ] sounds on opening; Wilkins, 2013).

In the overall appraisal, the dental hygienist should examine the patient's gait, eyes, lips, skin, and head and neck area. Check for lymphadenopathy or lymph nodes that are abnormal in size, consistency, or number. The TMJ also should be examined.

The overall assessment also includes determination of the patient's vital signs. Vital signs include blood pressure, pulse rate, and respiration rate and provide immediate evidence of the patient's basic physiologic functions. Vital signs should be taken at every dental appointment.

The intraoral examination involves screening for **oral cancer** by examining the tongue, gingiva, lining mucosa, and hard palate for color, bleeding, enlargements, and the presence of pain. It is not within the scope of this text to thoroughly discuss the components of the extraoral/intraoral examination.

Dental Evaluation

Dental evaluation begins with a general assessment of the dentition. **Dental charting** is done and analyzed not only for existing restorations, periodontal factors, and needed care but also for the impact of each finding on gingival health. The dental hygienist must examine overhangs, food impaction sites, crown contours, bridge abutments (a tooth or implant used for support and retention of a crown or removable partial denture), and pontics (a missing tooth that is replaced with a restoration and for which there are no roots) as possible biofilm-retention sites and evaluate the success of the patient in cleansing these areas. Box 14–1 lists the components of the dental evaluation. Identification of these areas and any resulting dental needs will allow for sequential planning, proper instrumentation, and continual recording and updating of the patient's clinical services.

Evaluate the Number of Teeth

The dental hygienist should begin by determining which teeth are present or missing in the dentition and charting the findings. Information provided by the past dental history, patient interview, and radiographic findings will enable the dental hygienist to determine whether missing teeth were missing at birth, are impacted, or have been extracted due to periodontal, endodontic, or restorative problems. The history of extractions should be discussed to determine the patient's attitude toward dental health and the incidence of dental disease.

Caries

The initial detection of caries starts with a process of careful examination. Clinical evidence of dental **caries** may be detected first visually, through a change in tooth color, radiographs, fiber optics, laser fluorescence, or other transilluminating devices. Avoiding damage created by explorers

---

Box 14–1: Components of the Dental Evaluation

- Number of teeth present or absent
- Evaluation of the teeth for dental and root caries
- Restorative status: presence and condition of existing restorations
- Dental implants
- Malpositioning and proximal contact relationships
- Occlusion/parafunctional habits
- Conditions of tooth wear
- Intraoral appliances
- Dental anomalies
- Dentinal hypersensitivity

Did You Know?

Just like fingerprints, everyone's tongue print is different.

is important to the dynamic process of demineralization and remineralization over time (Fejerskov, 1997; Rocklen & Wolff, 2011).

The standard method for classifying dental caries is G. V. Black's classification system. Types of dental caries are described by location. Pit and fissure caries frequently are found in the grooves and crevices of occlusal, lingual, and buccal surfaces. Smooth-surface caries is found on the facial, lingual, and interproximal surfaces of teeth.

Root-surface caries is found on the roots of teeth. This is of particular concern in periodontal therapy because of an increased accumulation of biofilm due to loss of anatomic tooth structure and difficulty in removing tooth-accumulated materials (e.g., bacterial biofilm, calculus, and stains) from that location. Several risk factors predispose to root caries: (1) gingival recession, which exposes the cementum to the oral environment (causes of gingival recession include periodontal disease and postperiodontal surgery; the number of teeth with gingival recession increases with age only because the teeth have been in the mouth longer); (2) xerostomia, particularly in the elderly due to systemic medication, which may decrease salivary flow; (3) head and neck radiation, resulting in xerostomia; (4) advanced age, because of age-related reduction in salivary gland function; (5) lack of fluoride; and (6) smoking and poor general health status or multiple medication use (smokers and patients on multiple medications have a significantly higher prevalence of root caries than nonsmokers and patients in good health; Page, 1998; Ravald & Birkhed, 1992).

Root caries is detected clinically by visual inspection and/or use of a blunt-ended instrument (e.g., periodontal probe). There are two classifications of root caries. Root caries either can be apparent on an exposed root surface (Figure 14–1 ■), where the gingival margin has receded onto the root surface below the caries or has developed in a pocket, with the gingival tissue covering the root area in a way that makes detection of the caries more difficult. Root caries is preventable with rigorous oral self-care and professional care.

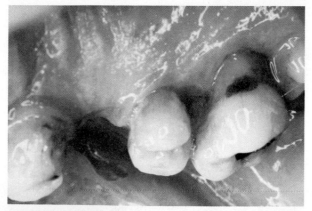

FIGURE 14–1 Gingival recession allows for visibility of root caries on the palatal surface of the maxillary first molar.

Rapid Dental Hint

Patients with rampant caries should be evaluated further for the cause. These caries may be due to methamphetamine use.

Did You Know?

Seventy-eight percent of Americans have had at least one cavity by age 17.

Restorative Status

Existing dental restorations should be evaluated for defective or undercontoured surfaces, overhanging margins, and proximal contacts. Ill-fitting removable prosthetic appliances, including clasps, also should be noted. Patients' complaints of floss breaking or shredding may indicate a defective restorative margin. Noting any inadequacies is of particular concern in the periodontal assessment. Any dental restoration should follow the contour of the original tooth, and there should be a tight, firm contact point between the restoration and the adjacent tooth. Overhangs and open margins are conducive to biofilm retention, impede oral hygiene, hinder proper scaling and root planing, affect probing accuracy, and can contribute to gingival inflammation and periodontal breakdown. At each appointment, the dental hygienist should update and record any changes that will influence ongoing treatment and continuity of care.

Dental Implants

Dental implants and their prosthetic suprastructures present a vast array of dental configurations conducive to biofilm retention. Survival rates for implants are good if the implants are well maintained and periodontal disease is well controlled prior to dental implant placement (Greenstein & Lamster, 1997). Methods of examination of dental implants and peri-implant tissues (Figure 14–2 ■) are reviewed later in the text.

Malpositioning and Proximal Contact Relationships

Evaluation of malposed teeth should include teeth that are in facial or lingual version when compared with the normal alignment of existing dentition. Malpositioning can have

Rapid Dental Hint

When root caries is recognized, determine the cause. Is it xerostomia due to medications?

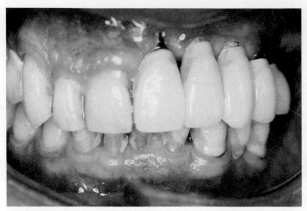

FIGURE 14–2 Dental implants replacing the maxillary left central and lateral incisor, canine, and first premolar. Note the tissues around the implants. Gingival recession is present on these teeth.

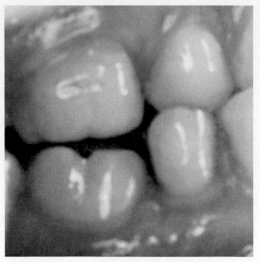

FIGURE 14–4 The maxillary first molar is ankylosed and never fully erupted. This tooth is intruded. The mandibular first molar is extruded above the occlusal plane. Uneven marginal ridges result from this occlusal problem.

an effect on oral hygiene and the integrity of a sound periodontium. Tooth crowding can occur anywhere in the dentition. Crowding of teeth may encourage food impaction and biofilm accumulation by compromising oral hygiene and consequently exacerbating gingival inflammation (Figure 14–3 ■). Crowding of teeth per se does not cause or accelerate periodontal tissue destruction, but crowding does make oral hygiene difficult, resulting in the accumulation of bacterial biofilm and calculus, and this can then start the process of tissue destruction.

Often a missing tooth may cause the adjacent tooth to tip mesially. When the crown tips or tilts into the edentulous space, causing the gingival on the mesial surface to bunch up, a biofilm trap is created. When proximal contact is lost, for example, after an extraction, teeth can drift or shift physiologically (both crown and root movement) into the edentulous space. Tipped (just the crown moves, whereas the root is stationary) and drifted teeth (the entire tooth has moved) can lead to uneven marginal ridges. If a tooth is missing, the opposing tooth may extrude into the edentulous space (Figure 14–4 ■). In such a situation,

the tooth will be coronal to the line of occlusion. When a tooth is apical to the occlusal plane, it is considered to be intruded. Frequently, a tilted or extruded tooth is associated with a plunger cusp, which is a pronounced cusp with steep inclined planes that causes a wedging effect on the interproximal area of the opposite arch. This may lead to food impaction and inflamed tissues.

Contacts between teeth should be checked using dental floss. The patient may complain of food impaction where there is an open contact or diastema between two adjacent teeth. Open contacts develop because of (1) congenital tooth abnormalities, (2) teeth that are extruded beyond the occlusal plane, (3) loss of support from an adjacent tooth, and (4) loss of bone support around a tooth (causing the tooth to move and lose adjacent tooth contact; Figure 14–5 ■).

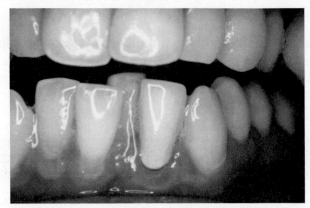

FIGURE 14–3 Crowding of the mandibular incisors decreases the efficiency of oral hygiene practices.

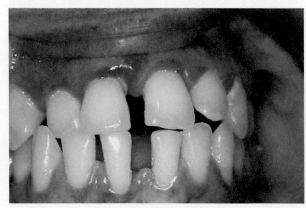

FIGURE 14–5 Numerous diastema in the maxillary arch were caused by loss of bony support.

Adjacent marginal ridges should be at the same level. Uneven marginal ridges due to extrusion or intrusion of a tooth produce a poor tooth contact relationship, which results in loss of protection of the interdental papillae from food impaction or trauma.

CONDITIONS OF TOOTH WEAR Conditions and situations that may account for loss of tooth structure include dental attrition, abrasion, and erosion. Usually, the intraoral examination coupled with a patient interview will reveal the type of **tooth wear** and its causes.

Attrition is the loss of tooth structure as a result of tooth-to-tooth contact. Causes include unconscious clenching or grinding of teeth, constant chewing of abrasive foods, the normal wear of tooth structure by physiologic masticatory (chewing) forces, or the mesial drifting of teeth due to the normal aging process. It is important to recognize a bruxing habit in patients who are undergoing restorative care. Contact between a natural tooth and a porcelain crown surface results in rapid wear of the tooth because porcelain is a very hard material. It is best to have tooth-to-artificial-crown contacts on a metallic surface or a highly polished porcelain surface. Attrition is found most often on the incisal/occlusal surfaces of teeth (Figure 14–6 ■) but also is found on proximal tooth surfaces that are flat, as seen with mesial drifting. Attrition also occurs as wear facets, which are small, smooth, polished, flat surfaces on the enamel where there is heavy tooth contact. Usually, wear facets are seen on the side of a tooth cusp.

Abrasion is the abnormal mechanical wearing away of tooth structure for reasons other than mastication. Frequently, it is evident on exposed cementum as a notch apical to the cementoenamel junction (Figure 14–7 ■). Examples of abrasion include excessive force from improper toothbrushing techniques (Dyer, Addy, & Newcombe, 2000), use of a hard-bristle toothbrush, and very abrasive dentifrices. Abrasion also can occur on the incisal/occlusal surfaces when an object such as a pin or pipe is held between the teeth for many years.

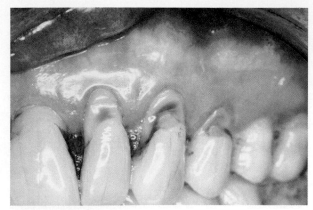

FIGURE 14–7 V- or U-shaped notching at the exposed cervical root surface just apical to the cementoenamel junction.

Abfractions are classified as a noncarious dental lesion. Numerous theories are found in dental literature concerning the etiology of abfraction including tooth fatigue, flexure (stress), and biomechanical loading of the tooth especially at the cervical area of the tooth. These lesions are usually wedge shaped with sharp line angles. Dental abfractions can occur alone or associated with toothbrush abrasion. Treatment involves observation or placement of a restoration.

Erosion is the chemical wearing away of tooth structure, usually enamel (Figure 14–8 ■). It is caused by

Rapid Dental Hint

When abrasion is recognized, first determine if it is localized or generalized. Generally, the patient's brushing technique, toothbrush, or dentifrice should be changed.

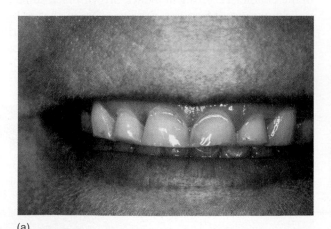

(a)

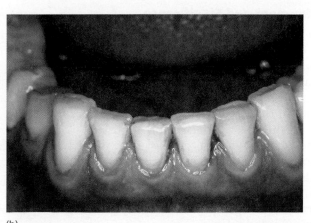

(b)

FIGURE 14–6 (a) Attrition of the maxillary teeth due to bruxism. (b) Note that the brownish dentin is exposed as a result of enamel loss.

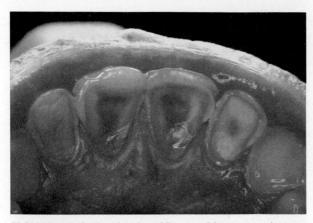

FIGURE 14–8 Erosion in a 35-year-old woman who was bulimic. Chronic vomiting wore away the enamel on the palatal surfaces of the maxillary anterior teeth, creating a shiny, smooth surface.

dietary acids (e.g., acidic beverages, lemons) and gastric juices coming from regurgitation or vomiting, as seen in bulimia. Location of the erosion cannot be considered pathognomonic (a direct cause) for certain etiologic factors, although if erosion is present on the palatal surfaces of maxillary incisors, it is most likely due to gastric juices. Traditionally, erosion is proportionally greater in younger patients, but erosion may increase with age as the salivary flow rate decreases.

Intraoral Appliances

Orthodontics, retainers, and splinting wires often present difficulty in cleansing the areas through normal toothbrushing and flossing techniques. Once biofilm builds around such appliances and the gingival tissue response occurs with edema and gingival overgrowth, the condition becomes even more difficult to manage. Determining the need for altered home care through a complete oral hygiene analysis can prevent future inflammatory responses.

Tooth Stain Evaluation

Development and Significance

Tooth stains are discolorations on or within tooth surfaces. Depending on its origin, the stain can be classified as exogenous or endogenous. Depending on its location, the stain can be intrinsic if it is internal to the hard tissue or extrinsic if it is external to the surface. Exogenous stains are derived from external sources and often are thought to reside on the outer surface of the tooth. They come from chromogenic (producing color or pigment) bacteria, foods, or chemicals. Endogenous stains are incorporated into the structure of the tooth and cannot be removed by surface polishing. Combinations of these classifications can exist, so stains can be exogenous and extrinsic or endogenous and intrinsic (Table 14–1 ■).

Types of Intrinsic Stains

Endogenous stains are always intrinsic because they come from within the tooth and therefore are incorporated into the tooth structure. Examples include (Goldstein & Garber, 1995):

- A nonvital tooth where the pulpal contents have discolored the enamel (this could have resulted from deep dental caries).
- An older patient in whom the teeth appear "yellowish brown" from dentin exposure (with aging, the enamel becomes thinner, exposing the darker color of the underlying dentin).
- Ingestion of excessive fluoride (fluorosis) between the third month of pregnancy and 8 years of age (the teeth appear as whitish opaque to brownish).
- Ingestion of the antibiotic tetracycline during calcification of the developing teeth.

Women should not take tetracycline after the second trimester of pregnancy, and children up to 8 years of age also should not be given tetracycline. Minocycline, a semi-synthetic derivative of tetracycline, can cause discoloration in adult teeth. Discoloration depends on concentration (the more tetracycline ingested, the more discoloration). Initially, a yellow fluorescent color is seen that changes to a nonfluorescent grayish brown color.

Extrinsic stains may become intrinsic if they are incorporated into the enamel or dentin, as in amalgam leakage or tobacco stain embedded into the enamel surface.

Types of Extrinsic Stains

Yellow stain can cause the tooth to appear yellowish or dull. It is associated with the color of the underlying biofilm and can be removed by biofilm removal. Brown-black stain can be seen in coffee or tea drinkers who do not brush enough to remove the tannin. Biofilm does not have to be present because the pellicle may take on the brown staining alone. Increasing brushing frequency or changing the toothpaste to a more abrasive one may be all that is needed to control the staining. Chewing tobacco often penetrates microcracks in the enamel, resulting in a dark brown-black stain.

Smoking tobacco can produce a stain that is light to dark brown and leathery. It will follow the distribution of the biofilm or lodge on the tooth surface most exposed to

Rapid Dental Hint

Removing a tetracycline stain is tough. Bleaching the teeth may help somewhat. The best treatment for tetracycline stains, however, especially if they are severe, is porcelain veneers.

Table 14–1 Classification of Common Tooth Stains

Stain	Origin	Treatment	Figure
Intrinsic stains			
Brownish red, bluish black	Nonvital pulp	Root canal treatment, tooth leaching	
Grayish brown	Tetracycline	Vital tooth bleaching, porcelain veneers	
Whitish brown Localized	Decalcification	Restore with a restoration; use sodium fluoride (0.05%) rinse	
Generalized	Excessive fluoride ingestion during enamel formation (fluorosis)	Restorative care or no treatment necessary	
Yellowish brown	Dentin exposure	No treatment necessary	
Extrinsic stains			
Brown	Tobacco (nicotine)	Remove with scaling and tooth polishing	
	Coffee or tea (tannins)	Remove with scaling and tooth polishing	
	Chlorhexidine oral rinse, stannous fluoride dentifrice or rinse	Remove with scaling and tooth polishing	
		Brush dorsal surface of tongue	

(*continued*)

Table 14–1 Classification of Common Tooth Stains (*continued*)

Stain	Origin	Treatment	Figure
Black-line	Gram-positive rods	Remove with scaling and tooth polishing	
Green stain	Chromogenic bacteria	No scaling; polish with mild abrasive	

the tar products of combustion. The stain can cover the cervical third of the tooth or expand to cover the central third as well. It is mostly on the lingual surfaces but can be in the pits and fissures as well. Some tobacco staining can be so severe that it will incorporate in the irregular surfaces of the enamel or exposed dentin. The exogenous, extrinsic stain becomes subsurface and intrinsic, and it increases with neglect. After removal of the extrinsic stain by polishing, increased frequency of biofilm removal is required for maintenance. Intrinsic stains may require bleaching for removal.

Black-line stain is a black line that follows in continuous fashion, the facial and lingual gingival margin. It has virtually no thickness and is only 1 mm wide. It usually traverses 1 mm above the gingival margin. This stain is associated with the gram-positive rod of *Actinomyces* species (Slots, 1974). Even though this bacterium is present, the stain is not associated with poor oral hygiene. The microorganisms embed in an adherent matrix and attach to the pellicle. The stain is common in women and children and occurs naturally. Meticulous home care is required to reduce the quantity or frequency of black stain.

Green stain is light or yellowish green to very dark green. The composition comes from chromogenic bacteria and fungi, decomposed hemoglobin (blood), and some inorganic elements. The stain is common in children, occurring on the gingival half of the facial surfaces of the maxillary anterior teeth and extending to the proximal surfaces. The stain can occur as a small curved line following the gingival margin or become a diffused smear covering the facial surface. The enamel under the stain is often rough and demineralized, which encourages biofilm retention. Biofilm and stain removal through polishing is necessary, yet prevention of recurrence depends on meticulous home care.

Chlorhexidine, used in oral rinses to control biofilm and gingivitis, discolors the teeth with a yellow-brown stain on the proximal surfaces, on restorations, and on the tongue (Löe & Schlott, 1970). In approximately 50% of patients, staining occurs within a few days after starting the rinse. The cause of the staining is unclear, but it may be the result of a reaction with foods containing aldehydes or ketones. Although the staining is not permanent, it is a significant side effect that may deter routine compliance. Polishing the

Rapid Dental Hint

Determine if the stain is intrinsic or extrinsic because the treatment options will vary.

enamel or exposed root surfaces removes the stain. Often a patient will have staining only interproximally and not on the direct facial or lingual surfaces. This indicates that the patient practices good oral self-care.

Significance of Stains

The significance of stains relates to the rough surfaces they may create and the resulting biofilm retention sites. Stains can adhere directly to a tooth, discolor the pellicle and biofilm, or become part of the tooth.

If either of the first two occurs, the tooth surface could have an overlay of stain. This is cosmetic at first until it increases in thickness. If biofilm adheres to the stain, the same gingival response occurs. The stain needs to be removed to promote oral cleanliness and eliminate possible biofilm retention sites.

The key to choosing a removal process is identification of the stain by source and location. Analysis of the color is not always the only determinant of source. Some colors, such as brown, may represent poor hygiene, tobacco use, tea or coffee consumption, or dental fluorosis. The analysis also must determine if the stain resides on the surface and can be removed by polishing or is intrinsic and must be removed by tooth bleaching.

Dentinal Hypersensitivity

Many patients experience **dentinal hypersensitivity** as a painful response to an irritation where roots are exposed. Dentinal hypersensitivity is a transient, sharp pain arising from exposed dentin in response to a stimulus; it does not last very long. Hypersensitivity will vary in intensity from very mild to excruciatingly painful. Some patients can tolerate the pain, whereas others simply cannot endure it.

Etiology of Dentinal Hypersensitivity

Although not all patients with exposed dentin experience dentinal or root surface hypersensitivity, an estimated 8% to 30% of people in the United States complain of some type of acute or chronic dentinal hypersensitivity resulting from vigorous toothbrushing, tooth whitening, thermal stimulus, mechanical periodontal debridement, or periodontal surgery that exposes the root surfaces. Higher prevalence has been reported in populations of peridontally involved patients (Wilkins, 2013; Taani & Awartani, 2002).

Although there are numerous theories explaining the etiology of hypersensitive tooth surfaces, the most prevalent theory is the hydrodynamic explanation (Paine, Slots, & Rich, 1998). This theory states that the fluid in the exposed dentinal tubules contracts or expands when an external stimulus is applied. The pain experienced is due to this minute fluid movement within the tubules.

The most common situation in which hypersensitivity occurs is as follows: Initially, gingival recession occurs, in which the gingival margin migrates apically as a result of trauma or forceful toothbrushing, and this exposes the underlying cementum. The thin cementum can be worn away easily by the abrasive agents in dentifrices or from mechanical root debridement, which exposes the underlying dentin and the open dentinal tubules. Usually, the pain is instigated by thermal changes such as cold air or cold foods (ice cream or a cold drink), a mechanical stimulus such as toothbrushing or touch with an instrument or other object, or a chemical stimulus such as sweets.

Identification

It is important to rule out any dental pathology. The dental hygienist can be among the first practitioners to recognize dentinal hypersensitivity. A patient usually complains of a tooth that hurts but will not say, "I have a hypersensitive tooth." If a patient cannot identify a specific tooth, then the problem probably is not a hypersensitive tooth but rather a root or crown fracture, leaking restorations, or teeth in hyperfunction. If the patient points to a tooth, the dental hygienist should ask further questions pertaining to various risk factors.

Testing for sensitivity should be a part of the initial examination and should include something that can be used as a baseline measurement of sensitivity. Using a brief blast of air is one method of assessing hypersensitivity. The area should be dried before using the air syringe. Most patients who have gingival recession should have sensitivity tests. It also may be important to do pretreatment sensitivity tests before periodontal therapy (e.g., instrumentation, periodontal surgery) so that it can be determined if any posttherapy sensitivity was present before treatment or has resulted from the treatment (Zapletalová, Peřina, Novotný, & Chmelíčková, 2007). Management of hypersensitivity is discussed in Chapter 20.

Dental Hygiene Application

The dental examination follows the medical/dental history and is an intricate step in assessing baseline data and dental care of the patient. With a thorough and systematic approach to the dental examination, risk factors can be identified that will aid in the appropriate treatment planning needs of the patient.

Key Points

- The dental examination involves identification of contributory local risk factors for periodontal diseases.
- Individual teeth and the entire dentition are examined for deviations.

- Dentinal hypersensitivity is a common complaint; identifying causes will help in its treatment.

Self-Quiz

1. Which one of the following risk factors is characteristic for root caries?
   a. Chlorhexidine
   b. Xerostomia
   c. Parafunctional habit
   d. Alcohol consumption

2. Which one of the following methods best detects root caries?
   a. Visual inspection or use of blunt-ended instrument (e.g., periodontal probe)
   b. Radiographs
   c. Rinsing with a disclosing agent
   d. Brushing with an abrasive dentifrice

3. Which of the following terms describes loss of tooth structure due to occlusion on an opposing porcelain crown?
   a. Abrasion
   b. Attrition
   c. Erosion
   d. Wear facet

4. For each type of stain listed, select the correct origin from the list provided. (Table 14–1)

Stain	Origin
1. Whitish brown	a. Bacteria
2. Yellowish brown	b. Fluorosis
3. Green	c. Dentin exposure
4. Brown	d. Cigarette smoking

5. All visible stains have to be removed from the tooth surfaces because stains are harmful to the teeth.
   a. Both the statement and the reason are correct and related.
   b. Both the statement and the reason are correct but not related.
   c. The statement is correct, but the reason is not.
   d. The statement is not correct, but the reason is correct.
   e. Neither the statement nor the reason is correct.

Case Study

Age: 67   Blood Pressure: 130/85
Gender: Male   Pulse Rate: 83
Height: 6'1"   Respiratory Rate: 18
Weight: 183

Medical History

Patient has no current physician. Complains of fatigue and recent weight loss. Also he "feels a low grade fever frequently and night sweats".

Medications

OTC allergy medication for seasonal allergies

Dental History

Patent visits the dentist every year. Has missed his last two appointments. Brushes one to two times a day and does not floss.

Social History

Patent has a high stress job. Has been in a long term relationship.

Nutrition History

Tries to eat a balanced diet

Chief Complaint

Teeth are very sensitive to hot, cold, and sweats.

Clinical Findings

Moderate plaque and calculus. White blemishes on tongue and throat that bleed when wiped off. Prominent palpable cervical lymph nodes. Inflamed gingiva with heavy bleeding upon probing.

Questions

1. Upon clinical oral examination the stains exhibited are most likely caused by?
   a. Smoking or chewing tobacco
   b. Coffee and tea stains
   c. Gram-positive rod of actinomyces
   d. Chromogenic bacteria
   e. A, B
   f. A, D
   g. All of the above

Answer: E.

2. The white blemishes in the patient's mouth are most likely?
   a. Linea alba
   b. Oral cancer
   c. Lichen planus
   d. Candidiasis

Answer: D

3. All of the symptoms displayed by the patient are indicative of HIV except:
   a. Lymphadenopathy
   b. Oral candidiasis
   c. Fatigue and weight loss
   d. Bleeding gums
   e. Periodontal disease

Answer: E.

4. Which of the following are factors in the patient's periodontal condition?
   a. Lack of oral hygiene
   b. Overhang on tooth #14
   c. High stress
   d. Patient's age
   e. HIV
   f. All of the above

Answer: F.

References

Dyer, D., M. Addy, and R. Newcombe. 2000. Studies in vitro of abrasion by different manual toothbrush heads and a standard toothpaste. *J Clin. Periodontal*. 27:99–103.

Fejerskov, O. 1997. Concepts of dental caries and their consequences for understanding the disease. *Community Dent. Oral Epidemiol*. 25:5–12.

Greenstein, G., and I. Lamster. 1997. Bacterial transmission in periodontal diseases: A critical review. *J. Periodontal*. 68:421–431.

Goldstein, R. E., and D. A. Garber. 1995. *Complete dental bleaching*, 2–13. Chicago: Quintessence.

Löe, H., and C. Schlott. 1970. The effect of mouthrinses and topical application of chlorhexidine on the development of dental plaque and gingivitis in man. *J. Periodont. Res*. 5:79–83.

Page, R. 1998. Risk assessment for root caries in adults. *Oral Care Rep*. 8:7.

Paine, M. L., J. Slots, and S. K. Rich. 1998. Fluoride use in periodontal therapy: A review of the literature. *J. Am. Dent. Assoc*. 129:66–69.

Ravald, N., and D. Birkhed. 1992. Prediction of root caries in periodontally treated patients maintained with different fluoride programmes. *Caries Res*. 26:450–458.

Rocklen, G. K., and M. Wolff. 2011. Technological advances in caries diagnosis. *Dent. Clin. N. Am*. 55:441–452.

Slots, J. 1974. The microflora of black stain on human primary teeth. *Scand. J. Dent. Res*. 82:484.

Taani, Q., and F. Awartani. 2002. Clinical evaluation of cervical dentin sensitivity (CDS) in patients attending general dental clinics and periodontal specialty clinics (PSC). *J. Clin. Periodontol*. 29(2):118–122.

Wilkins, E. M. 2013. *Clinical practice of the dental hygienist*, 11th ed., 144–149, 674–686. Philadelphia: Lippincott Williams & Wilkins.

Zapletalová, Z., J. Peřina, R. Novotný, and H. Chmelíčková. 2007. Suitable conditions for sealing of open dentinal tubules using a pulsed Nd:YAG laser. *Photomed Laser Surg*. 25(6):495–499.

Visit www.pearsonhighered.com/healthprofessionsresources to access the student resources that accompany this book. Simply select Dental Hygiene from the choice of disciplines. Find this book and you will find the complimentary study tools created for this specific title.

15

Clinical Examination: Gingival Assessment

Eva M. Lupovici

OUTLINE

Introduction
Objectives of a Gingival Assessment
Risk Factors for Gingival Diseases
Clinical Assessment Procedures
Dental Hygiene Application
Key Points
Self-Quiz
Case Study
References

EDUCATIONAL OBJECTIVES

Upon completion of this chapter, the reader should be able to:

- Describe the rationale for performing a gingival assessment as part of the patient evaluation.
- Describe the clinical features of the gingiva in health and disease.
- Evaluate the procedures used in performing a gingival assessment.
- Differentiate bleeding at the gingival margin from bleeding on probing.
- Recognize and discuss factors found in gingival assessment procedures that may be predictors of future disease activity.

GOAL: To provide knowledge of the clinical and histologic features of gingival changes in disease.

KEY WORDS

Introduction

Traditional diagnostic procedures are divided into two components: detection of inflammation and assessment of damage to periodontal tissues (Armitage, 1996). Detection of inflammation will be discussed in this subsection, and the next subsection addresses the resulting damage to the periodontium.

In considering the status of the periodontium, practitioners frequently state that the tissue is either "normal" or "diseased," with no in-between stage. In medicine as well as in dentistry, however, there is a range of normality. Slight deviations from the healthy norm can fall within the range of normality for an individual.

Objectives of a Gingival Assessment

The purpose of performing a **gingival assessment** is to evaluate the condition of the gingival tissues and to determine inflammatory and noninflammatory changes. Gingival assessment is one of the essential steps in identifying **inflammatory periodontal diseases**. The accurate recording of initial examination findings is essential in formulating an appropriate treatment plan, as a baseline comparison with future clinical findings after the initial phase of therapy is completed, and in subsequent periodontal maintenance visits.

Risk Factors For Gingival Diseases

The inflammatory process occurs in response to the presence of irritation to the tissues caused by dental plaque. Inflammation is the host's response to the irritation, which stimulates tissue repair. However, as noted in previous chapters, additional risk factors predispose a host to gingival or periodontal diseases. Host susceptibility to periodontal diseases should be considered if inflammation is not resolved after treatment. Knowledge of all the potential risk factors is important in providing the appropriate treatment.

Risk factors for gingival inflammation or gingival enlargement include the following:

* Poor home care
* Changes in hormone levels, as seen in pregnancy, menopause, puberty, or use of oral contraceptives
* Systemic diseases, such as diabetes mellitus, leukemia, or human immunodeficiency virus (HIV) infection
* Eruption of the permanent dentition
* Certain drugs, including phenytoin, valproate, cyclosporine, and calcium channel blockers

Clinical Assessment Procedures

When examining the interdental papillae and gingival margin, the dental hygienist should compare them with adjacent areas. These are the first areas that are affected clinically by inflammation. In the presence of inflammation, gingival tissue manifests some or all of the following five cardinal signs: redness (rubor), swelling (tumor), and heat (calor). Pain (dolor) and loss of function (functio laesa) may not be present until the advanced stages of periodontal disease. If inflammation is not resolved, then the inflammatory infiltrate progresses into the attached gingiva and alveolar mucosa. Because the alveolar mucosa is composed of loose connective tissue, the inflammatory infiltrate travels through it more quickly than through the attached gingiva, which is composed of dense connective tissue.

Color

The entire mouth should be examined visually, not just the anterior portions of the oral cavity. In health, the color of the gingiva is salmon pink. Color is determined by the degree of vascularity, epithelial keratinization, presence of melanin, and thickness of the epithelium. In the presence of inflammation, the color of the tissues can be various shades of red (erythema) or light to whitish pink, depending on the chronicity of the lesion. Initially, there is a bright red color, which can change to deeper red or bluish red (cyanotic) or pale white in severe periodontal disease. Tissue redness should not be used as the sole indicator of inflammation, nor is it strongly associated with or a predictor for future periodontal disease activity (PDA; Halazonetis, Haffajee, & Socransky 1989). However, the absence of gingival redness is more indicative of the absence of disease (Lang, Adler, Joss, & Nyman, 1990).

Gingiva color may appear to be healthy superficially at clinical examination and still be diseased because the site of inflammation is deep within the tissues and not seen at the gingival margin until after the disease progresses. Conversely, individuals with thin oral epithelium may have a healthy gingiva that is red in color.

Within the normal range, healthy gingiva varies in color. In certain dark-skinned individuals such as Asians, African descendants, and Mediterranean people, the gingiva will appear to have a light brown to black pigmentation due to the presence of melanin (Table 15–1 ■). Another cause for variation in gingival color may be an amalgam restoration. The metals from an amalgam restoration may absorb into the gingiva, causing a bluish-gray color. This is termed an amalgam tattoo. This condition causes discoloration

---

Did You Know?

The gingiva is a pink color due to keratin in the epithelium.

Rapid Dental Hint

When assessing the color of the gingival tissues, compare these tissues with adjacent areas.

Table 15–1 Clinical and Histologic Changes Seen in Health and Gingivitis

Clinical Features	Histologic Features	Figure
Color		
In *health*, the gingiva is salmon pink.	Presence of keratin.	 Salmon pink gingiva
Pigmentation	Indicates the production of melanin by melanocytes; this does not indicate the presence of inflammation or disease.	 Pigmented gingiva
In *acute inflammation*, the tissues exhibit various shades of red (fiery red); in *chronic inflammation*, the gingiva may be a bluish red (cyanotic or magenta) or pale white.	Redness is due to increased vasodilation (engorged blood vessels) resulting in locally increased blood flow. As the condition worsens, the bluish red color is due to stagnation of blood in the vessels. The pale white color is due to the repair process with excessive collagen formation.	 Inflamed gingiva
Contour		
Free gingival margin		
Knife-edged	Intact gingiva fibers brace the gingiva to the tooth.	 Knife-edged free gingival margins
Rolled or rounded	Destruction of gingival fibers.	 Rolled free gingival margins
Gingival cleft	Narrow slit in the gingiva starting at the gingival margin; probably associated with tooth position in the arch or the beginning of pocket formation; not related to occlusal forces, as once thought.	 Gingival cleft

Clinical Features	Histologic Features	Figure
Interdental papillae		
Pyramidal or pointed (flatter in posterior)	Papillae completely fill in gingival embrasure; no tissue destruction.	 Pyramidal papillae
Bulbous	Enlarged papillae due to accumulation of fluid in the tissue; the papilla is not tucked in the gingival embrasure but partly covers the enamel.	 Bulbous papillae
Blunted	Destruction of the tip of the papilla.	 Blunted papillae
Absent	Destruction of the entire papilla; occurs where there is a diastema.	 Absent papillae
Cratered	Destruction of the tissue between the papillae; a "concavity."	 Cratered papillae
Consistency		
Firm and resilient	Intact collagen fibers in the lamina propria give the gingiva its firm consistency. Tissues are easily compressed with a blunt instrument.	 Firm gingiva

(continued)

Table 15–1 Clinical and Histologic Changes Seen in Health and Gingivitis (*continued*)

Clinical Features	Histologic Features	Figure
Edematous	Loss of collagen and vascular permeability resulting in fluid accumulation in the surrounding tissue.	Edematous gingiva
Fibrotic	Reparative process whereby the fibroblasts in tissue in an attempt to heal produce and secrete excessive collagen. Tissue becomes hard and nonresilient. Tissue is not compressible.	Fibrotic gingiva
Retractable	Loss of collagen fibers. Papillae and margins are easily retracted by a blast of air.	Retractable gingiva
Surface Texture		
Stippling	Stippling results from the intersecting epithelial ridges on the undersurface of the epithelium. An excessive amount of stippling is seen in chronic inflammation.	Stippling
Shiny and smooth	Can occur in health or disease. In disease, loss of stippling occurs because of accumulation of fluid in the underlying gingival connective tissue.	Loss of stippling

of the gingiva (Figure 15–1 ■), but is not inflammatory in nature, and the gingiva is considered to be healthy.

Contour

Examining the contour of the gingiva is the next phase of the gingival assessment. Gingival contour is determined by the shapes and positions of the teeth, alignment of the teeth, location and size of the contact area, size of the gingival embrasure, and soft-tissue inflammation. Therefore, the contour of the gingiva will vary from anterior to posterior areas and between individual teeth.

MARGINAL GINGIVA AND INTERDENTAL PAPILLAE In health, the marginal gingiva (or free gingival margin) is knife-edged in contour. In disease, the margins become rolled or rounded due to destruction of the circular fibers.

Interdental papillae in healthy gingiva are tightly tucked into the gingival embrasures. Papillae of anterior teeth are pyramidal in shape because they follow the cementoenamel junction (CEJ) and contact areas, which are narrow. Papillae of posterior teeth are flatter because the CEJ is flatter and the contact areas are wider. In disease, the papillae become bulbous or enlarged because of edema.

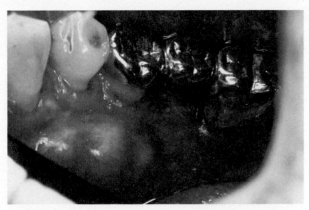

FIGURE 15–1 An amalgam tattoo is seen on the lingual surface near the second premolar. This is healthy gingiva.

The papillae may be cratered where there is a depression between the facial and lingual papillae or blunted where the tip of the papilla is absent and there is an open gingival embrasure. Blunting of the gingiva also may be due to non-inflammatory causes such as overuse or misuse of interdental cleaning aids. It may be caused in response to the use of an interdental brush in areas where the interdental papilla completely fills the gingival embrasure. Changes in the contour of the gingiva can reflect current or past periodontal tissue destruction.

GINGIVAL CLEFTS In examining gingival contour, the dental hygienist may observe a gingival cleft or a pseudocleft. A gingival cleft is a V-shaped slit that extends apically from the gingival margin. A gingival cleft may be caused by many factors, such as incorrect toothbrushing, improper flossing (flossing cleft), or a break through the gingiva around a tooth as a result of pocket formation. Gingival clefts can resolve spontaneously or may require periodontal surgery.

A pseudocleft is a gingival cleft that occurs when adjacent papillae become enlarged to the point that they join each other at the center of the tooth (see Table 15–1). This is not a true cleft because there is no marginal tissue destruction. Pseudocleft is seen commonly in patients with crowding of teeth or in patients with severely enlarged gingiva who are taking certain medications such as phenytoin, cyclosporine, or nifedipine. In addition, coronal migration of the gingival margin caused by the gingival overgrowth results in the formation of a pseudopocket or gingival pocket.

Consistency

The consistency of the gingiva is examined by lightly pressing the side of the periodontal probe against the marginal and interdental gingiva. Consistency refers to the firmness of the underlying connective tissue. In health, the gingiva is firm and resilient when pressed. As stated earlier, inflammatory changes occur within the vascular connective tissue of the gingiva, and when edema is present, the tissue will "pit" and not rebound quickly when the periodontal probe is applied lightly. Edema causes gingival enlargement, resulting in the formation of a gingival pocket or pseudopocket.

Firm, resilient gingiva may not be an indicator of health, however, as seen with fibrotic gingiva. Upon examination, fibrotic gingiva will be hard and will not show a "pit" when tested with a periodontal probe.

Recent studies have found that smokers have the same or less gingival inflammation than nonsmokers (American Academy of Periodontology, 1996; Stafne, 1997). However, the gingival consistency in smokers tends to be fibrotic with rolled gingival margins. Smoking or smokeless tobacco chewing causes the tissue to become hyperkeratinized with an abnormal whitish thickening of the keratin layer of the epithelium. Following smoking cessation, the gingiva returns to its condition prior to smoking (Haber, 1994).

During the disease process, the collagen fibers are destroyed, causing the gingiva to be retractable or flaccid (see Table 15–1). Once the inflammation is eliminated and controlled, the collagen fibers may reform and unite the gingiva to the tooth.

Surface Texture

Surface texture is assessed by drying the attached gingiva with gauze and observing the surface for stippling. Clinically, stippling is described as having an appearance similar to the outside peel of an orange. The presence or absence of stippling does not necessarily indicate the health status of the gingiva. Stippling is present in health and in chronic inflammation when the gingiva becomes fibrotic. In chronic inflammation, the presence of stippling represents tissue scarring. Edematous gingival tissue may retain stippling. In the absence of stippling, the gingiva is described as being smooth or shiny.

Size: Gingival Enlargement

The size of the gingiva is influenced by several factors, such as cellular and intercellular elements and vascular supply. In gingival overgrowth or enlargement, the free gingival margin is located coronal to its normal position at or slightly coronal to the CEJ. Gingival enlargement can be the result of a tissue response to inflammation caused by dental plaque, hormonal imbalance in pregnancy and puberty, side effects of certain medications, mouth breathing, and iatrogenic dentistry such as poorly contoured crowns.

The alternative drying and wetting of the gingiva during mouth breathing promotes an inflammatory response causing gingival enlargement from the maxillary canine to the canine. The appearance of the gingiva, especially the palatal surface, is usually shiny and red in color.

Gingival enlargement of the maxillary tuberosity is not considered to be a disease state. The enlargement is developmental in origin.

Hereditary gingival fibromatosis is a rare form of severe gingival enlargement seen commonly in children beginning with the eruption of either the primary or permanent dentition. The etiology is unknown, but heredity is most likely involved. Gingival enlargement is generalized throughout the mouth, involving both the papillae and the marginal gingiva. The teeth may be completely covered by tissue overgrowth, preventing eruption.

Hormonal and Drug-Influenced Gingivitis

HORMONAL CHANGES Clinically, gingivitis in pregnancy is characterized by either generalized or localized inflammation to the gingival papillae, which show a sharp demarcation from the attached gingiva. The inflammation or swelling can spread to involve the marginal gingiva. The gingiva is bright red and edematous, with a shiny, smooth surface. The molars show the most inflammation, followed by the premolars and the incisors (Silness & Löe, 1963).

In more severe cases, pregnancy tumors also may occur, but these are not considered a true neoplasm; they are an inflammatory reaction to the dental plaque. Actually, a pyogenicgranuloma occurring in a pregnant patient is called a pregnancy tumor. This swelling appears mainly in the anterior facial areas of the mouth. It is a mass of tissue that protrudes outward. It is deep red and edematous.

Postpartum, these gingival conditions usually regress to their status during the second month of pregnancy. Most of the gingival changes seen during pregnancy can be prevented by removal of plaque and meticulous home care.

Gingival inflammation during pregnancy is not exclusive to pregnancy. Similar gingival changes, except for pregnancy tumors, are seen in adolescents as puberty gingivitis. These patients develop massive gingival enlargement that recurs even in the presence of little plaque. After puberty, the enlargement regresses, but total disappearance only occurs after all local irritants are removed.

DRUG-INFLUENCED GINGIVAL ENLARGEMENT Clinically, drug-induced gingivitis is seen as a generalized overgrowth of the gingiva, especially of the interdental papillae on the facial gingiva, of the maxillary and mandibular teeth, particularly the anterior sextent, and does not often occur in edentulous areas (Figures 15–2 ■, 15–3 ■). Enlargement of the gingiva may result in malpositioning of teeth and interference with normal chewing, speech, and oral hygiene (Pihlstrom, 1990). The gingival tissue in cyclosporine-induced overgrowth tends to be more soft, red or bluish red, and fragile, and it bleeds more easily on probing than tissue undergoing phenytoin-induced overgrowth (Hallmon

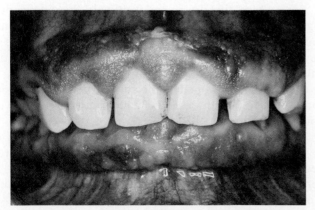

FIGURE 15–2 A 38-year-old woman taking phenytoin for seizures for the last 3 years. Note the generalized gingival enlargement, especially the interdental papillae.

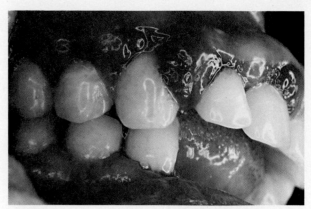

FIGURE 15–3 A 56-year-old woman taking nifedipine for hypertension. Note the enlargement of the interdental papillae. The enlarged papillae take on a lobulated or nodular appearance.

Rapid Dental Hint

Determine the cause when gingival inflammation and enlargement are recognized.

& Rossmann, 1999). Other medications that may cause gingival enlargement are the calcium channel blockers (e.g., nifedipine, amlodipine, diltiazem).

In most cases, maintaining strict plaque control can prevent this enlargement, but surgical intervention frequently is required to obtain physiologic gingival contours and aesthetics.

Gingival Bleeding

The next step in the gingival examination is to determine the presence of marginal bleeding. This can be done by several methods, including stroking the lining of the sulcus or inserting a wooden or plastic wedge to assess proximal bleeding (Caton & Polson, 1985). If the stroke method is used, the probe is placed within the gingival crevice and is dragged from one interproximal space to the other interproximal space on the same tooth. Any bleeding seen within 30 seconds is labeled as a bleeding site. Bleeding measured at the gingival margin or crevice is often indicative of gingival inflammation. On the other hand, **bleeding on probing** (BOP; bleeding coming from a pocket during periodontal probing) indicates a deeper inflammatory involvement. In private practice or a clinic setting, bleeding on probing usually is recorded as being either absent or present by placing a red dot over the site that bleeds. For research purposes, a bleeding index is used to standardize measurements. It is important to note that bleeding may be masked if the gingiva is fibrotic. Former heavy and current heavy smokers have been reported to show a significant suppression of high BOP compared to never smokers (Shimazaki et al., 2006). Many patients are taking low-dose aspirin for prevention of stroke and heart attack. It has been documented that aspirin intake of 325 mg/day for 7 days moderately increased the appearance of bleeding on probing in a patient population that had ≥ 20% BOP sites.

Bleeding occurs when there is disruption of the sulcular and junctional epithelium allowing for passage of blood or exudate from the lamina propria into the sulcus. The epithelium is avascular and receives its blood supply and nutrients from the underlying vascular lamina propria. When the epithelium becomes inflamed, it reacts by forming microulcerations. Thus, sweeping the lining of the crevice or probing allows for blood to pass through from the engorged and newly formed blood vessels in the lamina propria subjacent to the epithelium.

Bleeding traditionally is accepted as an objective clinical sign of inflammation; however, some visually inflamed gingival sites do not bleed. Therefore, it can be stated that bleeding is not always an early sign of gingival inflammation, and the actual mechanisms responsible for bleeding probably are not truly understood. In addition, the presence of bleeding from a periodontitis site is a poor predictor of future attachment loss (Armitage, 1996). On the other hand, the absence of bleeding is strongly indicative of low levels of inflammation (Lang et al., 1990) and high periodontal stability (Goodson, 1992). Thus, it can be stated that bleeding on probing is a poor positive predictor of periodontal disease, but conversely is a very strong negative predictor. The clinical interpretation of this research is that although BOP presence may not indicate periodontal disease, continued absence of BOP is a strong predictor (approximately 98%) of continued periodontal health. Gingival bleeding has been related to increased gingival crevicular fluid flow rate, which is associated with the presence of inflammation

Rapid Dental Hint

Bleeding on probing indicates clinical inflammation. This is similar to getting a splinter in your finger. The same inflammatory process occurs.

Rapid Dental Hint

The easiest way to record bleeding is either the site bleeds (+) or it doesn't

(Armitage, 1996). Another limitation of the use of bleeding as an inflammatory parameter is the possibility that healthy tissues may bleed on stimulation or probing (Lang et al., 1990) when excessive probing forces are used or improper toothbrushing methods or improper use of interdental cleaning aids has occurred. Also, healthy tissue may bleed if the patient is a smoker or taking certain medications such as warfarin, aspirin, or clopidogrel (Schrodi et al., 2002). Thus, the dental hygienist must discriminate between bleeding sites that are inflamed and those that bleed for other reasons. To eliminate bleeding, the pathologic process must be changed. Traditionally, altering plaque levels by periodontal debridement and improved oral hygiene has been successful, especially in the reduction of gingivitis.

Dental Hygiene Application

After the gingival assessment is completed, the findings are summarized according to location, distribution, and severity of the gingival changes. The findings can be either localized or generalized (localized to certain areas such as the mandibular lingual teeth or generalized throughout the entire mouth). Distribution is marginal, papillary, or diffuse. If the marginal gingiva is affected, it is called marginal inflammation. If the interdental papillae are affected, it is called papillary inflammation. If the free, attached, and/or alveolar mucosa is affected, it is referred to as diffuse. Severity is classified as mild, moderate, or severe.

Key Points

- The purpose of performing a gingival evaluation is to determine the status of the gingiva and the presence or absence of gingival inflammation and/or gingival enlargement.
- Gingival enlargement can be due to an inflammatory response to dental plaque or to certain drugs.

- The steps involved in a gingival evaluation include assessing for gingival color, contour, consistency, surface texture, size, and bleeding.
- The absence of bleeding indicates periodontal stability.

Self-Quiz

1. Which one of the following features describes the gingival appearance in a patient who is a 30 pack-years smoker?
   a. Red gingiva and cratered interdental papillae
   b. Red gingiva and bulbous gingival margins
   c. Whitish gingiva and absent interdental papillae
   d. Whitish gingiva and rolled, receded gingival margins

2. Which one of the following considerations must be addressed by the dental hygienist when performing a gingival assessment?
   a. Determine inflammatory changes.
   b. Evaluate periodontal disease activity.
   c. Assess destruction of supporting and alveolar bone.
   d. Evaluate probing depth changes.

3. Which one of the following statements is related to bleeding on probing or sulcular stimulation?
   a. The absence of bleeding is strongly indicative of low levels of inflammation.
   b. The presence of bleeding from a periodontitis site is a good predictor for future attachment loss.
   c. All visually inflamed gingival sites bleed.
   d. Bleeding occurs when there is disruption of the oral epithelium.

4. From the following list, select the items associated with gingival enlargement.
   a. Gingival inflammation
   b. Hormonal changes
   c. Cigarette smoking
   d. Mouth breathing
   e. Collagen
   f. Bruxism
   g. Medications
   h. Calcium channel blockers
   i. Cyclosporine

5. Tissue redness should be used as the primary indicator of inflammation because it is strongly associated with future periodontal disease activity.
   a. Both the statement and the reason are correct and related.
   b. Both the statement and the reason are correct but not related.
   c. The statement is correct, but the reason is not.
   d. The statement is not correct, but the reason is correct.
   e. Neither the statement nor the reason is correct.

6. Which of the following statements regarding bleeding on probing and disease activity is correct?
   a. Good positive indicator
   b. Poor negative indicator
   c. Strong negative indicator
   d. Is not correlated to disease activity

7. A patient is taking 325 mg/day of aspirin. Which of the following would be anticipated to occur while probing?
   a. Increased bleeding
   b. Decreased bleeding
   c. No effect on bleeding
   d. Should not probe a patient taking aspirin or other anticoagulants

8. Bleeding on probing is a clinical sign of
   a. disease activity.
   b. inflammation.
   c. clinical attachment loss.
   d. bone loss.

9. All of the following are drugs that can cause gingival enlargement *except* one. Which one is the exception?
   a. Aspirin
   b. Cyclosporine
   c. Nifedipine
   d. Diltiazem

10. Bleeding that occurs in the gingival crevice originates from the
    a. epithelium.
    b. lamina propria.
    c. alveolar bone.
    d. periodontal ligament.

Case Study

The dental hygienist is reading the chart entry describing the gingival condition for the 30 year old female about to be seen for a 6 month recall visit. The chart entry reads that there was inflammation of the gingival including the free and attached interdental gingival on lingual of teeth 23–26, and buccal of teeth 3 and 4. The tissue is described as edematous and red with probing depths of 3 mm in these areas.

1. What does the dental hygienist know about the gingival health of this patient?
   a. localized papillary gingivitis
   b. generalized diffuse gingivitis
   c. chronic fibrotic gingivitis
   d. within normal limits for patient

Answer: A. The chart entry indicates that the condition is limited to certain areas and is then localized. The dental hygienist must reassess this finding. The condition is papillary when it involves the interdental papilla and not the alveolar mucosa. Edematous tissue has lost collagen whereas fibrotic tissue has excessive collagen.

2. What will the dental hygienist assess when re-evaluating the gingival tissue?
   a. determine bleeding points
   b. assess for drug-induced gingival overgrowth
   c. ask if pregnant
   d. a and b
   e. all of the above

Answer: E. All of the above could be a factor in determining the gingival health. Hormonal changes can affect the gingival as well as drug-induced conditions for gingival overgrowth.

3. Upon re-probing the 3 mm sites do not bleed. What can be determined from this finding?
   a. Inflammation has progressed to the bone
   b. Inflammation is at low level of activity
   c. Probing force was too heavy
   d. The patient is a smoker

Answer: B. Bleeding is not always an early sign of inflammation however the absence of bleeding is a strong negative predictor of periodontal disease. Smokers may bleed even with healthy tissue. Increased probing force may cause bleeding.

References

American Academy of Periodontology. 1996. Tobacco use and the periodontal patient. *J. Periodontol.* 67:51–56.

Armitage, G. C. 1996. Periodontal diseases: Diagnosis. *Ann. Periodontol.* 1:37–215.

Caton, J., and A. Polson. 1985. The interdental bleeding index: A simplified procedure for monitoring gingival health. *Compend. Contin. Educ. Dent.* 6:88–92.

Goodson, J. M. 1992. Diagnosis of periodontitis by physical measurement: Interpretation from episodic disease hypothesis. *J. Periodontol.* 63:373–382.

Haber, J. 1994. Cigarette smoking: A major risk factor for periodontitis. *Compend. Contin. Educ. Dent.* 15:1002, 1004–1008, 1014.

Halazonetis, T. D., A. D. Haffajee, and S. S. Socransky. 1989. Relationship of clinical parameters to attachment loss in subsets of subjects with destructive periodontal diseases. *J. Clin. Periodontol.* 16:563–568.

Hallmon, W. W., and J. A. Rossmann. 1999. The role of drugs in the pathogenesis of gingival overgrowth. *Periodontology 2000* 21:176–196.

Lang, N. P., R. Adler, A. Joss, and S. Nyman. 1990. Absence of bleeding on probing: An indicator of periodontal stability. *J. Clin. Periodontol.* 17:714–721.

Pihlstrom, B. L. 1990. Prevention and treatment of Dilantin®-associated gingival enlargement. *Compend. Contin. Educ. Dent.* 11(Suppl. 14):S506–S510.

Schrodi, J., L. Recio, J. Fiorellini, et al. 2002. The effect of aspirin on the periodontal parameter bleeding on probing. *J. Periodontol.* 73:871–876.

Shimazaki, Y., T. Saito, Y. Kiyohara, et al. 2006. The influence of current and former smoking on gingival bleeding: The Hisayama Study. *J. Periodontol.* 77:1430–1435.

Silness, J., and H. Löe. 1963. Periodontal disease in pregnancy. *Acta Odontol. Scand.* 21:533–551.

Stafne, E. E. 1997. Cigarette smoking and periodontal disease: The benefits of smoking cessation. *Northwest Dent.* (September–October): 25–29.

Visit www.pearsonhighered.com/healthprofessionsresources to access the student resources that accompany this book. Simply select Dental Hygiene from the choice of disciplines. Find this book and you will find the complimentary study tools created for this specific title.

Clinical Examination: Periodontal Assessment

Theodore L. West

OUTLINE

EDUCATIONAL OBJECTIVES

Upon completion of this chapter, the reader should be able to:

- Describe the components of a periodontal assessment.
- Explain the clinical significance of each component of a periodontal assessment.
- Differentiate the significance of measuring clinical attachment level from probing depth.
- List several factors that can affect the accuracy of probe readings.
- Discuss the problems associated with a mucogingival defect.
- Describe the various causes of gingival recession.
- Discuss the concept of periodontal disease activity.

GOAL: To provide the basic elements for performing a periodontal examination.

KEY WORDS

Introduction

The periodontal examination performed by a dental hygienist has many purposes. First, large population groups in health fairs, schools, hospitals, clinics, and other institutions may need to be examined rapidly for periodontal diseases requiring further evaluation and subsequent treatment—the periodontal **screening**. For visual detection of periodontal diseases, rapid screening can be performed with as little instrumentation as two disposable wooden tongue blades and a flashlight to evaluate tooth loss, migration, and mobility; gingival recession, redness, suppuration, and swelling; and calculus and plaque levels. Essentially, screening is done in a single visit to differentiate between health and disease.

Rationale for Periodontal Assessment

A more thorough examination requires a mouth mirror, a periodontal probe, and radiographs. The periodontal assessment includes complete medical and dental histories and the recording of gingival findings, probing depths, clinical attachment levels, tooth mobility, tooth malposition, level of oral hygiene, occlusal relationships, and bone levels.

This **periodontal assessment** provides the baseline for the long-term monitoring of periodontal disease activity (Armitage, 2004). Such **monitoring** is often performed by the dental hygienist from one to four times a year at the periodontal maintenance visit. Such monitoring for increases in clinical attachment loss, gingival recession, swelling, bleeding, tooth mobility, and so on, because of the episodic and recurrent nature of periodontal diseases, is vitally necessary if the patient is to be maintained in a state of periodontal health. It often becomes the dental hygienist's responsibility to find and point out areas of recurrent periodontal disease activity in a patient's mouth.

Finally, the periodontal assessment examination should be used by the practitioner as an **outcome measure** to evaluate the success of periodontal treatment and the need for and frequency of periodontal maintenance visits (Douglas, 2006).

It seems likely that some general dental practices do not adequately assess periodontal diseases (McFall, Bader, Rozier, & Ramsey, 1988). In a study of almost 2,500 patient records from 36 general practices, radiographic bone loss was seen in over half the film sets. However, only one in five records showed a periodontal diagnostic entry or a notation about pocket formation. This random sample of adult patient records had very infrequent recordings of bleeding, recession, furcation invasions, pocketing, tooth mobility, and so on. These findings can be compared with an epidemiologic study in the same state of North Carolina (Bawden & DeFriese, 1981) that indicated 55% to 75% of the adult population was affected by periodontal disease.

If periodontal disease assessment in the general dental practice is inadequate, then it certainly must follow that the monitoring of periodontal disease progression becomes an impossibility. It seems probable that the burden for assessing and monitoring periodontal diseases in a general practice may fall, to a greater or lesser extent, on the shoulders of the dental hygienist.

Although periodontal diseases occur primarily in the adult population, they also can occur in young people, occasionally in a very severe form. Therefore, a periodontal evaluation should be performed for all patients regardless of age. A national survey of over 2,600 individuals 19 years of age and older, using a mouth mirror, explorer, and periodontal probe, showed 28% with periodontitis, 53.9% with gingivitis, and only 17.3% free of periodontal disease in the youngest group (19–44 years). In the 45- to 64-year-old age group, only 8.3% were free of periodontal disease, and 47.6% had pocket depths of 4 mm or more (Brown, Oliver, & Löe, 1989). Periodontal diseases have now been associated with increased risk for heart disease, stroke, diabetic complications, and premature, low-birth-weight babies. Because race, socioeconomic factors, nutrition, tobacco use, and various systemic diseases can further increase the prevalence of periodontal diseases at any age, the importance of the periodontal examination is obvious.

Periodontal disease severity represents the total destruction and healing that occur during the lifetime of a tooth (Jeffcoat, 1994). It is the status of the periodontium or extent of tissue damage at the time of the examination (Lamster, Celenti, Jans, Fine, & Grbic, 1993) and is determined by visual inspection, single measurements of probing depths, and evaluating radiographs for bone loss.

Periodontal disease activity, which is different from periodontal disease severity, is defined as the current or ongoing (at the time of the examination) loss of soft-tissue attachment, specifically destruction of the gingival fibers and apical migration of the junctional epithelium with subsequent alveolar bone loss. Periodontal disease activity is usually seen as episodic periods of exacerbation or active periodontal tissue destruction (loss of connective tissue attachment and alveolar bone) with intervening periods of quiescence or disease inactivity (Greenstein & Caton, 1990; Jeffcoat, 1994; Lamster et al., 1993). Periodontal disease activity is difficult to determine because it is a measurement of the continued breakdown of periodontal pockets between two points in time (separated by several weeks to months). Destruction must have occurred at some time between these two measurements.

Although periodontal probing and radiographic assessment are retrospective views of disease activity and cannot identify an active disease site from an inactive one (nor accurately predict future destruction), they are still the foundation on which the classification of the disease and its treatment is made (Haffajee, Socransky, & Goodson, 1983). The clinical importance of distinguishing between a progressive or active periodontal lesion and a stable or inactive lesion is apparent. Therefore, more sophisticated techniques and assessments have been introduced recently that are designed to determine current periodontal disease activity and/or if a site will break down in the future (Williams, Beck, & Offenbacher, 1996). For a review of these adjunctive assessment tests, refer to Chapter 18.

Periodontal Terminology

Periodontal Probing Depths

SCREENING METHOD Periodontal probing is the most commonly used physical screening method for measuring the depth of the gingival crevice and the **clinical attachment level**. Periodontal probing is a clinical approximation of the depth of a gingival sulcus or periodontal pocket (Armitage, 1995). Measurement of probing depths allows the practitioner to make certain presumptions about the state of health of the periodontium. Periodontal pockets are the result of the destruction of the coronal part of the junctional epithelium and the connective tissue attachment to the tooth surface at the apical aspect of the junctional epithelium (Figure 16–1 ■). The clinical significance of having pockets greater than 5 mm in depth is that such pockets may be difficult or impossible for the dental team to maintain in a state of health, even with a patient's best oral hygiene self-care efforts and frequent professional cleanings.

Clinically, probing depth is defined as the distance from the gingival margin to the most apical extent of the probe or where physical resistance of the probe is met. This approximates the level of soft tissue attachment (junctional epithelium) to the tooth. In healthy gingiva the free gingival margin is approximately 0.5 to 2 mm coronal to the cementoenamel junction (CEJ).

It should be noted that here we are using the term *probing depth* rather than *pocket depth* because what is being probed could be a pocket or a sulcus. This text will continue to use the term *probing depth* unless otherwise indicated.

Limitations of Probing. In health, the apical extent of the periodontal probe routinely penetrates the coronal to middle portion of the junctional epithelium (Listgarten, Mao, & Robinson, 1976; Robinson & Vitaek, 1979; Spray, Garnick, Doles, & Klawitter, 1978). When the gingiva is inflamed, the probe can transverse the junctional epithelium to deeper levels within the tissue. It can stop at, enter, or go through the lamina propria to the alveolar bone crest. Thus this measurement may be greater than the actual tissue destruction. Therefore, the clinical probing depth noted may be greater than the histologic probing depth due to probe penetration of inflamed tissue (Armitage, Svanberg, & Löe, 1977).

Probing depth measurements have several inherent limitations besides the degree of gingival inflammation (Robinson & Vitaek, 1979). The apical extent of probe penetration depends on the force used to probe (van der Velden, 1979), variations in placement and angulation of the probe, the site being probed, the type of probe used, the size of the probe (Keagle, Garnick, Searle, King, & Morse, 1989), and tooth anatomy. Other factors that influence the accuracy of probing include the presence of calculus, the visibility of the area, and the level of patient sensitivity. Despite these limitations, periodontal probing remains the most accurate and widely used method of assessing periodontal destruction. When done carefully, a probing difference of 2 mm or more can be clinically meaningful.

Disease Progression. Periodontal probing is important in determining past periodontal disease activity and is used to evaluate the results of periodontal treatment. Single probing measurements do not adequately reflect periodontal disease progression; they only signify past disease activity or the severity of attachment or bone loss at one point in time. Therefore, serial probing measurements must be done (e.g., at periodontal maintenance visits) and compared with previous measurements to determine whether the disease is progressing (Jeffcoat, 1994).

Probing depth measurements therefore are good for identifying areas that are potential therapeutic problems on a site-by-site basis (Armitage, 1995) and to determine the type of treatment needed. However, in longitudinal monitoring (e.g., at periodontal maintenance visits) for disease progression, probing depths are not reliable in determining the amount of detachment of the soft tissues from the root surface because the gingival margin may change its position over time due to gingival recession or gingival enlargement. This was first described in 1961 by Garguilo, Wentz, and Orban (Figure 16–2 ■).

LEVEL OF ATTACHMENT Clinical attachment level (CAL) is the distance from the CEJ to the most apical extent of the periodontal probe or where resistance is met. Clinical attachment level is a clinical approximation of the loss of connective tissue attachment from the root surface (Armitage, 1996). Measuring the level of attachment of the base of the pocket on the tooth surface gives a better indication of the severity of periodontal disease.

Because the position of the gingival margin changes over time, probing depth measurements are not reliable for

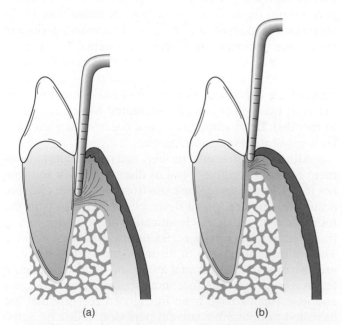

(a)   (b)

FIGURE 16–1 Probing depth measurement. (a) Deep pocket with apical migration of the junctional epithelium and bone loss. Probing depth is 6 mm. (b) Shallow probing depth (2 mm). There is no attachment loss or bone loss.

A. Sulcus depth
B. Attached epithelium
C. Apical point of epithelial attachment below cementoenamel junction
D. Bottom of sulcus from cementoenamel junction
E. Cementoenamel junction to alveolar bone
F. Deepest point of epithelial attachment to alveolar bone

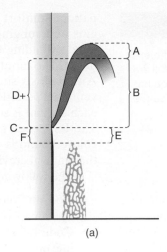

(a)

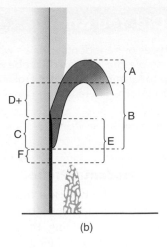

(b)

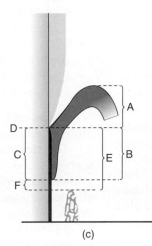

(c)

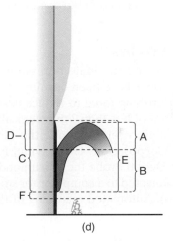

(d)

FIGURE 16–2 Schematic illustrations showing the different positions of the gingival margin. (a) Periodontal health. (b–d) The junctional epithelium has migrated onto the root surface.

determining the extent of detachment of soft tissue from the root surfaces. Measurement of the clinical attachment level is the reference method used to establish disease progression. The CEJ is a stable reference point that does not move over time. If the stationary point used is a part of the tooth other than the CEJ (e.g., cusp tip or restoration), the term used is *relative attachment level*. Although probing depth measurements are considered to be less valid for monitoring disease progression, they still should be considered as a clinical measure (Carlos, Brunelle, & Wolfe, 1987; Reddy, 1997).

When performing a periodontal charting, it is advisable to measure probing depths and to record the location of the free gingival margin. Future comparisons can then determine disease activity. In addition, the position of the gingival margin relative to the CEJ should be drawn on the chart.

Connective Tissue Attachment Loss. Attachment level measurements determine the amount of attachment loss if it has occurred on a tooth. **Attachment loss** is defined as the pathologic detachment of the gingival collagen fibers from

the root surface with the concomitant apical migration of the junctional epithelium along the root surface. Supporting and alveolar bone resorption also occurs as a result of the inflammatory events, but is a consequence of the attachment loss.

A significant increase in CALs is the gold standard for measurement of periodontal disease activity or a site that is actively losing connective tissue attachment at a given site (Goodson, 1986). Currently, a change in clinical attachment level of between 2 and 3 mm, measured at different examination visits, must occur before a site can be labeled disease-active (with attachment loss). Clinical attachment level measurements are important because over time it will determine if a site has experienced further connective tissue attachment loss or gain.

Individuals who have extensive attachment loss also may have gingival recession, but if they have shallow probing depths and no bleeding, they are considered to have a healthy periodontium and not periodontitis at that point in time. Such patients could have been treated successfully and the disease progression stopped, or they may be in remission with no disease activity present.

Other Uses of the Periodontal Probe

The periodontal probe can be used not only to determine the level of the soft tissue attachment to a tooth but also to establish the presence of bleeding, the location of the mucogingival junction, the amount of gingival recession, the width of keratinized/attached gingiva, and the consistency of the gingiva.

Controlled-Force Probes

Within the past decade, automated pressure-sensitive or controlled-force probes have been developed that provide a fixed 20 to 25 g probing force to reduce examiner error and to make changes of less than 2 mm clinically meaningful. Examples of these probes include the Florida probe (Florida Probe® Corporation, Gainesville, FL) and the Interprobe™ (The Dental Probe Inc., Richmond, VA). Most such probes are connected to a computer for storage of data (see Figure 16–3 ■). Automated recording of the CEJ also has been developed.

With automated probing, the loss of tactile sense inherent in manual probing has been shown to increase rather than decrease probing errors. This is especially true in probing the patient with untreated periodontitis in whom subgingival calculus deposits are present. In the treated patient, controlled-force probing has been shown to be more accurate in some studies but not in others (Armitage, 1996).

Although the Florida probe has been used in a number of research studies to reduce the interexaminer error, and the Interprobe was designed for routine clinical practice, their use has not been widely accepted. The automated probing examination may be more time consuming when compared with manual probing with no clear advantage of increased accuracy. It seems likely, however, that rapid, accurate, and easy-to-use automated probes will be available in the near future.

Periodontal Screening and Recording

The Periodontal Screening and Recording (PSR) system provides a rapid, 2- to 3-minute periodontal screening examination for detecting and monitoring periodontal diseases. This system was developed by the American Dental Association and the American Academy of Periodontology with financial support from the Procter & Gamble Company. PSR indicates when a more comprehensive full-mouth periodontal examination should be performed.

The key component of the system is a thin, plastic or metal, ball-end periodontal probe. The ball tip enhances patient comfort and aids in detecting overhanging margins and subgingival calculus. The probe has a colored band extending from 3.5 to 5.5 mm for classifying pocket depth. The mouth is divided into six sextants or sections. Although six sites are probed on each tooth as in a conventional periodontal examination, only the deepest site in each sextant is scored and recorded in the patient's chart. The PSR code score is determined by how much of the colored band is visible when the PSR probe is placed in the gingival crevice.

The following are the codes used:

- Code 0: Colored probe area completely visible; no bleeding; no calculus or roughness
- Code 1: Colored probe area completely visible; bleeding; no calculus or roughness
- Code 2: Colored probe area completely visible; bleeding; calculus and/or roughness
- Code 3: Colored probe area partially visible (4–5 mm depth)
- Code 4: Colored probe area submerged completely (5.5 mm depth)

An asterisk is used to denote a furcation defect, tooth mobility, mucogingival involvement, or soft tissue recession.

The treatment of patients is based on their sextant scores. A code 3 or code 4 indicates that a more comprehensive periodontal examination and charting of the affected sextant are required to determine the treatment. When this system is used in the long-term monitoring of periodontal patients whose deep probing sites are being maintained nonsurgically, recording the tooth number and attachment level alongside the PSR coding box facilitates rapid monitoring of these sites at each periodontal maintenance visit.

Examination Techniques

Periodontal Probing Depths

To assess the probing depth, six measurements are recorded for each tooth: three on the facial surface (mesiofacial, facial, distofacial) and three on the lingual surface (mesiolingual, lingual, distolingual). It is best to develop a standardized sequence when probing. For instance, probing should start on the facial tooth surfaces of the maxillary right quadrant, proceeding to the maxillary left quadrant, then to the palatal surfaces of the maxillary right quadrant, then to the maxillary left quadrant, and finally to the mandibular quadrants in the same sequence. The probe is "walked" in approximately 1 mm increments to follow the level of attachment. Spot probing is not adequate for a thorough periodontal examination. When a reading is between two millimeter marks on the probe, the higher reading is used.

Most errors occur in interproximal readings. When probing interproximal sites on posterior teeth, the probe is angled slightly so that the tip of the probe reaches the col area, just under the contact area of the tooth

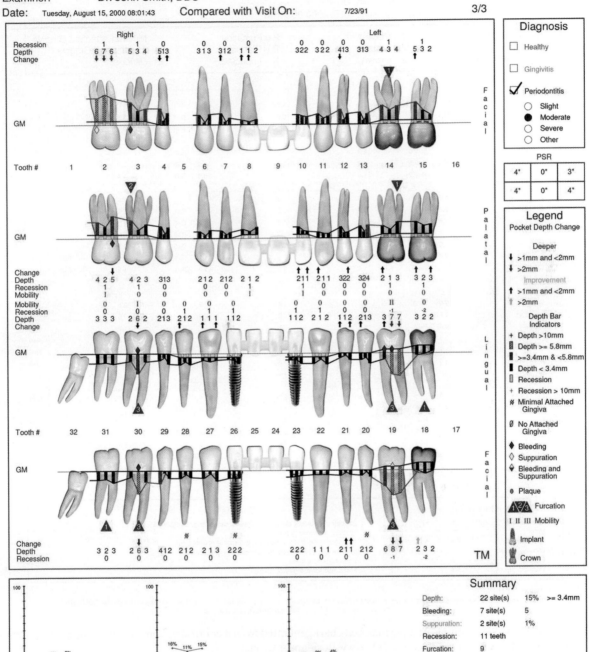

FIGURE 16–3A Example of a periodontal chart generated from a controlled-force probe. (Courtesy of Florida Probe Corporation, Gainesville, FL, www.floridaprobe.com.)

FLORIDA PROBE

Chart #:	1234567
Name:	Test Patient
Examiner:	Dr. John Smith, DDS
Date:	Tuesday, August 15, 2000 08:01:43

B = Bleeding	R = Recession	F = Furcation	~ = Minimal Attached Gingiva
S = Suppuration	M = Mobility	P = Plaque	? = No Attached Gingiva
I = Implant	C = Crown	X = Impacted	Br = Bridge

tooth		DB		B			MB		ML			L			DL			
1																		
2		6.2 S		7.2	R=1	F=0	6.2		5.0 B		F=0	2.2	R=1		3.4		F=0	M=I
3		5.0 B		2.8	R=1	F=0	3.4		2.8		F=0	1.4	R=1		3.8		F=2	M=0
4		4.4		1.2	R=0.0		3.2		3.0			1.2	R=0		3.2			M=0
5																		
6		2.6		0.6	R=0.0		2.8		2.2			0.8	R=0		1.8			M=0
7		3.0		0.8	R=0.0		1.8		1.6			1.0	R=0		2.0			M=0
8	Br	1.2		0.8	R=0.0		1.4		2.0			0.8	R=1		1.4			M=I

tooth		MB		B			DB		DL			L			ML			
9	Br	2.8		1.6	R=0.0		2.0		1.6			0.8			2.8			M=I
10	Br	2.6		2.2	R=0.0		2.0		0.8			1.0	R=1		2.0			M=I
11		2.8		1.6	R=0.0		2.2		1.2			1.2	R=0		1.6			M=0
12		4.0	F=0	1.2	R=0.0		2.8	F=0	1.6			1.4	R=0		3.0			M=0
13		3.2		1.0	R=0.0		2.8		3.4			1.6	R=0		3.2			M=0
14	C	4.0		2.8	R=1	F=1	3.8		3.2		F=1	1.2	R=1		2.2		F=0	M=0
15	C	4.8		2.6	R=1	F=0	1.4		2.6		F=0	2.2	R=1		3.2		F=0	M=0
16																		
17																		
18	C	2.2		3.0	R=-2	F=0	2.2		1.4			2.2	R=-2	F=1	2.6			M=0
19		5.4		7.8 BS	R=-1	F=3	7.2		7.2			6.8 B	R=-1	F=3	2.6 B			M=II
20		1.4		0.4	R=0	~	1.8		2.8			1.2	R=0		1.8			M=0
21		1.4		0.6	R=0		1.2		1.8			0.6	R=0		1.2			M=0
22		1.2		1.2	R=0		1.2		2.0			0.6	R=1		1.8			M=0
23	Br	1.8		1.6	R=0		1.4		1.8			0.8	R=1		0.8			M=0
24	Br	2.0		1.0	R=0.0		2.0		1.4			0.4			1.6			M=0

tooth		DB		B			MB		ML			L			DL			
25	Br	2.4		1.0		~	1.6		2.2			0.4			0.4			M=0
26	Br	2.0		2.0	R=0	~	2.0		1.8			0.8	R=1		0.6			M=0
27		2.0		0.8	R=0		2.8		0.8			1.2	R=1		0.8			M=0
28		2.0		1.0	R=0	~	1.8		2.0			1.2	R=1		2.0			M=0
29		3.4		0.6	R=0		2.0		2.8			1.0	R=0		1.8			M=0
30		1.6		6.2 B	R=0	F=3	3.0		2.2			5.4 B	R=0	F=3	2.0			M=I
31		2.4		2.2	R=0	F=1	3.2		2.8			2.4	R=0	F=0	2.6			M=0
32	X																	

Plaque Index Score		Summary
All Surfaces:	0%	24 Teeth 7 site(s) bleeding 2 site(s) suppurating, BOP = 17%
Molar:	0%	12 site(s) deepened by at least 1 mm
Interproximal:	0%	14 moderate site(s) with 4 progressing deeper by at least 1mm.
Buccal / Lingual:	0%	8 severe site(s) with 8 progressing deeper by at least 1mm.
Buccal:	0%	9 furcations were found
Lingual:	0%	5 teeth had some degree of mobility

FIGURE 16–3B Example of a periodontal chart generated from a controlled-force probe. (Courtesy of Florida Probe Corporation, Gainesville, FL, www.floridaprobe.com.)

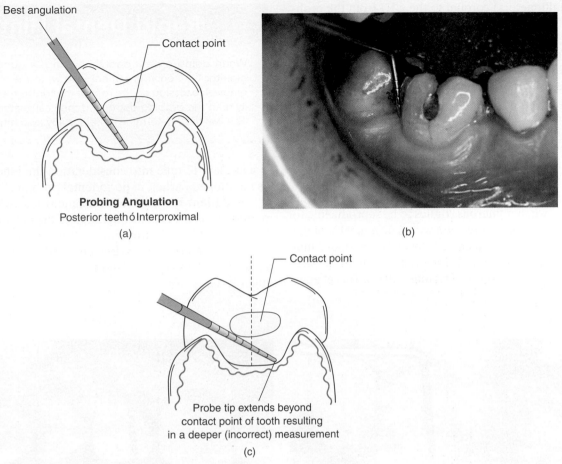

FIGURE 16–4 (a) Correct probe angulation on a posterior tooth. Probe inserts under the contact area into the col. (b) Clinically, the probe is angled to reach the col. (c) Incorrect probe angulation.

(Figure 16–4 ▪). When probing interproximal sites on anterior teeth, the probe needs to be parallel to the long axis of the tooth but at the same time should be as close to the interproximal area and not at the line angle (Figure 16–5 ▪). The probe is parallel to the long axis of all teeth on the facial and lingual surfaces.

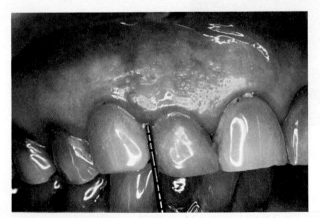

FIGURE 16–5 Correct probe placement on an anterior tooth. Probe is not angled, but it must reach interproximally with the shank against the teeth.

BLEEDING SITES In clinical practice, the primary value of bleeding on probing as a diagnostic sign is that its presence indicates that the tissues are inflamed and not healthy (Armitage, 1995). Bleeding points should be recorded on the chart with a small red dot over the probing depth measurement. Bleeding on probing indicates inflammation in the deeper tissues, whereas bleeding or stroking the gingival crevice indicates gingivitis. Sites that bleed with deep pockets and clinical attachment loss are at greater risk for future tissue destruction and should be monitored (Lang, Joss, & Nyman, 1990; Lang & Löe, 1993). Sites that do not bleed on probing are likely not breaking down.

Clinical Attachment Level

The CAL must take into account the probing depth and location of the gingival margin. To assess the CALs, two measurements are needed: probing depth and the distance of the gingival margin from the CEJ at each of the six sites around the tooth. If gingival recession is present (Figure 16–6a ▪), the CAL is determined by adding the gingival recession value and the probing depth. If there is gingival overgrowth or a pseudopocket (see Figure 16–6b), the CAL is determined by subtracting the amount of gingiva (in millimeters) coronal to the CEJ from the probing depth. If the free gingival margin is located at the CEJ (see Figure 16–6c), the CAL is equal to the probing depth. There is more tissue destruction or loss of attachment when gingival recession is present. When the attachment loss is 5 mm or greater with deep periodontal pockets, the patient should be referred to a specialist.

Another method to determine the CAL is to give a negative number to the amount of recession and then subtract it from the probing depth. A positive number is given to the amount of gingival overgrowth and then subtracted from the probing depth.

Repeated measurements, when done in this manner, have been shown in numerous studies to be reproducible to within 61 mm 90% of the time and within 62 mm 99% of the time (Armitage, 1996). Attachment loss of more than 2 mm has become the gold standard for the assessment of periodontal disease progression (Armitage, 1996). This change

is necessary to take into consideration the inherent errors, as mentioned earlier, in periodontal probing.

A patient has clinical attachment loss when there is periodontitis with apical migration of the junctional epithelium (Bouchard, Boutouyrie, Mattout, & Bourgeois, 2006; López, Fernández, Jara, & Baelum, 2001). Determination of attachment loss is part of the calculation of clinical attachment levels.

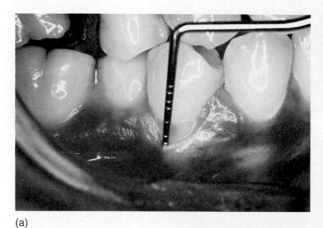

(a)

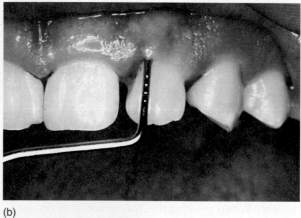

(b)

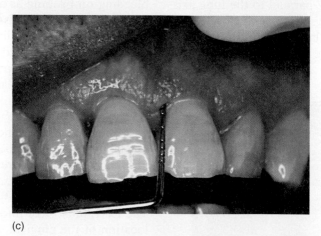

(c)

FIGURE 16–6 Probing depth versus clinical attachment level. Probing depth is the distance from the free gingival margin to the attached gingival tissues. Clinical attachment level is the distance from the CEJ to the attached gingival tissues. When the free gingival margin is apical to the CEJ (a), add the amount of recession to the probing depth (3 mm + probing depth [2 mm] = 5 mm clinical attachment level). When the free gingival margin is coronal to the CEJ (b), the distance to the CEJ is measured and subtracted from the probing depth (5 mm probing depth – 2 mm gingival enlargement = 3 mm clinical attachment level). (c) When the free gingival margin is at the CEJ, the probing depth equals the clinical attachment level (2 mm probing depth = 2 mm clinical attachment level).

Gingival Position

In health, the free gingival margin is located approximately 0.5 to 2 mm coronal to the CEJ. **Gingival recession** is defined as a shift in the gingival margin apical to the CEJ with exposure of the root surface to the oral environment. Actually, because the soft tissue margin may not always be composed of gingiva, the term *soft tissue recession* rather than *gingival recession* may be more appropriate. However, because this is currently not universally accepted, this text will continue to use gingival recession (Wennström, 1996). Gingival recession may be localized to one tooth or generalized throughout the mouth. Usually, the facial surface is involved, but all other tooth surfaces could be involved as well.

MEASUREMENT OF GINGIVAL RECESSION Visible recession, which is seen clinically, is measured from the CEJ to the gingival margin and represents the apparent position of the gingiva. Hidden recession, which is covered by the gingiva and therefore not visible, can only be measured by placing a periodontal probe at the level of attachment. This represents the actual position of the gingiva or the level of soft tissue attachment (junctional epithelium) to the tooth surface (Figure 16–7 ■). The visible recession added to the hidden recession equals the clinical attachment level. The clinical importance of measuring recession is often overlooked. There can be loss of attachment or gingival recession without a corresponding increase in probing depth. This often can be misleading, and it could be assumed that there is no tissue destruction occurring when actually there is.

ETIOLOGY OF GINGIVAL RECESSION The principal predisposing factor that determines whether recession occurs is the anatomy of the area, specifically the thickness of the alveolar bone and overlying gingiva. The etiology of gingival recession is multifactoral. Etiologic factors include the following:

1. Mechanical trauma: soft tissue trauma from overzealous toothbrushing (Figure 16–8 ■)
2. Orthodontic movement
3. Dental procedures
4. Crown margins
5. Clasps from partial dentures
6. Destructive inflammatory periodontal disease, where there is loss of attachment (destruction of gingival fibers and apical migration of the junctional epithelium; Figure 16–9 ■)

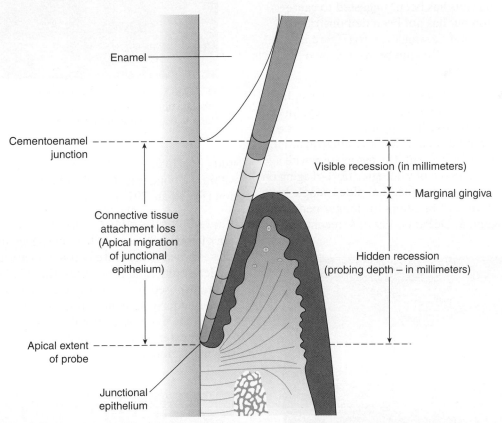

Enamel

Cementoenamel junction

Connective tissue attachment loss (Apical migration of junctional epithelium)

Apical extent of probe

Junctional epithelium

Visible recession (in millimeters)

Marginal gingiva

Hidden recession (probing depth – in millimeters)

FIGURE 16–7 Diagram showing visible and hidden recession. Clinically, visible recession is determined by measuring with a periodontal probe from the CEJ to the free gingival margin. Hidden recession corresponds to the probing depth. The visible recession measurement added to the hidden recession measurement equals the clinical attachment level (CAL).

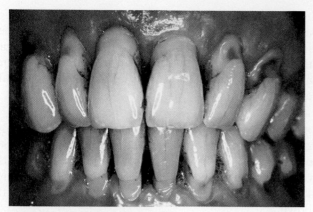

FIGURE 16–8 Generalized gingival recession due to overzealous toothbrushing.

7. Tooth malposition (rotated, lingually or facially displaced teeth), where the alveolar bone over a prominent root such as a maxillary canine is thin or absent
8. Periodontal therapy (periodontal debridement or surgery), where tissue shrinkage has occurred
9. Oral habits causing injury to the gingiva, such as fingernail biting
10. Anatomic variations that may accelerate gingival recession, including a high frenum attachment pulling the free gingival margin (Figure 16–10 ■).
11. Occlusal trauma (this has been suggested to cause gingival recession but has not been demonstrated)
12. Cigarette smoking and chewing tobacco (Figure 16–11 ■), but the exact mechanism has not been elucidated (Gunsolley et al., 1998)

It is imperative that the cause be determined in individual cases so that the progressive nature of the recession can be controlled and interceptive therapy initiated if necessary. Gingival recession can be seen in healthy gingiva; inflammation may or may not be present. The association with age does not necessarily suggest a physiologic effect of aging on recession. It may just reflect the fact that older people have been subject to the force of brushing for longer periods of time (Joshipura, Kent, & DePaola, 1994). A recent clinical

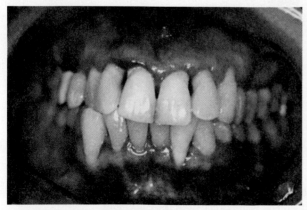

FIGURE 16–9 Gingival recession in a refractory periodontitis patient. Note the presence of inflammation. Gingival recession is due to the disease process.

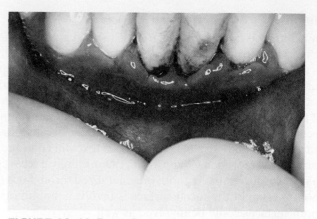

FIGURE 16–10 Recession on the mandibular incisors caused by the high frenum attachment pulling on the free gingival margin. Note the heavy accumulation of plaque and calculus.

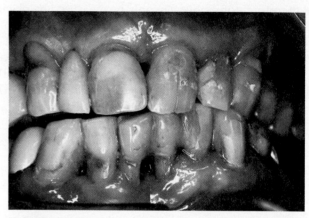

FIGURE 16–11 A 55-year-old man who placed chewing tobacco in the facial vestibule of the anterior teeth. Note the gingival recession on the anterior teeth.

study concluded that tooth volume and/or tooth position within the bone was strongly associated with gingival recession (Richman, 2011).

CLINICAL SIGNIFICANCE OF GINGIVAL RECESSION Identification of gingival recession has clinical significance. Root surfaces exposed to the oral environment are more vulnerable to the development of root caries. The thin layer of cementum on the exposed root surface may wear away easily, exposing the underlying dental tubules to the oral environment. Fluid in the exposed dentinal tubules contracts or expands when an external stimulus such as cold or touch is applied. This may stimulate nerves to produce pain. In addition, the

Rapid Dental Hint

Gingival recession should be documented on the periodontal chart. The cause of the recession must be determined to offer the appropriate treatment.

col shape changes when gingival recession is present. If the interdental area is open so that no col exists, the facial and palatal gingiva become continuous and keratinized. Thus interproximal recession may create areas of food impaction.

PATHOGENESIS The pathogenesis of gingival recession is debatable. As mentioned earlier, it has been considered perhaps to be a normal physiologic process that occurs with increasing age, but there is limited documentation to uphold this concept. Others consider it to be a pathologic condition. When the free gingiva is thin, the inflammatory lesion will occupy and degrade the entire connective tissue portion, resulting in collapse of the free gingiva (Wennström, 1994). If there is less than 1 mm or more of attached gingiva, the free gingival margin may be movable, which allows microorganisms to enter into the crevice, initiating an inflammatory response.

The amount of attached gingiva needed for gingival health is controversial. Experimental studies (Wennström & Lindhe, 1983a, 1983b) have failed to consistently support the concept of a minimal width of gingiva for maintenance of periodontal health.

Mucogingival Considerations

A mucogingival involvement or defect is defined as a discrepancy in the relationship between the free gingival margin and the mucogingival junction. Pathology or loss of attachment may not be involved. Common mucogingival conditions may be the result of

- Gingival recession, resulting in inadequate or diminished attached gingiva
- Probing depths extending to or beyond the mucogingival junction into the alveolar mucosa (Figure 16–12 ■)
- Anatomical variations that may complicate the management of these conditions, including a high frenum attachment pulling the gingival margin away from the tooth surface (surgical intervention may be necessary to augment the amount of attached gingiva and correct the mucogingival problem)

MUCOGINGIVAL EXAMINATION A thorough mucogingival examination using appropriate screening techniques and recording the free gingival margin and mucogingival junction on the chart is necessary to detect these conditions. This also enables the practitioner to monitor the progressive nature at future periodontal maintenance visits so that appropriate treatment can be rendered. Although radiographs are not used in the identification of mucogingival problems, appropriate radiographs may be used as part of a preoperative appraisal.

Recording the free gingival margin on the chart will identify the presence or absence of gingival recession or overgrowth. Recession on all six tooth surfaces should be recorded. It is important to measure the amount of recession (in millimeters) because it provides information for determining total attachment loss.

The next step in the mucogingival examination is to determine the total width or height of keratinized gingiva. The width of keratinized gingiva is determined by measuring with a periodontal probe the distance from the gingival margin to the mucogingival junction. The width of attached gingiva is determined by subtracting the probing depth (free gingiva) from the amount of keratinized gingiva (Figure 16–13 ■). Mucogingival involvement exists when no attached gingiva is present on a tooth. To establish the position of the mucogingival junction, move the side of the periodontal probe gently across the alveolar mucosa in an apical-coronal direction until the tissue stops moving (Figure 16–14 ■). At this point, elastic fibers are not present, and attached gingiva is coronal to the mucogingival junction. Other methods include the visual method. The problem with this technique is that with inflammation, the gingiva is red, and it will be difficult to differentiate between the red alveolar mucosa and the gingiva. Another method is to pull the lip outward, and the mucogingival junction is seen at the point of tension. This is sometimes misleading, and the actual location of the mucogingival junction is not always distinguished.

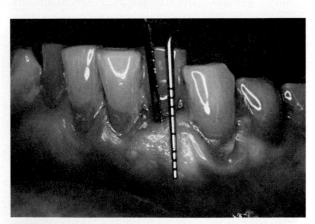

FIGURE 16–13 (*Left probe*) Determination of the amount of gingiva (free + attached) by measuring from the free gingival margin to the mucogingival junction. (*Right probe*) Determination of the amount of attached gingiva by subtracting the probing depth (right probe measurement) from the total width of gingiva (left probe measurement).

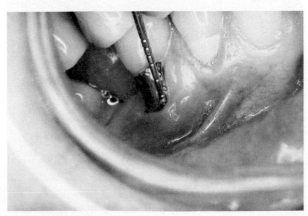

FIGURE 16–12 There is no attached gingiva present on this tooth. This is a mucogingival defect.

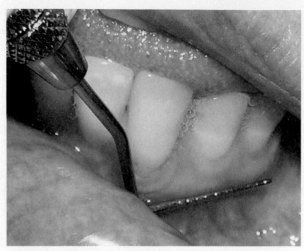

FIGURE 16–14 The periodontal probe is gently placed on the alveolar mucosa and moved coronally until the tissue does not move. This is the mucogingival junction.

Did You Know?

The alveolar mucosa is more movable than the attached/free gingiva because it contains loose connective tissue.

To determine if any frenal attachments are encroaching on the gingival margin, retract the cheeks and lips laterally by pulling with the thumb and index finger, and watch for movement of the gingival margin in the frenal attachment area.

DELAYED PASSIVE ERUPTION Delayed passive eruption occurs in adults when the free gingival margin failed to migrate apically toward the CEJ and still remains on or near the cervical bulge of the enamel, creating a "gummy smile" (Figure 16–15 ■). This condition is also seen in children up to the time of completed eruption of permanent teeth. This is a normal situation, and the process of passive eruption ultimately will move the free gingival margin apically.

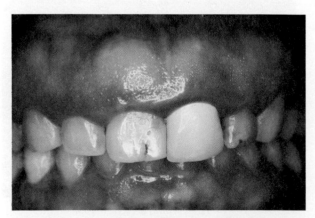

FIGURE 16–15 A 40-year-old patient exhibiting delayed passive eruption. Note that the gingival margin is located on the cervical bulge of the enamel.

Rapid Dental Hint

Patients with "gummy smiles" should be evaluated for delayed passive eruption.

Suppuration

Suppuration, also referred to as purulent exudate or pus, is a clinical feature of inflammation. Pus is composed of dead cells, polymorphonuclear leukocytes (PMNs or neutrophils), and tissue fluids. The presence of suppuration indicates an ongoing infection in the periodontal pocket. Pus can be detected visually coming from the pocket by either probing the gingival crevice or using digital pressure from the base of the crevice on the outer surface of the gingiva moving in a coronal direction (Figure 16–16 ■).

Tooth Mobility

Tooth mobility is classified as either physiologic or pathologic. Physiologic movement of a tooth is limited to the width of the periodontal ligament space. All teeth have some degree of physiologic mobility that occurs with normal function. The range of physiologic mobility varies according to the time of the day and the tooth. It is most evident on teeth with short roots, such as mandibular incisors, and early in the morning. Increased tooth mobility in the hours just after awakening is due to slight extrusion of the tooth as a result of limited occlusal contact during sleep.

Pathologic mobility of teeth results from bone loss, gingival inflammation, periapical pathology, hormonal imbalance (e.g., pregnancy gingivitis), or occlusal trauma, where excessive occlusal forces are placed on a tooth. Periodontal disease can be advanced without any evidence of increased tooth mobility. Therefore, the severity of tooth mobility is not always due to the amount of bone loss. Because tooth

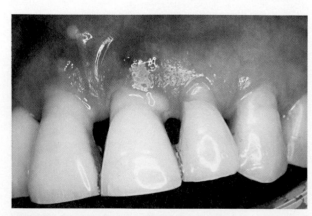

FIGURE 16–16 Suppuration detected from the maxillary central incisors. Deep probing depths were noted.

mobility may not result from periodontal problems, identification of the cause is important so that the appropriate treatment can be rendered.

MEASUREMENT OF TOOTH MOBILITY The degree of mobility can be measured either manually or with electronic devices. Although the most common classification for measuring pathologic tooth mobility is the Miller classification, it remains very subjective. Mobility is assessed by using the handles of two hand instruments on the facial and lingual aspects of the crown and applying force. The Miller classification is summarized in Box 16–1 (Miller, 1950). Mobility requires treatment when the patient feels discomfort or when the mobility increases over time.

Fremitus

Fremitus is the vibrational movement of a tooth under occlusal forces. Fremitus is determined by gently placing the index finger on the facial surfaces of the maxillary teeth while instructing the patient to tap the teeth together and grind them side to side. Only the maxillary teeth are checked for fremitus because the arch is fixed, whereas the mandibular arch is moving.

Rapid Dental Hint

When you detect mobility on a tooth, the next step is to determine the cause. Without knowing the cause, you cannot effectively treat the patient.

Box 16–1: Classification of Pathologic Mobility (Miller's Classification)

1. First distinguishable sign of tooth movement greater than normal in a facial/lingual direction

2. Movement of the tooth in a facial/lingual direction up to 1 mm

3. Movement of the tooth in a facial/lingual direction more than 1 mm and/or depressed in a vertical direction

The amount of fremitus is subjective, but the following guide can be used:

+ (slight vibrations can be felt);

++ (obvious, palpable vibrations can be felt, but movement of the tooth is barely visible); or

+++ (visible movement is seen).

Did You Know?

You can only check for fremitus on the maxilla because it is a fixed structure. The mandible moves.

Fremitus should be eliminated by occlusal adjustment by means of, say, selective grinding.

Pathologic Tooth Migration

Pathologic tooth migration is defined as the movement of teeth due to the disruption of forces that normally maintain physiologic tooth position. Tooth movement can occur in any direction. Clinically, this may be seen as increased spacing between teeth, dramatic overjet of anterior teeth (anterior flaring), rotation of teeth, or extrusion where tooth migration occurs in an occlusal or incisal direction (Figure 16–17 ■). Usually, tooth mobility is also present. Any of these symptoms is a common chief complaint of a patient that may prompt a professional evaluation. As part of the clinical examination, it is important to ask the patient if spaces between the teeth have increased over time or if they have always been present. It is important to recognize signs and symptoms of pathologic migration and determine the cause of the problem to render appropriate treatment as early as possible to prevent the situation from getting worse (Greenstein, Cavallaro, Scharf, & Tarnow, 2008).

Periodontal disease destruction of the attachment apparatus plays a major role in the etiology of pathologic migration (Towfighi et al., 1997). Other contributing factors include parafunctional habits such as tongue thrusting or bruxism, teeth adjacent to edentulous areas, and drug-induced gingival enlargement.

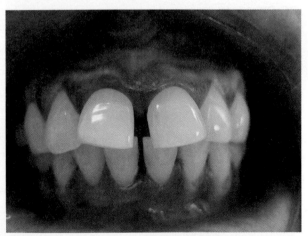

FIGURE 16–17 Pathologic tooth migration in a 26-year-old woman with rapidly progressive periodontitis. The patient complained of flaring and increasing space between the maxillary central incisors.

Furcation Involvement

A furcation or furca is the area of root division on multi-rooted teeth, including the maxillary first and second molars, maxillary first premolar, and mandibular first and second molars. The third molars usually have fused conical roots. Because the maxillary molars have three roots (mesiobuccal, distofacial, palatal), they are trifurcated. There are three furcation entrances: mesial, distal, and buccal. The mandibular molars are bifurcated; that is, they have two roots (mesial and distal). There are two furcation entrances: buccal and lingual. The maxillary first premolar is also bifurcated, having a buccal and lingual root (Figure 16–18 ■). There are two furcation entrances: mesial and distal.

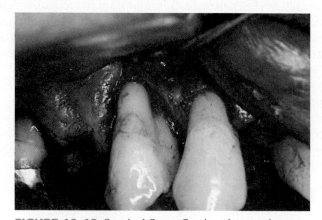

FIGURE 16–18 Surgical flap reflection shows a furcation defect on the maxillary first premolar. Fluting of the root is evident also.

Furcation involvement occurs when interradicular bone (bone between the root branches of the same tooth) destruction occurs. Furcation involvement is affected by factors such as the length of the root trunk and the presence of root concavities, which create a plaque trap. The root trunk is the area on the tooth from the CEJ to the roof or entrance of the furca (Figure 16–19 ■). As seen radiographically, high furcation with a short root trunk will have a greater chance of interradicular bone destruction early in the disease process than a low furcation with a long root trunk. The average root trunk length on a maxillary molar is about 4 mm at the mesial, 5 mm at the distal, and 4 mm at the buccal furcation. The root trunk length of the mandibular molar is 3 mm on the buccal aspect and 4 mm on the lingual aspect (Dunlap & Gher, 1985; Gher & Dunlap, 1985). This suggests that a minimum of 5 mm of attachment loss on a molar may result in early furcation involvement.

CLASSIFICATION OF FURCATION INVOLVEMENT The clinical detection of furcation involvements is important because it is difficult for both the patient and the dental hygienist to effectively clean these areas. Radiographic interpretation does not allow sufficient detection of furcation involvement. The anatomy of the tooth and location of the furca are determined from both the radiograph and clinical examination. The pattern of interradicular bone loss is both horizontal and vertical. Although many classifications

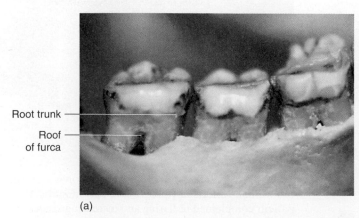

Root trunk

Roof of furca

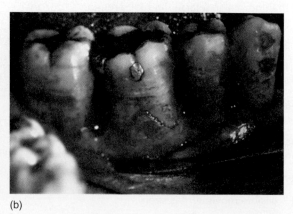

(a)　　　　　　　　　　　　　　　　　　(b)

FIGURE 16–19 (a) Dry-skull specimen of a furcation involvement on the mandibular molars. Root trunk length is the distance from the CEJ to the entrance (roof) of the furca. (b) Flap is reflected during surgery. There is bone loss around the molar but the furcation is intact without bone loss.

Rapid Dental Hint

Do not forget that the maxillary first premolar has furcas. When there is furcation involvement, that tooth most likely does not have a good prognosis because it has a long root trunk.

of horizontal furcation involvement have been suggested, Glickman's classification is described in Table 16–1 ■. Classification of vertical bone loss (Tarnow & Fletcher, 1984) is described in Figure 16–20 ■.

TECHNIQUE FOR LOCATING FURCATION INVOLVEMENTS A calibrated curved Nabers probe is used to clinically locate the furcation entrances and degree of horizontal pattern of bone destruction (Figure 16–21a ■). In the maxillary molar, the mesial furcation is not centered. The entrance is usually located about two-thirds of the buccal-lingual width toward the palatal aspect of the tooth (see Figure 16–21b). Thus, the mesial furcation is approached from the palatal side. The distal furcation is centered equally from the buccal and palatal aspects of the tooth (in the interproximal

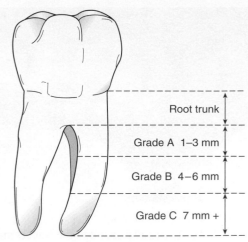

FIGURE 16–20 Schematic drawing of a mandibular molar demonstrating the vertical classification of furcation involvement. The amount of vertical bone loss is determined from the roof of the furca apically.

area), and thus the Nabers probe can be positioned from either the buccal or palatal side. The instrument handle is placed parallel to the long axis of the tooth. When a furcation defect is found, it is noted in the chart on the

Table 16–1 Glickman's Classification of Furcation Involvement (Horizontal Pattern of Bone Destruction)

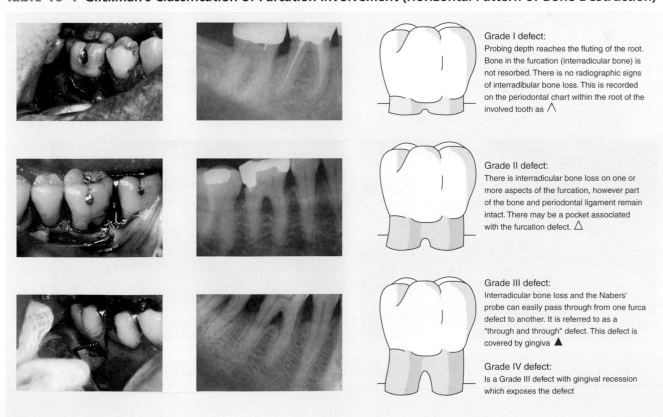

Grade I defect:
Probing depth reaches the fluting of the root. Bone in the furcation (interradicular bone) is not resorbed. There is no radiographic signs of interradibular bone loss. This is recorded on the periodontal chart within the root of the involved tooth as ∧

Grade II defect:
There is interradicular bone loss on one or more aspects of the furcation, however part of the bone and periodontal ligament remain intact. There may be a pocket associated with the furcation defect. △

Grade III defect:
Interradicular bone loss and the Nabers' probe can easily pass through from one furca defect to another. It is referred to as a "through and through" defect. This defect is covered by gingiva ▲

Grade IV defect:
Is a Grade III defect with gingival recession which exposes the defect

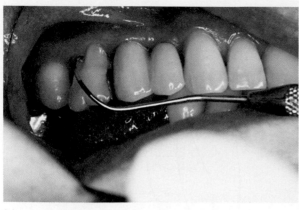

(a)

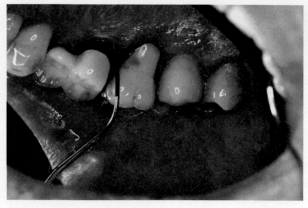

(b)

FIGURE 16–21 (a) Placement of the Nabers probe in determining the presence of a buccal furcation. Note that the handle is parallel to the occlusal plane. (b) Nabers probe placed to determine the presence of a mesial furcation of a maxillary molar. Note that the handle is parallel to the long axis of the tooth when probing interproximal furcations. (Reprinted with permission from the American Academy of Periodontology. Copyright 1984. Tarnow D., and P. Fletcher. Classification of the vertical component of furcation involvement. *J. Periodontol.* 1983;55:283–284.)

involved root. Furcations thus can be classified according to their horizontal and vertical component of bone loss, for example, IIA.

CERVICAL ENAMEL PROJECTIONS Cervical enamel projections (CEPs) are extensions of enamel toward and often into the furcation area. This area is thought to be a plaque trap, enhancing plaque accumulation. This area may be more prone to attachment loss because instead of a connective tissue attachment, the periodontal attachment on enamel will be via a junctional epithelium, which may not be as strong (Easly & Drennan, 1969). However, it has been demonstrated that an epithelial attachment may be just as resistant as a connective tissue attachment to inflammatory disease.

Did You Know?

The Nabers probe was named after a famous periodontist, Claude Nabers.

Palatogingival Groove

Palatogingival groove is a common developmental anomaly of maxillary incisors. A midpalatal groove usually extends apically into the root surface. Grooves allow for plaque accumulation and may contribute to the pathogenesis of periodontal and endodontic lesions (Figure 16–22 ■). Treatment involves periodontal and endodontic consultations to see the viability of keeping the tooth (Ballal, Jothi, Bhat, & Bhat, 2007).

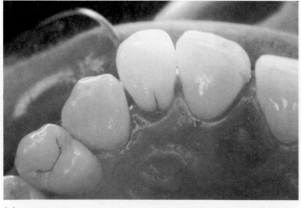

(a)

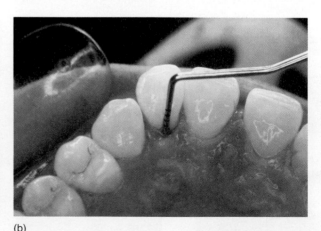

(b)

FIGURE 16–22 (a) Palatogingival groove on the maxillary lateral incisor. (b) Probing reveals a deep pocket that is difficult to maintain.

Dental Hygiene Application

Documentation of clinical findings is done on a periodontal chart. Many types of charts are available. It is important to accurately date and record all clinical findings for legal reasons and to permit the comparison of pretreatment measurements with posttreatment values. Documentation includes the medical and dental histories, chief complaint, oral hygiene evaluation (plaque index), and gingival and periodontal evaluations.

Findings from the periodontal examination should be interpreted together with the medical, dental, oral hygiene, gingival, and radiographic assessments. Recording of clinical attachment level is important for long-term monitoring of patients for periodontal destruction.

There may be a relationship between periodontal status of a patient and peri-implant health. A recent clinical study found that there may be a correlation in teeth and implants between biofilm and bone loss and pocket depths or bleeding. They found a higher percentage of implant failure when the bone loss of the associated teeth was ≥ 3 mm (Lopez-Piriz et al., 2012).

Another new theory that has recently surfaced in literature is the relationship between periodontal health and body mass index. Previously it has been reported that poor oral health was related to high body mass index (BMI). Now, studies have shown that plaque index, dental biofilm, and probing depths are statistically associated with periodontal inflammation and high BMI and obesity, independent of dietary habits and insulin resistance (Benguigui et al., 2012).

Key Points

- All new and maintaining patients should receive a periodontal examination.
- Probing depth is measured from the gingival margin to wherever the tip of the probe stops (in the junctional epithelium).

- Clinical attachment level is measured from the CEJ to the apical extent of the probe and is a more accurate long-term measurement for disease progression than probing depths.

Self-Quiz

1. Which one of the following reasons explains why measuring the clinical attachment levels (CALs) is a more reliable method for determining clinical attachment loss over time than probing depth measurements?
   a. Less penetration into the junctional epithelium occurs.
   b. Stable reference point is used (e.g., CEJ).
   c. More measuring points are used on the tooth.
   d. Less bleeding occurs at periodontal active sites.

2. From the following list, select the items associated with gingival recession.
   a. Pathologic condition
   b. Caused by malocclusion
   c. Can be seen in healthy gingiva
   d. Referred to as the sum of the visible recession plus the hidden recession
   e. Amount of attached gingiva is controversial

3. Which one of the following techniques describes how visible recession is recorded?
   a. Use a periodontal probe to measure from the cementoenamel junction to the free gingival margin.
   b. Use a periodontal probe to measure from the free gingival margin to the base of the pocket.
   c. Use an explorer to determine the location of the cementoenamel junction.
   d. Use an explorer to determine the apical extent of the junctional epithelium.

4. Which one of the following conditions is related to gingival recession?
   a. Grinding and clenching of teeth
   b. Tongue thrusting
   c. Tooth malposition
   d. Mouth breathing

5. Which one of the following is a cause of a mucogingival involvement or defect?
   a. Mouth rinses with high alcohol content
   b. Brushing with a hard-bristle toothbrush
   c. Inadequate amount or width of attached gingiva
   d. Inadequate amount or width of alveolar mucosa

6. Which of the following teeth with class II furca involvement has the worst prognosis?
   a. Mandibular first molar
   b. Mandibular second molar
   c. Maxillary first premolar
   d. Maxillary first molar

7. Loss of attachment indicates that the
   a. gingival fibers have been detached from the enamel.
   b. periodontal ligament fibers have regenerated.
   c. junctional epithelium has migrated apically along the root.
   d. circular fibers have detached from the root.

8. A mucogingival involvement or defect is defined as a discrepancy in the relationship between the mucogingival junction and the
   a. cementoenamel junction.
   b. free gingival margin.
   c. nonkeratinized epithelium.
   d. junctional epithelium.

9. Which of the following terms describes the current or ongoing (at the time of the examination) loss of soft-tissue attachment?
   a. Periodontal disease activity
   b. Periodontal disease severity
   c. Clinical attachment loss
   d. Furcation involvement

10. Visible recession added to the hidden recession equals the
    a. clinical attachment level.
    b. relative attachment level.
    c. probing depth.
    d. mucogingival defect.

Case Study

The dental hygienist is about to begin a clinical examination for returning 55 year old male who was last seen 6 months ago in the practice. There are radiographs from one year ago and probing depths from 6 months ago. The periodontal charting does not reflect if there is recession or the location of the gingival margin. The medical history does not indicate diabetes or heart disease. His BMI is within normal limits.

1. What do the radiographs and probing depths indicate?
   a. periodontal disease severity
   b. current tissue breakdown
   c. periodontal disease activity
   d. clinical attachment loss

Answer: B. The probing depths and radiographs show previous history of disease activity but do not identify active disease sites. Periodontal severity is the total destruction and healing that occurs in a lifetime. It is determined by visual inspection, single measurements of probing, and evaluating radiographs for bone loss. It does not determine if the site is actively breaking down.

2. What is required information in order to determine the clinical attachment level?
   a. current probing depths and the measurement from the CEJ to gingival margin
   b. current radiographs and current probing depths
   c. previous probing depths compared to new probing depths
   d. gingival margin or recession charted

Answer: A. The most recent information to record the clinical loss of attachment from the CEJ to the apical extent of the periodontal pocket or junctional epithelium. The location of the gingival margin must be related to the CEJ and the depth of the pocket.

3. What factors might influence the periodontal disease activity of this patient?
   a. furcation involvement
   b. pathologic mobility
   c. loss of attached gingiva
   d. b and c
   e. all of the above

Answer: E. All of the above factors could be conditions which will allow for more biofilm collection, loss of connective tissue attachment, or bone loss. All factors should be routinely monitored and compared to previous findings.

References

Armitage, G. C. 1995. Clinical evaluation of periodontal diseases. *Periodontology 2000* 7:39–52.

Armitage, G. C. 1996. Periodontal diseases: Diagnosis. *Ann. Periodontol.* 1:37–215.

Armitage, G. C. 2004. The complete periodontal examination. *Periodontology 2000* 34(1):9–21.

Armitage, G. C., G. K. Svanberg, and H. Löe. 1977. Microscopic evaluation of clinical measurements of connective tissue attachment levels. *J. Clin. Periodontol.* 4:173–190.

Ballal, N.V., V. Jothi, K. S. Bhat, and K. M. Bhat. 2007. Salvaging a tooth with a deep palotogingival groove: An endo-perio treatment—a case report. *Int. Endod. J.* 40(10):808–817.

Bawden, J. W., and G. H. DeFriese. (eds.). 1981. *Planning for dental care on a statewide basis: The North Carolina Dental Manpower Project.* Chapel Hill: The Dental Foundation of North Carolina.

Benguigui, C., V. Bongard, J. D. Ruidavets, et al. 2012. Evaluation of oral health related to body mass index. *Oral Dis.* April 5.

Bouchard, P., P. Boutouyrie, C. Mattout, and D. Bourgeois. 2006. Risk assessment for severe clinical attachment loss in an adult population. *J. Periodontol.* 77(3):479–489.

Brown, L. J., R. C. Oliver, and H. Löe. 1989. Periodontal diseases in the U.S. in 1981: Prevalence, severity, extent, and role in tooth mortality. *J. Periodontol.* 60:363–380.

Carlos, J. P., J. A. Brunelle, and M. D. Wolfe. 1987. Attachment loss versus pocket depth as indicators of periodontal disease: A methodologic note. *J. Periodont. Res.* 22:524–525.

Douglas, C. W. 2006. Risk assessment and management of periodontal disease. *JADA* 137 (suppl. 3):27S–32S.

Dunlap, R. M., and M. E. Gher. 1985. Root surface measurements of the mandibular first molar. *J. Periodontol.* 56:234–238.

Easly, J. R., and G. A. Drennan. 1969. Morphological classification of the furca. *J. Can. Dent. Assoc.* 35:105–107.

Garguilo, A. W., F. M. Wentz, and B. Orban. 1961. Dimensions and relations of the dentogingival junction in humans. *J. Periodontol.* 32:261–267.

Gher, M. E., and R. W. Dunlap. 1985. Linear variation of the root surface area of the maxillary first molar. *J. Periodontol.* 56:39–43.

Goodson, J. M. 1986. Clinical measurements of periodontitis. *J. Clin. Periodontol.* 13:446–455.

Greenstein, G., and J. Caton. 1990. Periodontal disease activity: A critical assessment. *J. Periodontol.* 61:543–552.

Greenstein, G., J. Cavallaro, D. Scharf, and D. Tarnow. 2008. Differential diagnosis and management of flared maxillary anterior teeth. *J. Am. Dent. Assoc.* 139:715–723.

Gunsolley, J. C., S. M. Quinn, J. Tew, C. M. Gooss, C. M. Brooks, and H. A. Schenkein. 1998. The effect of smoking on individuals with minimal periodontal destruction. *J. Periodontol.* 69:165–170.

Haffajee, A. D., S. S. Socransky, and J. M. Goodson. 1983. Clinical parameters as predictors of destructive periodontal disease activity. *J. Clin. Periodontol.* 10:257–265.

Jeffcoat, M. K. 1994. Current concepts in periodontal disease testing. *J. Am. Dent. Assoc.* 125:1071–1078.

Joshipura, K. J., R. L. Kent, and P. F. DePaola. 1994. Gingival recession: Intra-oral distribution and associated factors. *J. Periodontol.* 65:864–871.

Keagle, J. G., J. J. Garnick, J. R. Searle, G. E. King, and P. K. Morse. 1989. Gingival resistance to probing forces: I. Determination of optimal probe diameter. *J. Periodontol.* 60:167–171.

Lamster, I. B., R. S. Celenti, H. H. Jans, J. B. Fine, and J. T. Grbic. 1993. Current status of tests for periodontal disease. *Adv. Dent. Res.* 7:182–190.

Lang, N. P., A. R. Joss, and S. Nyman. 1990. Absence of bleeding on probing: An indicator of periodontal stability. *J. Clin. Periodontol.* 17:714–721.

Lang, N. P., and H. Löe. 1993. Clinical management of periodontal diseases. *Periodontology 2000* 2:128–139.

Listgarten, M. A., R. Mao, and P. J. Robinson. 1976. Periodontal probing and the relationship of the probe tip to periodontal tissues. *J. Periodontol.* 47:511–513.

López, R., O. Fernández, G. Jara, and V. Baelum. 2001. Epidemiology of clinical attachment loss in adolescents. *J. Periodontol.* 72(12):1666–1674.

Lopez-Piriz, R., A. Morales, M. J. Gimenez, et al. 2012. Correlation between clinical parameters characterising peri-implant and periodontal health: A practice-based research in Spain in a series of patients with implants installed 4–5 years ago. *Med. Oral Patol. Oral Cir. Bucal.* May 1.

McFall, W. T., Jr., J. D. Bader, G. R. Rozier, and D. Ramsey. 1988. Presence of periodontal data in patient records of general practitioners. *J. Periodontol.* 59:445–449.

Miller, S. C. 1950. *Textbook of periodontia*, 3rd ed., 125. Philadelphia: Blakiston.

Reddy, M. S. 1997. The use of periodontal probes and radiographs in clinical trials of diagnostic tests. *Ann. Periodontol.* 2:113–122.

Richman, C. 2011. Is gingival recession a consequence of an orthodontic tooth size and/or tooth position discrepancy? "A paradigm shift." *Compendium* 32:62–69.

Robinson, P. J., and R. M. Vitaek. 1979. The relationship between gingival inflammation and resistance to probe penetration. *J. Periodont. Res.* 14:230–243.

Spray, J. R., J. J. Garnick, L. R. Doles, and J. J. Klawitter. 1978. Microscopic demonstration of the position of periodontal probes. *J. Periodontol.* 49:148–152.

Tarnow, D., and P. Fletcher. 1984. Classification of the vertical component of furcation involvement. *J. Periodontol.* 55:283–284.

Towfighi, P. P., M. A. Brunsvold, A. T. Storey, R. M. Arnold, D. E. Willman, and C. A. McMahan. 1997. Pathologic migration of anterior teeth in patients with moderate to severe periodontitis. *J. Periodontol.* 68:967–972.

van der Velden, U. 1979. Probing force and the relationship of the probe tip to the periodontal tissues. *J. Clin. Periodontol.* 6:106–114.

Wennström, J. L. 1994. Mucogingival surgery. In eds. N. P. Lang and T. Karring, *Proceedings of the 1st European Workshop on Periodontology*, 193–199. London: Quintessence.

Wennström, J. L. 1996. Mucogingival therapy. *Ann. Periodontol.* 1:671–701.

Wennström, J. L., and J. Lindhe. 1983a. Plaque-induced gingival inflammation in the absence of attached gingiva in dogs. *J. Clin. Periodontol.* 10:266–276.

Wennström, J. L., and J. Lindhe. 1983b. The role of attached gingiva for maintenance of periodontal health: Healing following excisional and grafting procedures in dogs. *J. Clin. Periodontol.* 10:206–221.

Williams, R. C., J. D. Beck, and S. N. Offenbacher. 1996. The impact of new technologies on the diagnosis and treatment of periodontal disease: A look to the future. *J. Clin. Periodontol.* 23:299–305.

Visit www.pearsonhighered.com/healthprofessionsresources to access the student resources that accompany this book. Simply select Dental Hygiene from the choice of disciplines. Find this book and you will find the complimentary study tools created for this specific title.

Radiographic Assessment

Herbert Frommer and Jeanine J. Stabulas-Savage

OUTLINE

EDUCATIONAL OBJECTIVES

Upon completion of this chapter, the reader should be able to:

- Identify and discuss the periodontal structures seen on a radiograph.
- Discuss the rationale for utilizing radiographs in periodontics.
- Explain the features of conventional and digital imaging.
- List and discuss the benefits and limitations of radiographs used in periodontics.
- Explain the radiographic improvements aimed at decreasing patient radiation exposure.
- Discuss the types of radiographs used in the treatment planning and evaluation of implants.

GOAL: To provide a radiology background that is used in conjunction with clinical data to recognize and classify periodontal diseases.

KEY WORDS

Introduction

The proper classification, evaluation, and treatment of the periodontal diseases can be accomplished only with a combination of radiographic and clinical examinations. Therefore, we must be aware of the diagnostic limitations of radiographs because periodontal diseases have both soft tissue and bony components. Soft-tissue changes such as inflammation, gingival enlargement, and recession cannot be seen on radiographs because such tissues have decreased density and therefore appear radiolucent on a radiographic image. Due to the superimposition of the buccal and lingual alveolar bone plates, bone loss in some areas also may not be seen. Radiographs essentially portray a three-dimensional disease process in two planes. This point must be kept in mind when viewing radiographs because the appearance can be very misleading.

Despite these limitations, a proper periodontal classification cannot be made without the appropriate survey of radiographs. Radiographs serve to (1) identify predisposing factors, (2) detect early to moderate bone changes where treatment can preserve the dentition, (3) approximate the amount of bone loss and its location, (4) help in evaluating the prognosis of affected teeth and the restorative needs of these teeth, and (5) serve as baseline data and as a means to evaluate posttreatment results.

This chapter will discuss the role of conventional radiographs (i.e., radiographs taken on film with an X-ray machine) and computer-based image processing (i.e., the use of a computer to display and enhance images of teeth and bone).

Conventional Radiographs: Intraoral Technique

Parameters

The three parameters, or choices, that the dental professional selects at the control panel of an X-ray machine are kilovoltage, milliamperage, and exposure time. Understanding the effect of each of these parameters on the diagnostic X-ray beam is important and will help in making a correct classification of the disease process (i.e., dental hygiene assessment).

KILOVOLTAGE The amount of penetration of the X-ray beam is controlled by the kilovoltage. The suitable range for dental radiography is 65 to 100 kilovolt peak (kVp). This range is determined by the density of the objects to be radiographed (e.g., teeth, bone). Kilovoltage settings above 100 kVp result in overpenetration, and settings below 45 kVp would result in underpenetration. Kilovoltage settings in the range of 45 to 65 kVp, although producing a diagnostic beam, are never used because of the excess secondary radiation that results.

The question to be answered is: "Within the acceptable kilovoltage range, what kilovoltage is most appropriate for periodontal diagnosis?" The answer is determined by the degree of density and contrast that is most diagnostic for the clinician. Density is the degree of blackness on a film, and contrast is the difference in the degrees of blackness between adjacent areas.

Radiographs have a high degree of (short-scale) contrast when low kilovolt-peak settings are used. The X-ray photons either penetrate the tissue or are absorbed—a sort of yes-or-no, black-or-white reaction. When higher kilovolt-peak settings are used, there is less contrast, and the overall tone of the radiograph is gray. This occurs because there is much more partial penetration with the resulting long-scale contrast. Such low contrast is not as satisfying visually as high contrast, but early changes in object density such as early bone loss may be seen in the gradations of gray as a result of more selective penetration, which is not present in high-contrast films. Theoretically, therefore, higher kilovolt-peak settings with their resulting long-scale contrast produce better results in terms of periodontal diagnosis. A number of clinicians, however, feel that the human eye is not capable of seeing these very subtle gray changes and recommend using 75 kVp, where bony changes are distinguished more easily.

MILLIAMPERAGE The milliamperage setting controls the number of X-rays generated in a given exposure time. As noted earlier, the kilovoltage determines the quality (penetration) of the X-rays produced, but the milliamperage determines the quantity of X-rays produced.

It is more precise, however, to consider the concept of milliampere seconds (mAs) than milliamperage alone because the milliamperage setting and duration of exposure are interdependent values. To produce a diagnostic exposure, different types of film need different milliamperage-second settings, and this is determined by the sensitivity and the focal distance of the film. If the milliamperage setting is increased, then the exposure time can be reduced. For example, an exposure, at a given kilovolt-peak setting, of 1 s using 10 mA is 10 mAs. A 2 s exposure at the same kilovolt-peak setting using 5 mA would produce an identical film because the resulting exposure is again 10 mAs ($10 \times 1 = 10$ and $5 \times 2 = 10$). Both patients would receive the same amount of radiation. The only advantage of the higher milliamperage is the decrease in exposure time, which lessens the chance of patient movement. Common practice today is to use short exposure times at a magnitude of 6 impulses (1/10 s), so patient movement is less of a factor (see following discussion). This reduction in exposure time to 1/10 s alone, however, will not prevent patient movement or gagging; it just facilitates obtaining the radiograph before such movement occurs. Thus, it is apparent that it makes no diagnostic and little technical difference if we work at 5, 6, 7, 10, or 15 mA. It should be pointed out that conventional dental X-ray machines do not have milliamperage settings higher than 15 because of heat limitations within the tube.

Dental X-ray machines do not emit a continuous stream of radiation when an exposure is made; rather, they emit a series of radiation impulses. The number of impulses depends on the number of cycles per second in the electric current being used. With 60-cycle alternating current, which is standard, there are 60 X-ray pulses per second. Newer-generation X-ray machines have timer dials calibrated in impulses, not in seconds. On the timer dial, 15 would mean 15 impulses or 15/60 s exposure. These extremely short exposure times can only be controlled by an electric timer. The old mechanical timers are not this precise, and all X-ray machines should have electronic timers that are capable of delivering short, accurate exposure times.

It should also be noted that many of the newer dental x-ray units have preset mA and kVp settings. Therefore, the operator is only responsible for adjusting the time setting for each exposure rather than having to monitor the appropriate mA and kVp settings as well.

Film Type

Even with the introduction of digital radiographs, conventional film remains in use as an image receptor in dentistry. In periodontal diagnostic radiology, the most commonly used sizes are number 1 (narrow anterior), number 2 (adult size), and number 3 (long bitewing). Adult films (#2 size) with the appropriate film-holding devices are often utilized for bitewing exposures in lieu of the long bitewing (#3 size film).

The film sensitivity, or speed, determines how much radiation and exposure time (e.g., milliampere seconds) are necessary to produce an image on the film. The speed of the film is determined mainly by the size of the silver halide crystals and presence of radiosensitive dyes in the film emulsion.

Films are designated by American National Standards Institute (ANSI) categories, with category A film being the slowest and category F film being the fastest. Presently, category F speed film is being utilized in dentistry as it decreases radiation exposure to the patient when compared to E- and D-speed film. The early objections to F-speed film based on decreased definition and lack of contrast is not substantial enough to disregard the obvious reduction of radiation exposure to the patient.

Paralleling versus the Bisecting Technique

In periodontal radiographic diagnosis, use of the **paralleling technique** with a 16-inch film focal distance for periapical radiographs is the method of choice. In this technique, the teeth and the film are parallel to each other, and the central ray of the X-ray beam is directed perpendicular (right angle) to both. With proper use of this technique, there will be no dimensional distortion or false and misleading indications of bone levels. The 16-inch focal distance, the so-called long cone, is used to compensate for the image enlargement caused by the increase in tooth-to-film (object–film) distance necessary to achieve the parallelism between the teeth and the film.

In the bisecting technique, the film is placed as close to the tooth as possible, and the central ray of the X-ray beam is directed perpendicular to an imaginary line between the angle formed by the long axis of the tooth and the plane of the film. This technique is not recommended for periodontal diagnosis because it results in a distortion and exaggeration of the alveolar bone level. Excess vertical angulation (i.e., distortion of the length of the teeth, either foreshortening or elongation) may lead to a perception of early furcation involvement when there is actually no interradicular bone loss.

Conventional Radiographs Used in Periodontics

Table 17–1 ■ reviews the different types of intraoral and extraoral radiographs used in conjunction with clinical data to recognize and classify periodontal diseases (Hodges, 1997). Many radiographs are available, but

Table 17–1 Selection Criteria of Conventional Radiographs for Periodontics

Type of Film	Indications	Limitations
Periapical	Viewing the apex of the root for any pathology (i.e., periapical radiolucency) Determining morphology (shape) of roots and root length Recognizing horizontal and vertical patterns of bone loss Evaluating implants Viewing interproximal dental caries	Technique errors may reduce the ability to detect crestal bone loss. Detection of incipient interproximal dental caries. Detection of pathologic lesions in the mandible and maxilla. Evaluation of other structures such as sinuses and the mandibular canal.
Bitewing	Viewing the alveolar crest bone height (use vertical bitewings) Evaluation of defective restorations (i.e., overhang)	Cannot view the apical area of a tooth. Evaluation of the morphology and length of roots.
Panoramic	Viewing the area of the maxilla and mandibular arches (i.e., impacted teeth, sinuses, and pathologic lesions)	Not used for recognizing periodontal diseases or dental caries.

periapical, bitewing, and panoramic radiographs are used most commonly in periodontics to evaluate periodontal structures.

Conventional radiographs give a history of past periodontal disease destruction but do not provide information on current periodontal disease status. As mentioned earlier, radiographs represent a two-dimensional view of three-dimensional objects, so it is difficult to recognize the slight changes in alveolar bone that would indicate early or mild periodontal disease. Other limitations and benefits of radiographs are discussed in Box 17–1. As a result, radiographs are used primarily in periodontics to determine the severity and pattern of bone loss, the morphology (i.e., length and shape) of roots, root proximity, pathologic lesions such as a cyst or an abscess, and the effects of occlusion.

Just as a single periodontal probing recording only provides information on past disease activity, it is important to compare several sets of full-mouth radiographs over a period of time to evaluate for periodontal disease progression (Hollender, 1992; Jeffcoat & Reddy, 1991). In addition, radiographic findings always should be correlated with the corresponding probing depth measurements.

Periapical Radiographs

A periapical radiograph shows the entire area around a tooth, including the apex of the root. Periapical radiographs are part of the full-mouth survey and are taken of anterior and posterior teeth. The number of periapical films taken for a full-mouth survey varies generally from 14 to 20.

Film technique errors occur quite often with periapical radiographs as a result of improper alignment of the film with the tooth and the X-ray beam with the film.

Box 17–1: Benefits and Limitations of Conventional Radiographs

Radiographs do show

- Crestal alveolar bone levels
- Clinical crown-to-root ratio
- Calculus on proximal tooth surfaces
- Metallic restorations
- Morphology of roots (i.e., root length, root shape)

Radiographs do not show

- Periodontal pockets
- Buccal and lingual plates of bone
- Hard-to-soft-tissue relationship
- A successfully treated patient
- Bone loss until about 30% to 50% of loss of mineralization occurs

Rapid Dental Hint

It is best to take vertical bitewings on a patient with bone loss. The crest of bone may not be seen on horizontal bitewings.

Excessive vertical angulation causes foreshortening (roots appear shorter and the alveolar crest appears to be closer to the cementoenamel junction than it truly is) and occlusal surfaces to be cut off. This can result in inaccurate recording of the crestal alveolar bone level. Insufficient vertical angulation causes elongation and roots to be cut off from the radiograph. Overlapping of proximal tooth surfaces is caused by improper horizontal angulation of the radiographic beam.

Bitewing Radiographs

The bitewing radiograph is by far the best radiograph to interpret posterior alveolar bone levels and bone loss with the least amount of distortion or technique error. Bitewing radiographs show the crowns of the maxillary and mandibular teeth and the alveolar crest. Identification of carious lesions is best with bitewing radiographs. Posterior bitewing radiographs are part of the full-mouth survey and can include up to four views. Bitewing films can be placed either horizontally or vertically. Vertical bitewing radiographs are especially useful in periodontal patients with moderate to severe bone loss (this is determined by periodontal probing and previous radiographs, if available) to evaluate crestal bone. Horizontal bitewing radiographs do not show the entire bone height. Two posterior vertical bitewing radiographs may be sufficient, however, for visualization of both maxillary and mandibular teeth. The radiographs are taken perpendicular to the alveolar crest so that the crestal bone is depicted accurately. Anterior vertical bitewing radiographs can also be taken.

Panoramic Radiology

The image on a panoramic film shows the entire dentition and supporting bone structure from condyle to condyle on one film. The resulting image, however, does not have the same degree of definition seen on an intraoral periapical or bitewing radiograph. This shortcoming is inherent to the pantomographic process and is also caused by the use of intensifying screens.

Rapid Dental Hint

Remember, panoramic radiographs are not used to recognize periodontal disease.

Many diagnostic problems in dentistry require a high degree of radiographic definition. Early detection of such conditions as disruption of the periodontal ligament, loss of crestal alveolar bone, a thickened periodontal ligament, and ongoing caries requires the maximum amount of radiographic definition. Because of this, panoramic films have very limited value in the diagnosis of periodontal disease. If a panoramic film is used instead of a full-mouth survey, it must be augmented with both anterior and posterior bitewing radiographs and selected periapical films where indicated. Many technique errors can occur with panoramic radiographs, including improper patient positioning and operator errors.

Periodontal Structures

To recognize disease, the normal anatomy must be understood. Periodontal anatomy identified on radiographs includes the supporting structures such as the alveolar bone, periodontal ligament space, and cementum (Figure 17–1 ■). Because gingiva is a noncalcified soft tissue structure, the X-rays go completely through it and are not absorbed, thus the gingiva is not seen as a radiopaque structure.

Interdental Septum

The normal crest of interproximal bone runs parallel to a line drawn between the cementoenamel junctions on adjoining teeth at a level approximately 2.0 mm apical to the cementoenamel junction (Figure 17–2 ■). The shape of the alveolar crest is determined primarily by the contact area of adjacent teeth and the shape of the cementoenamel junction. The alveolar crest is flatter in posterior areas and more convex and pointed anteriorly. The width of the interdental septum can be determined by viewing a radiograph. The interdental septum can be narrow in cases of close root proximity. In some instances, the roots of adjacent teeth are so close that there may be little to no cancellous bone. Teeth that frequently show close root proximity include

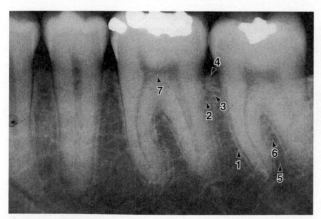

FIGURE 17–1 Radiograph of the periodontal structures (1 = lamina dura; 2 = periodontal ligament space; 3 = interproximal bone; 4 = alveolar bone crest; 5 = trabecular bone; 6 = interradicular bone; 7 = pulp).

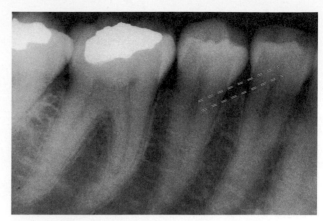

FIGURE 17–2 Radiograph showing the normal relationship of the crestal bone level being parallel with the cementoenamel junctions of adjacent teeth. No bone loss is depicted in this radiograph.

Did You Know?

Approximately 50% of bone must be demineralized before it is evident on an X-ray.

the distobuccal root of the maxillary first molar and the mesiobuccal root of the maxillary second molar and the mandibular anteriors.

Radiographically, a thin radiopaque line surrounds the entire root and is continuous with the alveolar crest (see Figure 17–1). This is referred to as the lamina dura. Clinically, it represents the alveolar bone that lines the tooth socket.

Periodontal Ligament Space

The periodontal ligament fibers (or principal fibers) transverse from the cementum to the alveolar bone. Because these fibers are soft tissue, they are not evident on radiographs. Instead, the space where the fibers are located appears as a radiolucent area surrounding the entire tooth (see Figure 17–1). On one side of the space is the cementum, and the other border is the lamina dura. Evaluating the width of the periodontal ligament (space) is important during the occlusal examination. If a tooth has excessive occlusal loads placed on it, the periodontal ligament compensates for the resulting tooth mobility by becoming thicker. This shows up on a radiograph as a widened periodontal ligament (Figure 17–3 ■).

Did You Know?

Fibroblasts from the periodontal ligament are responsible for regeneration of lost periodontal structures. This concept is called guided tissue regeneration.

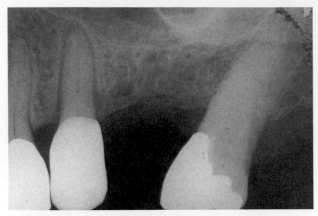

FIGURE 17–3 The maxillary second premolar shows a widened periodontal ligament space due to an excessive occlusal load placed on it.

Periodontal Interpretation

Using radiographs as an evaluation tool in the recognition of periodontitis has several limitations that are listed in Box 17–1. It is difficult to determine changes in bone simply by viewing radiographs. For this reason, clinical data must be incorporated with radiographic findings in an assessment of periodontal status. For example, a patient's radiographs may show moderate bone loss, but previously the patient may have had periodontal surgery for pocket reduction. Thus, the radiographs still show bone loss, but the periodontal charting shows probing depths from 1 to 3 mm without bleeding on probing. At this time the patient does not have periodontitis. The radiographs show past disease activity, not what is presently occurring.

Bone Loss

Conventional radiographs represent an insensitive technique in detecting early, small bony defects (bone loss). Before bone loss is identified on a radiograph, approximately 30% to 50% loss of mineralization must occur (Jeffcoat, 1992; Jeffcoat & Reddy, 1991). In addition, radiographically, the cortical bone plates may hide slight bone loss.

Radiographic evaluation of alveolar bone loss associated with periodontitis is based on the status of the interdental septum (Kasaj, Vasiliu, & Willershausen, 2008). Fuzziness or breaks in the continuity of the lamina dura have been described as the earliest radiographic signs of bone loss. However, the radiographic observation that the loss of crestal lamina dura is a sign of periodontitis is not totally accurate (Armitage, 2004). Clinical studies have shown that sites did not break down, even though there was a break in the lamina dura. Moreover, absence of crestal lamina dura is a common radiographic finding in normal, nondiseased interproximal sites (Rams, Listgarten, & Slots, 1994). Thus, it is more accurate to state that the presence of an intact crestal lamina dura represents a stable site than that the absence of a crestal lamina dura indicates a disease site (Armitage, 2004; Rams et al., 1994).

PATTERNS OF BONE LOSS The severity, distribution, and pattern of bone loss can be determined from radiographs. Clinically, as measured with a periodontal probe, two types of bony pockets exist: suprabony and infrabony. A gingival pocket or pseudopocket is not associated with bone loss. These bony pockets are associated with two patterns of bone loss: horizontal and vertical. In horizontal bone loss, interdental bone is destroyed equally along the surfaces of adjacent teeth (Figure 17–4a ■). Suprabony pockets,

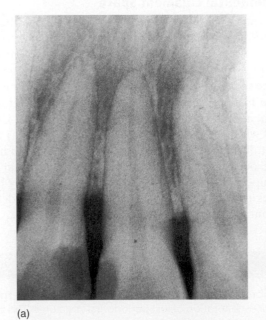

(a)

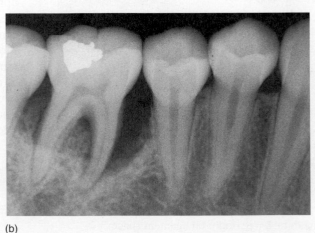

(b)

FIGURE 17–4 (a) A periapical radiograph showing a horizontal pattern of bone loss. (b) Vertical or angular bone loss on the mesial surface of the first molar with furcation involvement.

where the base of the pocket is coronal to the alveolar bone crest, are characterized by horizontal bone loss. In vertical (angular) bone loss, the resorption on one tooth sharing the septum is greater than on the other tooth (Figure 17–4b). Infrabony pockets, where the base of the pocket is apical to the alveolar crest, are associated with vertical bone loss.

SEVERITY OF BONE LOSS The severity, or amount, of bone loss is classified as mild, moderate, or severe. One way to determine the amount of bone loss is to determine the percentage of bone loss. This is done by measuring the length from the cementoenamel junction to the tip of the root and the distance from the cementoenamel junction to the alveolar crest. The percentage of bone loss is calculated by dividing this number by the root length and multiplying by 100 (Hodges, 1997). Bone loss of less than 20% is usually classified as mild; bone loss between 20% and 50% is moderate; and bone loss of more than 50% is severe. It also should be remembered that 30% to 50% bone loss must be present before it is evident radiographically.

DETERMINATION OF BONE LOSS The first step in determining if there is radiographic bone loss is to draw an imaginary line connecting the cementoenamel junction of adjacent teeth and then a line on the alveolar crest. If the alveolar crest is more than approximately 2 mm apical to the cementoenamel junction, there is bone loss. The next step is to determine if the pattern of bone loss is horizontal or vertical. In vertical bone loss, the bone level is not parallel to the cementoenamel junctions of adjacent teeth. In horizontal bone loss, the bone level is parallel to the cementoenamel junctions of adjacent teeth. If a tooth is not in the normal occlusal plane (e.g., extruded, intruded, or tipped), the bone level will not be in a straight line, but neither will the cementoenamel junctions, so the lines will still be parallel to each other (Figure 17–5 ■).

> **Did You Know?**
>
> Teeth with furcation involvement can be seen on a radiograph, but clinical assessment is also necessary.

Despite these limitations, **conventional radiographs** are still mandatory in the recognition and treatment of periodontal diseases. They provide an excellent measurement of the history of periodontal disease in a patient and provide important information about the interproximal bone changes that occur over time (Academy of Periodontology, 2011). The detection of predisposing factors is one of the most important roles of radiography in periodontal diseases, and the detection and elimination of local irritants are essential steps in prevention or actual periodontal therapy.

Calculus

Early deposits, small and not fully calcified, are not seen radiographically. Even calcified supragingival calculus, which is seen most often on the lingual surfaces of lower anterior teeth and the buccal surfaces of upper molars, is not seen clearly in its early stage because of superimposition of tooth structure (e.g., roots) and cortical plates. Subgingival calculus on the proximal surfaces is more easily detected in the early calcified stages. Calculus appears as an irregularly pointed radiographic projection from the proximal root surface (Figure 17–6 ■).

Anatomic Configurations

Only through radiographic examination can information about the size, shape, and positions of the roots of periodontally involved teeth be obtained. It is important to document the lengths of the root trunks of multirooted teeth to ensure tooth survival. A tooth with a short root trunk has "higher" furcation entrances and longer roots. A tooth with a long root trunk has shorter roots, but the

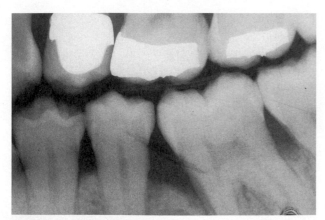

FIGURE 17–5 The area between the premolar and molar shows uneven crestal alveolar bone that parallels the uneven cementoenamel junctions. There is horizontal bone loss but not angular bone loss.

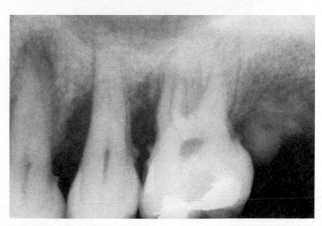

FIGURE 17–6 Calculus spurs evident on all tooth surfaces.

furcation entrance is more apical. Therefore, more bone has to be destroyed in the development of a furcation involvement.

Another important factor in the overall periodontal prognosis is the shape of the roots. The space between the roots is also important. Roots of multirooted teeth can be diverging, converging, or conical. Diverging roots have a larger surface area for periodontal attachment including bone. Teeth with thicker, diverging, longer roots have a better prognosis than conical or converging roots. Roots also can be long and tapered or short, bulbous, and conical. These factors are important in evaluating the present condition and planning periodontal and restorative therapy.

In restorative case planning, the crown-to-root ratio is an important factor. This ratio is the relationship of the length of the root embedded in bone compared with the length of the rest of the tooth. The greater the length of the tooth embedded in bone, the better is the prognosis for support of a fixed or removable prosthesis. A 2:1 crown-to-root ratio is desirable. Teeth with bulbous roots have more area for attachment than those with fine tapered roots.

Radiographically Detectable Periodontal Changes

Gingivitis

Because gingivitis is a soft-tissue change, there are no radiographic findings other than the presence of predisposing or contributing factors (e.g., condition of restorations).

Slight (Mild) Periodontitis

This stage of periodontal disease is characterized radiographically by changes in the crest of the interproximal bone septum and triangulation of the periodontal ligament space (Figure 17–7 ■). Triangulation is widening of the periodontal ligament space at the crest of the interproximal septum that gives the appearance of a radiolucent triangle to what is normally a radiolucent band. Fading of the density of the crest with cup-shaped defects appears in the early stages of periodontitis.

Moderate Periodontitis

In this stage, bone loss may be apparent in both horizontal and vertical planes. Radiolucencies appear in the furcations of multirooted teeth, indicating interradicular bone loss. This is a furcation involvement and is confirmed clinically using a probe designed for the purpose of measuring this specific area of bone loss. In this stage, horizontal bone loss on the buccal or lingual surface may go undetected because of superimposition. Careful examination of the radiograph in most cases reveals a difference in density indicating different levels of bone on the buccal and lingual surfaces (Figure 17–8 ■).

Severe Periodontitis

This stage of periodontal disease is easily identified radiographically by the advanced vertical and horizontal patterns of bone loss, furcation involvement, thickened periodontal ligament, and indications of changes in tooth position (Figure 17–9 ■).

Periodontal Abscess

The radiographic signs of a periodontal abscess may vary greatly. Such a diagnosis is dictated by an acute clinical manifestation. Clinically, a deep periodontal pocket is usually found. The periodontal abscess is caused by the occlusion of an existing pocket; therefore, the radiograph of the acute episode may not vary greatly from previous radiographs of the existing condition that produced the pocket. In other instances, there may be signs of rapid and extensive bone destruction.

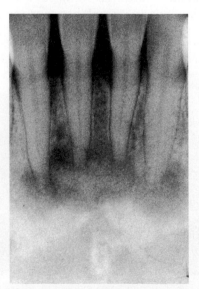

FIGURE 17–7 Slight (mild) chronic periodontitis. Generalized slight horizontal bone loss of less than 20%.

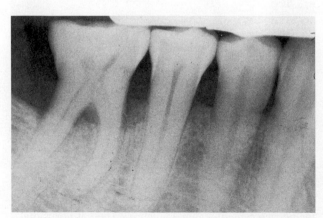

FIGURE 17–8 Moderate chronic periodontitis. Localized furcation involvement on the mandibular molar.

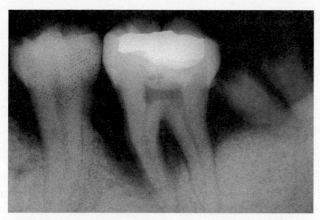

FIGURE 17–9 Severe chronic periodontitis. Generalized extensive horizontal and vertical bone loss of more than 50% and furcation involvement.

Frequency of Radiographs (Selection Criteria)

Among the many methods of reducing a patient's radiation exposure (e.g., rectangular collimation, filtration, fast film, and digital sensors), selection criteria also are very important and are the responsibility of the dentist. Selection criteria are descriptions of clinical conditions and historical data that identify patients who are most likely to benefit from a particular radiographic examination. These guidelines help the practitioner select which patient needs radiographs and determine which radiographs are needed. The final decision rests with the individual dentist and is determined by professional judgment.

The practice of taking radiographs based on a time interval rather than patient needs, as determined by clinical examination and dental history, is not considered the appropriate way to practice dental radiology. In relation to periodontal care, there should never be a policy, for example, that mandates a new full-mouth survey every 2 years or bitewing radiographs every 6 months. The radiographic needs of each patient are different and should not be based on the calendar but rather on a complete clinical examination, the patient's radiation history and the history of previous periodontal therapy or signs and symptoms of the disease (i.e., the patient's risk factors for dental disease).

An expert panel of dentists under the auspices of the Public Health Service (U.S. Department of Health and Human Services, 2004) has developed guidelines for the prescription of dental radiographs. One of the patient categories is "Periodontal disease or a history of periodontal treatment." The recommendations call for a full-mouth survey for every new patient, comprised of periapical and bitewing films. For the recall examination, radiographs should be taken for evaluation of previous periodontal therapy (e.g., surgery, bone grafting, implants, or when there is a dramatic change in the probing depth measurement). In any patient, radiographs should never be taken before there is a complete clinical examination. Based on this examination, a radiographic prescription is formulated, the films are taken, and a final classification and treatment plan are determined.

Digital Imaging

Radiographic improvements are designed to reduce patient radiation exposure and to simplify identification and measurement of changes in alveolar bone height. The most recent addition to dental radiology is **direct digital radiography**. Presently, there are various digital systems available on the market, each with its own variations. Many clinicians are converting from film to digital imaging. With digital imaging, there is up to a 90% reduction in radiation exposure when compared with D-speed conventional radiographic film (Jeffcoat, 1998). Direct digital radiography replaces the film used in a conventional intraoral radiograph with an electronic sensor. This sensor, the approximate size of intraoral film, is placed in the patient's mouth in the same manner as one would place film. The exposure is made, and the sensor sends impulses based on the penetration of the object by the X-ray photons to a computer. These impulses are then digitized and formed into an image by the computer. The image can be stored, printed in hard copy, darkened or lightened, reversed, colorized, magnified, measured, or transmitted to a remote site.

A computer monitor creates an image using pixels or tiny dots that become a recognizable form when projected on the screen. Viewing the digital radiograph allows the clinician to determine bone loss through the percentage of lightness and darkness of pixels. White, the lightest shade, indicates the maximum amount of bone mineral, whereas black, the darkest shade, indicates absence of bone mineral.

From a periodontal standpoint, all the diagnostic criteria mentioned previously in terms of conventional radiographs stay the same. The instant imaging is a time advantage and the substantial reduction in patient exposure is desirable, and the periodontal diagnostic capabilities, when compared with film, are about equal. There may be some advantage in determining bone levels by image reversal or colorization, but this varies among practitioners. These systems are available for commercial in-office use.

Digital Subtraction Radiology

Digital subtraction radiology (DSR) magnifies images, allowing detection of osseous changes (bone loss) that are too small to be seen in a visual examination of conventional film. As mentioned earlier, comparing radiographs from different time periods is important in detecting progressive bone loss. Because of the superimposition of cortical plates and roots of teeth, it is almost impossible to detect changes in the bone level unless there was a dramatic loss of bone (Jeffcoat, 1998). In digital subtraction radiology, two images taken at two different visits are compared, and all structures that do not change, such as cortical plates and roots of teeth, are not shown on (subtracted from) the image. Any changes in bone level are indicated by a color-shaded area; red is for bone loss, and green is for bone gain. DSR has not been used much in clinical practice because it is a difficult technique to master, but it is used frequently in clinical research.

Radiographs in Implantology

At the present time, the basic diagnostic radiographs used in screening implant patients are conventional radiographs such as periapical, occlusal, and panoramic films. In addition, **computed tomographic (CT) scans** are used for a three-dimensional view of the bone. It is most important to realize that to diagnose and plan for implant placement, one must be able to view the implant site in three dimensions or planes. As dental professionals, we are used to seeing objects in two planes, mesiodistal and incisoapically. We do not see objects in a three-dimensional view except with occlusal films in the buccolingual plane, and this information is critical in implant planning. Of the techniques used, only CT images can supply this information.

Periapical/Occlusal Films

If the film can be placed parallel to the ridge and the field size allows for visualization of the entire proposed alveolar area, then periapical films can be used. Unfortunately, there are very few patients who fit this criterion, and thus periapical views are of limited value. Occlusal films, if they can be positioned, can augment the periapical film to view the third dimension.

Pantomograms (Panoramic Films)

The panoramic film is currently the most commonly used radiograph in treatment planning for an implant patient. Pantomograms are ideal for showing the structures of the mandible and maxilla, including the locations of nerves. Although the field size is large enough in panoramic films, there is still no cross-sectional visualization. There is also an uneven amount of magnification (27%) in different areas of the mouth, and this can be very misleading in interpreting the radiograph. The exact location of the mandibular canal is difficult to determine on a pantomogram. Thus, pantomograms should not be used as the only method for evaluating osseous structures.

Conventional Tomograms

Cross-sectional tomograms are an excellent way to obtain the necessary field visualization. Tomograms are cross-sectional images perpendicular to the edentulous ridge. Images are often blurry or indistinct, and this procedure is time consuming. Because very few offices have tomographic units, referral to medical radiologists or hospitals is necessary. If a dental professional is to refer a patient to this type of facility, it is probably better to refer for CT imaging.

Computed Tomography (CT Scanning)

TRADITIONAL CT Three-dimensional computed tomography (CT) imaging is essentially digitized tomography that results in an enhanced image in all three dimensions or planes that is much easier to read than a conventional tomogram. The CT scanner makes a 1.0 to 1.5 mm thick slice or cut of the edentulous area (Figures 17–10 ■, 17–11 ■). The tomogram measures the amount of energy transmitted through the object. The information is transmitted to a computer, which displays the image on a monitor.

CT scans are ideal for locating the amount and quality of bone available for implant placement above the mandibular canal (this is where the mandibular nerve is located) in the posterior area of the mandible. When maxillary areas are being used as implant sites, CT scans should be used to locate the sinuses and determine the amount and quality of available bone.

CONE BEAM CT Limitations of CT include radiation, machine size, and cost. However, in dental imaging cone beam computed tomography (CBCT) has now been

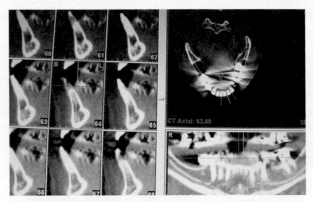

FIGURE 17–10 CT scan showing cross sections or "slices" of the mandible.

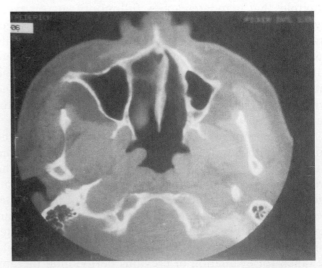

FIGURE 17–11 Axial CT at the level of the maxillary sinus.

introduced (Misch, Yi, & Sarment, 2006). It uses smaller, cheaper machines with high-quality results. Cone beam CT imaging system also allows pinpointing the exact location and dimensions of an area of interest in the jaw. CBCT can take images of both the maxilla and mandible at the same time and emits less radiation than a panoramic radiograph. Typical CT scans require separate scans for the maxilla and mandible. There is much less radiation with cone beam CT; each typical CT scan subjects the patient to 200 to 300 times the radiation required for a panoramic radiography. When both jaws need to be scanned, the patient is collectively receiving 400 to 600 times the radiation dose for a panoramic radiograph. These machines not only are used for implant placement but can also measure periodontal defects and image the temporomandibular joint. CBCT scanners utilize a narrow, columninated cone beam of radiation that requires only two to eight times the amount of radiation used in a panoramic radiograph. In addition, CBCT is accurate to one-tenth of a millimeter (0.1 mm), whereas traditional CT scanners are off by 0.5 mm or more.

Postoperative Implant Evaluation

Baseline radiographs are taken to verify the fit of the abutment to the fixture head and document bone levels around an implant. After placement of implants, clinical and radiographic evaluations are necessary at continuing care or supportive periodontal therapy visits (Degidi, Nardi, & Piatelli, 2008; Joly, Martorelli de Lima, Carvalho da Silva, 2003; Pontes et al., 2008). Periapical and panoramic films are used for posttreatment evaluation. The primary reason for taking radiographs postoperatively is to help monitor the bone level around the implant. Periapical films are best for this purpose. For the edentulous patient, follow-up radiographs should be taken annually for 3 years and then once every other year. Pantomograms are also used to determine bone changes and the status of the abutment and fixture. Alveolar bone loss of less than 0.2 mm per year after the first year of placement is considered acceptable for a successful implant (Rosenlicht & Ansari, 2010). CT scans cannot be used because the metallic implants produce image "noise" that interferes with proper interpretation.

Dental Hygiene Application

Adequate radiographs and imaging systems are necessary for a complete periodontal and implant examination. Many techniques and systems are available. Conventional radiographs are adequate for visualizing the tooth and surrounding tissues. Conventional radiographs are also used to determine the amount and quality of bone available for implant placement in the anterior sextant of the mandible and maxilla. However, CT scans are necessary to evaluate the implant site in the maxilla and posterior areas of the mandible for its osseous status and proximity to vital structures (e.g., sinuses and mandibular canal).

Key Points

- Radiographic interpretation is used to supplement clinical findings from the periodontal assessment (e.g., probing depths, clinical attachment levels).
- Posterior vertical bitewing radiographs are ideal for visualizing the level of the alveolar bone crest.

- Radiographs do not show gingival and periodontal pockets or mobile teeth.
- The CT and cone beam CT scan is the most commonly used imaging system for visualizing implant sites in the maxilla and posterior areas of the mandible.

Self-Quiz

1. The radiographic evaluation of alveolar bone loss associated with periodontitis is based on the status of which one of the following structures?
   a. Interdental septum
   b. Cementoenamel junction
   c. Periapical bone
   d. Periodontal ligament fibers

2. Which one of the following radiographic structures is described as a thin radiopaque line surrounding the entire root and is continuous with the alveolar crest?
   a. Dentin
   b. Cementum
   c. Lamina dura
   d. Periodontal ligament fibers
   e. Gingival fibers

3. Which one of the following types of imaging systems is recommended for use before implant placement and can be used to measure periodontal defects as well?
   a. Panoramic
   b. Periapical
   c. Cone beam CT
   d. Vertical bitewing

4. Which one of the following types of radiographs is best used to evaluate the alveolar bone crest for moderate to severe bone loss?
   a. Periapical
   b. Horizontal bitewing
   c. Vertical bitewing
   d. Panoramic
   e. Computed tomography

5. Which one of the following periodontal changes can be seen on radiographs?
   a. Gingival recession
   b. Periodontal pockets
   c. Furcation involvement
   d. Tooth mobility

6. All the following types of radiographs are currently used in the treatment planning of implants except one. Which one is the exception?
   a. Periapicals
   b. Bitewings
   c. Panoramic
   d. CT scan

7. Which one of the following features does the computed tomographic (CT) process provide?
   a. A three-dimensional view of the area of interest
   b. A two-dimensional view of the area of interest
   c. A global view of all oral structures
   d. A close-up view of the periapical structures

8. All the following are reasons for using radiographs in periodontics except one. Which one is the exception?
   a. Identify predisposing factors.
   b. Detect early to moderate bone changes.
   c. Determine the shape and depth of periodontal pockets.
   d. Serve as baseline data and as a means of evaluating posttreatment results.

9. The normal crest of interproximal bone is located at a level
   a. 2.0 mm apical to the cementoenamel junction.
   b. 3.0 mm coronal to the cementoenamel junction.
   c. 2.0 to 3.0 mm coronal to the cusp tip of the crown.
   d. 3.5 mm apical to the cusp tip of the crown.

10. Which one of the following types of radiographs is used primarily in clinical research rather than clinical practice?
    a. Panoramic films
    b. Direct digital radiography
    c. Digital subtraction radiography
    d. Computed tomography

Case Study

A 60-year-old male returns for his periodontal maintenance visit. The dental hygienist reviews the radiographs available from previous visits to determine the current state of his periodontal condition. From the most recent radiographs the dental hygienist notes that the crestal bone level is 3 mm below the CEJ on teeth 29, 30, 31. Tooth #32 was extracted.

1. If the bone loss in the mandibular molar region is not parallel to the CEJ the bone loss is defined as
   a. Radicular
   b. Horizontal
   c. Vertical
   d. Furcation

Answer: C. Vertical bone loss is not parallel while horizontal bone loss is parallel to the CEJ. There was no indication given about other types of bone loss.

2. What is the current periodontal disease activity?
   a. Gingivitis
   b. Moderate active periodontitis
   c. Chronic periodontitis
   d. Cannot be determine without other clinical data

Answer: D. The patient may have been treated for periodontal disease yet might not be currently active in the disease. Probing depths and bleeding points as well as the clinical attachment level are needed for a full assessment.

3. What type of radiograph would give the shape and length of the roots as well as the horizontal bone loss?
   a. bitewing
   b. periapical
   c. panoramic
   d. occlusal

Answer: B. Periapical radiographs show both the root apex and the patterns of bone loss. Bitewings do not show the apex of the root. Panoramic films are not utilized for periodontal disease recognition. Occlusal films can augment a periapical but not replace it in use.

References

Academy of Periodontology. 2011. Comprehensive periodontal therapy: A Statement by the Academy of Periodontology. *J. Periodontol.* 82(7):943–949.

Armitage, G. C. 2004. Periodontal diagnoses and classification of periodontal diseases *Periodontoogy 2000* 34: 9–21.

Degidi, M., D. Nardi, and A. Piattelli. 2008. Peri-implant tissue and radiographic bone levels in the immediately restored single-tooth implant: A retrospective analysis. *J. Periodontol.* 79(2): 252–259.

Hodges, K. O. 1997. Recommendations for radiographs. In ed. K. O. Hodges, *Concepts in nonsurgical periodontal therapy*, 118–149. Albany, NY: Delmar.

Hollender, L. 1992. Decision making in radiographic imaging. *J. Dent. Educ.* 56:834–843.

Jeffcoat, M. K. 1992. Imaging techniques for the periodontium. In eds. T. J. Wilson, K. S. Kornnan, and M. G. Newman, *Advances in periodontics*, 47–57. Chicago: Quintessence.

Jeffcoat, M. K. 1998. Periodontal diseases: Epidemiology and diagnosis. Consensus reports from the 1996 World Workshop in Periodontics. *J. Am. Dent. Assoc.* 129:9S–14S.

Jeffcoat, M., and M. S. Reddy. 1991. A comparison of probing and radiographic methods for detection of periodontal disease progression. *Curr. Opin. Dentistry* 1:45–51.

Joly, J. C., A. F. Martorelli de Lima, and R. Carvalho da Silva. 2003. Clinical and radiographic evaluation of soft and hard tissue changes around implants: A pilot study. *J. Periodontol.* 74(8):1097–1103.

Kasaj, A., C. H. Vasiliu, and B. Willershausen. 2008. Assessment of alveolar bone loss and angular bony defects on panoramic radiographs. *Eur. J. Med. Res.* (January 23) 13(1):26–30.

Misch, K. A., E. S. Yi, and D. P. Sarment. 2006. Accuracy of cone beam computed tomography for periodontal defect measurements. *J. Periodontol.* 77(7):1261–1266.

Pontes, A. E. F., F. S. Ribeiro, V. C. da Silva, R. Margonar, et al. 2008. Clinical and radiographic changes around dental implants inserted in different levels in relation to the crestal bone, under different restoration protocols, in the dog model. *J. Periodontol.* 79(3):486–494.

Rams, T. E., M. A. Listgarten, and J. Slots. 1994. Utility of radiographic crestal lamina dura for predicting periodontitis disease activity. *J. Clin. Periodontol.* 21:571–576.

Rosenlicht, J. L., and R. Ansari. 2010. Contemporary radiographic evaluation of the implant candidate. In eds. C. A. Babbush, J. A. Hahn, J. T. Krauser, and J. L. Rosenlicht, *Dental implants: The art and science*, 2nd ed., 110–123. St. Louis, MO: Elsevier.

U.S. Department of Health and Human Services. 2004. *The selection of patients for x-ray examinations*. Washington, DC: U.S. Government Printing Office.

Visit www.pearsonhighered.com/healthprofessionsresources to access the student resources that accompany this book. Simply select Dental Hygiene from the choice of disciplines. Find this book and you will find the complimentary study tools created for this specific title.

Advances in Detecting and Monitoring Periodontal Diseases

Denise Estafan

OUTLINE

EDUCATIONAL OBJECTIVES

Upon completion of this chapter, the reader should be able to:

- Evaluate the role of using adjunctive diagnostic aids as a predictor for periodontal breakdown.
- Explain the advantages and disadvantages of the various adjunctive diagnostic methods for detecting periodontal disease activity.
- Distinguish the type of patient who may benefit from adjunctive diagnostic testing.

GOAL: To introduce diagnostic methods that can be used as a supplement to conventional periodontal assessments for recognizing and monitoring periodontal diseases.

KEY WORDS

Introduction

Currently, identifying inflammatory periodontal diseases involves recognizing disease severity. Such traditional tests as visual inspection, probing depths, clinical attachment levels, and radiographs have not changed in the last 40 years and are considered the foundation for a periodontal examination. However, newer examination techniques may provide additional information beyond what can be obtained from a clinical examination. Such information may offer predictions about the future of periodontal disease progression and patient evaluation. Approximately 30% of periodontal diseases are recurrent, so it is necessary to monitor the patient to identify problem sites before further tissue damage occurs. Research is ongoing to determine the overall plausibility and effectiveness of these tests. Ultimately, the screening of at-risk patients may allow for improved treatment and prevention of periodontal diseases.

The past decade has seen the evolution of several diagnostic methods designed to be used as an adjunct or in combination with the clinical examination (Estafan, Weinberg, & Estafan, 1999). These methods help in identifying **periodontal disease activity** or patients at risk for an episode of active disease and are designed to help determine the most appropriate mode of treatment. The present standard for periodontal disease activity is a change in clinical attachment level of 2 to 3 mm. Various methods are used to analyze the products of the host response to dental biofilm and to identify specific microbial (bacterial) species. The greatest value of diagnostic testing may lie in the ability to identify the cause of the disease or tissue destruction (e.g., bacterial infection or host response—over- or under-responsive). Hopefully, appropriate testing will allow the practitioner to make therapeutic decisions before the onset of disease activity or at an early stage in its development. The initial determination of the need for active periodontal therapy still depends on use of a periodontal probe, gingival inspection, and radiographs (Bader, 1995). Therefore, these new assessment methods shift the focus from determining disease severity to evaluating disease progression or the risk of future periodontal breakdown—in essence, quantifying ongoing disease activity.

Adjunctive tests for the evaluation of periodontal diseases are divided into three main groups: gingival crevicular fluid assays, microbial tests, and genetic assays (Estafan et al., 1999; Box 18–1). Only a few of the tests are available in the United States for in-office use. Table 18–1 ■ reviews the advantages and disadvantages of various tests.

Gingival Crevicular Fluid Assays

Of the three most common fluids found within the oral cavity (**gingival crevicular fluid** [GCF], serum, and saliva), GCF has been the focus of most research in recent years. GCF is a fluid that originates from the gingival connective tissue (lamina propria) and flows into the gingival crevice. As a result of inflammation, GCF is formed when fluids leak from dilated blood vessels within the lamina propria.

Box 18–1: Supplemental Diagnostic Tests in Periodontics

Methods of detecting bacteria:

- Culture and sensitivity techniques
- DNA probe (Micro-IDent® and Micro-IDent® Plus; Hain Diagnostics, Arizona)
- Dark-field or phase-contrast microscopy (available commercially)
- Immunologic assays (not available commercially)
- Enzyme-based assays (not available commercially)

Methods of detecting sites actively breaking down or at risk for future destruction:

- Gingival crevicular fluid assays (not commercially available)
- Collagenase
- Aspartate aminotransferase

Genetic susceptibility test:

- Interleukin-1 genotype (PST™ Genetic Test; Advanced Dental Diagnostics, Franklin TN)

As this fluid flows through the inflamed connective tissue, it picks up tissue breakdown products, enzymes, and other substances involved in the immune response. In this regard, it is an "inflammatory soup" containing subgingival bacteria, inflammatory cells, and a vast array of other substances (mediators) produced by bacteria and host cells. GCF is relatively easy to collect by placing paper strips into selected pockets. It is these features that make GCF a good source of potential markers of periodontal destruction (Sorsa et al., 2010; Pradeep, Manjunath, Swati, Shikha, & Sujatha, 2007).

In areas affected by periodontal disease, GCF is an abundant source of substances (e.g., inflammatory mediators) that appear to play a central role in the tissue breakdown processes associated with periodontitis. This idea has led to the investigation of certain inflammatory mediators and their possible role as markers for active periodontitis (Armitage, 1992). Although these investigations have, over the past 20 years, resulted in the evolution of many techniques for assessing various aspects of disease, currently none are commercially available. Among the mediators that have been looked at most closely are host-derived enzymes (enzymes produced by host cells), inflammatory mediators, and tissue breakdown products.

Host-Derived Enzymes

During the disease process, certain host cells found in the body, such as polymorphonuclear leukocytes (neutrophils), release certain enzymes, including β-glucuronidase and elastase. These **host-derived enzymes** are components of GCF and have been reported to be associated with an increased

Table 18–1 Advantages and Limitations of Selective Adjunctive Tests

Test	Advantages	Limitations
Culture	• Identifies specific microorganisms • Determines antibiotic sensitivity	• Expensive and time-consuming; takes a long time to get results back from lab • Technique sensitive; diverse data from different labs (use of different media, sampling, transport) • Cell vitality must be preserved during transportation to lab • Some organisms may be lost through sampling
DNA probe assays	• Highly sensitive and specific for targeted periodontal pathogens • Viable organisms not needed • Samples sent by mail after collection chair-side • Rapid identification (18 hours)	• Need special disposal procedures for radioactive waste • Certain bacterial species may not be detected due to highly sensitive nature of the test • Performed in a lab
Microscopic test (phase-contrast microscopy)	• Good for chair-side patient awareness of the importance of bacteria in periodontal disease • Not suitable to monitor disease activity • Motivational tool for patient's biofilm-control habits	• Does not specifically identify bacterial species (e.g., spirochetes), only shape, size, and mobility
GCF enzyme assays	• Rapid and inexpensive • Technique insensitive, so easy to perform chair-side • Good for screening purposes • In-office use	• Cannot identify specific bacteria, but allows for rapid assessment of bacterial enzymatic activity • Need sufficient amount of enzymes

risk of clinical attachment loss and bone loss (Lamster, Holmes, et al., 1995; Lamster, Oshrain, et al., 1988). Elevated levels of these enzymes in the GCF, which can be used as markers for periodontitis, are most evident 6 months before the occurrence of disease (Palcanis et al., 1992).

Aspartate aminotransferase (AST) is an intracellular enzyme (e.g., it stays inside the cell) that indicates cell death when it is present extracellularly (e.g., outside the cell). Cell death leads to the release of the contents of the cell into the extracellular fluid. When AST is present at elevated levels in GCF, it has been shown to predict clinical attachment loss (Persson, DeRouen, & Page 1990), but over a shorter period than β-glucuronidase and elastase. Evidence from studies on AST in the GCF of patients at risk for periodontal disease indicates that elevated levels of the enzyme can predict clinical attachment loss an average of 3 months in advance of detection by more traditional means (Chambers et al., 1991). Currently, however, no test is available commercially.

Collagenase is an enzyme that breaks down collagen and is responsible for normal collagen remodeling. Collagenase-2 (MMP-8) is a biomarker in periodontitis and cardiovascular diseases (Sorsa et al., 2011). In the presence of inflammation, however, excessive amounts of collagenase are produced that cause periodontal tissue destruction during periodontal inflammation. Collagenase is produced by and released from host cells such as neutrophils (Overall, Sodek, McCulloch, & Birek, 1991). Fibroblasts also produce and release collagen and collagenase, but this occurs during normal tissue remodeling. Currently, however, no test is available commercially to detect "high" collagenase levels in the GCF.

Prostaglandin E$_2$

Prostaglandin E$_2$ (PGE$_2$) is a metabolite of arachidonic acid that is associated with many inflammatory effects, including bone loss. PGE$_2$ concentrations in the GCF of patients with clinical attachment loss of 3 mm or more have been shown to be significantly higher than in patients without this level of attachment loss (Offenbacher, Odler, & van Dyke, 1986). Identification of high levels of PGE$_2$ in GCF can indicate an increased risk of periodontal disease up to 6 months prior to its appearance clinically. Currently, however, no test is available commercially in the United States.

Microbial Tests

Bacterial biofilm is the primary cause of the initiation and progression of inflammatory periodontal diseases. Suggested **periodontal pathogens** include *Aggregatibacter actinomycetemcomitans, Porphyromonas gingivalis, Tannerella* *forsythensis, Prevotella intermedia, Campylobacter rectus, Eikinella corrodens, Fusobacterium nucleatum, Capnocytophaga sputigena, Peptostreptococcus mitis, Selenomonas* spp., *Eubacterium* spp., and *Haemophilus* spp. (Loomer, 2004; Socransky & Haffajee, 1991; Tanner, 1992).

Over the past few decades, the understanding of periodontal diseases has changed dramatically. Because specific bacterial types have been well documented to cause periodontal diseases, including localized and generalized aggressive periodontitis, and refractory cases, treatment of periodontal diseases is best aimed at identification of the periodontal pathogens responsible. Although no single one of these pathogens has been indicated as the organism responsible for disease progression, all the preceding bacteria are considered potential periodontal pathogens when identified in subgingival biofilm samples. Identification of these pathogens allows for faster and better treatment aimed at eliminating or reducing bacterial levels.

Because gingivitis and chronic periodontitis are not commonly associated with specific bacteria, identification of these diseases probably would not benefit from the use of microbial testing.

Many methods for bacterial testing are available for research and clinical use. These include culturing, microscopic DNA and probe, and immunologic techniques.

Culture Techniques

Culturing allows for the growth of certain microorganisms found in periodontal pockets. Specific in-office procedures must be followed. After removal of supragingival biofilm, samples of subgingival bacteria are taken from the biofilm with a curet, placed in a transport fluid, and sent to a licensed clinical laboratory within a day or two to maintain bacterial viability (bacteria must be alive on reaching the laboratory). The laboratory then disperses the sample, dilutes it, and plates it on selective and nonselective media. The most common pathogens are identified, and antibiotic susceptibility is determined. A detailed report of the findings is then sent back to the dental office, including the systemic antibiotics to which the cultured bacteria are sensitive. Knowing the susceptibility or resistance of specific microorganisms to these antibiotics provides important guidelines for antibiotic use in conjunction with periodontal therapy.

Cost and time constraints limit the use of such a process, so it is not appropriate for all patients. However, culture analysis may be useful for patients who do not respond to conventional therapy, especially if they have taken antibiotics previously (Armitage, 1993). In addition, culturing is limited in that it can only detect living bacteria; some bacteria may not survive transportation to the laboratory.

Microscopic Techniques

Identification of subgingival biota also may be accomplished through various microscopic techniques such as phase-contrast and dark-field microscopy. Rather than identifying specific bacteria, phase-contrast microscopy categorizes bacteria by motility (e.g., spirochetes), and dark-field microscopy identifies the morphology or shape

(e.g., cocci, rods; Sixou, 2003). Bacterial shifts from nonmotile to motile species often indicate a change from health to disease (Listgarten & Levin, 1981). Genus and species determination, as well as antibiotic susceptibility, is not possible using these techniques. Many dental offices use microscopic techniques solely for patient education. Clinically, a digital camera and monitor are attached to the microscope.

Nucleic Acid (DNA) Probe Analysis

All living organisms contain DNA (deoxyribonucleic acid), which carries all genetic information needed for the coding for proteins, the basic building blocks of life (Papapanou, Engelbretson, & Lamster, 1999). The DNA of each species consists of a specific sequence that is unique to that organism. Nucleic acid probe analysis identifies DNA sequences specific for certain subgingival periodontal pathogens. In the dental office, biofilm samples are collected by inserting a special sterile paper point into the base of a pocket. This paper point is then placed in an air-filled vial and mailed to a testing service. Bacterial DNA is so stable that no special transport fluid is required before mailing the sample, and the bacteria do not have to be living. This is a key advantage to using DNA as a biochemical marker in the identification of periodontal pathogens. The microorganism's DNA is cut into single-strand fragments. The DNA probe is made in the laboratory and labeled with either a radioactive or enzyme marker. If binding of the labeled DNA probe strands occurs, the test organism is thus identified. DNA probe reports are rapid, are relatively inexpensive, and can detect nonviable species (Loesche, 1992; Sonnier, 1996). This test (Micro-IDent® and Micro-IDent® Plus; Hain Diagnostics, Arizona) identifies eleven pathogens, including *Aggregatibacter actinomycetemcomitans* (Aa), *Prevotella intermedia* (Pi), *Porphyromonas gingivalis* (Pg), *Eikenella corrodens* (Ec), *Campylobacter rectus* (Cr), *Tannerella forsythensis, Treponema denticola* (Td), and *Fusobacterium nucleatum* (Fn). *P. gingivalis, T. forsythensis,* and *A. a.* are very strongly considered to be pathogenic for periodontal disease. A sterile paper point is inserted into the pocket for 10 seconds. This test also gives a list of antibiotics that the bacteria are susceptible to.

Currently, there is no reason to use DNA probes routinely in every patient. DNA probes should be reserved for difficult refractory cases in which previous treatments have failed to control disease progression. It can also be used to monitor therapy outcome after the disease is controlled and to evaluate implant sites. Because certain antibiotics are almost always effective against anaerobic pathogens (infections), these infections are usually treated empirically or hypothetically.

Immunologic Assays

The enzyme-linked immunosorbent assay (ELISA) is based on the specific binding of an antibody to an antigen on the surface of a periodontal pathogen. The primary antibody is detected by labeling with a fluorescent secondary antibody. ELISA is able to identify specific bacteria. It is an expensive test and currently used only in research.

Enzyme-Based Assays

The enzymatic approach is based on the ability to screen for the presence of an enzyme unique to one or more bacterial species. In this assay, a biofilm sample is exposed to a substance that is degraded by the specific enzyme in question. For example, *Treponema denticola, Porphyromonas gingivalis*, and *Tannerella forsythensis* produce a trypsin-like enzyme that degrades a substance called BANA (benzoyldi-arginine-2-naphthylamide). A positive test indirectly indicates the presence of one or more of the three bacteria (Papapanou et al., 1999).

Genetic Assays

Numerous established and potential risk factors are associated with periodontal diseases, including smoking, smokeless tobacco, systemic diseases, age, medications, stress, and genetics (heredity). All these factors, except for genetics and age, are acquired or environmental and can be controlled or eliminated. (Kornman and colleagues 1997) addressed the first association between **genetics** and periodontal diseases. Interleukin-1 (IL-1) is a cytokine produced and secreted by inflammatory cells such as macrophages as a result of accumulation of bacterial biofilm. IL-1 is responsible for inflammation and bone loss. Some individuals produce too much IL-1 in response to bacterial challenge. These individuals are more susceptible to the onset and rapid progression of periodontal diseases than individuals who do not show an IL-1 genotype (gene). IL-1 does not cause periodontal disease directly, but it predisposes the patient to the disease process by increasing inflammation when bacteria are present (Newman, 1998). This information allows the patient to be monitored more closely and helps dental practitioners recommend optimal preventive therapy and supportive care programs (Newman, 1998).

A saliva-based genetic test is available that determines if a patient has an IL-1 genotype. This test, which is the first genetic test for periodontal disease susceptibility, is called Genotype PST™ Plus (Periodontal Susceptibility Testing; Advanced Dental Diagnostics, Franklin, TN). The test is performed by collecting saliva from the patient. The sample is analyzed in a licensed medical laboratory to determine if the patient is positive or negative for the IL-1 genotype. An IL-1 gene-positive patient is about seven times more likely to develop or have advanced periodontal disease than a gene-negative patient, and this genotype occurs in approximately 30% of the population (Alexander, 2012).

MyPerioID® PST® (OralDNA Labs, Brentwood, TN) is another salivary assay used to determine the patient's genetic susceptibility to periodontal disease.

Salivary Diagnostic Assays

Salivary DNA test (OralDNA Labs, Brentwood, TN) can determine the presence, type, and concentration of specific periodontal pathogens. The results of this assay reports on the presence of pathogenic bacteria above the threshold and identifies the risk for attachment loss.

Clinical Applications

Although at present a good clinical judgment of the presence of periodontal disease can be made using existing diagnostic procedures, this decision may be very subjective and sometimes unreliable. Therefore, there is a need for more precise decision making, and care should be taken in evaluating and using these new systems. However, presently, there are no completely validated assessment procedures that can identify progressing or active periodontitis.

Because the etiology of and risk factors for periodontal diseases are multifaceted, the most important steps for patient evaluation include a comprehensive clinical and radiographic analysis and identification of modifying systemic risk factors, including cigarette smoking and diabetes mellitus. In addition, the host response contributes to the development and progression of the disease. Therefore, no microbial or host response test will definitively determine the initiation or progression of disease.

It is without foundation to use these tests on all periodontal patients. A critical factor that needs to be considered when a practitioner chooses to introduce diagnostic testing as part of patient care is when to use the tests. At a time when there is great pressure to reduce healthcare costs, judicious application is critical (Lamster, 1996).

Culture and sensitivity testing can provide guidelines for antibiotic selection in certain cases, including periodontitis patients who are refractory to previous treatment. Such patients probably have been treated previously with numerous antibiotics, and bacterial resistance could have developed. DNA probe analysis can be helpful in these patients, providing rapid results within 24 hours. Assessment of the genetic susceptibility of a patient or of children of parents with advanced periodontal disease may soon prove to be an important tool in the initiation of preventive measures.

Dental Hygiene Application

Traditional clinical assessments usually will detect inflammatory lesions and direct practitioners to areas requiring therapy and possible additional testing (Greenstein & Rethman, 1998). Presently, *microbial assays and host-response diagnostic tests (including tissue destruction)* appear to have meager use and limited applicability in routine diagnosis in periodontics. These adjunctive diagnostic tests may improve clinical decision making but require further confirmation followed by controlled clinical studies. Additional testing may be beneficial at specific sites or for individual patients when there is diagnostic uncertainty regarding the absence or presence of diseases or when the medical or dental history suggests that a patient is at risk of developing periodontitis (Greenstein & Rethman, 1998). Currently, however, few of these tests are available commercially, and no test is available that will definitively determine if a site is actively losing attachment and bone or will lose attachment in the future. There are no specific guidelines to follow, but some factors to consider include cost of testing, age of the patient, patient motivation, and systemic health of the patient.

Key Points

- No clinical test is available that will currently determine if a site is actively breaking down or predict periodontal breakdown; more research is needed.
- A combination of traditional and new diagnostic testing can, in some cases, provide more complete information for treatment planning.
- Additional bacterial tests are used for site-specific treatment, for additional information to assist treatment, and to rule out other causes of disease.

- Bacterial tests include culture, DNA probe, and microscopic.
- Host response tests include GCF assay and genetic susceptibility test.

Self-Quiz

1. From the list provided, select the items associated with determining the susceptibility of certain bacteria to antibiotics.
   a. Phase-contrast microscopy
   b. DNA probe
   c. Dark-field microscopy
   d. Temperature
   e. GCF assay
   f. Bacterial culture

2. All the following types of patients could have adjunctive periodontal diagnostic testing be of greatest use except one. Which one is the exception?
   a. New patients who have not received therapy previously
   b. Treated patients who initially present with advanced periodontal disease
   c. Patients not responding to periodontal treatment
   d. Patients with previously treated gingivitis

3. Which one of the following statements may indicate that a genetic risk factor is contributing to a patient's periodontal condition?
   a. Destruction of bone early in life
   b. Production of excessive amounts of interleukin-1
   c. Demonstration of high levels of bacteria in childhood
   d. Presentation with highly inflamed soft tissues

4. Which of the following indications is for using host-based diagnostic periodontal tests?
   a. Determine the need for future maintenance care
   b. Identify periodontal sites that are bleeding
   c. Evaluate the need for more aggressive periodontal treatment
   d. Distinguish between active and inactive disease sites

5. Which one of the following tests is highly sensitive for specific periodontal pathogens present in a subgingival sample of biofilm?
   a. Culture
   b. DNA probe
   c. GCF enzyme assay
   d. Microscopic technique

6. In which one of the following secretions are high levels of host-derived enzymes found?
   a. Whole saliva
   b. Crevicular fluid
   c. Sweat
   d. Serum

7. Which one of the following statements is related to adjunctive periodontal tests?
   a. Eventually they will replace conventional periodontal assessment techniques.
   b. They are used on all periodontal patients presenting in the office.
   c. Established guidelines need to be determined.
   d. They are cost effective and easy to perform.

8. Which one of the following tests identifies the motility of bacteria?
   a. Enzyme-linked immunosorbent assay (ELISA)
   b. Phase-contrast microscopy
   c. DNA probe
   d. GCF enzyme
   e. Temperature

9. Which one of the following host cells synthesizes and releases beta-glucuronidase and elastase?
   a. Mast cells
   b. Lymphocytes
   c. Neutrophils
   d. Eosinophils
   e. Fibroblasts

10. All of the following statements are correct concerning the use of DNA probe assays except one. Which one is the exception?
    a. They are highly sensitive and specific for targeted periodontal pathogens.
    b. Samples are sent to an outside laboratory.
    c. They require viable microorganisms.
    d. They provide rapid identification.

Case Study

A female patient in for a periodontal maintenance visit will receive an updated probing, periodontal tissue re-examination, and assessment of clinical attachment levels. The dental hygienist is concerned that the patient sometimes has pocket areas which bleed and there was an increase in the pocket depth of the mesial of #3 from 4 to 6 mm last visit. The dental hygienist is considering other options in the care plan.

1. Adjunctive tests such as cultures will provide which of the following?
   a. Quantify disease severity
   b. Determine need for initial therapy
   c. Evaluate potential risk of new breakdown
   d. All of the above

Answer: C. The initial determination still depends upon probing, gingival inspections, and radiographs which give the disease severity. Adjunctive tests may help determine disease progression or risk of future breakdown.

2. Which of the following adjunctive test is utilized for detecting sites actively breaking down?
   a. Culture and sensitivity test
   b. Gingival crevicular fluid assays
   c. Dark-field or phase-contrast microscopy
   d. Genetic susceptibility tests

Answer: B. GCF assays show enzymatic to predict activity. Cultures and dark-field show specific microorganisms. Susceptibility tests show the possibility of the disease based upon genetics.

3. What is the advantage of the dental hygienist collecting the information from the adjunctive tests?
   a. None as they have not been validated to predict progression
   b. Microbial or host response test will definitively determine disease progression
   c. So many tests are available commercially
   d. The tests are low cost and easy to use

Answer: A. No clinical test is available that will currently determine if a site is actively breaking down or predict periodontal breakdown; more research is needed.

References

Alexander, D.C. 2012. A conversation with Kenneth S. Kornman, DDS, PhD. *Inside Dentistry* 8(3).

Armitage, G. C. 1992. Diagnostic tests for periodontal diseases. *Curr. Opin. Dent.* 21(1):53–62.

Armitage, G. C. 1993. Periodontal diagnostic aids. *Calif. Dent. Assoc. J.* 21(11):35–46.

Bader, H. I. 1995. Contemporary periodontics and a vision for the future: Diagnostics and monitoring the treated case. *Dentistry Today* 1:42–45.

Chambers, D. A., P. B. Imrey, R. L. Cohen, J. M. Crawford, M. E. Alves, and T. A. McSwiggin. 1991. A longitudinal study of aspartate aminotransferase in human gingival cervical fluid. *J. Periodont. Res.* 26:65–74.

Estafan, D., M. A. Weinberg, and A. Estafan. 1999. Adjunctive diagnostic methods for monitoring progressive periodontal diseases. *Gen. Dent.* (Jul–Aug) 47(4):374–380.

Greenstein, G. S., and M. P. Rethman. 1998. Diagnosing destructive periodontal diseases. In eds. M. Nevins and J. T. Mellonig, *Periodontal therapy: Clinical approaches and evidence of success*, Vol. 1. Chicago: Quintessence.

Kornman, K. S., A. Crane, H.-Y. Wang, et al. 1997. The interleukin-1 genotype as a severity factor in adult periodontal disease. *J. Clin. Periodontol.* 24:72–77.

Lamster, I. B. 1996. In-office diagnostic tests and their role in supportive periodontal treatment. *Periodontology 2000* 12:49–55.

Lamster, I. B., L. G. Holmes, K. B. Gross, R. L. Oshrain, D. W. Cohen, et al. 1995. The relationship of β-glucuronidase activity in crevicular fluid to probing attachment loss in patients with adult periodontitis: Findings from a multicenter study. *J. Clin. Periodontol.* 22:36–44.

Lamster, I. B., R. L. Oshrain, D. S. Harper, R. S. Celenti, C. A. Hovliaras, and J. M. Gordon. 1988. Enzyme activity in crevicular fluid for detection and prediction of clinical attachment loss in patients with chronic adult periodontitis: Six-month results. *J. Periodontol.* 59:516–523.

Listgarten, M. A., and S. Levin. 1981. Positive correlation between the proportions of subgingival spirochetes and motile bacteria and susceptibility of human subjects to periodontal deterioration. *J. Clin. Periodontol.* 8:122–138.

Loesche, W. J. 1992. DNA probe and enzyme analysis in periodontal diagnostics. *J. Periodontol.* 63:1102–1109.

Loomer, P. M. 2004. Microbiological diagnostic testing in the treatment of periodontal diseases. *Periodontology 2000* 34(1):49–56.

Newman, M. 1998. Genetic, environmental, and behavioral influences on periodontal infections. *Compend. Contin. Educ.* (special issue) 19(1):25–31.

Offenbacher, S., B. M. Odler, and T. E. van Dyke. 1986. The use of crevicular fluid prostaglandin E_2 as a predictor of periodontal attachment loss. *J. Periodont. Res.* 21:101–112.

Overall, C. M., J. Sodek, C. A. G. McCulloch, and P. Birek. 1991. Evidence for polymophonuclear leukocyte collagenase and 92-kilodalton gelatinase in gingival crevicular fluid. *Infect. Immun.* 59:4687–4692.

Palcanis, K. G., I. K. Larjara, B. R. Wells, K. A. Suggs, J. P. Landis, et al. 1992. Elastase as an indicator of periodontal disease progression. *J. Periodontol.* 63:237–242.

Papapanou, P. N., S. P. Engelbretson, and I. B. Lamster. 1999. Current and future approaches for diagnosis of periodontal diseases. *N. Y. State Dent. J.* (April):32–38.

Persson, G. R., T. A. DeRouen, and R. C. Page. 1990. Relationship between gingival crevicular fluid levels of aspartate aminotransferase and active tissue destruction in treated chronic periodontitis patients. *J. Periodont. Res.* 25:81–87.

Pradeep, A. R., S. G. Manjunath, P. P. Swati, C. Shikha, and P. B. Sujatha. 2007. Gingival crevicular fluid levels of leukotriene B_4 in periodontal health and disease. *J Periodontol.* 78:2325–2330.

Sixou, M. 2003. Diagnostic testing as a supportive measure of treatment strategy. *Oral Dis.* 9 (Suppl 1):54–62.

Socransky, S. S., and A. D. Haffajee. 1991. Microbial mechanisms in the pathogenesis of destructive periodontal diseases: A critical assessment. *J. Periodont. Res.* 26:195–212.

Sonnier, K. E. 1996. Microbial testing: Present and future. *Clin. Update* 18(4):7.

Sorsa, T., M. Hernandez, J. Leppilahti, et al. 2010. Detection of gingival crevicular fluid MMP-8 levels with different laboratory and chair-side methods. *Oral Dis.* 16:39–45.

Sorsa, T., T. Tervahartiala, J. Leppilahti, et al. 2011. Collagenase-2 (MMP-8) as a point-of-care biomarker in periodontitis and cardiovascular diseases. Therapeutic response to non-antimicrobial properties of tetracyclines. *Pharmacol. Res.* 63(2):108–113.

Tanner, A. 1992. Microbial etiology of periodontal diseases: Where are we? Where are we going? *Curr. Opin. Dent.* 2(1):12–24.

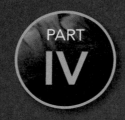

Periodontal Diseases: Treatment Planning, Implementation, and Evaluation Phase

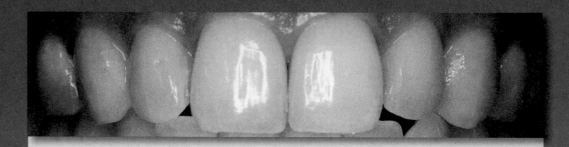

OUTLINE

19

Problem-/Evidence-Based Treatment Planning

Michael P. Rethman and Jill Rethman

OUTLINE

EDUCATIONAL OBJECTIVES

Upon completion of this chapter, the reader should be able to:

- Describe the problem-based approach to treatment planning.
- Formulate a problem list for each patient.
- Formulate an action plan for each problem listed.
- Describe treatment guidelines for periodontal patients.
- Explain when more aggressive forms of therapy are needed and thus appropriate times for referral to or comanagement with a periodontist.
- Describe periodontal prognostic signs.

GOALS: To provide an understanding of problem-based learning (PBL) in developing a periodontal treatment plan.

KEY WORDS

Introduction

Controlling inflammation is the initial treatment objective of therapies for the periodontal diseases. The key to controlling inflammation is to eliminate, reduce, or change the makeup of microbes residing in the mouth. Of course, once inflammation is brought under control, the prevention of recurrent periodontitis is essential (Hancock, 1996; Van Dyke, 2007).

Research findings have shown that plaque microbes and their by-products are responsible for the initiation and progression of the periodontal diseases (Haffajee & Socransky, 2006; Ismail, Morrison, Burt, Caffesse, & Kavanagh, 1990; Kolenbrander et al., 2006). Additional research has found that the host's immune response to infection plays an important role in determining how periodontal destruction manifests itself by producing chemical modulators that actually may accelerate periodontal destruction (Grossi et al., 1994, 1995; Van Dyke & Serhan, 2003). Therefore, comprehensive periodontal therapy may include tactics to modulate the host's immune response in addition to traditional efforts to suppress periodontal pathogens.

This chapter explores current concepts of periodontal treatment planning with a focus on **problem-based** learning.

Problem-Based Learning (PBL) Approach to Treatment

A problem-based recording system is designed to introduce the student to a technique for developing an individualized treatment plan for each patient. Problem-based learning (PBL) initially identifies significant problems from the patient's medical/dental history from which a differential dental hygiene diagnosis (or interpretation) will be made for each sign and/or symptom on the problem list. The problem list will be used as a guide to develop a treatment plan and a comanagement or a referral system. A decision-making tree can be also be used to help decide on the proper treatment in each case. Therapeutic decision making refers to the process of the use of the decision theory, which is the study of the best possible outcomes for decisions made under varying conditions, in making decisions about treatment of individual cases.

Tables 19–1 ■ through 19–3 ■ provide an overall concept of therapeutic decision making when treatment planning a periodontal case.

The American Academy of Periodontology has developed practice parameters on the diagnosis and treatment of periodontal diseases. The *Parameters of Care* (American Academy of Periodontology, 2000a) are strategies to assist oral healthcare practitioners in making clinical decisions from a range of treatment options to achieve a desired outcome.

For many years, periodontitis was thought to be the inevitable result of poor oral hygiene along with uncontrolled dental plaque biofilm and calculus accumulation.

This was termed the nonspecific plaque hypothesis (Loesche, 1976). In recent decades, research has suggested instead that there are microbial species whose presence tends to signal a greater likelihood of progressive periodontal destruction (Haffajee et al., 1991). Furthermore, for most patients, evidence suggests that procedures aimed at suppressing these species will improve clinical outcomes (American Academy of Periodontology, 2000b; Haffajee & Socransky, 2006). However, for adults, frontline periodontal therapy remains largely nonspecific in design—because conventional clinical and self-care procedures often succeed among this predominating group of patients with periodontal diseases. For periodontal diseases in young people, for refractory disease in adults, and in special situations, periodontal therapy may include procedures aimed at specific putative periodontal pathogens.

Goals of Periodontal Therapy

The ideal goal of periodontal therapy is to restore the periodontium to a comfortable and functional state of health for the balance of the patient's life. Therefore, most periodontal therapy aims to prevent the initiation, progression, or recurrence of periodontal diseases, termed arrestive periodontal therapy. The first step in developing a treatment plan should be to determine individual treatment goals for each patient.

Periodontal Therapy: Ongoing Care

The management of most patients with periodontal diseases demands continued reassessments and adjustments to ongoing care. Reassessment and adjustments are necessary because periodontal care is not permanent in the sense that many other highly successful dental therapies are considered permanent (e.g. the permanent crown on a decayed tooth). For most cases of chronic periodontitis, the only permanent periodontal end point is tooth (or implant) loss. Furthermore, no single periodontal treatment produces ideal outcomes for all patients.

Once a patient is practicing thorough daily oral hygiene, the ideal interval between patient appointments—even for patients in periodontal maintenance programs—may be as brief as every 2 to 3 months (American Academy of Periodontology, 2000b; Axelsson & Lindhe, 1981). For patients who are not engaged in thorough daily oral hygiene and/or who continue to demonstrate signs of periodontal attachment loss, professional maintenance intervals may be even shorter. Frequent reexaminations, reevaluations, and adjustments to therapy often are necessary for many years.

Did You Know?

The most frequently performed periodontal surgical procedure by periodontists is flap surgery to provide access for root debridement.

Table 19–1 Diagnostic Decision Making for Periodontal Diseases

Diagnostic Test	When to use	Features of Test
Periodontal screening and recording	For all patients in clinical practice	It is a screening tool; entire dentition is not probed but it is quick and easy to perform.
Gingival assessment	For all patients in clinical practice	Assessing for gingival inflammation. Bleeding on probing is indicative of inflammation; absence of bleeding is indicative that there is no inflammation.
Periodontal probing	For all patients in clinical practice	Comparing clinical attachment levels at separate time intervals can show if there is attachment loss. Cannot predict future attachment loss from a single probing depth at a visit.
Radiographic assessment	For all patients in clinical practice	Absence of bone loss may be indicative that there is a low-risk for future periodontal disease activity but use clinical probing depths and radiographic assessment together when diagnosing periodontal disease.
Microbial testing	Refractory patients; high-risk patients	Has limitations; expensive, but may be used to determine pathogens and antibiotic sensitivity.

Table 19–2 Nonsurgical Treatment Choices for Periodontal Diseases

Nonsurgical Treatment	Procedure Performed	Notes
Periodontal debridement	Scaling and root planing using hand and power-driven instruments	Mainstay for periodontal diseases. Treatment outcome is reduction in probing depths, reduction in bleeding and gain in clinical attachment; reevaluation is completed at 4 to 8 weeks after initial therapy.
Adjunctive therapy with antimicrobials	Use of rinses (e.g., chlorhexidine) in conjunction with periodontal debridement	In some patients, using a rinse with high substantivity such as chlorhexidine may be beneficial to reduce gingival inflammation. Not to be used in place of periodontal debridement.
Controlled-release drug delivery	Subgingival placement of an antimicrobial	Indicated for localized chronic periodontitis. As an adjunctive therapy to periodontal debridement when there are residual bleeding probing sites ≥ 5 mm. Outcomes include reduction in probing depths and bleeding and gain in clinical attachment levels.
Systemic antibiotics	Systemic antibiotics prescribed with periodontal debridement/surgery	Indicated for recurrent periodontitis and aggressive periodontitis.

Table 19–3 Surgical Treatment Choices for Periodontitis

Surgical Therapy	Procedure Performed	Notes
Open flap debridement	Surgical flap reflected; gain access; debride root surface; close flap	For pocket elimination/reduction or gaining access to underlying root surface for easy debridement. Healing by long junctional epithelium
Gingivectomy/ gingivoplasty	Remove and reshape gingiva without a flap	Indicated for psuedopockets or gingival enlargement; not for areas with vertical/angular bone loss

Surgical Therapy	Procedure Performed	Notes
Guided tissue regeneration (GTR)	Flap surgery with use of bone grafts/bone substitutes and a barrier membrane to allow regeneration of bone, PDL. and cementum rather than a long junctional epithelium	Periodontal sites with infrabony defects (vertical bone loss) or ideally mandibular teeth with Class II furcation defects
Root coverage	Autogenous soft tissue grafts, barrier membrane, or ascellular dermal matrix (Alloderm)	Grafts used to cover roots to decrease root sensitivity, enhance esthetics
Dental implants	Use of titanium fixtures and crown	Indicated for missing teeth; careful selection of patients — look for closeness of vital structures such as the maxillary sinus and mandibular canal.

Given this context, practitioners need to comply with their ethical and medical/legal responsibilities to refer periodontitis patients to specialists, provide comparable periodontal care in the general practice, or partner with a specialist to share responsibilities for periodontal patients. Suggestions governing what, when, and why to refer are made where appropriate throughout this chapter.

Problem List

A problem list should be set up for individual periodontal patients (Table 19–4 ■). The problem list will identify the patient's problems by reviewing the chief complaint and medical, social (habit), and dental histories. For each problem identified, a solution should be written, and expected outcomes (the result of taking care of the problem), prognosis (predication of recovery), and any major concerns must be addressed. Identified problems may have multiple solutions.

Risk Assessment for Periodontal Diseases

An important aspect of treatment planning is to perform **risk assessment** to determine either predisposition for developing periodontal conditions or for susceptibility for further breakdown. Numerous risk factors have been identified that predispose an individual to periodontitis. Risk factors that cannot be modified — known as risk indicators or determinants — include increased age, male gender, lower socioeconomic status, and genetics. Modifiable risk factors include the presence of plaque biofilm and microbiota, poor oral hygiene, and the use of tobacco products. Indeed, the primary risk factor for developing periodontitis is tobacco smoking, whereas certain systemic conditions — most notably diabetes — are also factors (American Academy of Periodontology, 2008). Risk assessment for the periodontal diseases typically consists of the patient filling out a form indicating specific habits or conditions. The clinician then subjectively interprets the findings to determine disease susceptibility. Unfortunately, research has shown that such methods are not accurate and can lead to inappropriate treatment (Persson, Mancl, Martin, & Page, 2003). An objective, computer-based tool could result in more uniform and accurate periodontal clinical decision making, improved oral health, reduction in the need for complex therapy, and reduction in healthcare costs. One such tool is the Oral Health Information Suite® (PreViser Corporation, Mount Vernon, WA). Risk scores calculated using the periodontal risk calculator (PCR) and information gathered during a standard periodontal examination predict future periodontal status with a high level of accuracy and validity (Page, Martin, Krall, Mancl, & Garcia, 2003). Clinically validated periodontal disease risk and severity analysis, as well as suggested treatment options for a patient, are calculated by entering 23 data points. Risk is reported on a clinically validated numeric scale (1 indicating very low risk to 5 indicating very high), whereas disease severity is described on a validated 1 (health) to 100 (severe periodontitis) numeric scale. Reports are generated while the patient is still in the chair. Patients are given this analysis as simple-to-understand numeric scores that demonstrate improvement or deterioration in their periodontal health status.

Frequent and regular patient education in self-diagnosis and self-care techniques (Axelsson, Nystrom, & Lindhe, 2004; Douglass 2006) can also be used as a risk assessment tool for periodontal diseases.

Rapid Dental Hint

Developing the problem list, solutions, and expected outcomes not only addresses the clinical concerns of the patient but also helps identify the patient's subjective concerns.

Table 19–4 Periodontal Problem List

Problems	Solutions (Plan)	Expected Outcome/Prognosis/ Major Concerns
Chief Complaint	Address chief complaint	Treat the chief complaint first
Risk Factors		
Medical History (e.g., diabetes, HIV)	• Detailed assessment • Consultations required • Advise patient of relationship between systemic diseases and periodontal disease	Concern with possible delayed healing
Dental History (e.g., previous periodontal care)	• Detailed assessment • Previous periodontal surgery and/or repeated deep scaling and root planing procedures • Frequency of maintenance care	Compliance is a deciding factor in prognosis
Genetics	Blood test determines possible susceptibility to periodontal diseases. Unfortunately tests are imperfect in predicting subsequent periodontal status.	If determined to be susceptible, patient must be compliant with periodontal care
Smoking	Smoking cessation program	• Concerned with periodontal and systemic diseases • Good prognosis if patient is willing to quit
Iatrogenic dentistry	Look for open margins, overhangs, and open contacts, and replace or modify existing restorations	Concerned with food impaction and plaque biofilm traps
Poor oral hygiene	Patient education, monitoring, technique modulation as needed and encouragement	Nonadherence may increase incidence or progression of periodontitis
Soft Tissues		
Gingival inflammation	Eliminate/reduce gingival inflammation with mechanical debridement and oral hygiene	Concerned with development/ progression of gingivitis and permits more useful subsequent clinical assessments
Soft-tissue recession	Determine etiology; may need periodontal surgery (mucogingival)	Improved esthetics and/or greater comfort and facilitates better oral hygiene and mitigation of the risk of future recession.
Abnormal tissue architecture: Gingival overgrowth	Determine etiology; drug-induced or hereditary or plaque-induced inflammation; may need periodontal surgery to correct	Difficulty performing optimal oral hygiene
Lack of attached gingiva	Determine etiology; determine if prosthetics will be done; may need gingival plastic surgery to correct	Is site prone to inflammation, discomfort, recession?
Probing depths	Deep probing depths: mechanical debridement followed by reevaluation and if needed periodontal surgery	Deep probing depths limit the effectiveness of oral hygiene and mechanical debridement; future attachment loss is more likely

Problems	Solutions (Plan)	Expected Outcome/Prognosis/Major Concerns
Hard Tissue		
Ridge defects	Surgical intervention; planning for implants	Implant placement/esthetics
Teeth		
Missing teeth	Replacement of missing teeth	Concerned with short- and long-term ramifications with regard to esthetics, speech, masticatory function, and comfort
Mobility	Determine etiology: bone loss, occlusal trauma, inflammation, and treat accordingly	Concerned with patient comfort as well as increasing mobility, less favorable responses to oral hygiene, scaling/root planing or periodontal surgery
Fremitus, occlusal wear, abfractions	Determine etiology: bone loss, occlusal interferences, and treat accordingly to eliminate fremitus	Concern with patient comfort and continued occlusal trauma
Parafunctional habits	Eliminate parafunctional habits; counseling or appliances	Concerned with occlusal trauma/good prognosis if eliminated
Radiographic Findings		
Horizontal bone loss	With deep probing depths surgery is often indicated to reduce probing pocket depths and facilitate oral hygiene	Prognosis depends on several factors including amount of bone remaining, mobility, furcation involvement
Vertical bone loss	Surgical intervention is often useful, especially at sites thought likely to progress	Prognosis depends on several factors including amount of bone remaining, mobility, furcation involvement
Root proximity	Identify teeth and monitor for periodontal breakdown	Concerned with amount of interproximal bone remaining
Pathology		
Mucosal lesions	Determine size, shape, color, and location; refer to specialist; excisional biopsy	Primarily concerned with oral cancer, although mucosal abnormalities may signal both local and systemic pathologies.
TMD/pain	Excercises/appliances/referral to specialist	Reduced function, pain

Did You Know?

Risk assessment is commonplace for medical conditions, yet its potential for oral conditions remains largely untapped.

Treatment Planning

Once the examination and risk assessment are completed, the data must be analyzed. Data include the patient's medical and dental history, complete radiographs, detailed periodontal data, tooth conditions (including vitality, caries, and morphologic abnormalities), and dental awareness.

Patient Comanagement and Referral to a Periodontist

Although patients experiencing periodontal problems may be referred to a periodontist at any time, preliminary phases of periodontal therapy often are performed in the general practice. Sometimes, especially for mild cases, this is all that is necessary to achieve the goal of periodontal therapy (Dockter et al., 2006). However, even for patients who are ultimately referred, the benefits of self-care training, motivation, and emphasis on team building in the general practice increase the likelihood of treatment success by the periodontist. Hygienists, general practitioners, and periodontists who function as a team maximize the likelihood of optimal outcomes.

Although a licensed general practitioner legally may provide comprehensive periodontal therapy to any informed and consenting patient, he or she is ethically and legally required to meet the same standard of care for such therapy as a specialist. Therefore, with the welfare of periodontal patients in mind, the following comanagement and referral guidelines are proposed—with the knowledge that exceptions occur.

Guidelines for Referral and Comanagement

Any patient who has one or more periodontal sites that show persistent signs of inflammation should be considered for referral. Often these patients fit in one or more of the following categories:

1. Chronic periodontitis with deeper probing depths, furcation involvement, and/or problematic gingival recession
2. Aggressive (localized, generalized) periodontitis
3. Periodontitis associated with systemic diseases (such as diabetes mellitus)
4. Periodontitis with significant or increasing tooth mobility
5. Periodontal lesions adjacent to necrotic (or endodontically treated) teeth
6. Refractory (considered nonresponsive to treatment) or recurrent periodontitis (responsive, but still headed downhill)
7. Patients who have aesthetic concerns about the interplay between teeth, restorations, and the gingiva or alveolar arches
8. Patients with mucocutaneous disorders affecting the oral soft tissues (e.g., pemphigus, lichen planus)

In 2006, the American Academy of Periodontology released the *Guidelines for the Management of Patients with Periodontal Diseases* (American Academy of Periodontology, 2006). This document was developed to assist clinicians in identifying individuals most at risk for developing periodontal diseases. Along with the practitioner's skill and judgment, the *Guidelines* can help identify patients at risk as early as possible, thus hopefully preventing more severe conditions. The *Guidelines* are not mandates, nor do they specify treatment modalities. When used as a framework for patient management, they can enhance communication among all members of the oral healthcare team and determine those patients most appropriate for specialty care. Box 19–1 contains the *Guidelines* document.

PHASES OF TREATMENT Ideal **treatment planning** incorporates a logical interplay between periodontal and nonperiodontal procedures. This is because successful management of the periodontal diseases is a multifaceted discipline that can be affected by other dental conditions and treatments. Box 19–2 depicts four sequential phases that are guidelines for overall case management. In addition to developing a "best case" treatment plan, reasonable alternatives should be considered and presented to the patient. Flowcharts may help delineate the general route a patient takes during treatment (Boxes 19–3 through 19–8). It is important for practitioners to remember that the phases described here do not imply that every needful patient will go through the phases only once, indeed, because of the chronicity of many periodontal diseases, patients may go through the following phases repeatedly over a lifetime.

Phase I: Nonsurgical/Initial Preparation. The goal of Phase I therapy is to reduce all etiologic and risk factors to the maximum extent possible—short of surgical intervention. Conditions associated with pain, such as a periodontal abscess, necrotizing ulcerative gingivitis, or traumatic injury, should be treated at this time. Nonrestorable and periodontally hopeless teeth should be identified and extracted. Teeth needing endodontic therapy should be treated.

Oral hygiene instruction and patient education are performed. Patients need to learn that diligent self-care is the critical foundation for successful periodontal treatment. Boxes 19–5 through 19–10 emphasize self-care training, professional analyses, and technique refinement to a degree some may consider excessive. However, failure to provide

Box 19–1: Guidelines for the Management of Patients with Periodontal Diseases

LEVEL 3: PATIENTS WHO SHOULD BE TREATED BY A PERIODONTIST

Any patient with:

Severe chronic periodontitis
Furcation involvement
Vertical/angular bony defect(s)
Aggressive periodontitis (formerly known as juvenile, early-onset, or rapidly progressive periodontitis)
Periodontal abscess and other acute periodontal conditions
Significant root surface exposure and/or progressive gingival recession
Peri-implant disease
Any patient with periodontal diseases, regardless of severity, whom the referring dentist prefers not to treat.

LEVEL 2: PATIENTS WHO WOULD LIKELY BENEFIT FROM CO-MANAGEMENT BY THE REFERRING DENTIST AND THE PERIODONTIST

Any patient with periodontitis who demonstrates at reevaluation or any dental examination one or more of the following risk factors/indicators* known to contribute to the progression of periodontal diseases:

Periodontal Risk Factors/Indicators

Early onset of periodontal diseases (prior to the age of 35 years)
Unresolved inflammation at any site (e.g., bleeding upon probing, pus, and/or redness)
Pocket depths > 5 mm
Vertical bone defects
Radiographic evidence of progressive bone loss
Progressive tooth mobility
Progressive attachment loss
Anatomic gingival deformities
Exposed root surfaces
A deteriorating risk profile

*It should be noted that a combination of two or more of these risk factors/indicators may make even slight to moderate periodontitis particularly difficult to manage (e.g., a patient under 35 years of age who smokes).

Medical or Behavioral Risk Factors/Indicators

Smoking/tobacco use
Diabetes
Osteoporosis/osteopenia
Drug-induced gingival conditions (e.g., phenytoins, calcium channel blockers, immunosuppressants, and long-term systemic steroids)
Compromised immune system, either acquired or drug induced
A deteriorating risk profile.

LEVEL 1: PATIENTS WHO MAY BENEFIT FROM CO-MANAGEMENT BY THE REFERRING DENTIST AND THE PERIODONTIST

Any patient with periodontal inflammation/infection and the following systemic conditions:

Diabetes
Pregnancy
Cardiovascular disease
Chronic respiratory disease

Any patient who is a candidate for the following therapies who might be exposed to risk from periodontal infection, including but not limited to the following treatments:

Cancer therapy
Cardiovascular surgery
Joint-replacement surgery
Organ transplantation

FREQUENTLY ASKED QUESTIONS (FAQS) (UPDATED IN 2012)

The American Academy of Periodontology's Guidelines for the Management of Patients with Periodontal Diseases

1. What are the *Guidelines*?
   - The *Guidelines* provide information to assist in the timely identification of patients who would benefit from co-management by the referring dentist and the periodontist.
2. Why did the Academy develop the *Guidelines*?
   - The Academy's objective is to encourage referring dentists and periodontists to work together to optimize the health of patients. Determining if and when a patient should be referred to a periodontist are sometimes difficult issues. These *Guidelines* are intended to help the general practitioner in the rapid identification of those patients at greater risk for the consequences of periodontal inflammation and infection and, therefore, those patients most appropriate for specialty referral.
   - Despite recent advancements in periodontal therapy, periodontal diseases continue to present significant challenges for the public and dental profession. Periodontal diseases remain a major cause of tooth loss in adults. In addition, periodontal diseases are associated with systemic conditions, such as cardiovascular disease, diabetes, adverse pregnancy outcomes, and respiratory disease. Periodontists are experts in assessing and treating periodontal diseases.
   - Accumulating evidence, including recent literature, suggests that an increasing number of patients would benefit from periodontal specialty care. This evidence also suggests that these patients are being referred later in the disease process than in the past.

Box 19–1: Guidelines for the Management of Patients with Periodontal Diseases (*cont.*)

3. Who needs/benefits from the *Guidelines*?
   - All dental teams and their patients can benefit from using the *Guidelines*.
4. How were the *Guidelines* developed, and who developed them? Did the Academy collaborate with organized dentistry or any other groups or individuals on these *Guidelines*?
   - A Board of Trustees–appointed task force consisting of periodontal practitioners, academicians, and researchers developed the *Guidelines*.
   - The Academy distributed a draft version of the *Guidelines* to all members, the American Dental Association, Academy of General Dentistry, and American Dental Hygienists' Association for commentary.
   - All organizations and more than 375 members provided commentary.
   - The task force revised the *Guidelines* based on the comments received.
5. What are the benefits of using the *Guidelines*?
   The *Guidelines* will:
   - Help the practitioner in triaging patients who currently have or who are at risk for the development of periodontal diseases.
   - Help the general practitioner more effectively address the association of periodontal diseases and systemic diseases/conditions.
   - Assist the general dentist and hygienist in the management of periodontal diseases.
   - Result in appropriate and timely treatment of periodontal diseases.
   In addition, the *Guidelines*:
   - Should enhance the restorative outcomes by establishing and maintaining a healthy periodontal foundation.
   - Are clear, concise, and should be easy to incorporate into daily practice and will enhance the partnership between periodontists and referring dentists.
6. Where do the *Guidelines* fit in the process of care?
   - The *Guidelines* will become an integral part of patient management.
   - The *Guidelines* do not replace the knowledge, skills, and abilities of the dental team.
7. The *Guidelines* mention the concept of risk assessment. What is risk assessment, and why is it so important?
   - Risk assessment is the process of determining the qualitative or quantitative estimation of the likelihood of adverse events that may result from exposure to specified health hazards or from the absence of beneficial influences. Upon dental examination, many practitioners incorrectly assume that a patient in a state of periodontal health is not at risk for developing periodontitis. Indeed, the patient may have risk factors/indicators (e.g., a smoking habit, diabetes, and young age) that could increase the probability of the occurrence of periodontitis in the future. Therefore, risk assessment helps predict a patient's disease state at some future point in time or the rate of progression of current disease.

8. Why are patients with furcation involvement considered among those patients who "should be treated by a periodontist"?
   - Periodontists are specialists trained to assess and treat the more advanced forms of periodontal diseases and associated lesions. Furcation involvements are among the most problematic periodontal lesions. Therefore, it is often appropriate that earlier manifestations of these complex lesions be evaluated and managed by a periodontist.
9. The *Guidelines* suggest that certain patients can only be treated by a periodontist. Is this true?
   - No. Some patients can be well managed within the general dental practice, whereas others would benefit from co-management with a periodontist. The Academy understands that the education, experience, and interests of individual general practitioner dentists vary, and, therefore, specialty referral may occur at different stages of a patient's disease state and risk level. Referral is not only associated with treatment but also includes consultation.
10. Do all patients who are referred to periodontists require surgery?
    - No. Comprehensive care by a periodontist includes nonsurgical and/or surgical therapies depending on the needs of the individual patient.
11. Dental implants, oral reconstructive and corrective procedures, and tissue engineering are not included in the *Guidelines*. Why aren't these procedures included?
    - These *Guidelines* are focused on the management of patients with periodontitis. They do not include all areas of periodontal specialty care or specific treatment modalities. Dental implants, periodontal plastic surgery, oral reconstructive surgery, and tissue-engineering procedures are currently performed by periodontists. The American Academy of Periodontology continually develops useful diagnostic and patient treatment recommendations that are available at perio.org.
12. Where is the research to support statements made in the *Guidelines*?
    - The Academy's Web site includes many resources that support the *Guidelines for the Management of Patients with Periodontal Diseases*. These resources are located at www.perio.org/resources-products/posppr2.html.
13. Is the Academy implying a medicolegal standard with the dissemination of these *Guidelines*?
    - This document is intended to serve as a guide for the dental team in managing patients with periodontal diseases.
    - The Academy believes that all dentists have the right to practice according to their education, training, and experience. Clearly, each dentist has an obligation to render treatment in the best interests of the patient. It is hoped that this document will help dentists identify patients at greatest risk for periodontal diseases so that these patients receive appropriate and timely periodontal care.

Explanation of Terms

- May: A choice to act or not; indicates freedom or liberty to follow a suggested alternative.

- Should: A highly desirable direction but does not mean mandatory.

- Must: Used to express a command; indicates an imperative or duty. This term does not appear in the document and is provided as a comparison to the terms "may" and "should."

- Co-management: A shared responsibility for patient care between a periodontist and referring dentist. This patient management may consist of consultation and/or treatment.

- Reevaluation: Assessment of a patient's periodontal status and risk profile after therapy to be used as a basis for subsequent patient management.

- Deteriorating risk profile: Adverse changes in risk factors/indicators suggestive of disease onset or progression.

- Disease definitions: For disease definitions such as severe chronic periodontitis, aggressive periodontitis, and acute periodontal conditions, please refer to volume 4 of the *Annals of Periodontology* at www.perio.org/resources-products/classification.htm.

- Peri-implant disease: Chronic inflammation and/or bone loss around dental implants that may influence implant status.

- Periodontal inflammation: Most periodontal diseases including chronic and aggressive periodontitis are inflammatory diseases. Chronic periodontitis has an infectious etiology from the endogenous plaque biofilm. This type of opportunistic infection results in a chronic release of inflammatory cytokines, prostaglandins, and destructive enzymes from neutrophils and mononuclear cells in the periodontium. The ensuing chronic inflammation in the tissue is what leads to the pathologic anatomic changes clinically detectable as periodontal pockets and alveolar bone loss. Furthermore, some microorganisms of the biofilm and inflammatory mediators from the affected tissue may adversely affect systemic chronic inflammatory diseases and pregnancy outcomes.

- Significant root surface exposure: Gingival recession of sufficient magnitude that results in the loss of tooth structure, sensitivity, esthetic concerns, or attachment loss.

Source: Reprinted with permission from the American Academy of Periodontology. The *Guidelines* were approved by the Board of Trustees of the American Academy of Periodontology in August 2006. Any citation of this document must be to the *Journal of Periodontology* as: American Academy of Periodontology. Guidelines for the management of patients with periodontal diseases. *J Periodontol* 2006;77:1607–1611. The *Guidelines* will be updated periodically. The most current version of the *Guidelines* is available online at www.perio.org/resources-products/posppr3-1.html.

Box 19–2: Phases of Periodontal Treatment

Phase I or initial therapy: Disease control

- Emergency care; relief of acute symptoms*

- Oral hygiene instruction*

- Nutritional counseling*

- Correction of inadequate restorations (e.g., overhang or poorly contoured restorations,* open proximal contacts)

- Periodontal debridement*

- Antimicrobial therapy (oral rinses, oral irrigation for patient self-care, controlled-release products)*

- Systemic antibiotics, if indicated, in aggressive cases

- Fluoride application (varnish or other) for caries control or desensitization, if indicated*

- Smoking cessation*

- Minor orthodontic movement

- Occlusal therapy (including night guards)*

- Extraction of hopeless teeth

- Reevaluation of initial therapy*

Phase II therapy: Surgical access, sometimes inducing sustained anatomic alterations

Phase III therapy: Restorative/prosthetic care

- Final restorations fabricated

Phase IV therapy: Maintenance care

- Evaluation of patient's oral hygiene*

- Smoking cessation*

- Treatment depends on the condition of the periodontium

*Procedures that may be performed by dental hygienists in some jurisdictions. Check with individual state practice regulations.

Box 19–3: Periodontal Health

Gingival tissues are healthy, and there is no bleeding after gentle probing.

First appointment: 45 minutes to 1 hour

- Comprehensive oral evaluation (new patients) or periodic oral evaluation (existing patients)—consisting of a medical and dental history update, vital signs, head and neck examination, and oral cancer screening

- Complete X-ray series, including vertical bitewings (new patients) or indicated radiographs (existing patients)

- Oral hygiene instruction

- Oral prophylaxis

- Selective polishing, if needed

- Nutritional counseling for the control of dental caries

- Fluoride application (varnish or other) for moderate or high caries risk individuals

- Tobacco counseling for the control and prevention of oral disease, if indicated

- Suitable maintenance interval established (3, 6, or more months)

compulsive clinical emphasis on patient motivation and self-care techniques invites treatment failures that might be avoided.

Oral prophylaxis and periodontal debridement are often performed. The tissue responses to in-office and improved self-care may be assessed as soon as a week later. Frequent reassessment is commonplace insofar as the chronic nature of most forms of periodontitis necessitates that ongoing care be based on the responses observed to previous therapies.

Multiple appointments during this phase help the patient better understand his or her role as cotherapist. They also help build the key concept of a patient–hygienist–dentist team—organized to fight together against periodontitis on a site-by-site basis.

As this phase draws to a close, if signs of inflammation persist at deeper probing sites—especially those the patient is keeping free of supragingival plaque—the need for periodontal surgery is often obvious to everyone.

Phase II: Periodontal Surgery. Although evidence exists suggesting an approximate equivalence between arrestive outcomes of closed debridement procedures and open (surgical) procedures in many types of periodontal defects, practitioners need to know that the design of these nonsurgical studies (e.g., 20 minutes of root planing per tooth) is clinically unrealistic (Froum, Weinberg, & Tarnow, 1998; Lindhe et al., 1984; Pihlstrom, McHugh, Oliphant, & Ortiz-Campos, 1983; Ramfjord et al., 1987). In addition,

root anatomy (such as concavities), furcations, and deep probing depths can compromise the ability to effectively instrument areas via root planning (American Academy of Periodontology, 2001).

Many periodontal surgical procedures are performed to provide the practitioner with better and faster access to deep periodontal pockets. These surgeries may be arrestive or regenerative. A single surgical procedure may incorporate both elements. For example, an osseous (bone) graft may be placed in a deep infrabony defect on one tooth, whereas bone in adjacent areas may be reduced to facilitate the placement of a pocket-eliminating apically positioned surgical flap that establishes a maintainable gingival form.

Other periodontal surgical procedures may be performed to address gingival recession. The indications for such surgery include dentinal sensitivity, aesthetic complaints, or continuing recession. Many times these procedures are both arrestive and regenerative in character.

Additional periodontal surgical procedures may be performed to maximize the aesthetic results associated with new restorative dentistry. Examples include ridge augmentation and crown lengthening. Procedures performed for aesthetics alone are usually termed periodontal plastic surgery.

Phase III: Restorative Care. Restorative dentistry is performed in this phase. Ideally, periodontal and prosthetic dentists work together to design restorations that satisfy aesthetic, comfort, and functional needs without compromising future periodontal health.

Phase IV: Maintenance Care. Phase IV consists of periodontal maintenance (also termed recall or continuing care). The goal of periodontal maintenance is to prevent continued periodontal destruction. Maintenance care includes reexamination and assessment of the periodontal condition and patient self-care. It often includes an oral prophylaxis and may include periodontal debridement and other local therapies that target persistently inflamed sites. Phase IV is similar to Phase I in many ways and based on what's observed, may result in patients returning to Phase II or Phase III.

The frequency of periodontal maintenance visits is individualized and depends on the patient's periodontal status, medical condition, and self-care motivation and effectiveness. Regular periodontal maintenance care is especially important following surgical procedures to facilitate treatment success (DeVore et al., 1986).

Rapid Dental Hint

Tailor the appointment to the needs of the patient. Certain procedures may or may not be provided based on the individual's presentation at the time.

Box 19–4: Gingivitis

Probing depths of less than 4 mm; plaque and calculus present; no bone loss or mobility.

First appointment: 1 hour

- Comprehensive oral evaluation (new patients) or periodic oral evaluation (existing patients)—consisting of a medical and dental history update, head and neck examination, and oral cancer screening. Make referrals to appropriate physicians if necessary.

- Periodontal examination.

- Complete X-ray series, including vertical bitewings (new patients) or indicated radiographs (existing patients).

- Note and record sites that bleed on gentle probing.

- Oral hygiene instruction after staining for plaque and relating stained areas to bleeding sites.

- Full-mouth instrumentation.

- Nutritional counseling for the control of dental caries.

- Tobacco counseling for the control and prevention of oral disease, if indicated.

Second appointment: At least 45 minutes, scheduled 7 to 10 days after first appointment

- Review medical and dental history.

- Stain for plaque and record results.

- Note and record sites that bleed on gentle probing.

- Evaluate tissue response to previous treatment on a site-by-site basis. If inflammation persists, determine the cause. If plaque or calculus are present, debride the area(s) and reinforce oral hygiene. Adjunctive antimicrobial mouth rinses may be recommended.

- Reinforce plaque control instruction.

- Selective polishing, if indicated.

- Nutritional counseling for the control of dental caries, if needed.

- Fluoride application (varnish or other) for moderate or high caries risk individuals.

- Tobacco counseling for the control of oral disease, if needed.

- If gingival health has been achieved, a suitable maintenance interval is established (3 to 6 months), or after 7 to 10 days, a third appointment is scheduled if needed.

- Referral to periodontist, if necessary, with alternating maintenance visits planned.

Informed Consent

Before examination and treatment, the patient must give consent. For medicolegal reasons, **informed consent** is usually recorded using a document signed by the patient and the practitioner because any treatment provided without consent legally may constitute a battery. Furthermore, a valid consent requires that the patient be made reasonably knowledgeable about the risks and benefits associated with the proposed treatments, alternative treatments, as well as no treatment. Some individuals cannot execute a legally valid consent, including minor children.

For periodontal patients, the informed consent form should clearly reflect that the patient understands and accepts the need for periodontal maintenance and oral hygiene self-care.

Treatment Guidelines

The following treatment guidelines were written for new patients but can be adapted for existing patients. Although treatment-planning guidelines are helpful, it is important to remember that treatment must be tailored to each patient and can change for individual patients based on what's observed over time. Experience and the scientific literature have demonstrated that responses to therapy can vary from one patient to another or even in the same patient at different sites and at different times. Therefore, each patient may respond uniquely to the therapy provided.

This section contains guidelines for treating typical periodontal patients and patients with other periodontal conditions, including medication- and hormone-influenced gingivitis, gingivitis and periodontitis related to systemic conditions, aggressive periodontitis, and acute periodontal conditions.

As discussed previously, these guidelines include intensive and continual emphasis on self-care, self-care assessment (by the practitioner), and professional reassessments (of tissue status) on a site-by-site basis. For many patients, these are essential for long-term treatment success. Furthermore, the suggested time allowance for each appointment is subject to change based on the patient's response to care. Of course, these are only guidelines. The ultimate decision and responsibility for how to treat a patient rests with the individual practitioner.

Periodontal Health

Patients presenting with no bleeding on gentle probing and light to no supragingival plaque biofilm and calculus only require an oral prophylaxis (see Box 19–2). Subgingival root

Box 19–5: Slight (Mild) Chronic Periodontitis

Probing depths of 4 to 5 mm; clinical attachment loss (CAL) of 1 to 2 mm; slight horizontal bone loss (up to 20%); no mobility or furcation involvement; supra- and subgingival deposits; bleeding on probing.

First appointment: 1 hour

- Comprehensive oral evaluation (new patients) or periodic oral evaluation (existing patients)—consisting of a medical and a dental history update, head and neck examination, and oral cancer screening. Make referrals to appropriate physicians if necessary.

- Supragingival debridement, if needed, to facilitate a periodontal examination.

- Periodontal examination. Sites that bleed on probing should be recorded.

- Complete X-ray series, including vertical bitewings (new patients) or indicated radiographs (existing patients).

- Stain for plaque and relate stained areas to bleeding sites as part of oral hygiene instruction (patient learns cause and effect).

- Periodontal debridement by quadrant (use of local anesthesia is determined by the practitioner; local anesthesia is a big part of successful treatment).

- Adjunctive antimicrobial irrigation or mouth rinse, if indicated.

- Nutritional counseling for the control of dental caries.

- Tobacco counseling for the control and prevention of oral disease, if indicated.

- Application of desensitizing medicaments, if needed.

Second, third, and fourth appointments: At least 45 minutes (each scheduled 7 to 10 days after previous appointment)

- Review medical and dental history.

- Evaluate tissue response from previous treatment.

- Stain for plaque.

- Relate stained areas to any bleeding sites as part of oral hygiene instruction (patient learns cause and effect).

- Reinforce plaque biofilm-control instruction.

- Continue debridement procedures by quadrant.

- Nutritional counseling for the control of dental caries.

- Tobacco counseling for the control and prevention of oral disease, if indicated.

- Sustained, slow-release, local-delivery antimicrobials may be used at sites not fully responsive to self-care and

debridement (as long as clinical parameters are promptly reassessed and nonresponders are referred, this tactic should offer little or no risk).

- Application of desensitizing medicaments, if needed.

Fifth appointment (reevaluation of therapy): At least 45 minutes (scheduled 4 to 8 weeks after previous appointment) (Segelnick & Weinberg, 2006)

- Review medical and dental history.

- Evaluate tissue response from previous treatment.

- Oral and dental examination.

- Periodontal examination; record sites that bleed on probing.

- Stain for plaque and relate stained areas to any bleeding sites as part of oral hygiene instruction (patient learns cause and effect; sites that persist in bleeding on probing, despite not staining positive for supragingival plaque, suggest more aggressive therapy may be needed at that site).

- Coronal polishing, as indicated.

- Nutritional counseling, if needed.

- Fluoride application (varnish or other) for moderate or high caries risk individuals.

- Tobacco counseling, if indicated.

- Application of desensitizing medicaments, if needed.

At this time, the patient may be put on a suitable maintenance interval of every 2 to 4 months if inflammation appears arrested (e.g., no bleeding on probing from deep pockets at sites that patient is maintaining plaque-free) and there is no other reason to refer to a specialist (e.g., unresolved dentinal hypersensitivity, gingival recession, desire or need for periodontal plastic surgery). Over time, this interval can be increased in patients who remain inflammation-free.

If there are nonresponsive sites characterized by deep (4 mm or more) probing depths that bleed on probing or at sites of previous attachment loss, referral to or comanagement with the periodontist is appropriate. Given the potential for rapid loss of attachment at any susceptible site, a decision to engage in "watchful waiting" is ethically and legally problematic.

If bleeding on probing persists at shallower sites (gingivitis), the practitioner should reevaluate the patient's self-care techniques and remove any subgingival calculus from suspect sites. Bleeding at sites with shallow pockets that are being kept plaque-free by patients may indicate potentially serious systemic diseases. Referral to the periodontist is an option for these patients as well.

Box 19–6: Moderate Chronic Periodontitis

Probing depths of 6 to 7 mm; clinical attachment loss (CAL) of 3 to 4 mm; moderate horizontal/vertical bone loss (20% to 50%); mobility and early furcation involvement; supra- and subgingival deposits; bleeding on probing.

First appointment: 1 hour

- Comprehensive oral evaluation (new patients) or periodic oral evaluation (existing patients)—consisting of a medical and dental history update, head and neck examination, and oral cancer screening. Make referrals to appropriate physicians if necessary.

- Complete X-ray series, including vertical bitewings (new patients) or indicated radiographs (existing patients). Referral to the periodontist depends on the type and amount of bone loss.

- Supragingival debridement, if needed, to facilitate a periodontal examination.

- Periodontal examination. Sites that bleed on probing should be recorded.

- Stain for plaque and relate stained areas to bleeding sites as part of oral hygiene instruction (patient learns cause and effect).

- Nutritional counseling for the control of dental caries.

- Tobacco counseling for the control and prevention of oral disease, if indicated.

- Application of desensitizing medicaments, if needed.

Second, third, and fourth appointments: 1 hour (each scheduled 7 to 10 days after previous appointment)

- Review medical and dental history.

- Evaluate tissue response from previous treatment.

- Stain for plaque and relate stained areas to any bleeding sites as part of oral hygiene instruction (patient learns cause and effect; sites that persist in bleeding on probing, despite not staining positive for supragingival plaque, suggest more aggressive therapy may be needed at that site).

- Reinforce plaque biofilm-control instruction.

- Periodontal debridement by quadrant (local anesthesia may be indicated). Periodontal endoscopy may facilitate the success of this procedure.

- Recommend home adjunctive antimicrobial irrigation or mouth rinse, if indicated.

- Nutritional counseling for the control of dental caries.

- Tobacco counseling for the control and prevention of oral disease, if indicated.

- Application of desensitizing medicaments, if needed.

Fifth appointment (reevaluation of therapy): 1 hour (scheduled 4 to 8 weeks after previous appointment) (Segelnick & Weinberg, 2006)

- Review medical and dental history.

- Evaluate tissue response from previous treatment.

- Oral and dental examination.

- Periodontal examination; record sites that bleed on probing.

- Stain for plaque and relate stained areas to any bleeding sites as part of oral hygiene instruction (patient learns cause and effect; sites that persist in bleeding on probing, despite not staining positive for supragingival plaque, suggest more aggressive therapy may be needed at that site).

- Periodontal debridement by quadrant (local anesthesia may be indicated).

- Recommend home adjunctive antimicrobial irrigation or mouth rinse, if indicated.

- Sustained, slow-release, local-delivery antimicrobials may be used at nonresponsive sites. (If clinical parameters are promptly reassessed and nonresponders are referred, this tactic should offer little or no risk.)

- Coronal polishing, as indicated.

- Nutritional counseling, if needed.

- Fluoride application (varnish or other) for moderate or high caries risk individuals.

- Tobacco counseling, if indicated.

- Application of desensitizing medicaments, if needed.

At this time, the patient may be put on a suitable maintenance interval of 2 to 4 months if inflammation appears arrested (e.g., no bleeding on probing from deep pockets at sites that patient is maintaining plaque-free) and there is no other reason to refer to a specialist (e.g., unresolved dentinal hypersensitivity, gingival recession, desire or need for periodontal plastic surgery).

However, if bleeding on probing persists at sites with deeper (4 mm or more) probing depths or at sites of previous attachment loss, referral to the periodontist is indicated—probably for periodontal surgery at those sites. Persistent bleeding on probing at sites that the patient is keeping plaque-free suggests that the local cause of refractory inflammation hasn't been fully addressed. Persistent bleeding on probing at sites thought to be free of local etiological factors is suggestive of a number of serious systemic maladies. Such circumstances strongly suggest prompt referral to a specialist.

If no bleeding on probing is present and deep pockets persist, referral to the periodontist may be considered. Research suggests that deep pockets will not break down further if they repeatedly fail over time to demonstrate bleeding on probing. However, this should be viewed in light of other research showing that deeper pockets are more likely than shallower pockets to experience additional attachment loss due to periodontitis.

Box 19–7: Severe Chronic Periodontitis

Probing depths of more than 8 mm; clinical attachment loss (CAL) of > 5 mm; horizontal and vertical bone loss (> 50%); mobility and furcation involvement.

First appointment: 1 hour

- Comprehensive oral evaluation (new patients) or periodic oral evaluation (existing patients)—consisting of a medical and dental history update, head and neck examination, and oral cancer screening. Make referrals to appropriate physicians if necessary. If the patient does not want to be referred to the periodontist, document the refusal in the patient's chart.

- Complete X-ray series, including vertical bitewings (new patients) or indicated radiographs (existing patients). If severe bone loss and heavy deposits exist, consider immediate referral to the periodontist for legal ramifications. If it is decided that initial therapy is to be done in the general practitioner's office, the following steps should be performed.

- Supragingival debridement, if needed, to facilitate a periodontal examination.

- Periodontal examination. Sites that bleed on probing should be recorded.

- Stain for plaque and relate stained areas to bleeding sites as part of oral hygiene instruction (patient learns cause and effect).

- Nutritional counseling for the control of dental caries.

- Tobacco counseling for the control and prevention of oral disease.

- Application of desensitizing medicaments, if needed.

Second appointment: 1 hour (scheduled as soon as possible after initial visit)

- Review medical and dental history.

- Stain for plaque and relate stained areas to bleeding sites as part of oral hygiene instruction (patient learns cause and effect; sites that persist in bleeding on probing, despite not staining positive for supragingival plaque, suggest more aggressive therapy may be needed at that site).

- Reinforce plaque biofilm-control instruction.

- Periodontal debridement by quadrant (use of local anesthesia may be indicated).

- Recommend home adjunctive antimicrobial irrigation or mouth rinse, if indicated.

- Nutritional counseling for the control of dental caries.

- Tobacco counseling for the control and prevention of oral disease, if indicated.

- Application of desensitizing medicaments, if needed.

Third, fourth, and fifth appointments: 1 hour (scheduled every 7 to 10 days)

- Review medical and dental history.

- Evaluate tissue response from previous treatment.

- Stain for plaque and relate stained areas to bleeding sites as part of oral hygiene instruction (patient learns cause and effect; sites that persist in bleeding on probing, despite not staining positive for supragingival plaque, suggest more aggressive therapy may be needed at that site).

- Reinforce plaque-control instruction.

- Continue debridement procedures by quadrant. Using a periodontal endoscope may facilitate better access and improve the chances of treatment success.

- Recommend home adjunctive antimicrobial irrigation or mouth rinse, if indicated.

- Sustained, slow-release, local-delivery antimicrobials may be used at nonresponsive sites (if clinical parameters are promptly reassessed and nonresponders are referred, this tactic should offer little or no risk).

- Nutritional counseling for the control of dental caries.

- Tobacco counseling for the control and prevention of oral disease, if indicated.

- Application of desensitizing medicaments, if needed.

Sixth appointment (reevaluation of therapy): 1 hour (scheduled 4 to 8 weeks after previous appointment) (Segelnick & Weinberg, 2006)

- Review medical and dental history.

- Evaluate tissue response from previous treatment.

- Periodontal examination; record sites that bleed on probing.

- Stain for plaque and relate stained areas to bleeding sites as part of oral hygiene instruction (patient learns cause and effect).

- Reinforce plaque-control instruction.

- Selective polishing, if indicated.

- Sustained, slow-release, local-delivery antimicrobials may be used at nonresponsive sites (if clinical parameters are promptly reassessed and nonresponders are referred, this tactic should offer little or no risk).

- Nutritional counseling for the control of dental caries.

- Fluoride application (varnish or other) for moderate or high caries risk individuals.

- Tobacco counseling for the control and prevention of oral disease, if indicated.

- Application of desensitizing medicaments, if needed.
- At this time, referral to the periodontist is necessary for legal ramifications.

Only rarely will the procedures outlined here result in resolution of inflammation in pockets deeper than 8 mm. (If successful, treat as for moderate chronic periodontitis.)

Therefore, these patients are often referred early on to a periodontist. Many periodontal patients have areas that vary from severe periodontitis to mere gingivitis. Good treatment results may be observed at some sites and not others. The worst-performing site(s) is what determines the need for referral or nonreferral—one or more such sites define a patient as refractory.

Box 19–8: Refractory Periodontitis (Nonresponsive Cases)

The patient does not fully or partially respond to conventional therapy.

First appointment: 1 hour

- Comprehensive oral evaluation (new patients) or periodic oral evaluation (existing patients)—consisting of a medical and dental history update, head and neck examination, and oral cancer screening. If this is an existing patient and previous treatment in the office has been ineffective, immediate referral to the periodontist is appropriate.
- If the patient does not want to be referred to the periodontist and wants treatment in the general practitioner's office, document the patient's informed refusal in the chart.
- Complete X-ray series, including vertical bitewings (new patients) or indicated radiographs (existing patients). If severe bone loss and heavy deposits, consider immediate referral to a periodontist for legal ramifications. Even though referral is indicated, if it is decided that therapy is to be done in the general practitioner's office, the following steps should be performed.
- Supragingival debridement, if needed, to facilitate periodontal examination.
- Periodontal examination. Sites that bleed on probing should be recorded.
- Stain for plaque and relate stained areas to bleeding sites as part of oral hygiene instruction (patient learns cause and effect; sites that persist in bleeding on probing, despite not staining positive for supragingival plaque, suggest that the etiology at that site has not been fully addressed.
- Periodontal debridement by quadrant (use of local anesthesia is determined by the practitioner) in conjunction

with systemic antibiotics (four to five appointments). A periodontal endoscope may facilitate better outcomes.

- Consider adjunctive diagnostic/bacteriologic tests (e.g., genetic test, culture, DNA probe).
- Nutritional counseling for the control of dental caries.
- Tobacco counseling for the control and prevention of oral disease, if indicated.
- Application of desensitizing medicaments, if needed.
- Referral to a periodontist.

Third, fourth, and fifth appointments: 1 hour (scheduled every 7 to 10 days)

- Review medical and dental history.
- Evaluate tissue response from previous treatment.
- Chart sites that bleed on gentle probing.
- Stain for plaque and relate stained areas to bleeding sites as part of oral hygiene instruction (patient learns cause and effect).
- Reinforce plaque-control instruction.
- Continue debridement procedures by quadrant.
- Nutritional counseling for the control of dental caries.
- Fluoride application (varnish or other) for moderate or high caries risk individuals.
- Tobacco counseling for the control and prevention of oral disease, if indicated.
- Application of desensitizing medicaments, if needed.

These patients are best treated by a periodontist.

debridement is contraindicated. Once oral hygiene efficacy is ensured, a suitable periodontal maintenance schedule is determined, usually every 6 to 12 months.

The motivated and periodontally healthy patient is often "dentally aware." Indeed, past dental therapy may be responsible for the healthy state the patient now enjoys. Such patients generally like discussing new advancements in dentistry. They usually welcome improvements in professional care and self-care and may question the practitioner about new treatment concepts. Oral hygiene instruction time may be used to discuss new oral hygiene products and their applications. The patient must be reminded of the need for future examinations (because problems may occur even though the patient currently appears healthy).

Gingival Diseases

DENTAL-PLAQUE-INDUCED GINGIVITIS Most cases of gingivitis are plaque-related and are best treated by instrumentation and oral hygiene instructions (see Box 19–4). Dental-plaque-induced gingival diseases can be related to dental plaque only or can be modified by systemic factors, medications, or malnutrition (Armitage, 1999). An example of a dental-plaque-induced gingival disease modified by systemic factors is hormone-associated gingivitis. Pregnancy, oral contraceptives, and puberty can contribute to gingival inflammation. Treatment of hormone-influenced gingivitis is aimed at lowering dental biofilm levels by maintaining meticulous oral hygiene. Frequent periodontal maintenance also may help.

With all cases of gingivitis, the therapeutic goal is to establish gingival health by eliminating the etiologic factors. The ultimate objective is to prevent sites from progressing to periodontitis, and initial periodontal debridement and oral hygiene instructions are the key to minimizing microbial plaque accumulation.

Because we are unable to predict which sites will progress, the entire mouth must be treated. Patients need to be aware of the need for adequate toothbrushing and the use of interdental cleaning aids. Supplemental use of antimicrobial agents (e.g., as mouth rinses or used as home irrigation agents) is recommended in certain patients, such as those with severe bleeding that interferes with debridement procedures or those with poor manual dexterity. Following treatment, the patient is placed on a well-monitored periodontal maintenance program.

For all types of gingival diseases, sulcular sites that bleed on gentle probing should be noted and recorded and pointed out to the patient. Plaque staining will reveal areas of dental biofilm accumulation. These should be recorded as well. Bleeding often occurs at these sites. The patient needs to understand this relationship. The patient also needs to appreciate that if a site bleeds as a result of self-care, that site usually needs more self-care attention, not less. This runs counter to the intuition of most patients, whose common response to bleeding is to "leave the area alone."

If the patient is taught to understand that the destructive process is at an early stage and that proper professional care and self-care likely will return the tissues to health, treatment is more likely to succeed. Involve your patients as cotherapists.

NON-PLAQUE-INDUCED GINGIVAL DISEASES This category of gingival diseases was included in the latest classification of periodontal diseases and conditions (Armitage, 1999). It includes gingival conditions where the primary etiologic agent is not dental plaque biofilm, but where plaque biofilm is a modifying factor. These include gingival diseases of bacterial, viral, fungal, and genetic origin. Also included are manifestations of systemic conditions, traumatic lesions, and foreign body reactions. One of the more commonly encountered non-plaque-induced gingival diseases is drug-induced gingival disease.

DRUG-INDUCED GINGIVAL DISEASE Gingival enlargement is sometimes seen in patients taking certain medications. Removal of dental plaque biofilm and calculus by meticulous oral hygiene and regular professional mechanical debridement may help to prevent or slow gingival overgrowth. Therefore, initial treatment should focus on improved self-care and professional plaque and calculus removal. Unfortunately, gingival enlargement still may occur, making it difficult to perform effective self-care and may even interfere with chewing, speech, and appearance. For patients with drug-induced gingival enlargement, overgrowth usually requires surgical intervention. Recurrence is common if the drug is continued. Therefore, it is important to inform the patient's physician about the oral condition and inquire if an alternative drug could be prescribed.

Gingival overgrowth may also be seen in patients with orthodontic appliances. For orthodontic patients, surgical removal of fibrotic pseudopockets can be performed at any time, but recurrence is likely if orthodontic appliances remain.

Periodontitis

The current list of periodontitis classifications includes chronic, aggressive periodontitis as a manifestation of systemic conditions; necrotizing periodontal diseases; abscesses of the periodontium; periodontitis associated with endodontic lesions; and developmental or acquired deformities and conditions (Armitage, 1999). Chronic periodontitis (formerly termed adult periodontitis) is the most common form of periodontitis seen in otherwise healthy patients. Aggressive periodontitis (formerly termed early-onset periodontitis) is less common but more difficult to treat and should be referred to the periodontist. A brief overview of chronic, aggressive, and necrotizing diseases follows as well as peri-implantitis. Other chapters cover these conditions in greater detail.

CHRONIC PERIODONTITIS In general, the treatment of patients with chronic periodontitis begins with oral hygiene instructions and periodontal debridement, followed by surgical therapy if needed. Patients are then monitored, and treatment is modified as necessary as part of an ongoing periodontal maintenance program. Repeated surgeries sometimes are necessary.

Periodontal patients who demonstrate attachment loss and probing pocket depths of 4 to 5 mm (slight periodontitis) often respond adequately (e.g., elimination of bleeding on probing) to meticulous periodontal debridement and effective oral self-care (see Box 19–5). In moderate periodontitis (attachment loss with probing depths of 6 to 7 mm; see Box 19–6) and severe periodontitis (attachment loss with probing depths of more than 8 mm; see Box 19–7), periodontal debridement is less predictable (Stambaugh, Dragoo, Smith, & Carasali, 1981). Following oral hygiene instruction and periodontal debridement, such patients are usually referred to the periodontist—often for periodontal surgery at nonresponsive sites.

Patients with gingival recession should be evaluated. If the recession causes tooth pain, is progressing, or interferes with aesthetics, gingival grafting may be indicated. Sometimes watchful waiting is a useful approach. Intraoral photography can be useful to help compare changes over time.

It should be noted that chronic periodontitis is site-specific. Some patients demonstrate clinical attachment loss and/or probing depths that are normal at some sites, suggestive of slight periodontitis at other sites, and indicative of moderate or severe periodontitis at others. Therefore, periodontal debridement and improved self-care may be adequate at some sites but inadequate at others in the same patient. The most problematic sites guide ideal patient management. In other words, the persistence of even one diseased site is sufficient to justify referral for more aggressive therapy. Locally applied antibiotics are sometimes used in conjunction with periodontal debridement and can produce short-term improvements in clinical parameters. However, it remains unclear how often or how successful this approach may be over longer periods of time.

Refractory periodontal patients who do not respond to proper periodontal treatment (see Box 19–8) despite quality self-care and participation in a well-monitored periodontal maintenance program should be referred to a periodontist.

AGGRESSIVE PERIODONTITIS Apparently healthy young people (younger than 30 years of age) can have underlying immune system irregularities that may manifest as periodontitis with rapid attachment loss and bone destruction (American Academy of Periodontology, 2003; Tonetti & Mombelli, 1999). Treatment of this type of periodontitis is similar to that for chronic forms of periodontitis except that surgical intervention and/or antibiotic therapy often are used immediately. Therefore, these patients should be referred promptly to a periodontist.

Necrotizing Periodontal Diseases

Necrotizing ulcerative gingivitis (NUG) and necrotizing ulcerative periodontitis (NUP) are collectively referred to as necrotizing periodontal diseases. Necrotizing ulcerative gingivitis (NUG) is an infection localized to the gingiva. Contributory risk factors include emotional stress, poor oral hygiene, cigarette smoking, and HIV infections (Rowland, 1999). NUP involves the attachment apparatus and is seen primarily in individuals with systemic conditions including, but not limited to, HIV infection, severe malnutrition, and immunosuppression (Novak, 1999). Treatment includes periodontal debridement and analgesics. Because NUG and primary herpetic gingivostomatis often occur in young adults, clinicians need to be able to discriminate between the two insofar as the herpes infection is highly contagious. Because both NUG and primary herpes cause gingivitis, the most reliable way to rule out herpes is to look for small round ulcerations on the hard palate. The presence of such ulcerations indicates a herpetic infection as would ulcerations on the lips. Very rarely, herpes infection and NUG occur simultaneously, probably with the herpetic infection setting the state for NUG. Although a key therapeutic approach to NUG includes debridement, patients with oral herpetic infections should not be debrided. Referral to a periodontist may be indicated for treatment of NUG or to help rectify any resulting untoward potentially permanent periodontal effects.

Peri-Implantitis

Treatment of peri-implant diseases may include periodontal debridement, oral hygiene instructions, mouth rinses, systemic antibiotics, arrestive and regenerative periodontal surgery, and/or implant removal. Referral to a periodontist is recommended.

Prognosis

Prognosis is a prediction of the future course of a malady with or without treatment. All aspects of the patient's history, data from the clinical examination, and the patient's healing capacity are factors.

Common clinical factors used in assigning a prognosis are reviewed in Box 19–9 (McGuire & Nunn, 1996). This checklist can be reviewed as part of developing a prognosis for each patient. The more unfavorable factors noted, the worse the prognosis. Furthermore, prognosis determination and risk assessment help develop a more appropriate treatment plan both before and after active therapy.

Prognosis is usually reported using a graded scale. This may be a simple scale such as good, guarded, or poor or a scale with more intervals such as good, fair, poor, questionable, or hopeless (Box 19–10; McGuire & Nunn, 1996).

Determination of prognosis is important in treatment planning so that the practitioner and patient can agree on a plan that best satisfies the patient's overall goals while minimizing disappointments if setbacks occur. Realistic prognoses are of amplified importance in complex cases that combine periodontal and restorative therapies. This is because in these patients, the unexpected loss of a key abutment tooth may necessitate replacement of complicated and expensive crown and bridge prosthetics.

Box 19–9: Individual Tooth and Overall Periodontal Diagnosis: Signs and Symptoms

Factors involved with individual tooth prognosis

- Probing depths
- Amount of alveolar bone remaining (not lost)
- Pathologic tooth mobility (and cause of mobility)
- Pattern of bone destruction (horizontal, vertical— and number of bony walls remaining)
- Root anatomy (short or long roots; tapered or bulbous)
- Crown: root ratio
- Pulp involvement: tooth restorability
- Furcation defects; location

Factors involved with overall (entire mouth) prognosis

- Age of patient (younger has worse prognosis)
- Medical history involvement (systemic diseases)
- Smoking
- Family history of periodontal disease (genetics)
- Oral home care (adherence)

Box 19–10: Classification of Prognosis of Teeth

- Good prognosis: Not much periodontal destruction including probing depths so that the sites can be easily maintained by the patient and the clinician.
- Fair prognosis: Once a furcation defect occurs the tooth as a fair prognosis; Class I defect that can be easily maintained. About 75% of bone remains around the tooth.
- Poor prognosis: Approximately 50% of bone remains around the tooth; Class II furcation defects that may become more difficult to maintain.
- Questionable prognosis: Less than 50% of bone remains around the tooth; Class III furcation defects are present; cannot be maintained with possible extraction.
- Hopeless prognosis: No bony support remains and tooth must be extracted.

Use of mouth rinses is an adjunct to oral self-care and should not be as a substitute.

Geriatric Patients

Although the same general guidelines already provided for chronic periodontitis patients apply to the elderly, geriatric patients often have special needs. They may present with uncontrolled dental plaque biofilm and/or xerostomia. Other oral pathologies, including oral cancers, are more common among members of this age group.

Plaque Control

Age-related factors may limit the ability of a patient to perform adequate oral self-care. Using a toothbrush or dental floss may be impossible for patients with arthritis or stroke-related impairments. Dementia may affect an individual's ability or motivation to perform daily oral hygiene procedures. Virtually any debilitating systemic illness may predispose patients to periodontitis—and many of these maladies are seen more commonly in aged populations. Most important, periodontal treatment may be complicated by multiple medical conditions.

Xerostomia

Decreased saliva production occurs with advancing age (Ghezzi & Ship, 2003). Furthermore, many of the hundreds of medications known to decrease salivary flow are used by older people. Antidepressants, antihistamines, antihypertensives, antipsychotics, diuretics, antiparkinsonians, and antianxiety agents all may contribute to xerostomia (Brangan, 1994). Older patients, with decreased protective properties of saliva, are at increased risk for dental caries and periodontal diseases (Rees, 1998).

If a patient complains of xerostomia, or if dryness seems to be contributing to oral problems, relevant systemic

Adjunctive Treatment

Antimicrobials

Systemic antibiotics often are prescribed as part of the treatment of aggressive periodontitis or of periodontitis patients with systemic maladies. For example, administration of a systemic antibiotic, debridement, and surgery constitute an appropriate course of therapy for a patient with a localized aggressive periodontitis. Systemic antibiotics are not generally used in patients with chronic periodontitis or gingivitis. In the case of refractory periodontal diseases, systemic antibiotics are commonly utilized.

The regimens governing the use of systemic antibiotics in patients with periodontitis are frequently changing. Therefore, clinicians who consider using systemic antimicrobials to treat aggressive and refractory periodontitis must remain very up-to-date with the appropriate biomedical literature.

Controlled-release antimicrobial drug systems as supplements to periodontal debridement may be indicated when clinical signs of inflammation (bleeding on probing) persist in pockets of 5 mm or greater at localized sites. However, continuing reassessment is needed to determine if other therapies are indicated.

Chlorhexidine gluconate rinses are prescribed frequently for specified periods when mechanical plaque control is not feasible (e.g., after surgery, after acute infection). Antimicrobial rinses are not indicated in patients with periodontitis because rinses are only delivered supragingivally.

medications should be identified and alternatives considered. Saliva substitutes may be recommended, but these have limited effectiveness and can be expensive. Antimicrobial rinses may make sense in these patients as do fluoride-containing mouth rinses aimed at inhibiting dental caries either on crowns or exposed tooth roots.

Treatment Considerations

When treating geriatric patients, the practitioner must consider systemic concerns that may complicate the management of periodontal conditions. It may be important for the dentist and hygienist to consult with a patient's physician to review pertinent details of the patient's medical conditions.

Treatment goals for the elderly are the same as for the young, that is, the preservation (or restoration) of an aesthetic, comfortable, and functional dentition. This is not to suggest that age should not be a factor in planning how best to achieve these goals; indeed, conservative therapy may be more appropriate in older patients for a number of reasons. Whatever treatment is planned, it should be flexible and adapted to each patient's particular needs. As these needs change, so should the therapy.

Successful treatment of the elderly often requires a high degree of cooperation between the practitioner, patient, and other supporting caregivers. Modified self-care routines may be necessary, such as use of a toothpick or interdental brush instead of floss, a toothbrush with a modified handle such as a tennis ball, and the frequent use of antimicrobial agents (such as fluorides or chlorhexidine) along with mechanical plaque control. Automated oral hygiene devices may facilitate more effective plaque control.

Dental Hygiene Application

Research supports the majority of procedures routinely performed by the dental hygienist to prevent or arrest the progression of the common periodontal maladies. Science, combined with clinical experience and inferential skills, has produced the periodontal parameters of care for today. As time passes, continued scientific testing of new and old therapeutic tactics along with clinical experience will continue to underpin future parameters for periodontal care.

Periodontal treatment planning remains complicated. For now, ongoing periodontal care should be modulated based on the response of the patient to self-care and treatment rendered previously. If a desired and optimal response is not achieved, another reasonable approach must be considered and assessed. Critical analyses of outcomes will sometimes suggest that referral to a specialist is in the best interest of the patient.

Quality assessment has been defined as "a measure of care provided in a particular setting" (Burt & Eklund, 1992). Quality assurance is a broader concept that encompasses assessment of care along with the "implementation of any necessary changes to either maintain or improve the quality of care rendered" (Burt & Eklund, 1992).

Dental hygienists have the professional responsibility to promote the oral health of the public in the most effective ways possible. As excerpted from the American Dental Hygienists Association's (2007–2008) Code of Ethics*, "We acknowledge the following responsibilities to patients or clients:

- Provide oral health care utilizing high levels of professional knowledge, judgment, and skill.
- Maintain a work environment that minimizes the risk of harm.
- Serve all clients without discrimination and avoid action toward any individual or group that may be interpreted as discriminatory.
- Hold professional client relationships confidential.
- Communicate with clients in a respectful manner.
- Promote ethical behavior and high standards of care by all dental hygienists.
- Serve as an advocate for the welfare of clients.
- Provide clients with the information necessary to make informed decisions about their oral health and encourage their full participation in treatment decisions and goals.
- Refer clients to other healthcare providers when their needs are beyond our ability or scope of practice.
- Educate clients about high-quality oral heath care."

Key Points

- Evidence-based periodontal treatment based on dental literature focuses on the recognition of risk, prognosis, and treatment factors.
- The evidence-based approach is a good model for evaluating the results of periodontal therapy; however, as is the case in many biomedical fields, research is limited.
- Problem-based learning identifies a patient's dental problems.

- The ideal goal of periodontal therapy is to restore the periodontium destroyed by disease to a comfortable and functional state of health.
- Periodontal treatment involves ongoing care and demands continued reassessments.

*Reprinted by permission of the American Dental Hygienist Association.

Self-Quiz

1. Which one of the following factors improves the treatment decisions made by dental/medical practitioners?
   a. Clinical experience of the practitioner and use of scientific literature
   b. Following the advice of fellow dental practitioners
   c. Following the advice of fellow medical practitioners
   d. Consulting with the dental companies

2. Which one of the following statements is the ideal goal of periodontal therapy?
   a. Control or eliminate and prevent the initiation, progression, or recurrence of periodontal diseases.
   b. Promote tissue healing by regeneration or replacement of the lost tissue with new bone, cementum, and periodontal ligament.
   c. Restore the periodontium to an attractive, comfortable, and functional state of health for the balance of the patient's life.
   d. Allow the attachment apparatus to relax.
   e. Remove all microbial plaque every day.

3. Which one of the following steps should be first in developing a plan to treat a patient?
   a. Teach proper use of oral hygiene aids.
   b. Perform risk assessment.
   c. Discuss the case with the patient.
   d. Decide on the proper maintenance interval.
   e. Obtain informed consent for periodontal maintenance.

4. All of the following are phases of treatment except one. Which one is the exception?
   a. Phase I: disease control
   b. Phase II: surgical correction
   c. Phase III: restorative/prosthetic care
   d. Phase IV: maintenance care
   e. Phase V: implant care

5. In which one of the following phases of treatment is reevaluation of initial therapy completed?
   a. I
   b. II
   c. III
   d. IV
   e. V

6. Which one of the following treatment steps is most appropriate in controlling pregnancy-associated gingivitis?
   a. Surgical intervention
   b. Oral irrigation with chlorhexidine
   c. Plaque control with toothbrushing and flossing
   d. Systemic antibiotics
   e. Estrogen supplements

7. Which one of the following treatments is most appropriate for patients with localized aggressive periodontitis?
   a. Periodontal debridement, systemic antibiotics, and surgery
   b. Periodontal debridement and surgery
   c. Oral rinsing and periodontal debridement
   d. Oral irrigation and periodontal debridement
   e. Improved oral hygiene and watchful waiting

8. Which one of the following sequences is the best initial treatment for a patient with gingival enlargement caused by phenytoin?
   a. Oral hygiene instructions, periodontal debridement, systemic antibiotics, and surgery
   b. Oral hygiene instructions and periodontal debridement
   c. Periodontal debridement and systemic antibiotics
   d. Periodontal debridement and surgery
   e. Discontinuation of phenytoin

9. Which one of the following definitions best describes the term *prognosis*?
   a. Prediction of the future course of a condition with or without treatment
   b. Prediction of the future course of a condition without treatment
   c. Identification and naming of the type of condition present
   d. Patient's healing capacity

10. Which one of the following is the most important consideration when treating geriatric patients?
    a. Therapy may be complicated by multiple medical conditions.
    b. The ability to properly understand oral hygiene instructions may be impaired.
    c. Anxiety level is higher in this age group.
    d. Severe frailty inhibits normal maneuvering in the dental office.
    e. Physical impairments are possible.

Case Study

A 35-year-old male is scheduled with the dental hygienist in a general practice dental office. The patient has probing depths to 7 mm in the molar region and clinical attachment loss of 4 mm in some areas. There is moderate horizontal bone loss and a few areas of vertical bone loss on the maxillary molars. There is both supra and subgingival plaque and calculus and some bleeding upon probing. The periodontal classification is moderate chronic periodontitis.

1. The dental hygienist is planning a first series of non-surgical care before re-assessment for further therapies. The first visit would include which of the following procedures?
   a. scaling and root planning of maxillary arch
   b. comprehensive data collection, radiographs if indicated, and oral hygiene instruction
   c. ultrasonic scaling entire mouth and polishing
   d. ultrasonic scaling mandibular right quadrant

Answer: B. Before any scaling is performed a complete medical, dental, periodontal and radiographic assessment is completed and evaluated for patient risks, diagnosis, and prognosis.

2. How should the following visits be scheduled to remove the deposits?
   a. 4 visits to scale each quadrant
   b. 2 visits to scale each arch
   c. 5 visits to scale by quadrant and return to evaluate healing
   d. 3 visits more to scale by arch and return to polish and fluoride

Answer: C. Although it depends upon patient response the plan should include quadrant scaling at 7–10 day intervals to allow for healing and re-evaluation before the last visit at 4–8 weeks after previous appointment to evaluate tissue response.

3. The dental hygienist evaluated the tissue after all scaling and root planning has occurred. At this visit there is still bleeding upon probing and the pocket depth has not improved. What is considered as the next phase?
   a. Do a deep scaling of the areas by hand instead of ultrasonic
   b. Recall patient in four months to re-assess
   c. Provide fluoride and anti-microbial rinses
   d. Refer to a periodontist for co-management

Answer: D. Referral is indicated when there is unresolved inflammation at any site, the age of the patient at 35 years old, and CAL as indicated. Other adjunctive therapies might have been included in the previous appointments; however, if inflammation persists, other surgical treatment may be required.

References

American Academy of Periodontology. 2000a. Parameters of care. *J. Periodontol.* 71 (Suppl.):847–883.

American Academy of Periodontology. 2000b. Parameter on periodontal maintenance. *J. Periodontol.* 71:849–850.

American Academy of Periodontology. 2001. Academy Report: Treatment of plaque induced gingivitis, chronic periodontitis, and other clinical conditions. *J. Periodontol.* 72:1790–1800.

American Academy of Periodontology. 2003. Position paper: Periodontal diseases of children and adolescents. *J. Periodontol.* 74:1696–1704.

American Academy of Periodontology. 2006. Guidelines for the management of patients with periodontal diseases. *J. Periodontol.* 77:1607–1611.

American Academy of Periodontology. 2008. Position paper: Risk assessment. *J. Periodontol.* 79:202.

American Dental Hygienists' Association. 2007. *2007–2008 Bylaws and code of ethics.* Chicago: Author.

Armitage, G. 1999. Development of a classification system for periodontal diseases and conditions. *Ann. Periodontol.* 4: 1–6.

Axelsson, P., and J. Lindhe. 1981. The significance of maintenance care in the treatment of periodontal disease. *J. Clin. Periodontol.* 8:281–294.

Axelsson, P., B. Nystrom, and J. Lindhe. 2004. The long-term effect of a plaque control program on tooth mortality, caries, and periodontal disease in adults: Results after 30 years of maintenance. *J. Clin. Periodontol.* 31(9):749–57.

Brangan, P. 1994. Dental hygiene care for the older adult. In eds. M. L. Darby and M. Walsh, *Dental hygiene theory and practice*, 873–912. Philadelphia: W. B. Saunders.

Burt, B., and S. Eklund. 1992. *Dentistry, dental practice and the community*. Philadelphia: W. B. Saunders.

DeVore, C. H., D. M. Duckworth, F. M. Beck, M. J. Hicks, F. W. Brumfield, and J. E. Horton. 1986. Bone loss following periodontal therapy in subjects without frequent periodontal maintenance. *J. Periodontol.* 57:354–359.

Dockter, K. M., K. B. Williams, K. S. Bray, et al. 2006. Relationship between prereferral periodontal care and periodontal status at time of referral. *J. Periodontol.* 77:1708–1716.

Douglass, C. W. 2006. Risk assessment and management of peri-odontal disease. *JADA* 137(3):27S–32S.

Froum, S. J., M. A. Weinberg, and D. Tarnow. 1998. Compari-son of bioactive glass and open debridement. *J. Periodontol.* 68:698–709.

Ghezzi, E. M., and J. A. Ship. 2003. Aging and secretory reserve capacity of major salivary glands. *J. Dent. Res.* (October) 82(10):844–848.

Grossi, S. G., R. J. Genco, E. E. Machtei, A. W. Ho, G. Koch, et al. 1995. Assessment of risk for periodontal disease: II. Risk indi-cators for alveolar bone loss. *J. Periodontol.* 66:23–29.

Grossi, S. G., J. J. Zambon, A. W. Ho, G. Koch, R. G. Dunford, et al. 1994. Assessment of risk for periodontal disease: I. Risk indicators for attachment loss. *J. Periodontol.* 65:260–267.

Haffajee, A. D., and S. S. Socransky. 2006. Introduction to micro-bial aspects of periodontal biofilm communities, development and treatment. *Periodontology 2000* 42(1):7–12.

Haffajee, A. D., S. S. Socransky, J. Lindhe, R. L. Kent, H. Okamoto, and T. Yoneyama. 1991. Clinical risk indicators for periodontal attachment loss. *J. Clin. Periodontol.* 18:117–125.

Hancock, E. B. 1996. Prevention. *Ann. Periodontol.* 1:223–249.

Ismail, A. I., E. C. Morrison, B. A. Burt, R. G. Caffesse, and M. T. Kavanagh. 1990. Natural history of periodontal disease in adults: Findings from the Tecumseh Periodontal Disease Study, 1959–1987. *J. Dent. Res.* 69:430–435.

Kolenbrander, P. E., R. J. Palmer, A. H. Rickard, et al. 2006. Bac-terial interactions and successions during plaque development. *Periodontology 2000* 52(1):47–79.

Lindhe, J., E. Westfelt, S. Nyman, S. S. Socransky, I. L. Heij, and G. Bratthall. 1984. Long-term effect of surgical/nonsurgical treatment of periodontal disease. *J. Clin. Periodontol.* 11:448–458.

Loesche, W. 1976. Chemotherapy of dental plaque infections. *Oral Sci. Rev.* 9:65–107.

McGuire, K. M., and M. E. Nunn. 1996. Prognosis versus actual outcome: II. The effectiveness of clinical parameters in devel-oping an accurate prognosis. *J. Periodontol.* 67:658–665.

Novak, M. J. 1999. Necrotizing ulcerative periodontitis. *Ann. Periodontol.* 4:74–77.

Page, R. C., J. Martin, E. A. Krall, L. Mancl, and R. Garcia. 2003. Longitudinal validation of a risk calculator for periodontal disease. *J. Clin. Periodontol.* 30(9):819–827.

Persson, G. R., L. A. Mancl, J. Martin, and R. C. Page. 2003. Assessing periodontal disease risk: A comparison of clinicians' assessment versus a computerized tool. *J. Am. Dent. Assoc.* (May) 134(5):575–82.

Pihlstrom, B., R. McHugh, T. Oliphant, and C. Ortiz-Campos. 1983. Comparison of surgical and nonsurgical treatment of periodontal disease: A review of current studies and additional results after 6 1/2 years. *J. Clin. Periodontol.* 10:524–541.

Ramfjord, S. P., R. G. Caffesse, E. C. Morrison, R. W. Hill, G. J. Kerry, et al. 1987. Four modalities of periodontal treat-ment compared over 5 years. *J. Clin. Periodontol.* 14:445–452.

Rees, T. D. 1998. Drugs and oral disorders. *Periodontol 2000* 18:21–36.

Rowland, R. W. 1999. Necrotizing ulcerative gingivitis. *Ann. Periodontol.* 4:65–73.

Segelnick, S., and M. A. Weinberg. 2006. Reevaluation after initial therapy. When is the appropriate time? *J. Periodontol.* (September) 77(9):1598–601.

Stambaugh, R. V., M. Dragoo, D. M. Smith, and L. Carasali. 1981. The limits of subgingival scaling. *Int. J. Periodont. Restor. Dent.* 1(5):31–41.

Tonetti, M. S., and A. Mombelli. 1999. Early-onset periodontitis. *Ann. Periodontol.* 4:39–52.

Van Dyke, T. 2007. Control of inflammation and periodontitis. *Periodontology 2000* 45(1):158–166.

Van Dyke, T. E., and C. N. Serhan, 2003. Resolution of inflam-mation: A new paradigm for the pathogenesis of periodontal diseases. *J. Dent. Res.* 82(2): 82–90.

Visit www.pearsonhighered.com/healthprofessionsresources to access the student resources that accompany this book. Simply select Dental Hygiene from the choice of disciplines. Find this book and you will find the complimentary study tools created for this specific title.

20

Oral Hygiene for the Periodontal Patient: Beyond the Basics

Judith Kreismann and Khalid Almas

OUTLINE

EDUCATIONAL OBJECTIVES

Upon completion of this chapter, the reader should be able to:

- Describe measures to prevent and control the progression of periodontal diseases.
- Introduce protocols for different types of hygiene care recommended to the patient with periodontal diseases.
- Discuss the consideration of the patients' goals for their oral and systemic health.
- Discuss the importance of interdental cleaning in maintaining periodontal health.
- Discuss the significance of halitosis; how to control, and cure, and the role of the dental hygienist in patient care.
- Describe the standards for plaque-control regimen following periodontal and implant surgery.

GOAL: To provide information about the fundamentals of counseling patients with periodontal disease on oral hygiene self-care.

KEY WORDS

Introduction

There is no alternative to well-performed oral hygiene self-care as a preventive measure. The willingness and ability of patients to keep dental plaque below the threshold for disease is essential. Preventive measures are important for a healthy periodontium as well as to achieve a successful outcome of periodontal therapy. Preventive measures in periodontics depend on the removal of supra- and subgingival dental plaque biofilm. The most common preventive methods involve both personal and professional mechanical plaque control. Preventive measures should control or eliminate etiologic factors as well as eliminate risk factors for inflammatory periodontal diseases (Hancock, 1996). The control of supragingival plaque in conjunction with professional tooth cleaning subgingivally forms the basis for the management of progressive periodontal diseases (Corbet & Davies, 1993). Supragingival plaque control contributes to preventing or moderating subgingival microbial recolonization. This chapter focuses on fundamental information related to oral hygiene self-care for the periodontal patient.

Definition of Oral Hygiene Self-Care

Oral hygiene self-care, also known as oral physiotherapy or oral home care, is defined as physical therapy for the mouth or oral cavity. It refers to daily oral healthcare practices employed by the patient to prevent dental and gingival diseases and maintain optimal oral health. The rationale for oral hygiene self-care as well as professional periodontal debridement is to eliminate or suppress harmful microorganisms found in supragingival biofilm. Consequently, plaque control prevents the potential detrimental effects of pathogenic microorganisms on the teeth and periodontium. The primary method of oral hygiene self-care is the use of such mechanical oral hygiene measures as a toothbrush and interdental cleaning devices. Because not all bacteria in biofilms are pathogenic (disease-producing), the objective of treatment is not total elimination of all bacteria but rather control of the bacteria.

Periodontal Health: Motivation and Behavior

Because dental and periodontal health is taking on increasing importance for both patients and family members, evaluation of a patient's motivation and behavior in terms of oral self-care is important in the overall treatment plan.

In the process of evaluating a patient's oral hygiene, it is necessary to assess the clinical aspects of oral hygiene as well as relate the patient's attitude toward oral hygiene and his or her commitment to oral hygiene practices.

Did You Know?

In 200 CE, the Romans used a mixture of bones, eggshells, oyster shells, and honey to clean their teeth.

Periodontal Disease Control

It is well known that the accumulation of supragingival dental plaque on tooth surfaces near the free gingival margin is associated with the development of gingivitis. Thus, removal of dental plaque from tooth surfaces is a basic step in the prevention and treatment of gingivitis. Subgingival bacteria are derived from the supragingival dental plaque. If supragingival plaque is not removed, subgingival plaque develops. Subgingival bacteria play an important role in the progression of periodontal diseases. Therefore, meticulous mechanical supragingival plaque control can reduce the risk for the development of periodontitis or for disease recurrence after periodontal therapy or prevent further loss of attachment if periodontitis is already present (Addy & Adriaens, 1998; Westfelt, 1996). Clinical trials have shown that professionally delivered and frequently repeated supragingival tooth cleaning, combined with optimal self-performed plaque control, has a marked effect in controlling subgingival microbiota in moderate to deep periodontal pockets (Hellström, Romberg, Krok, & Lindhe, 1996).

Patient Education

Informing the periodontal patient about oral hygiene self-care is one of the most important roles of the dental hygienist. **Patient education** provides the patient with the necessary information and skills for the prevention of dental caries and periodontal diseases. A thorough knowledge of oral hygiene self-care is essential for dental hygienists to help plan successful preventive strategies related to a patient's individual plaque-control needs.

One way to highlight the presence of dental plaque is by using disclosing agents. The purpose of using disclosing tablets or liquid is for supragingival plaque detection. The most commonly used disclosing agent is erythrosin, which is FD & C Red No. 28. Erythrosin stains newly formed dental plaque, making it visible to the naked eye.

Oral hygiene instructions can be given personally by the dental hygienist, and/or the patient may be provided with a self-instruction manual, pamphlet, or videotape.

Preventive Measures

The primary goal of prevention is to achieve the lowest plaque level possible. Total elimination of bacteria is neither possible nor desirable because a number of beneficial bacteria exist in the oral cavity that are necessary for a balanced oral environment.

Preventive measures are classified into two main groups, depending on when mechanical plaque control is instituted during the disease process. **Primary prevention** describes preventive measures taken to prevent disease from occurring. It aims at reducing plaque in all individuals regardless of their susceptibility to disease. On the other hand, if periodontal disease is already present in an individual, the goal of treatment changes from preventing the occurrence of disease to preventing the disease from progressing further or preventing the recurrence of the disease after treatment. This is **secondary prevention** (Garmyn, van Steenberghe, & Quirynen, 1998).

Mechanical Plaque Control

Plaque control involves the regular removal of **oral or dental biofilms** from the teeth and adjacent oral tissues and the prevention of its accumulation. Because dental plaque may not be visible to the naked eye, patients may be unaware of it prior to disclosing. For this reason, a disclosing agent is recommended for patient education and prior to the patient's daily oral hygiene self-care regimen.

EVALUATION Exposure of plaque is a necessary first step in evaluation and can be accomplished with either disclosing tablets or liquid. Disclosing solutions show only gross changes and the quantity of stainable plaque. Disclosing agents do not differentiate between food and plaque, nor do they reveal the presence of microorganisms. The disclosing dye in the form of a solution or tablet absorbs into the dental plaque. The red solution does not contain FD&C red #3 or saccharin. The dental hygienist can use this visual resource to demonstrate the appropriate techniques of oral hygiene self-care to the patient. It is important to show the patient areas where plaque accumulates in proximity to the gingiva. Patients can self-disclose dental biofilms periodically to determine the effectiveness of their oral hygiene self-care techniques. However, merely teaching patients about the use of disclosing agents in their dental health education instruction is frequently not sufficient to motivate them to clean their teeth more effectively. Visual feedback may play an important part in health education. Photographs can be taken before treatment and after treatment to show the patient the results.

Oral Hygiene Self-Care Methods

Proper oral hygiene self-care accomplishes plaque control, improves appearance, refreshes the breath, and provides a sense of oral cleanliness. The oral hygiene plan designed for the patient should be based on the patient's specific oral hygiene needs. Numerous mechanical cleansing devices, including toothbrushes and interdental aids, are available commercially in today's highly competitive product market. The dental hygienist should be familiar with the particular characteristics of each product to make an appropriate recommendation for each patient. Oral health promotions can improve oral hygiene and gingival health (Watt & Marinho, 2005).

Toothbrushes

MANUAL TOOTHBRUSHES: DESIGN Clinical evaluation of the efficiency of toothbrushes and other oral hygiene devices is constrained by such factors as the time devoted to the method, the patient's hand pressure and dexterity, patient motivation, and the criteria used for measuring plaque (Yankell & Saxer, 1999). Therefore, toothbrush recommendations should be based on the toothbrushing

method prescribed, the patient's intraoral characteristics, patient motivation, the patient's manual dexterity, and product cost.

The standard manual toothbrush consists of a handle and head with bristles and/or filaments. Toothbrush designs vary greatly depending on the desired characteristics. The handle may be straight (conventional) or angled, have a double angulation of the neck, come with or without thumb rests, and/or have a wavelike contour. The shank may be conventional (straight), offset, twisted, or curved. The head may have any of the following features: diamond shaped, squared, rounded, and of variable sizes for infants, children, young adults, and adults. The bristles/filaments (bristles are made of individual filaments) are most often made from nylon. Compared with natural bristles, nylon bristles have shown certain superior qualities, such as bristle durability, cleanliness, and resistance to the accumulation of bacteria and fungi. Bristle stiffness is classified as soft, medium, and hard. Soft bristles are the most highly recommended. Hard bristles have been shown to cause gingival recession and excessive tooth wear, resulting in cervical abrasion (Figure 20–1 ■). Toothbrush bristle planes vary greatly in design. The flat (conventional), dome, bilevel, rippled, and tuft profiles are unique to each toothbrush. Frandsen (1986) reported that daily brushing with a conventional flat-bristle brush removes only 50% of plaque from tooth surfaces, with removal of plaque from interproximal surfaces especially lacking. Newer brush designs using more tapered and narrow bristles of varying lengths have been shown to more

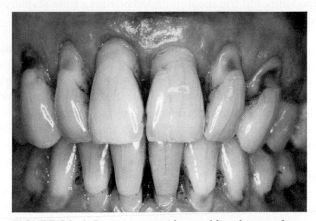

FIGURE 20–1 Improper use of a toothbrush caused gingival recession and tooth abrasion, identified by a notching in the cervical area of the maxillary lateral incisors and canines.

effectively reach interproximal areas, but more research and data evaluation is required. Research on toothbrush bristles has focused much attention on end rounding of the bristles. End-rounded bristles aid in reducing damage to the gingival tissue. Despite manufacturers' attempts to fabricate tooth-brushes with a high percentage of acceptable end-rounded bristles, studies have shown that poorly rounded, sharp and pointed, or flat bristle tips may be present in significant numbers even among brushes making claims of superior end rounding (Dellerman, Hughes, & Burkett, 1994; Checchi, Minguzzi, Franchi, & Forteleoni, 2001). Alternatives to conventional toothbrushes have been studied. One example is a disposable polyester foam sponge on a stick impregnated with a nonfoaming dentifrice. These sponge-like brushes have been used in hospitals and nursing homes and are shown to possess plaque-preventive capabilities. The spongelike brush was found to be effective in retarding accumulation of plaque from a plaque-free baseline on both facial and lingual tooth surfaces (Lefkoff, Beck, & Horton, 1995). It is especially useful after periodontal surgery.

FREQUENCY OF TOOTHBRUSHING Toothbrushing must be carried out on a regular basis. Because the frequency of brushing is tailored to meet individual needs, it is difficult to determine the number of times a day an individual must brush (Savolainen et al., 2005). It is recommended that an individual brush as many times a day as it takes to effectively remove dental plaque. Factors that affect the recommendations for frequency of toothbrushing include the rate of dental plaque formation, plaque visibility, state and susceptibility of oral disease, diet, and presence of contributory factors. Low-risk patients should be directed to brush at least twice a day. High-risk patients need to brush more frequently, especially after meals. The use of disclosing agents is highly recommended because it promotes meticulous removal of visible plaque from the teeth. The patient should individualize his or her own brushing technique to optimize plaque control. Current data on toothbrushing time suggests that people think they brush longer than they actually do. The average time spent on brushing is between 24 and 60 seconds, but the recommended brushing time actually is about 3 minutes (Cancro & Fischman, 1995).

POWERED TOOTHBRUSHES Alternatives to manual tooth-brushes include powered toothbrushes. A new generation of sonic and ultrasonic toothbrushes has become available. Powered toothbrushes were originally designed to simulate the action produced using a manual brush. However, effectiveness still depends on brush and bristle placement. Powered toothbrushes were originally recommended for patients lacking fine motor skills or for patients with physical or mental impairments, but recent innovations in technology have increased their usefulness for patients with periodontal disease, as well as patients with dental implants.

MECHANISM OF ACTION There are many types of powered sonic and ultrasonic toothbrushes on the market today.

Variations in brush head, bristle design, and brush movement exist. The various mechanical motions occur in rapid, short strokes in one or a combination of the following directions: reciprocating (in and out or up and down), rotational, counterrotational, or oscillating (vibrational). A newer generation of powered toothbrushes works by sonic waves and ultrasonic action.

EFFECTIVENESS Various studies with conflicting results have examined the effectiveness of powered toothbrushes compared with conventional brushes in plaque removal. Most studies in the 1960s and 1970s failed to show that powered toothbrushes removed plaque better than manual tooth-brushes. In the 1996 World Workshop in Periodontics it was concluded that limited evidence supports the fact that powered toothbrushes offer additional benefits compared with manual toothbrushes (Hancock, 1996).

A few powered toothbrushes may be superior in removing plaque from interproximal areas than conventional manual toothbrushes (Bader, 1992; Saxer & Yankell, 1997). One study suggests that the sonic toothbrush (Sonicare®, Phillips Electronics) is more beneficial in resolving inflammation and reducing pocket depths in patients with moderate periodontal disease (O'Beirne, Johnson, Rutger Persson, & Spektor, 1996). However, other randomized, controlled clinical studies have not proven conclusively any differences in the efficacy of plaque removal between manual and powered toothbrushes (Preber, Ylipaa, Bergström, & Ryden, 1991; Van der Weijden, Danser, Nijboer, Timmerman, & Van der Velden, 1993). A recent clinical study using 62 adult patients with significant amounts of plaque, calculus, and inflammation demonstrated that brushing with either a manual or ultrasonic toothbrush significantly reduced bleeding and gingival inflammation. Neither toothbrush showed superiority over the other in removing plaque (Forgas-Brockmann, Carter-Hanson, & Killoy, 1998). The novelty of using a new device may in part increase self-care efforts, thus improving oral hygiene.

Powered toothbrushes have been found to be superior in removing tooth stains (Grossman, Cronin, Dembling, & Proskin, 1996). The Braun Oral-B® Plaque Remover (Braun, Oral-B, MA) and Sonicare® have been shown to be superior to a manual toothbrush in removal of chlorhexidine stains (Moran & Addy, 1995). The Braun Oral-B 3D Excel power toothbrush more effectively removed calculus and stain compared to a manual toothbrush and the Sonicare Plus (Sharma, Galustians, Qaqish, Cugini, & Warren, 2002).

RECOMMENDING A POWERED TOOTHBRUSH Factors to consider when recommending a powered toothbrush include the toothbrush design, brushing motion, patient's interest and motivation, and the costs and benefits. Placement of bristles and the head of the toothbrush are important to avoid tissue trauma. The powered toothbrush should be moved slowly in sequence around the mouth using less pressure than with a manual toothbrush, thus producing less cervical abrasion and tissue trauma. Evaluation of a patient's ability to improve his or her plaque and gingival indices over time is the best method for determining the success of a specific powered toothbrush. Use of powered toothbrushes is safe on titanium dental implants.

The use of powered toothbrushes by patients with poor self-care compliance has shown some advantages (Hellstadius, Asman, & Gustafsson, 1993). Use of a powered toothbrush (counterrotational) in periodontal patients in a periodontal maintenance program has proved to be helpful in reducing plaque levels and enhancing gingival conditions (Yukna & Shaklee, 1993). Other patients that may benefit from the use of powered toothbrushes include those with limited manual dexterity, orthodontic patients, and children (parental brushing of children's teeth).

Interdental Care

Interdental cleaning is a primary area of neglect. A major factor in disease initiation and control is the anatomy of the interdental area. Cleansing of these interproximal areas depends on tooth alignment and tissue configuration. Supplemental aids are necessary because, despite new toothbrush designs, brushing alone is ineffective in the removal of interproximal plaque. Additional factors such as an individual's dexterity and compliance contribute to the

effectiveness of plaque removal and need for improvement (Paraskevas, 2005).

Various considerations are appropriate when recommending interdental cleaning devices. These factors are as follows:

- The presence or absence of interdental papillae
- Alignment of teeth
- Shape of teeth
- Tissue contour
- Condition of restorations
- Tightness of contact area
- Presence of bridges, dental implants, and orthodontic appliances
- Patient motivation and interest in interproximal cleaning
- Effectiveness of patient's self-care
- Size of gingival embrasure

TYPES OF GINGIVAL EMBRASURES There are three types of gingival embrasures (Figure 20–2 ■): Type I, in which the embrasure is completely filled with gingiva; Type II, in which there is slight to moderate recession of the interdental papillae; and Type III, in which there is extensive or complete loss of interdental papillae.

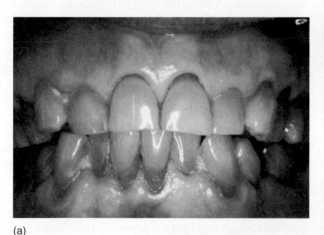
(a)

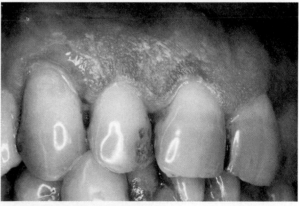
(b)

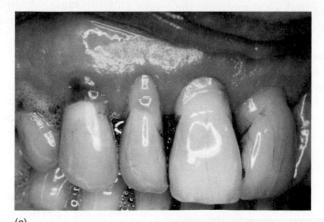
(c)

FIGURE 20–2 Three types of gingival embrasures. Interdental cleaning devices are specific for each type of embrasure. (a) Type I embrasure is completely filled with interdental gingiva. (b) Type II embrasure has partial loss of interdental gingiva (mandibular anterior teeth). (c) Type III embrasure has complete loss of interdental gingiva.

Dental Floss and Dental Tape. Numerous types of nylon dental floss are available: waxed, unwaxed, flat, round, colored, flavored, shred resistant, and impregnated with substances such as fluoride, baking soda, and tetrasodium pyrophosphate. Floss is indicated for use in Type I gingival embrasures, where the embrasures are completely filled with interdental papillae. It is also effective around implants. Dental floss is 80% effective in removing interproximal dental plaque (Lewis et al., 2004). Waxed dental floss may be more resistant to tearing or shredding but may be too bulky for tight contacts. Teflon-coated floss is made of polytetrafluoroethylene and is inserted easily into difficult access areas and resists fraying (Ciancio, Shibly, & Farber, 1992). Unwaxed floss is thin and easily manipulated through tight contact areas. Even though patients prefer to use waxed floss rather than unwaxed floss (Beaumont, 1990), there is actually no difference between the two flosses in efficacy in removing interproximal plaque (Hill, Levi, & Glickman, 1973). Floss may fray and tear where teeth are crowded or in areas where restorations are defective. Dental tape is broad and flat and should be used in open interdental spaces or between teeth without tight contacts and for polishing proximal tooth surfaces. The major advantage of colored floss is patient appeal and the patient's ability to see what is removed by flossing. This factor may help motivate the patient to floss regularly (Hague & Carr, 2007). A recent study found that four different floss products (unwaxed, woven, and shred-resistant floss and a powered flosser) in combination with a manual toothbrush removed plaque significantly better than the toothbrush alone. Clinical data also show that properly and frequently used dental floss may be effective in reducing interproximal gingivitis (Zimmer et al., 2006). The powered flosser was superior to the traditional floss products but there were no significant treatment differences between the three traditional floss products (Terézhalmy, Bartizek, & Biesbrock, 2008).

A floss modification called tufted dental floss, made by many manufacturers, has a stiff straight end with a section of unwaxed floss and an area of thicker nylon meshwork. The stiff end allows the floss to be passed easily under bridges, around implant abutments, through exposed furcations, or between orthodontic appliances.

The floss holder is a yoke-like device with a space between the two prongs of the yoke. The floss is secured tightly between the two prongs designed to facilitate movement of the floss interproximally. It is recommended for patients with limited manual dexterity.

The floss threader is a needle-like device to facilitate floss use under pontics and splinted crowns, between orthodontic appliances, through a gingival embrasure, or between teeth with tight contacts. It is used by threading approximately 12 inches of floss through the loop and then drawing it through the interproximal space. The floss is then engaged against the tooth surface.

An article (Segelnick, 2004) reported that daily flossing was practiced 2.4 times more often in patients seen in a private periodontal practice (19.3%) than in a hospital dental clinic (7.9%). It was concluded that patients who do floss most likely are not using the proper technique. Looking at the flossing technique, the average number of times patients reported to floss with an up-and-down motion was 2.6 times. There is a statistically significantly higher floss frequency among middle-aged patients as compared to older and younger patients. Women flossed significantly more frequently than men, which was seen only at the hospital clinic. Almost 40% of the individuals who reported flossing are not practicing the proper technique of flossing around the tooth.

Caution is necessary in flossing to avoid injury to the gingiva. The floss may cut the gingiva if it is pulled too quickly past the contact and/or if it is positioned too forcefully beneath the gingiva. Damage to the junctional epithelium may occur, especially in healthy gingiva. The patient should be instructed to perform flossing procedures in a systematic fashion (hence all mandibular and maxillary teeth are included). Mastering the flossing technique requires time and patience. Patients are discouraged and less motivated to incorporate the flossing regimen into their oral hygiene program when they have difficulties with manual dexterity or when they do not have the patience to do the job well (Lewis et al., 2004).

Today, resistance to flossing is prevalent among patients, as an alternative to manual tooth brushing and flossing, the daily use of oral irrigation and toothbrush effectively reduces the by-products of the host inflammatory response (Barnes et al., 2005). Home irrigation with a water jet and toothbrush has been shown to be as effective as the use of a manual or power toothbrush and floss for the reduction of bleeding and gingival inflammation (Darby & Walsh, 2010).

A specific floss also has been designed for cleaning implant supported dentures. The denture has to be removed before cleaning the abutments. The floss is looped from facial to lingual around the abutment and gently placed subgingivally until resistance is met. It is then crisscrossed and used in a sliding back-and-forth, up-and-down motion. Implant floss is made of braided nylon filaments and can be washed off after each use.

Interdental and Single-Tuft Brushes. Exposed furcations, root concavities (e.g., mesial concavity on the maxillary first premolar), and Type II and III gingival embrasures are best cleaned with an interdental or single-tuft brush (also called end-tuft brush; Figure 20–3 ■). Other uses for such brushes include the distal surface of the terminal molar, around pontics and maligned teeth, and around orthodontic appliances or dental implant abutments. The premoistened brush is inserted interproximally and used in an in-and-out direction. However, such brushes should not be forced to fit into gingival embrasures.

Interdental brushes consist of nylon filaments twisted onto a metal wire or a nylon-coated plastic wire that does not scratch or cause tissue trauma. This special brush is recommended for titanium surfaces. Interchangeable brushes come

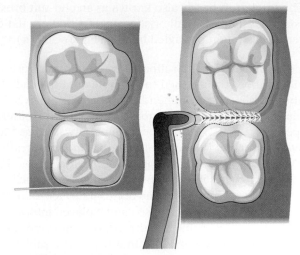

FIGURE 20–3 Floss is not as effective as an interdental brush in removing interdental plaque from tooth concavities.

in a variety of sizes and shapes, such as cylindrical (large and small) and tapered (Figure 20–4 ■). A unique wireless soft foam insert is available for postoperative periodontal care, medicament applications, and implant maintenance.

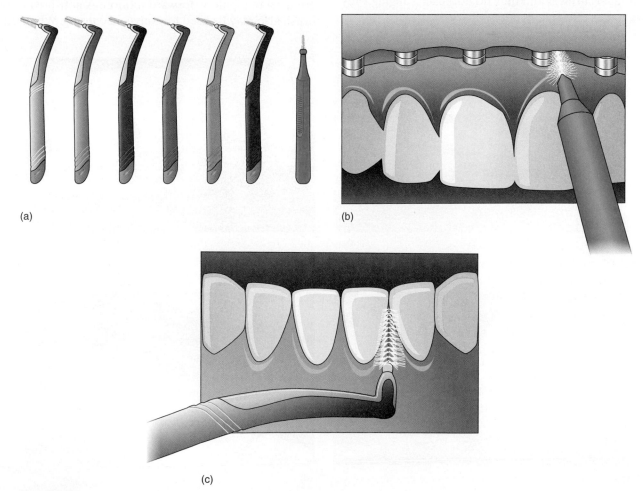

(a)

(b)

(c)

FIGURE 20–4 (a) Variations in types of interdental brushes. Uses of an interdental brush (b) in a Type II embrasure and (c) around implant abutments.

The single-tuft brush, also known as an end-tuft brush, consists of a group of small bristles or tufts that are flat or tapered on a straight or angled handle (Figure 20–5 ■).

Rubber-Tip Stimulator. The rubber-tip stimulator consists of a flexible rubber tip attached to a handle or at the end of a toothbrush. It is not recommended for healthy gingiva that completely fills the gingival embrasure, but it can be useful in Type II or Type III embrasures. Generally, it is used for removing plaque at the gingival margin, exposed furcation areas, concave surfaces, and open interdental areas. The tip is inserted gently into the interdental area and inclined approximately 45° away from the occlusal surface following the contour of the gingiva. It also can be placed interproximally at a 90° angle. A back-and-forth or rolling motion is used. In the past it was thought that use of the rubber tip increased keratinization and vascular function through gingival stimulation, but no clinical evidence exists to support this (Rounds & Tilliss, 1999).

Wooden Toothpicks. Wooden toothpicks are available as either a toothpick-in-holder or a triangular balsa wood stimulator. These devices are designed to be used where interdental papillae are missing (Type II and Type III embrasures). Because wooden toothpicks are difficult to use on lingual surfaces and they do not reach subgingivally, they are not as effective as dental floss.

The triangular stimulator should be moistened with saliva and then inserted interproximally, flat side toward the gingiva, moving in an in-and-out burnishing stroke. Discard the wedge if it becomes splayed.

The toothpick-in-holder is a plastic-handled instrument with a tapered, conical opening at one end where the toothpick is inserted; the excess portion is broken off. It is used for plaque removal along the gingival margin, within the sulcus, in root concavities, in furcation areas, and around orthodontic appliances; it may also be used for the application of medicaments (e.g., fluoride or a desensitizing agent). The blunt point and sides of the toothpick are placed in the sulcus to engage, debride, and dislodge adherent plaque.

Electric Interdental Cleaning Devices. One of the more recent advances in interdental cleaning is the Braun Oral-B Interclean®, an electric interdental cleaning device that consists of a thin, flexible cleaning filament (Figure 20–6 ■). This device has been shown to reduce plaque, gingivitis, and bleeding equal to or better than floss (Gordon, Frascella, & Reardon, 1996). Other automated interdental cleaners are available and include sonic devices, filament tips, brush tips, and flossers.

Tongue Cleansing

A number of tongue cleansing devices are available. These are used in a pull or forward motion. A soft-bristle toothbrush also may be used for tongue cleansing. When using a

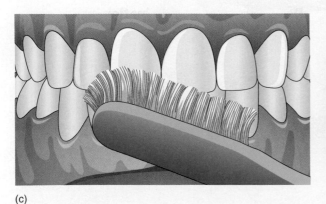

(a)

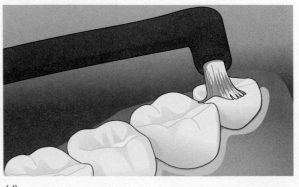

(b)

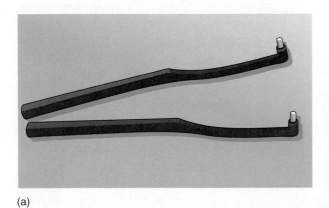

(c)

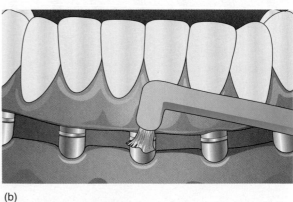

(d)

FIGURE 20–5 (a) Variations in single-tufted brushes (tapered and nontapered). Use of a single-tufted brush (b) around orthodontic appliances, (c) dental implants, and (d) the distal surface of the terminal tooth.

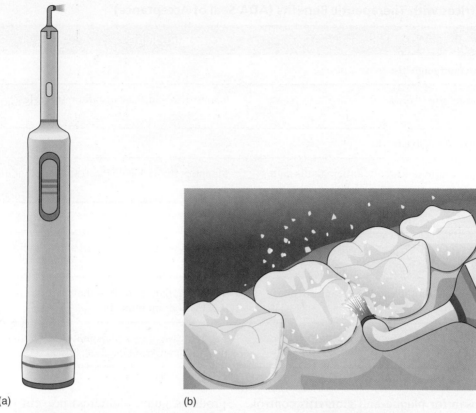

(a) (b)

FIGURE 20–6 (a) Braun Oral-B Interclean®. (b) Interproximal use of the device.

toothbrush, a brushing stroke starting on the posterior-most aspect of the dorsum of the tongue is performed with a roll to the tip of the tongue. Tongue brushing will improve tongue appearance and halitosis by removing coatings associated with bacteria, food, and smoking.

Dentifrices

A **dentifrice** is a toothpowder, toothpaste, or gel used in conjunction with a toothbrush to help remove plaque, materia alba, and stain from teeth. The word is derived from the Latin words *dens* ("teeth") and *fricare* ("to rub"). Although the mechanical action of brushing and flossing is the primary means of plaque removal, a dentifrice facilitates the oral hygiene process.

Dentifrices are considered to be either cosmetic or therapeutic. Cosmetically, they function in cleaning and polishing teeth, removing extrinsic stains, and freshening the oral cavity. There is a continuing effort by manufacturers to obtain additional dental benefits from dentifrices through the inclusion of agents designed to have a therapeutic action. Therapeutic agents are included in dentifrices to reduce caries; control gingivitis, plaque, and calculus formation; and reduce dentinal hypersensitivity (Table 20–1 ■).

Rapid Dental Hint

Remind patients to brush their tongue.

The main limitation of dentifrices as a therapeutic agent is the issue of patient compliance. Dental hygienists cannot control the frequency of use or amount or type of dentifrice used by a patient. Dentifrice selection is based most often on cosmetic qualities such as flavor, texture, appearance, and dispensability rather than therapeutic value. The public looks to dental professionals for specific recommendations. The dental hygienist must be up to date with product information and be able to recommend a dentifrice that will provide oral health benefits yet appeal to the patient for continued use. Dentifrices should be chemically stable, effective, and nontoxic. Products with the ADA Seal of Acceptance have sustained scrutiny and testing and can be safely recommended by dental hygienists.

Dentifrice Tube Contamination

Cross contamination and disease transmission may occur from toothbrushes that come in contact with an uncapped open dentifrice tube that may be shared by several family members. To prevent transmission of disease among the group, each should have his/her own tube of toothpaste that meets the individual's personal oral health needs (Darby & Walsh, 2010).

DENTIFRICE COMPONENTS Dentifrices contain basic components along with an active ingredient for its intended use. The active agent provides the therapeutic benefit and can include fluoride for anticaries effect, potassium nitrate or strontium chloride for desensitization (reducing or eliminating dentin sensitivity), sodium pyrophosphate for calculus

Table 20–1 Dentifrices with Therapeutic Benefits (ADA Seal of Acceptance)

Product Name	Active Ingredients
Anticavity/antiplaque/antigingivitis:	
Colgate® Total™ Toothpaste (Colgate-Palmolive Co., New York, NY)	0.30% triclosan, 0.24% sodium fluoride
Anticavity/antigingivitis/sensitive teeth:	
Crest® ProHealth Toothpaste (anticavity, antigingivitis and sensitive teeth)	Stannous fluoride 0.454%, 0.16% sodium fluoride
Prevention of calculus	
Colgate® Tarter Control Gel/Toothpaste (Colgate-Palmolive Co., New York, NY)	Tetrasodium pyrophosphate, 0.15% sodium fluoride
Aquafresh® Tartar Control Toothpaste (GlaxoSmithKline, PA)	Tetrapotassium pyrophosphate, tetrasodium pyrophosphate, 0.221% sodium fluoride
Crest® Tartar Protection Fluoride Gel/Toothpaste (Procter & Gamble, Cincinnati, OH)	Tetrapotassium pyrophosphate, disodium pyrophosphate, tetrasodium pyrophosphate, 0.15% sodium fluoride

inhibition, or triclosan for plaque and gingivitis control. Recent formulations have incorporated a combination of these active ingredients for maximal patient benefits.

In addition to water (15% to 50%), a typical dentifrice contains additional ingredients, including an abrasive (20% to 60%). Abrasives clean and polish to smooth lustrous tooth surfaces, allowing resistance to bacterial reaccumulation. The powders and pastes contain abrasives such as silicon oxides, chalk, hydrated aluminum oxide, and sodium bicarbonate. Commercial dentifrice powders are more abrasive than pastes. Abrasives usually do not damage the enamel, but may dull tooth luster. Therefore, a polishing agent is incorporated into most dentifrices, forming an abrasive system (Fischman & Yankell, 1999). Although the use of abrasive toothpastes may result in tooth wear, additional factors such as brushing habits, including technique used, pressure, direction, and frequency of brushing, and toothbrush bristle stiffness can influence the incidence of tooth surface abrasion. The more abrasive the dentifrice, the more likely it is to cause tooth wear in the cervical area. This area is more prone to abrasion because enamel is approximately 20 times harder than dentin or cementum (Fischman & Yankell, 1999). There is no valid reason to use a dentifrice with a greater abrasiveness or polishing effect than necessary to remove soft deposits, and stains on the teeth.

Humectants (20% to 40%) are a vehicle into which agents are incorporated to prevent hardening of the dentifrice when exposed to air. Common humectants are glycerin, sorbitol, mannitol, and polyethylene glycol. Surfactants (1% to 2%) act as detergents by contributing to the foaming action, lowering surface tension, and loosening deposits from the teeth. Sodium lauryl sulfate is the most commonly used detergent. Binders (1% to 2%; cellulose products, gums, alginates) prevent the separation of the solids and liquids in the dentifrice, maintain firmness and thickness, and ensure stability. Gels contain more binders to give the product a thicker quality. Flavoring and sweetening agents mask the poor-tasting ingredients and provide a pleasant flavor to the dentifrice. Flavorings include essential oils (peppermint, cinnamon, and wintergreen) and sodium saccharin. Colorants (1%) are dyes added to the dentifrice to enhance its attractiveness without staining or discoloring teeth or oral tissues or causing harm on ingestion.

FLUORIDE DENTIFRICES Dentifrices are the most widely used form of self-applied fluoride. Recommended for both children and adults, fluoride dentifrices can reduce caries by 20% to 30% when used twice daily on a regular basis. First introduced in the 1950s, fluoride dentifrices contained stannous fluoride as the anticaries agent. Current fluoride dentifrices contain sodium fluoride (0.24%) or sodium monofluorophosphate (0.76%). The anticaries efficacy of these two fluoride agents continues to be evaluated (Proskin & Volpe, 1995). Although some analyses indicate that there is no statistically or clinically significant difference between the two fluoride agents (Volpe, Petrone, Davies, & Proskin, 1995), it has been shown that the therapeutic benefit of fluoride depends on a dose-response relationship (Stephen, 1994) and a decrease in caries with increasing dose of fluoride. Sodium fluoride dentifrices appear to be retained longer, however, when compared with dentifrices containing sodium monofluorophosphate (Shellis & Duckworth, 1994) and thus may be more effective clinically (Duckworth, Jones, Nicholson, Jacobson, & Chestnutt, 1994).

Indications for fluoride gels include rampant caries, patients susceptible to caries, root caries, orthodontic appliances, dentinal hypersensitivity, and patients undergoing radiation therapy. Because over 95% of dentifrices contain fluoride and the benefits have been shown clinically for decades, issues of safety are of minor concern. Numerous studies have evaluated fluoride therapies for their impact on dental fluorosis (Stookey, 1994). Dentifrices have been identified as a causative factor in the increased prevalence of mild enamel fluorosis. For this reason, young children must be monitored for inadvertent dentifrice ingestion.

The mechanism of fluoride's anticaries effect in root caries is not well understood. Fluoride gels may have a beneficial effect in the prevention of caries on exposed root surfaces. An example of a home-applied gel prescription product is 1.1% sodium fluoride (Prevident® 5000 Plus Gel, Colgate Oral Pharmaceuticals; Neutracare®, Oral-B). These gels should be applied daily after home-care procedures. The gel is applied either by brushing it on the root surface for 1 minute or using a custom-made or disposable tray for 4 minutes.

STANNOUS FLUORIDE DENTIFRICES Before the introduction of sodium fluoride and sodium monofluorophosphate, stannous fluoride was incorporated into dentifrices. Stannous fluoride, in concentrations of greater than 0.3%, has been the most widely studied fluoride in controlling plaque and gingivitis. Clinical studies of caries and plaque prevention showed mixed results; therefore stannous fluoride does not have the ADA Seal of Acceptance.

Commonly reported adverse side effects include extrinsic tooth staining caused by the tin molecule and a metallic, bitter taste (Wilkins, 2012). Recent dentifrice formulations contain flavoring agents that mask the taste. Removal of stains caused by stannous fluoride is no more difficult than stain removal resulting from other product use (Beiswanger et al., 1995). Stannous fluoride is available as a brush-on gel, a mouth rinse, and a dentifrice.

TRICLOSAN-CONTAINING DENTIFRICES Triclosan is another therapeutic dentifrice. It is a phenolic compound with antiplaque/antigingivitis properties. It is a broad-spectrum antibacterial agent effective against gram-positive and gram-negative bacteria. Used as an antibacterial agent in soaps, deodorants, and cosmetics, triclosan recently became available in the United States in a dentifrice formulation (Total™, Colgate Oral Pharmaceuticals, New York, NY).

Colgate Total contains 0.3% triclosan and 2.0% polyvinylmethylether maleic acid (PVM/MA), which enhances its retention (substantivity) on hard and soft oral surfaces and adds anticalculus properties (Ciancio, 1997). Triclosan binds to plaque, resulting in a sustained impact on bacteria for over 12 hours after brushing (Volpe, Petrone, DeVizio, & Davies, 1996). Triclosan affects the quality of existing plaque (Lindhe, Rosling, Socransky, & Volpe, 1993) and plaque regrowth (Binney, Addy, McKeowns, & Everatt, 1996). When compared with other dentifrices, triclosan is as effective as stannous fluoride (Binney, Addy, Owens, & Faulkner, 1997) and sodium fluoride dentifrices (Binney, Addy, McKeowns, & Everatt, 1995) in inhibiting plaque. In addition, this product is also claimed to prevent caries. No adverse effects have been reported, and it is safe for oral use. Triclosan has the ADA Seal of Acceptance for antiplaque/antigingivitis properties. Few if any dentifrices have been shown to be effective in reducing carious lesions in interproximal areas. Colgate Total liquid toothpaste's (less viscous than traditional dentifrices) light foaming properties and lower surface tension may in theory, allow the liquid into interproximal spaces, deep grooves, and fissures better than traditional dentifrices. Further studies are necessary. This triclosan-containing liquid dentifrice may aid in reducing interproximal caries more than a standard fluoride dentifrice (Silva, Giniger, Zhang, & DeVizio, 2004).

SODIUM BICARBONATE/HYDROGEN PEROXIDE DENTIFRICES
Sodium bicarbonate (baking soda) has been used as a cleansing agent for many years and has been the primary abrasive agent in dentifrices. The therapeutic benefit of sodium bicarbonate dentifrices results from reduction of plaque and gingivitis and stain removal (Koertge, 1996; Zambon, Mather, & Gonzales, 1996). The mechanism of action is disruption of the bacterial cell membrane (Drake, Vargas, Cardenzana, & Srikantha, 1995). Even though baking soda disintegrates quickly during brushing (so that its abrasive action is not sustained), it still removes stains (Koertge, 1996). An additional benefit of baking soda dentifrices is their control of oral malodor (Brunette, 1996).

Hydrogen peroxide is added to dentifrices for its antigingivitis properties. Some manufacturers claim that hydrogen peroxide–containing dentifrices were developed to whiten teeth by decolorizing stains. Others claim that hydrogen peroxide freshens the mouth because of its bubbling action. Consumers often view these agents as more "natural." The concept of combining sodium bicarbonate with hydrogen peroxide is based on the regimen supported by the Keyes technique. Most dentifrices contain a low level of hydrogen peroxide (< 1%) that causes no harm to tissues (Marshall, Cancro, & Fischman, 1995).

The Keyes technique, was originally developed by Dr. Paul Keyes in the late 1970s for the treatment of periodontal disease without surgical intervention. It is based on monitoring of the disease with phase-contrast microscopy and treatment. The first phase involves mechanical therapy and is followed by local antimicrobial therapy. In this phase the patient uses a toothpaste composed of 3% hydrogen peroxide, salt, and sodium bicarbonate. Oral irrigation at home and in the office is also included. In the last phase of treatment, a systemic antibiotic such as tetracycline is prescribed. The Keyes technique was found to be no more effective than conventional periodontal therapy (Pihlstrom et al., 1987). In addition, oral ulcerations have been reported to result from short-term use of 3% hydrogen peroxide in combination with a salt solution (Levine, 1987).

Research findings on the efficacy of sodium bicarbonate/peroxide are mixed. One study concluded that after 3 months of using a sodium bicarbonate/peroxide dentifrice there was a 52% reduction in bleeding sites (Fischman, Kugel, Truelove, Nelson, & Cancro, 1992). Dentifrices containing hydrogen peroxide may decrease plaque and gingivitis, but mechanical access to submarginal sites is required for them to deliver a therapeutic effect (Marshall et al., 1995). When applied with a sulcular brush and an interproximal toothpick, sodium bicarbonate/hydrogen peroxide had no benefit in reducing the microbiota in 4 to 7 mm pockets (Cerra & Killoy, 1982). No antimicrobial benefits were exhibited when compared with conventional dentifrices (sodium fluoride, stannous fluoride) and mouth rinses (essential oils; Bacca et al., 1997). Arm and Hammer Dental Care Advanced Cleaning Mint toothpaste has the ADA Seal of Acceptance for anticaries properties.

TARTAR-CONTROL DENTIFRICES Calculus, although not a primary causative factor for periodontal disease, does play a contributing role in dental plaque retention due to its porous surface. The introduction of soluble pyrophosphates into dentifrices provides a chemical means of reducing supragingival calculus formation. Calcium and phosphorus from saliva are prevented from incorporating into the plaque matrix to form calculus.

Pyrophosphates act as crystal growth inhibitors, especially large, organized crystals that may delay mineralization of the plaque and make it more susceptible to mechanical removal. Once calculus has formed into an organized matrix, pyrophosphates are ineffective. Their effectiveness is limited to new supragingival calculus. For this reason, recommendations for use are appropriate after prophylaxis or scaling/root planing.

Many studies have evaluated the effectiveness of pyrophosphates on calculus formation (Addy & Koltai, 1994; Gaengler, Kurbad, & Weinert, 1993). Not only is there a reduction in new calculus formation, but also the number of sites in the mouth that are calculus-free is increased (Lobene, 1989). Results after 3 and 6 months indicated significant reductions in supragingival deposits (Schiff, 1987) by 35.5% and 45.9%, respectively. Calculus inhibitors cause the newly formed deposits to be softer and easier for the clinician to remove. The amount of force and number of strokes by the dental hygienist are reduced (White et al., 1996). The addition of a copolymer (methoxyethylene and maleic acid) to a pyrophosphate dentifrice enhances the anticalculus effect (Singh, Petrone, Volpe, Rustogi, & Norfleet, 1990).

In addition to the effect on hard deposits, anticalculus dentifrices may also exhibit antimicrobial activity by killing or inhibiting bacterial growth (Drake, Grigsby, & Drotz-Dieleman, 1994). Pyrophosphates have been found to reduce chlorhexidine-induced extrinsic stain (Bollmer, Sturzenberger, Vick, & Grossman, 1995).

Tissue irritation has been reported in the form of tissue sloughing (peeling) and tooth surface sensitivity. Pyrophosphates in dentifrices also have been thought to interact with the fluoride compounds and interfere with the remineralization process. Fluoride uptake is not altered by pyrophosphates. The anticaries benefits are similar for regular-formula and tartar-control dentifrices. The ADA Seal of Acceptance has been given to tartar control dentifrices based on their anticaries properties.

ZINC CITRATE–CONTAINING DENTRIFICES Viadent™ Advanced Care (Colgate Oral Pharmaceuticals, Canton, MA) has as its active ingredients 2% zinc citrate trihydrate, which is an antibacterial agent, and 0.8% sodium monofluorophosphate, which has anticaries properties. This formulation is also available as an oral rinse.

OTHER DENTIFRICE CATEGORIES Herbal-based and "natural" dentifrices are attractive alternatives to some patients interested in maintaining oral hygiene. Although these products have been documented to perhaps be as effective as conventional dentifrices in their ability to control plaque and gingivitis (Mullaby, James, Coulter, & Linden, 1995), their efficacy remains questionable. As long as these "natural" toothpastes contain fluoride, patients receive anticaries benefit. Patients must be informed of the limitations of their choice of dentifrice. The primary benefit of some of these alternatives is motivational, in that patients may be encouraged to brush more regularly with their chosen dentifrice.

Dentifrices containing a lactoperoxidase system (Biotene®, Laclede Professional Products, Rancho Dominguez, CA) may be beneficial for special patient groups. Patients with xerostomia were relieved of their symptoms after a 4-week daily use of a lactoperoxidase dentifrice and mouth rinse (Kirstila, Lenander-Lumikari, Soderling, & Tenovuo, 1996). Biotene does not have the ADA Seal of Acceptance.

Oral Home Care for Patients with Periodontal Disease

Because not every patient has the same type and severity of periodontal disease, the hygienist must customize an oral hygiene self-care plan for every patient. Patients who have gingivitis with intact interdental papillae are going to have a different hygiene strategy than a patient with generalized chronic periodontitis with blunted and absent papillae (Table 20–2 ■).

Postperiodontal Surgical Home Care

The important role of oral hygiene in controlling dental plaque growth and recolonization immediately after periodontal surgery cannot be overestimated (Sanz & Herrera, 1998). The degree of oral hygiene maintained by the patient

---

Did You Know?

Ninety-four percent of Americans say they brush nightly; 81% say they brush their teeth first thing in the morning.

Table 20–2 Oral Home Care for the Patient with Periodontal Disease

Type of Disease	Clinical Features	Toothbrush	Interdental Care and Adjunctive Care	Reasoning
Periodontal health	No clinical attachment loss or gingival recession. Intact interdental papillae. No bleeding.	Soft-bristled toothbrush; modified Bass technique.	Floss. If crowns are present, waxed floss may be easier for patient.	Because no disease is present, no modifications to home care are necessary. Observe proper technique and frequency of practice.
Gingivitis	Red and slight bleeding gingiva. No clinical attachment loss. Moderate to heavy plaque. Light/medium/heavy calculus. Most likely will have type I gingival embrasures.	Soft-bristled toothbrush; modified. Bass technique. If gingival recession is present, use the Charter's technique. For areas of edema use the Stillman's technique. *Antimicrobial toothpaste and rinses.*	Floss for type I gingival embrasures. Chemotherapeutics for rinsing or oral irrigation.	Emphasize brushing and flossing technique. Modify technique and frequency of practice. May include a mouth rinse as an adjunct to help reduce bacterial load.
Chronic periodontitis	Numerous sites with blunted or absent papillae. Plaque and calculus accumulations. Bleeding may be evident except if the patient is a smoker.	A soft-bristled toothbrush with a modified Bass technique. Stillman's technique for gingival recession or blunted papillae. *Antimicrobial and fluoride toothpaste, desensitizing toothpaste for recession.*	Floss for type I gingival embrasures and interdental brush for type II and III. Oral irrigators and mouth rinses for reduction of microbial load in pockets. Local delivery of antibiotics (Arestin, Atridox).	Adjunctive use of mouth rinse or other chemotherapeutics and oral irrigators.
Aggressive periodontitis	Lack of clinical inflammation with normal appearance. Deep pockets in affected areas, absence of heavy plaque or calculus formation. Rapid bone destruction.	A soft-bristled toothbrush with a modified Bass technique. *Antimicrobial and fluoride toothpaste.*	Floss for type I gingival embrasures, interdental brushes for open embrasures. Adjunctive use of systemic antibiotics, chemotherapeutic agents and mouth rinses.	Goal to slow progress of disease. Individualized instruction for plague control and positive reinforcement for client. Antimicrobial therapy.
Periodontitis associated with immune dysfunction	Severe bone loss and tooth loss resulting from body's lack of resistance to bacterial infections.	A soft-bristled toothbrush with modified Bass technique. For gingival recession use Stillman's technique. *Antimicrobial and fluoride toothpaste.*	Floss for type I gingival embrasures. Interdental brushes for type II and III embrasures. Adjunctive use of chemotherapeutic agents and mouth rinses.	Goal is to slow progress of periodontal disease exacerbated by the immune dysfunction.

(continued)

Table 20–2 Oral Home Care for the Patient with Periodontal Disease (*cont.*)

Type of Disease	Clinical Features	Toothbrush	Interdental Care and Adjunctive Care	Reasoning
Necrotizing ulcerative gingivitis (NUG)	Marginal gingiva is bright red, inflamed spontaneous bleeding, cratered punched out necrotic papillae, grayish-white pseudomembrane covering the gingiva, may include burning sensation, fetid odor, fever, enlarged lymph nodes.	Soft-bristled toothbrush with simple self-care. Gentle rolling strokes with minimal tissue movement. After inflammation begins to subside, more sulcular cleansing, gentle oral irrigation and microbials.	Careful slow addition of any products that could cause additional gingival irritation such as anticalculus toothpaste, rinses with high alcohol content. Gentle flossing after tissue healing begins appropriate to embrasures. Chemotherapeutics to complement antibiotic therapy.	Goal to allow for healing while adding in plaque-removal techniques.
Necrotizing ulcerative periodontitis (NUP)	Extensive necrosis of gingiva, red band around marginal gingiva, severe pain, spontaneous bleeding, extensive clinical attachment loss with deep periodontal pockets.	Soft-bristled toothbrush with gentle rolling strokes with minimal tissue movement. After inflammation begins to subside, more sulcular cleansing, gentle oral irrigation and microbials	Interdental brush for type II and III gingival embrasures. Oral irrigators and mouth rinses for microbial load in pockets.	Emphasize gentle brushing while healing, then add auxiliary plaque removal aides appropriate for embrasures.
Hormonal pregnancy gingivitis	Inflamed papillae, bright red, edematous tissue with a shiny smooth surface. Pregnancy tumors (pyogenic) in more severe cases.	Soft-bristled toothbrush; modified. Bass technique after symptoms recede.	Floss for type I gingival embrasure and interdental brush for type II and III gingival embrasures. Adjunctive use of chemotherapeutic mouth rinses.	Because inflammation will usually regress postpartum plaque removal and meticulous home care must be stressed

also influences the healing response after periodontal surgery (Flores-de-Jacoby & Mengel, 1995; Palcanis, 1996). Presently, it is unknown if the healing response results from the improvement in and maintenance of low plaque levels by the patient (Westfelt, 1996) or is related to the increased frequency of periodontal maintenance visits after surgery (Ramfjord, 1987).

If a periodontal dressing was used, the patient should be informed not to dislodge it. It is likely that the patient will be inclined to avoid brushing the area, but he or she should be instructed to lightly brush the exposed tooth surfaces and all other areas of the dentition with a soft or ultrasoft toothbrush. The Bass method should be avoided; other methods that do not place the bristles directly into the gingival crevice are recommended to prevent trauma to the healing tissue. Chlorhexidine is usually recommended after periodontal surgery.

Patients with periodontal disease frequently have localized or generalized blunted papillae due to the disease process or as a consequence of periodontal surgery. Because of the open embrasures, the use of interdental brushes and single-tuft brushes is recommended. A fluoride dentifrice should be used. Assess the need for an antimicrobial rinse.

The patient's plaque control must be closely monitored postsurgery.

Implant Home Care

Diligent home care around tissue-integrated implant prostheses is imperative for long-term success. Plaque-control procedures must start immediately after uncovering the implants. It is important that the dental hygienist customize a home-care regimen based on the patient's awareness and ability and the type of prosthesis present (Orton, Steele, & Wolinsky, 1989).

A multitude of home-care devices exist to assist in mechanical oral hygiene regimes. These devices include various manual (Figure 20–7 ■) or powered toothbrushes (Figure 20–8 ■) and specific interdental aids (Balshi, 1986).

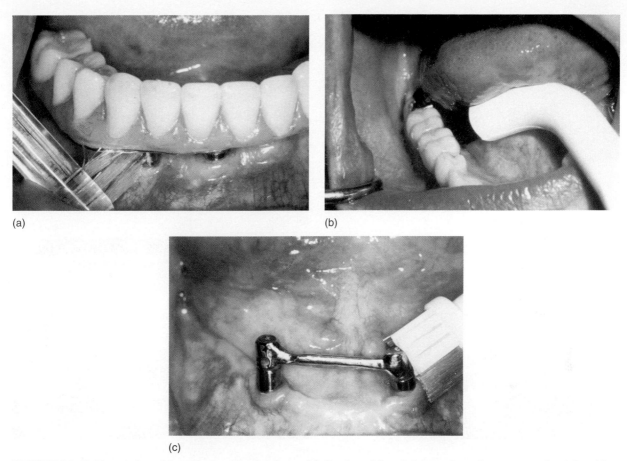

(a)

(b)

(c)

FIGURE 20–7 Types of toothbrushes used on implants. (a) Single-tuft brush (also referred to as an end-tuft brush). (b) Powered brush used with fixed partial denture superstructure. (c) Powered brush used with overdenture abutments and retention bar.

Soft or ultrasoft manual toothbrushes are the traditional means of plaque removal. However, toothbrush heads come in many different shapes and sizes, and brushes should be prescribed individually depending on the implant type and the patient's abilities. An excellent area-specific soft nylon brush is the single-tufted brush for use with individual implants, one implant at a time; the shaft can be bent for better access.

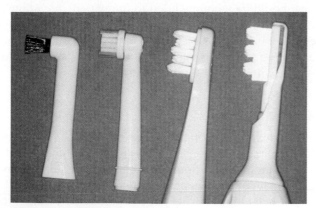

FIGURE 20–8 Various types of powered brush heads. Many clinicians recommend powered brushes for use around dental implants.

Various interdental devices are available, including interdental brushes, rubber-tip stimulators, wooden cleaners, numerous types of dental floss, and a plastic toothpick (Ultradent, Oral B). The brush attachment for interdental brushes is available as a plastic or nylon-coated wire rather than a metal wire to prevent scratching of implant surfaces. Interdental brushes are used only if the interdental papilla is blunted or absent. Various floss types, such as tufted floss or floss cords (PostCare™, Sunstar Americas Inc., Chicago), along with folded gauze or traditional floss, are effective and safe interproximal plaque-removal aids (Figure 20–9 ■).

Clinical use of antimicrobials (chemotherapeutic agents) can help to inhibit plaque and gingivitis around implants. These agents may be delivered by rinsing or applied topically (via toothbrush, floss, or cotton-tipped applicator). Rinsing with chlorhexidine gluconate

Did You Know?

Americans spend $2 billion a year on dental products such as toothpaste, mouthwash, and dental floss.

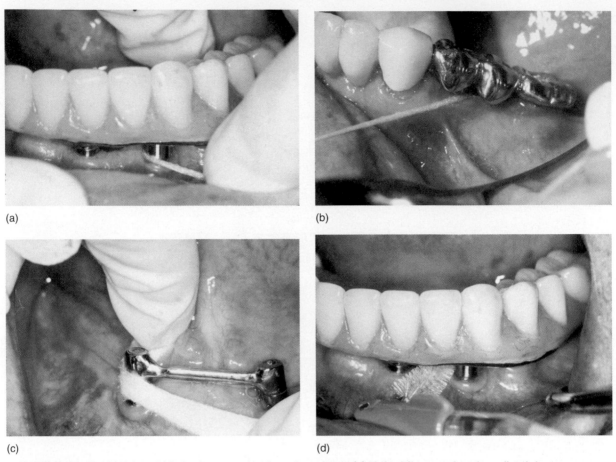

FIGURE 20–9 Oral hygiene aids for interproximal tooth surfaces. (a) Tufted floss used under a fixed denture. (b) Tufted floss used under a fixed bridge. (c) Folded gauze strip can be efficient when access is good. (d) Interdental brush used under a fixed partial denture.

(Peridex®, Omni or PerioGard®, Colgate Oral Pharmaceuticals) and Listerine® (McNeil-PPC) has been shown to be advantageous in the inhibition of bacterial plaque with patients with implants (Ciancio et al., 1995). Irrigation can be used if pathologic changes are present (Meffert, Langer, & Frutz, 1992). A study conducted by Felo, Shibly, Ciancio, Lauciello, and Ho (1997) investigated the effects of subgingival irrigation with chlorhexidine gluconate diluted with water on peri-implant gingival health compared with rinsing with chlorhexidine when used as an adjunct to routine peri-implant maintenance. Results suggested that powered subgingival irrigation with chlorhexidine may be better than rinsing in implant maintenance. However, even though the results of this study were favorable toward the use of irrigation at home, patients should not irrigate around implants until more controlled clinical studies can support its use.

Although rinsing with antimicrobials has been proven to be beneficial, some rinses do have unwanted side effects, such as staining, altered taste, and increased calculus formation. Because of the potential side effects, patients may prefer alternative delivery by applying the solution in a site-specific fashion to avoid undesirable effects.

Orthodontic Home Care

Orthodontic appliances tend to increase the accumulation of supragingival plaque on the teeth leading to the development of gingival inflammation and bleeding. Meticulous oral hygiene is important to control the development of gingival inflammation. During orthodontic treatment, the patient should be evaluated regularly. A soft-bristled toothbrush designed specifically for orthodontic appliances should be recommended to the patient, including an oral rinse if needed to supplement brushing. The Charters method of brushing is used to clean the brackets of cervical areas of the teeth. For interdental home care, use of a floss threader with floss or tufted floss is recommended.

Advice to the Patient

Noncompliance with oral hygiene self-care is a major factor in the recurrence of periodontal diseases. One role of the dental hygienist is to determine the patient's enthusiasm and manual dexterity in performing plaque control (Baker, 1995), which entails having good professional communication skills and patience because it is not easy for patients to change their habits. Besides lack of motivation, other reasons for plaque control failure include poor technique, lack of knowledge, and inconsistent performance (Van Dyke, Offenbacher, Pihlstrom, Putt, & Trummel, 1999).

Oral hygiene self-care programs are based on a patient's individual needs. Keeping the program simple will increase patient compliance. Try to adapt the oral hygiene program to the patient's lifestyle. Establishing good oral hygiene habits involves having patients clean their teeth in a systematic pattern (e.g., starting on the maxillary right and ending on the mandibular right). However, strict adherence to one approach may not always be in the best interests of thorough plaque removal and improved gingival health.

Oral physiotherapeutic products have limitations. Brushing and flossing are effective in the mechanical removal of most supragingival plaque but are limited in removing subgingival plaque due to the design of the devices and the contour of the gingiva. A periodontal patient may be able to access the subgingiva only slightly. The techniques described in this chapter can be modified to permit cleansing of all accessible areas of the dentition. A different regimen is applied after periodontal surgery, and the patient must be familiar with the various cleaning aids needed. The dental hygienist must introduce these new aids to the patient.

The iatrogenic effects of dentistry need to be eliminated prior to setting expectations for plaque removal. For example, unpolished amalgam restorations retain more plaque than polished ones. Composite materials may accumulate plaque greater than amalgam. Ill-fitting margins, overhangs, and rough surfaces on restorations should be evaluated for replacement or finishing because of plaque-retentive possibilities.

Effects of Improper Use of Oral Hygiene Devices

Once the importance of oral hygiene is explained to the patient and he or she begins to use numerous oral hygiene devices, the next step is to ensure that the patient is using each device correctly.

Toothbrushing

Factors that can cause acute or chronic tissue problems include incorrect bristle angulation or placement, heavy or long brushing strokes, a toothbrush with hard bristles, extremely abrasive toothpaste, and loss of concentration. Acute soft tissue lesions appear as small ulcers, red areas, or denuded gingiva. Chronic, long-standing gingival lesions present as gingival recession, rolled marginal gingiva, or gingival clefting. Gingival recession was found to occur mostly on the buccal surfaces of maxillary first molars, premolars, and canines (Björn, Andersson, & Olsson, 1981). Hard tissue lesions present as toothbrush abrasions occurring at the cervical area of teeth (see Figure 20–11). Tooth abrasion in most cases is due to the combined effect of toothbrushing and the use of dentifrices containing abrasives (Sangnes, 1976). Cervical abrasion may occur once the root surface has been exposed by gingival recession. Thus, for cervical abrasions to occur, they must be preceded by gingival recession.

Interdental Devices

Dental floss, interdental brushes, and single-tufted brushes can cause injury to the gingiva if improper techniques are used. Each device is indicated in different types of gingival embrasures. Gingival ulcers, cuts, and clefts can result from improper technique.

Floss should not be forced too deeply into the gingival crevices (Figure 20–10 ■). When floss is used as part of the daily plaque-control routine, the junctional epithelial cells adhering to the enamel are in a continuous state of disruption and healing (Waerhaug, 1981). Interdental brushes and single-tufted brushes should not be forced into gingival with intact papilla.

Interdental cleaning is easy to master if the dental hygienist provides proper teaching and supervision to the patient.

Dentinal Hypersensitivity

Maintaining plaque control is of utmost importance in reducing the sensitivity of exposed root surfaces. Often patients have difficulty complying with oral hygiene

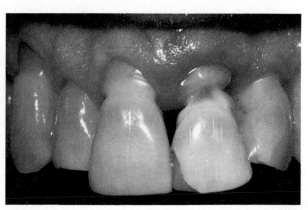

(a)   (b)

FIGURE 20–10 (a) Soft tissue trauma cause by improper flossing. (b) Soft tissue trauma caused by improper toothbrushing.

procedures because of the discomfort experienced during toothbrushing. Identification of hypersensitive areas is difficult, and frequently, toothbrushing is a major factor in localizing the sensitivity. Accordingly, root surfaces must be desensitized and an adequate oral hygiene self-care program maintained. In patients with good oral hygiene but with dentinal hypersensitivity, use of a desensitizing agent is recommended (Orchardson & Gillam, 2006).

Gingival recession as a result of the disease process (attachment loss), tooth malposition, faulty toothbrushing, or periodontal surgery can result in exposed dentin, which can result in hypersensitivity near the cervical area of the tooth. Usually, movement of fluid within the dentinal tubules causes discomfort in the exposed areas.

Root sensitivity occurs in approximately half of the patients following subgingival scaling and root planing (von Troil, Needleman, & Sanz, 2002). The intensity of root sensitivity increases for a few weeks after therapy, after which it decreases. In clinical practice, it may be recommended that patients should be made aware of the potential for root sensitivity prior to treatment (von Troil et al., 2002). A clinical study reported that scaling and root planing procedures in periodontal therapy resulted in an increase of teeth that respond to painful stimuli. However, pain experiences in general appeared minor, and only a few teeth in a few patients developed highly sensitive root surfaces following instrumentation (Tammaro, Wennström, & Bergenholtz, 2000).

Assessing the Patient's Need for Desensitization

The following steps are recommended to assess the type of desensitization needed:

1. Use the air syringe to assess whether there is sensitivity. Write on the tooth being evaluated a "+" if the tooth has a positive response to the stimulus.
2. Recommend use of a desensitizing dentifrice for about 4 to 6 weeks. The patient is instructed to brush two times a day for 1 minute.
3. Instruct the patient on proper brushing so that the situation does not get worse. The patient's brushing technique must be corrected if treatment is to be successful.
4. Discuss the role of diet with the patient. Acidic and citrus foods should be limited in the patient's diet. If the patient frequently consumes acidic foods or juices, he or she should be instructed to rinse the mouth with sodium bicarbonate to help neutralize the acidity.
5. At the next examination, do the air syringe test again, and if the sensitivity is gone, the patient can go back to his or her regular dentifrice. If the sensitivity reappears later, the patient can use the desensitizing dentifrice again. If the sensitivity is still present, an in-office treatment should be tried.

Treatment

A number of treatments are available for sensitive teeth. The type of treatment depends on the severity of the problem and the history of prior intervention. Treatment of dentin hypersensitivity focuses on blocking the opened dentinal tubules to prevent transmission of the noxious external stimuli and decreasing the intradental nerve excitability. Therapeutic products can be applied either professionally or by the patient. Most of the patient-applied over-the-counter (OTC) products must be used for a prolonged period of time (up to several months) for greatest effect. Manufacturers have added fluoride to the formula for its anticaries effect. It must be stressed to patients that optimal plaque control will help to reduce the sensitivity.

Table 20–3 ■ lists the more commonly used dentifrices for dentinal hypersensitivity. Potassium nitrate is effective in reducing cold and tactile sensitivity as compared with regular toothpaste (Silverman et al., 1996). Potassium nitrate acts quickly and directly on the pulpal nerves. Potassium nitrate–containing dentifrices are ADA approved for the relief of dentin sensitivity. Application of fluoride to the dentinal surface is a treatment option for dentinal hypersensitivity (Bartold, 2006; Jacobsen & Bruce, 2001).

Patient-Applied Treatment

Basically, potassium nitrate and stannous fluoride products are available for patient-applied treatments (Table 20–3).

DENTIFRICES Patient-applied medicaments are available as dentifrices, gels, and rinses. Dentifrices are helpful when many tooth surfaces are sensitive. For patients with mild sensitivity without loss of substantial tooth structure, a densensitizing dentifrice is recommended. Because it can take several weeks to see results, fluoride has been added to most dentifrices. It appears that a potassium nitrate–containing dentifrice works the fastest.

The longer the dentifrice is in contact with the dentin surface, the greater is its success. Thus, more frequent applications are advised. Instead of using a dentifrice in the usual manner, it may be more effective if the undiluted dentifrice is applied with a cotton applicator directly on the tooth surface.

FLUORIDES Of all the fluorides, stannous fluoride shows the most promise for topical application in periodontal therapy as an antibacterial and desensitizing agent. Application of stannous fluoride (gel: 0.4%, rinse: 0.63%, toothpaste: 0.454%) on a daily basis, after some time, can be therapeutic in reducing dentinal hypersensitivity. However, it often stings the gingiva, and patients may not comply with treatment. In addition, stannous fluoride can cause a yellowish or light brown stain on dentin (Ellingsen, Eriksen, & Rölla, 1982) more than enamel because of its porous nature, making it unaesthetic (Terézhalmy, Chaves, Bsoul, Baker, & He, 2007).

In-Office Treatment

If therapeutic dentifrices are not successful, in-office application of medicaments is recommended. Several products are available, including ferric oxalate, fluoride (with or without iontophoresis), bonding agents, varnishes, and glass ionomers (Table 20–4 ■).

Table 20–3 Patient-Applied Desensitizing Agents

Product	Active Ingredient	Method of Use
Crest Sensitivity Protection® (Procter & Gamble, Cincinnati, OH)	5% potassium nitrate, 0.15% sodium fluoride	Apply to toothbrush
Crest Pro-Health Toothpaste	Stannous fluoride 0.454%, 0.16% sodium fluoride	Apply to toothbrush
Gel-Kam® gel (Colgate Oral Pharm.,)	0.4% stannous fluoride	Apply to toothbrush and brush teeth. This product is available over-the-counter without a prescription. Available in 4.3 oz tubes or a pack with 2 to 3.5 oz tubes.
Gel-Kam® Oral Care Rinse (Colgate Oral Pharm.)	0.63% stannous fluoride	Patient places 1/8 fluid oz of concentrate in marked mixing vial (included in box) and adds water as directed to prepare a 0.1% stannous fluoride rinse. Rinse over a 3-week period.
STANIMAX™ Perio Rinse (SDI Labs, Glenview, IL)	0.63% stannous fluoride	1/8 fluid oz is diluted with warm water to make 1 oz of the rinse in a measuring cup that is provided.
STANIMAX™ Brush-on Gel (SDI Labs, Glenview, IL)	0.4% stannous fluoride	Apply gel to toothbrush and brush teeth.
Sensodyne® Toothpaste (GlaxoSmithKline)	5% potassium nitrate, sodium fluoride	Apply to toothbrush and brush teeth
Soothe Rx (Omni)	calcium, sodium, phosphorus, and silica	Prescription toothpaste. Tube-Stage 1: Use twice daily for 2 weeks. Packets-Stage 2: Use once weekly for 24 weeks. Apply a ribbon on toothrush. Brush for 2 minutes. Do not eat or drink for 30 minutes.

OXALATE SALTS Most oxalates (ferric oxalate and potassium oxalate) are available as acidic solutions. Oxalates are capable of blocking the dentinal tubules when they are placed on an area of exposed dentin. Often the patient brushes the oxalate off. Thus the patient must be instructed to not brush too vigorously so that the dentin will not be removed. It is best to evaluate the patient's brushing technique in the office.

FLUORIDES Stannous fluoride is applied topically on the exposed dentin, forming a sort of granular layer over the dentin surface that does not come off with brushing, so it seals or decreases dentin permeability.

Sodium fluoride is available as a paste (33% sodium fluoride, 33% kaolin, 33% glycerin). Sodium fluoride works best for about 7 to 14 days, and then its effects dissipate.

Various sodium fluoride solutions have been tried with limited success. When iontophoresis is used to allow the fluoride ion to penetrate into the dentinal tubules, longer-lasting effects, up to 3 to 4 months, are seen. A second application usually is necessary.

RESTORATIVE MATERIALS/RESTORATIONS Methacrylate resins, such as Seal and Protect, are used to seal the affected area but may provide relief for up to 6 months and then need to be reapplied. If all treatments discussed have failed to resolve the hypersensitivity, a restoration can be placed, but the restoration is usually finished with a diamond bur, which may open up new tubules below the restoration, recreating sensitive dentin. Because the restoration is located at the cervical third of the tooth, overhangs or rough surfaces may create more problems.

If the sensitivity can be narrowed down to just one or two teeth, a glass ionomer can be used.

Halitosis

Halitosis is the general term used to describe unpleasant breath, regardless of its sources, oral or nonoral (e.g., expired air). *Oral malodor* is the term especially used to describe the odor from the oral cavity.

Oral malodor, bad breath, or halitosis is a common complaint encountered by dental practitioners. It may be due to poor oral hygiene, local factors, or systemic involvement.

Table 20–4 Chair-Side Desensitizing Products

Product	Active Ingredient	Method of Use
Seal & Protect® (Dentsply, PA)	Methacrylate resins, PENTA, nanofillers, triclosan (a broad-spectrum antibacterial agent), and acetone	Isolate area, rinse and dry. Apply product and keep wet for 20 seconds.
		A gentle stream of compressed air is used to volatilize the acetone solvent and the material is light cured for 10 seconds. A second coat is then applied, dried, and light activated. Dentsply/Caulk claims the product provides symptomatic relief for up to 6 months.
Gel-Kam Dentinbloc® (Colgate Oral Pharm.)	1.09% sodium fluoride, 0.40% stannous fluoride, 0.14% hydrogen fluoride	Saturate a cotton pellet and apply to dry exposed dentin. Do not burnish; use light pressure.
Sensodyne® Sealant	6% ferric oxalate	Saturate a cotton pellet and apply to dry exposed dentin. Do not burnish; use light pressure.
STANIMAX-PRO™ (SDI Labs, Glenview, IL)	3.28% stannous fluoride	Can be used as a gel or diluted one-to-one with water to form a 1.64% stannous fluoride rinse.
Duraflor® (Pharmascience Inc., Montréal, Canada), Duraphat® (Colgate Oral Pharm., NY)	50 mg sodium fluoride varnish 5% sodium fluoride varnish	Apply to affected area with a cotton pellet. Apply to affected area with a brush that comes with kit or with a cotton pellet.
Denclude™ Dental Cream (Ortek-Therapeutics, NY)	Calcium carbonate, hydrated silica, arginine bicarbonate	Apply a thick ribbon to a soft toothbrush. Brush twice daily and expectorate. Don't eat of drink for 30 minutes afterward.
Proclude™ Prophylaxis Paste (Ortek-Therapeutics, NY)	Hydrated silica, calcium carbonate, arginine bicarcarbonate	Use as a polishing paste post-scaling and root planning to reduce sensitivity especially at cervical areas. Rinse after application.
NuCare™ Root Conditioner with NovaMin (SunStar-Butler)	Calcium, sodium, phosphorus, and silica	Tooth remineralization.
NuCare™ Prophylaxis Paste with Novamin (Sunstar-Butler)	Calcium, sodium, phosphorus, and silica	Tooth remineralization. Can apply after periodontal surgery.

Oral malodor affects a large proportion of the population and may cause a significant social or psychological handicap to those suffering from it.

It has been estimated that 10% to 30% of the U.S. population suffers from bad breath on a regular basis (Meskin, 1996). In other studies, 20% to 60% of the population suffers from chronic oral malodor, and in approximately half of these individuals, the problem becomes serious enough to create personal discomfort and social embarrassment (Bosy, 1997; Brunette, Proskin, & Nelson, 1998). There is potential impact of oral malodor on personal life, so sufferers often make desperate attempts to mask their oral malodor with mints and chewing gum, compulsive brushing, and repeated use of mouth rinses. In most cases, the problem of oral malodor has been shown to originate in the oral cavity, where conditions that favor the retention of anaerobic, mainly gram-negative bacteria, lead to the development of bad breath (Ratcliff & Johnson, 1999). In addition to the periodontal pockets, the most important retention site is the dorsum of the tongue with its numerous papillae (Delanghe et al., 1999; Scully, El-Maaytah, Porter, & Greenman, 1997). There are various compounds that produce unpleasant smells in the human oral environment, such as hydrogen sulfide, methanethiol, dimethylsulfide, n-dodecanol, n-tetradecanol, phenol, indole, diphenylamine, pyridine, and others (Kostelc, Preti, Zelson, et al., 1980). Especially volatile sulfur compounds

(VSC; hydrogen sulfide, methylmercaptan, and dimethyl sulfide), which arise from bacterial metabolism of amino acids, mainly contribute to oral malodor. It has been demonstrated that the intensity of clinical bad breath is significantly associated with amount of intraoral VSC level (Replogle & Beebe, 1996). The periodontal pocket is an ideal environment for VSC production with respect to the bacterial profile and sulfur source. In addition, VSC also accelerate periodontal tissue destruction. This may explain why patients with periodontal diseases often complain of oral malodor (Morita & Wang, 2001). Many people still believe that bad breath originates in the stomach. Halitosis is rarely a gastrointestinal condition (Page, 1997). Research reports now agree that, in the vast majority of cases, halitosis (80% to 90%) originates within the oral cavity, where anaerobic bacteria degrade sulfur-containing amino acids to the foul-smelling volatile sulfur compounds (Rosenberg, 1996; Tonzetich, 1997). The oral and systemic factors predisposing toward bad breath are given in Boxes 20–1 and 20–2.

Classification of Patients with Halitosis

Although halitosis involves oral, systemic, and psychological pathologies, a clear classification has not been established, and mismanagement of psychological or systemic cases of halitosis can occur. The classification system reported by Miyazaki and colleagues (1999) has three categories: genuine halitosis, pseudo-halitosis, and halitophobia. Genuine halitosis is subclassified as physiologic halitosis and pathologic halitosis. Pathologic halitosis is categorized as oral pathologic halitosis and extraoral pathologic halitosis (Table 20–5 ■).

Pseudo-halitosis and halitophobia both involve a psychosomatic condition. Patients complain of the presence of bad breath, but offensive malodor is not perceived by

---

Box 20–1: Oral Conditions That May Cause Bad Breath

- Periodontal pockets
- Xerostomia (dryness of mouth)
- Carious lesions
- Bacterial biofilms
- Interdental areas debris
- Spaces between the papillae of the tongue
- Poor restorations
- Calculus
- Erupting wisdom teeth (pericoronitis)
- Remaining roots
- Gangrenous pulps (necrosed pulp tissue)
- NUG (necrotizing ulcerative gingivitis)

Box 20–2: Causes to Consider in a Patient with Halitosis

Nonpathologic causes
Oral: morning breath, xerostomia due to mouth breathing and medications
Hunger
Tobacco
Foods: onion, garlic, pastrami, other meats
Alcohol

Pathologic causes
Periodontal disease, xerostomia (underlying illness), gingivitis, stomatitis, glossitis, cancer, candidiasis, parotitis

Gastrointestinal disorders
Gastroesophageal reflux, hiatal hernia, cancer

Nasal
Rhinitis, sinusitis, tumors, foreign bodies

Pulmonary
Bronchitis, pneumonia, tuberculosis, cancer

Systemic
Diabetes, uremia, hepatic disease, blood dyscrasias, rheumatologic disease, dehydration, fever

Psychiatric
Delusions

---

others. Improvement of the condition of pseudo-halitosis is expected by the explanation of examination results, counseling, and simple treatment measures, such as tongue cleaning. Thus, pseudohalitosis is treatable by dental practitioners. In contrast, patients who are halitophobic believe that there are definite physical or social factors that contribute to their belief in having halitosis, and they cannot be convinced that they do not have malodor. Because of the difficulty in treating halitophobia, it is not considered within the realm of dentistry (Yaegaki & Coil, 2000b). Treatment needs for breath odor are described in detail in Table 20–6 ■.

DIAGNOSIS AND ASSESSMENT OF ORAL MALODOR There are many methods available for examination, diagnosis, and assessment of oral malodor (Nachnani, 2011):

1. **Self-Assessment** Patients have been found to be incapable of scoring their own malodor in an objective fashion. Inability to smell one's own oral malodor has been attributed to adaptation or dulling of sensation resulting from continued exposure.
2. **Gas Chromatography** A few halitosis clinics use a gas chromatography (GC) equipped with a flame photometric detector for diagnosing halitosis (Yaegaki & Coil, 2000a). GC is the gold standard for oral malodor measurement (Miyazaki et al., 1999; Yaegaki & Coil, 2000a). It is an objective means to obtain exact values

Table 20–5 Classification of Halitosis with Corresponding Treatment Needs (TN)

Classification	Subdivision and Treatment Needs	Description
I. Genuine Halitosis A. Physiologic Halitosis	TN–1	• Obvious malodor intensity beyond socially acceptable level. • Malodor arises through putrefactive process within the oral cavity. • Neither specific disease nor pathologic condition that could cause halitosis is found. • Origin is mainly the dorso posterior region of the tongue. (Temporary halitosis as a result of dietary factors [e.g., garlic bread] should be excluded)
B. Pathologic Halitosis	1. Oral Pathologic TN-1 and TN-2	• Halitosis caused by disease, pathologic condition, or malfunction of oral tissues. • Halitosis derived from tongue coating modified by pathological condition (e.g., periodontal disease, xerostomia) is included in this subdivision.
	2. Extraoral Pathologic TN-1 and TN-3	• Malodor originates from nasal, paranasal, and laryngeal regions. • Malodor originates from pulmonary tracts. • Malodor originates from upper digestive tracts. • Malodor originates from disorders anywhere in the body whereby the odor is blood-borne and emitted via lungs (diabetes mellitus, hepatic cirrhosis, uremia, internal bleeding, etc.).
II. Pseudo-Halitosis	TN-1 and TN-4	• Obvious malodor is not perceived by others, although a patient stubbornly complains of the existence of his or her halitosis. • Improvement of this condition is highly promising by explanation of examination results, counseling, and simple treatment measures.
III. Halitophobia	TN-1 and TN-5	• After treatment for genuine halitosis or pseudo-halitosis, a patient persists in believing that he or she has halitosis, although no physical or social evidence exists.

Source: Yaegaki and Coil, 2000a; Miyazaki et al., 1999.

Table 20–6 Treatment Needs (TN) for Breath Odor

Category	Description
TN-1*	Explanation of halitosis and instruction for oral hygiene. Support and reinforcement of the patient's self-care for further improvement of his or her oral hygiene.
TN-2	Oral prophylaxis, professional cleaning, and treatment for oral diseases, especially periodontal diseases.
TN-3	Referral to a physician or medical specialist.
TN-4	Explanation of examination data, further professional instruction, education, and reassurance for improvement.
TN-5	Referral to a clinical psychologist, psychiatrist, or other psychological specialist.

*TN-1 is applicable to all cases requiring TN-2 through TN-5.

for the various odorous volatiles. It is a very sensitive method. A flame photometer detector is usually employed for the detection of VSC. Gas chromatography may also be combined with mass spectrometry (an instrument used to identify chemicals in a substance by their mass and charge) enlarging the scope of the method (Preti et al., 1992).

3. **Halimeter**   The Halimeter (Interscan, CA), using an electrochemical gas sensor cell, has become the primary tool in chronic halitosis research and diagnosis. The Halimeter is twice as sensitive to hydrogen sulfides as it is to methylmercaptan. Halimeter measurements are significantly influenced by other oral gases such as from chewing gum, strong mouthrinse odors, alcohol, shampoo, body lotion, smoking, and even water vapor.

4. **Organoleptic Measurement**   Organoleptic (the taste and aroma properties of a food or chemical) scoring (Miyazaki et al., 1999) is simply done by smelling the patient's breath and assigning a score of oral malodor (Yaegaki, 2000). A translucent tube is inserted into the patient's mouth. The patient exhales as the clinician smells the breath. When the recognition threshold (score 2 or over) is identified, a diagnosis of genuine halitosis is made.

   The patient is required to refrain from drinking coffee, tea, or juice; smoking; eating garlic; and using scented cosmetics before the assessment. The clinician must have a normal sense of smell. The clinician can regularly check his or her specific sense of smell by sniffing VSC from a freshly boiled egg or nori (seaweed that can be purchased in an Oriental food store; Yaegaki, 2000).

5. **Simple Determination of Oral Malodor**   When a simple determination of oral malodor is required, the spoon test is preferred. In the spoon test, the posterior area of the dorsal surface of the tongue is assessed by thorough scraping, using a disposable plastic spoon. Afterward, the spoon can be smelled; it has a very repulsive odor in patients with severe oral malodor (Yaegaki & Coil, 2000b).

6. **Psychological Assessment**   Halitophobia patients and many pseudo-halitosis patients have a psychosomatic condition (Miyazaki et al., 1999; Yaegaki, 2000). Because halitophobia is easily diagnosed using the halitosis classification of Miyazaki and colleagues (1999), corresponding patient management is improved. Psychological assessment is facilitated by specified, tested, and established questionnaires used to acquire medical history as a routine practice.

7. **Tongue Sulfide Probe**   Recently, a tongue sulfide probe for detecting oral malodor has been developed (Morita, Musinski, & Wang, 2001). The tongue sulfide level on the tongue dorsum (VSC level) is determined by using the tongue sulfide probe (Diamond General Development Corporation, Ann Arbor, MI). The probe is applied on the anterior, the middle, or

the posterior part of the tongue along the median groove of the tongue dorsum with a light pressure for 30 seconds. The probe is composed of an active sulfide-sensing element and a stable reference element. The sulfide-sensing element generates an electrochemical voltage proportional to the concentration of sulfide ions present. This voltage is measured relative to the operating point of the reference element.

TREATMENT OF ORAL MALODOR   The first step in treating oral malodor is to assess and treat all oral diseases and conditions that may contribute to oral malodor. The following treatment methods have proven their effectiveness to a variable level (Roldán et al., 2005) for treating oral malodor.

1. **Tongue Cleaning**   Treatment needs (TN) corresponding to the classification of halitosis in dental practice has been categorized into five levels (see Table 20–6; Miyazaki et al., 1999). Practical management of physiologic halitosis requires TN-1 with cleaning the tongue being more essential than mouth rinsing, because the origin of physiological halitosis is mainly the dorso posterior region of the tongue. Tongue coating is comprised of desquamated epithelial cells, blood cells, and bacteria. Cleaning the tongue reduces VSC. Tongue brushing is preferred over tongue scraping (Yaegaki & Coil, 2000a). It is postulated that brush bristles sweep between papillae and remove microorganisms (Kleinberg & Codipilly, 2001). Tongue cleaning should be carried out before toothbrushing because mint flavor in toothpaste sensitizes the oropharyx to an elevated gag reflex (Yaegaki & Coil, 2000b). The middle and posterior parts of the tongue dorsum should be focused for a cleaning, as high proportional sulfide (pS) levels are found there (Morita et al., 2001).

2. **Oral Hygiene and Mouth Rinses**   Mechanical reduction of microorganisms through improved oral hygiene procedures has been associated with reductions in oral malodor.

   Additional treatments in TN-1 include routine oral hygiene procedures and mouth rinsing. Some clinical trials of mouth rinses claim to reduce VSC determined by gas chromatography or Halimeter (Yaegaki & Coil, 2000a). Mouth rinses containing cetylpyridinium chloride (CPC), chlorhexidine, or hydrogen peroxide have very limited role in controlling VSC. Currently, it has been recommended that patients use a zinc-containing mouthwash (Yaegaki & Coil, 2000b) such as BreathRx because zinc strongly inhibits bacterial cysteine proteinase and inhibits the destruction of shed epithelial cells and blood cells (Yaegaki & Suetaka, 1989).

3. **Toothpastes** Toothpastes containing triclosan and a copolymer or sodium bicarbonate were reported to reduce certain amounts of VSC, and these toothpastes also may be recommended (Niles et al., 1999). Such toothpastes include Colgate Total® and Arm and Hammer® Toothpaste.

4. **Chewing Gums** When people are concerned with oral malodor, approximately 70% use chewing gum (Yaegaki & Coil, 2000a). Chewing gum containing sugar was shown to reduce VSC in mouth air through an active pH change in the oral cavity (Kleinberg & Westbay, 1992). However, sugarless gum only masks halitosis with its flavors, producing a short-term effect (Reingewirtz, Girault, Reingewirtz, Senger, & Tenenbaum, 1999).

5. **Periodontal/Restorative Dental Treatment and Xerostomia** Periodontal treatment is frequently required as TN-2 because periodontal diseases contribute to oral pathologic halitosis. The reduction of salivary secretion may cause oral pathologic halitosis; the treatment of xerostomia may reduce oral malodor. Increased salivary flow may contribute to decreased oral malodor. Although dental caries may not be a significant cause of oral malodor, caries treatment may be recommended (Yaegaki & Coil, 2000b).

MANAGEMENT OF PATIENTS WITH PSEUDO-HALITOSIS (PATIENT WITH EXTRAORAL HALITOPHOBIA) Because extraoral pathologic halitosis treatments are out of the realm of dental clinicians, patients with extraoral halitophobia should be referred to medical practitioners (TN-3; Yaegaki & Coil, 2000b). Patients with pseudo-halitosis are able to accept the clinician's diagnosis that oral malodor does not exist after receiving literature support, education, and explanation of examination results (TN-4). If a patient is not able to accept the diagnosis of pseudo-halitosis or if a patient with halitosis believes that halitosis exists after the halitosis was treated, the patient should be diagnosed as halitophobic by the dentist. The patient/client should be referred to a psychological specialist (TN-5; Yaegaki & Coil, 2000b).

OVER-THE-COUNTER (OTC) PRODUCTS Over-the-counter oral health products are numerous in the market. The products include tongue brushes, tongue scrapers, mouth rinses, chewing gums, chewable aromatic tablets, mouth fresheners, oral sprays, and gels. Some OTC products may be genuinely effective as a result of actually reducing the number of bacteria, whereas others may mask the odors, though their masking effect may only last for a brief period (Loesche & Kazor, 2002).

Did You Know?

Upper-class Romans added expensive imported urine to their teeth whitening mix (unaware that it was the ammonia molecules that were brightening their teeth).

Dental Hygiene Application

The primary reference standard for detection of oral malodor is the human nose (organoleptic assessment) because it provides an overall evaluation of the existing malodor condition. For the treatment of bad breath, improved oral hygiene, especially tongue cleaning, has been shown to reduce VSC significantly.

The incorporation of diagnosis and management of oral malodor should be considered part of comprehensive dental care. Although most oral malodor have a simple cause, no single therapy is always effective. A team approach to diagnosis and treatment may involve the dentist; periodontist; ear, nose, and throat specialist; dietition; pharmacist; internal medicine specialist; and psychologist.

Supragingival and subgingival dental plaque biofilms play a major role in the initiation of periodontal diseases. Because the subgingival microbiota is derived originally from supragingival plaque, it is necessary to disrupt both groups of bacteria. This is accomplished through mechanical supragingival plaque removal by the patient using toothbrushes and interdental devices and by the dental hygienist by removing subgingival plaque.

It would seem that gingivitis should be treated easily with plaque removal. Unfortunately, many obstacles prevent the timely removal of plaque. Besides lack of motivation to learn and perform toothbrushing and flossing skills, many patients also perform inconsistently, lack knowledge, and employ poor technique.

Added to a daily regimen patients may benefit from topical antimicrobial chemotherapeutic agents to reduce biofilm and help prevent periodontal diseases. The rinses reduce plaque and gingivitis and reduce reservoirs of pathogens that may be unaffected by oral hygiene self-care strategies. An over-the-counter ADA accepted antiseptic mouth rinse is Listerine® (fixed combination of essential oils); Peridex®, a prescription rinse, has also been found to be effective (Guernlian, 2007).

Fluorides have successfully decreased the rate of dental caries. However, few advances in chemical plaque control (dentifrices) have been achieved in recent years, except for the introduction of triclosan. Tartar-control dentifrices offer a cosmetic benefit. Desensitizing toothpastes may aid in the alleviation of dentinal hypersensitivity. Baking soda/hydrogen peroxide dentifrices have not been shown to consistently elicit antiplaque/antigingivitis effects. Triclosan is the first chemical agent used in dentifrices that can claim benefits to periodontal health.

Key Points

- Plaque removal prevents gingivitis.
- The removal of plaque through daily plaque-control practices and professional cleanings is important in controlling subgingival plaque formation.
- There are numerous periodontal, dental, and medical causes of bad breath that need to be explored to effectively treat halitosis.
- The main goal of prevention is to achieve the lowest plaque level possible.

- Plaque-control measures by the patient and professional maintenance appointments are both important in maintaining gingival health and are essential parts of primary and secondary prevention of periodontitis.
- Dental floss is indicated for interproximal plaque removal in Type I gingival embrasures.
- There is no difference in efficacy of plaque removal with waxed or unwaxed dental floss.

Self-Quiz

1. Which one of the following statements describes the rationale for periodontal oral hygiene self-care?
   a. Reduction in the risk for development of dental caries
   b. Augmentation of the immune reaction to a bacterial insult
   c. Elimination or suppression of harmful microorganisms found in supragingival plaque biofilms
   d. Disruption of the number of subgingival microbial biota with a delay in the repopulation of pathogens

2. Which one of the following oral hygiene regimens is best for a patient after periodontal surgery?
   a. Resume regular brushing and flossing regimens.
   b. Use a soft-bristle toothbrush and an antimicrobial mouth rinse.
   c. Use powered toothbrush and floss.
   d. Use oral irrigation with chlorhexidine.

3. A patient says that he is doing the best he can with his home care, but he still has moderate to heavy supragingival deposits. Which of the following recommendations should the dental hygienist give to this patient?
   a. Don't worry because everyone gets some accumulations.
   b. Use an antimicrobial mouth rinse.
   c. Improve or change method of home care.
   d. Refer to a specialist.

4. Waxed dental floss has proven to be more effective in interdental cleaning than unwaxed dental floss because it is easier for the patient to handle.
   a. Both the statement and the reason are correct and related.
   b. Both the statement and the reason are correct but not related.
   c. The statement is correct, but the reason is not.
   d. The statement is not correct, but the reason is correct.
   e. Neither the statement nor the reason is correct.

5. From the following list, select the items associated with testing for halitosis on your patient.
   a. Self-assessment
   b. Tongue sulfide probe
   c. Chew gum test
   d. Psychological assessment
   e. Simple determination of oral malodor

6. From the following list, select the items associated with recommending interdental cleansing devices.
   a. Amount of plaque
   b. Manual dexterity
   c. Presence of a bridge
   d. Type of embrasure
   e. Severity of inflammation

7. Which one of the following methods best evaluates for effectiveness of a patient's oral hygiene?
   a. Show and tell
   b. Feedback
   c. Disclosing agents
   d. Self-documentation

8. For each oral hygiene aid listed, select the correct device for the appropriate gingival embrasure.

1. Interdental brush	a. Type I
2. Rubber-tip stimulator	b. Type II
3. Wooden wedge	c. Type III
4. Dental floss	

9. Which one of the following steps should be done first when treating a patient for dentinal hypersensitivity?
   a. Recommend a desensitizing dentifrice for 4 to 6 weeks.
   b. Instruct the patient on the proper toothbrushing method.
   c. Identify the tooth/teeth that is (are) painful.
   d. Apply sodium fluoride.

10. Which of the following oral hygiene aids is best used for interdental removal of plaque from implants?
    a. Toothbrush
    b. Powered toothbrush
    c. Interproximal brush with plastic core
    d. Interproximal brush with metal core

Case Study

A 35-year-old male is scheduled with the dental hygienist in a general practice dental office. The patient has probing depths to 7 mm in the molar region and clinical attachment loss of 4 mm in some areas. There is moderate horizontal bone loss and a few areas of vertical bone loss on the maxillary molars. There is both supra and subgingival plaque and calculus and some bleeding upon probing. The periodontal classification is moderate chronic periodontitis.

1. The dental hygienist is planning a first series of nonsurgical care before re-assessment for further therapies. The first visit would include which of the following procedures?
   a. scaling and root planning of maxillary arch
   b. comprehensive data collection, radiographs if indicated, and oral hygiene instruction
   c. ultrasonic scaling entire mouth and polishing
   d. ultrasonic scaling mandibular right quadrant

Answer: B. Before any scaling is performed a complete medical, dental, periodontal, and radiographic assessment is completed and evaluated for patient risks, diagnosis, and prognosis.

2. How should the following visits be scheduled to remove the deposits?
   a. 4 visits to scale each quadrant
   b. 2 visits to scale each arch
   c. 5 visits to scale by quadrant and return to evaluate healing
   d. 3 visits more to scale by arch and return to polish and fluoride

Answer: C. Although it depends upon patient response, the plan should include quadrant scaling at 7–10 day intervals to allow for healing and re-evaluation before the last visit at 4–8 weeks after previous appointment to evaluate tissue response.

3. The dental hygienist evaluated the tissue after all scaling and root planning has occurred. At this visit there is still bleeding upon probing and the pocket depth has not improved. What is considered as the next phase?
   a. Do a deep scaling of the areas by hand instead of ultrasonic
   b. Recall patient in four months to re-assess
   c. Provide fluoride and anti-microbial rinses
   d. Refer to a periodontist for co-management

Answer: D. Referral is indicated when there is unresolved inflammation at any site, the age of the patient at 35 years old, and CAL as indicated. Other adjunctive therapies might have been included in the previous appointments however if inflammation persists other surgical treatment may be required.

References

Addy, M., and P. Adriaens. 1998. Epidemiology and etiology of periodontal diseases and the role of plaque control in dental caries: Consensus report of group A. In eds. N. P. Lang, R. Attström, and H. Löe, *Proceedings of the European Workshop on Mechanical Plaque Control*, 99–101. Chicago: Quintessence.

Addy, M., and R. Koltai. 1994. Control of supragingival calculus. Scaling and polishing and anticalculus toothpastes: An opinion. *J. Clin. Periodontol.* 21:342–346.

Bacca, L. A., M. Leusch, A. C. Lanzalaco, D. Macksood, O. J. Bouwsma, et al. 1997. A comparison of intraoral antimicrobial effects of stabilized fluoride dentifrice, baking soda/hydrogen peroxide dentifrice, conventional NaF dentifrice and essential oil mouthrinse. *J. Clin. Dent.* 8:54–61.

Bader, H. J. 1992. Review of currently available battery operated toothbrushes. *Compend. Contin. Educ. Dent.* 13:1163–1169.

Baker, K. 1995. The role of dental professionals and the patient in plaque control. *Periodontology 2000* 8:108–113.

Balshi, T. J. 1986. Hygiene maintenance procedures for patients treated with the tissue integrated prosthesis (osseointegration). *Quintessence Int.* 17:95–102.

Barnes, C. M., C. M. Russell, R. A. Reinhardt, et al. 2005. Comparison of irrigation to floss as an adjunct to toothbrushing: Effect on bleeding, gingivitis, and supragingival plaque. *J. Clin. Dent.* 16:71–77.

Bartold, P. M. 2006. Dentinal hypersensitivity: A review. *Australian Dental Journal* 51(3):212–218.

Beaumont, R. H. 1990. Patient preference for waxed or unwaxed dental floss. *J. Periodontol.* 61:123–125.

Beiswanger, B. B., P. M. Doyle, R. D. Jackson, et al. 1995. The clinical effect of dentifrices containing stabilized stannous fluoride on plaque founa and gingivitis. A six-month study with adlibtum brushing. *J. Clin. Dent.* 6:46–53.

Binney, A., M. Addy, S. McKeowns, and L. Everatt. 1995. The effect of commercially available triclosan-containing toothpaste compared to a sodium-fluoride containing toothpaste and a chlorhexidine rinse on 4-day plaque regrowth. *J. Clin. Periodontol.* 22(1):830–834.

Binney, A., M. Addy, S. McKeowns, and L. Everatt. 1996. The choice of controls in toothpaste studies: The effect of a number of commercially available toothpastes compared to water on a 4-day plaque regrowth. *J. Clin. Periodontol.* 23(5):456–459.

Björn, A. L., U. Andersson, and A. Olsson. 1981. Gingival recession in 15-year-old pupils. *Swed. Dent. J.* 5:141–146.

Bollmer, B. L. V., O. P. Sturzenberger, V. Vick, and E. Grossman. 1995. Reduction of calculus and Peridex stain with Tarter Control Crest. *J. Clin. Dent.* 6(4):185–187.

Bosy, A. 1997. Oral malodor: Philosophical and practical aspects. *J. Can. Dent. Assoc.* 63:196–201.

Brunette, D. M. 1996. Effects of baking soda–containing dentifrices on oral malodor. *Compend. Contin. Educ. Dent.* 17(Suppl. 19):22–31.

Brunette D. M., H. M. Proskin, and B. J. Nelson. 1998. The effects of dentifrice systems on oral malodor. *J. Clin. Dent.* 9:76–82.

Cancro, L. P., and S. L. Fischman. 1995. The expected effect on oral health of dental plaque control through mechanical removal. *Periodontology 2000* 8: 60–74.

Cerra, M. B., and W. J. Killoy. 1982. The effect of sodium bicarbonate and hydrogen peroxide on the microbial flora of periodontal pockets: A preliminary report. *J. Periodontol.* 53:599–603.

Checchi, L., S. Minguzzi, M. Franchi, and F. Forteleoni. 2001. Toothbrush filaments end-rounding: Stereomicroscope analysis. *J. Clin. Periodontol.* 28(4):360–371.

Ciancio, S. G. 1997. Triclosan: A new antigingivitis agent. *Biol. Ther. Dent.* 13:23–26.

Ciancio, S. G., C. Lauciello, O. Shibly, et al. 1995. The effect of an antiseptic mouth rinse on implant maintenance: Plaque & peri-implant gingival tissues. *J. Periodontol.* 66(11):962–965.

Ciancio, S. G., O. Shibly, and G. A. Farber. 1992. Clinical evaluation of the effect of two types of dental floss on plaque and gingival health. *Clin. Prevent. Dent.* 14:14–18.

Corbet, E. F., and W. I. R. Davies. 1993. The flow of supragingival plaque in the control of progressive periodontal disease: A review. *J. Clin. Peridontol.* 20:307–313.

Darby, M., and Walsh M. 2010. *Dental hygiene theory and practice*, 3rd ed. St. Louis, MO: Saunders Elsevier.

Delanghe, G., J. Ghyselen, C. Bollen, D. van Steenberghe, B. Vanderkerckhove, and L. Feenstra. 1999. An inventory of patients' response to treatment at a multidisciplinary breath odor clinic. *Quintessence Int.* 30:307–310.

Dellerman, P. A., T. J. Hughes, and T. A. Burkett. 1994. A comparative evaluation of the percent acceptable end-round bristles in the Crest Complete, the Improved Crest Complete and the Oral-B Advantage toothbrushes. *J. Clin. Dent.* 5:74–81.

Drake, D. R., B. Grigsby, and D. Drotz-Dieleman. 1994. Growth-inhibitory effect of pyrophosphate on oral bacteria. *Oral Micro. Immunol.* 9(1):25–28.

Drake, D., K. Vargas, A. Cardenzana, and R. Srikantha. 1995. Enhanced bacterial activity of Arm and Hammer Dental Care. *Am. J. Dent.* 8(6):308–312.

Duckworth, R. M., Y. Jones, J. Nicholson, A. P. Jacobson, and I. G. Chestnutt. 1994. Studies on plaque fluoride after use of F-containing dentifrices. *Adv. Dent. Res.* 8(2):202–207.

Ellingsen, J. E., H. M. Eriksen, and G. Rölla. 1982. Extrinsic dental stain caused by stannous fluoride. *Scand. J. Dent. Res.* (Feb) 90(1):9–13.

Felo, A., O. Shibly, S. G. Ciancio, F. R. Lauciello, and A. Ho. 1997. Effects of subgingival chlorhexidine irrigation of peri-implant maintenance. *Am. J. Dent.* 10:107–110.

Fischman, S. L., G. Kugel, R. B. Truelove, B. J. Nelson, and L. P. Cancro. 1992. Motivational benefits of a dentifrice containing baking soda and hydrogen peroxide. *J. Clin. Dent.* 3:88–94.

Fischman, S. L., and S. Yankell. 1999. Dentifrices, mouth rinses, and tooth whiteners. In eds. N. O. Harris and F. García-Godoy, *Primary preventive dentistry*, 5th ed., 103–125. Stamford, CT: Appleton and Lange.

Flores-de-Jacoby, L., and R. Mengel. 1995. Conventional surgical procedures. *Periodontology 2000* 9:38–54.

Forgas-Brockmann, L. B., C. Carter-Hanson, and W. J. Killoy. 1998. The effects of an ultrasonic toothbrush on plaque accumulation and gingival inflammation. *J. Clin. Periodontol.* 25:375–379.

Frandsen, A. 1986. Mechanical oral hygiene practices. In eds. H. Löe and D. V. Kleinman, *Dental plaque control measures and oral hygiene practices*, 93–116. Oxford: IRL Press.

Gaengler, P., A. Kurbad, and W. Weinert. 1993. Evaluation of anti-calculus efficacy: An SEM method of evaluating the effectiveness of pyrophosphate dentifrice on calculus formation. *J. Clin. Periodontol.* 20:144–146.

Garmyn, P., D. van Steenberghe, and M. Quirynen. 1998. Efficacy of plaque control in the maintenance of gingival health: Plaque control in primary and secondary prevention. In eds. N. P. Lang, R. Attström, and H. Löe, *Proceedings of the European Workshop on Mechanical Plaque Control*, 107–120. Chicago: Quintessence.

Gordon, J. M., J. A. Frascella, and R. C. Reardon. 1996. A clinical study of the safety and efficacy of a novel electric interdental cleaning device. *J. Clin. Dent.* 7:70–73.

Grossman, E., M. Cronin, W. Dembling, and H. Proskin. 1996. A comparative study of extrinsic tooth stain removal with two electric toothbrushes and a manual brush. *Am. J. Dent.* 9:25–29.

Guernlian, J. R. 2007. The role of dental plaque biofilm in oral health. *J. Dent. Hyg.* 81:116.

Hague, A. L., and M. P. Carr. 2007. Efficacy of an automated flossing device in different regions of the mouth. *J. Periodontol.* 78(8):1529–1537.

Hancock, E. B. 1996. Prevention. *Ann. Periodontol.* 1:223–249.

Hellstadius, K., B. Asman, and A. Gustafsson. 1993. Improved maintenance of plaque control by electric tooth brushing in periodontitis patients with low compliance. *J. Clin. Periodontol.* 20:235–237.

Hellström, M. K., P. Romberg, L. Krok, and J. Lindhe. 1996. The effect of supragingival plaque control on the microflora in human periodontitis. *J. Clin. Periodontol.* 23:934–940.

Hill, H. C., P. A. Levi, and I. Glickman. 1973. The effects of waxed and unwaxed dental floss on interdental plaque accumulation and interdental gingival health. *J. Periodontol.* 53:411–414.

Jacobsen, P. L., and G. Bruce. 2001. Clinical dentin hypersensitivity: Understanding the causes and prescribing a treatment. *J. Contemporary Practice.* 2(1):1–8.

Kirstila, V., M. Lenander-Lumikari, E. Soderling, and J. Tenovuo. 1996. Effects of oral hygiene products containing lactoperoxidase, lysozyme, and lactoferrin on the composition of whole saliva and on subjective oral symptoms in patients with xerostomia. *Acta Odontol. Scand.* 54:391–397.

Kleinberg, I., and M. Codipilly. 2001. Cysteine challenge testing as a method of determining the effectiveness of oral hygiene procedures for reducing oral malodor. *J. Dent. Rest.* 79(special issue):425.

Kleinberg, I., and G. Westbay. 1992. Salivary and metabolic factors involved in oral malodor formation. *J. Periodontol.* 63:768–775.

Koertge, T. E. 1996. Management of dental staining: Can low-abrasive dentifrices play a role? *Compend. Contin. Educ. Dent.* 17(Suppl 19):33–38.

Kostelc, J. G., G. Preti, P. R. Zelson, et al. 1980. Salivary volatiles as indicators of periodontitis. *J. Periodont. Res.* 15:185–192.

Lefkoff, M. H., F. M. Beck, and J. E. Horton. 1995. The effectiveness of a disposable tooth cleansing device on plaque. *J. Periodontol.* 66:218–221.

Levine, R. A. 1987. The Keyes technique as a cofactor in self-inflicted gingival lesions: A case report. *Compend. Contin. Educ. Dent.* 8:266–269.

Lewis, M. W., C. Holder-Ballard, R. J. Selders, Jr., M. Scarbecz, H. G. Johnson, and E. W. Turner. 2004. Comparison of the use of a toothpick holder to dental floss in improvement of gingival health in humans. *J. Periodontol.* 75(4): 551–556.

Lindhe, J., B. Rosling, S. S. Socransky, and A. R. Volpe. 1993. The effect of a triclosan containing dentifrice on established plaque and gingivitis. *J. Clin. Periodontol.* 20:327–334.

Lobene, R. R. 1989. A study to compare the effects of two dentifrices on adult dental calculus formation. *Clin. Dent.* 1:67–69.

Loesche, W. J., and C. Kazor. 2002. Microbiology and treatment of halitosis. *J. Periodontol.* 28:256–79.

Meffert, R., B. Langer, and M. Frutz. 1992. Dental implants: A review. *J. Periodontol.* 63:859–870.

Meskin, L. H. 1996. A breath of fresh air. *J. Am. Dent. Assoc.* 127:1282–86.

Miyazaki, H., M. Arao, K. Okamura, K. Yaegaki, and T. Matsuo. 1999. Tentative classification of halitosis and its treatment needs. *Niigata Dent. J.* 32:7–11.

Moran, J. M., and M. Addy. 1995. A comparative study of stain removal with two electric toothbrushes and a manual brush. *J. Clin. Dent.* 6:188–193.

Morita M., D. L. Musinski, and H. L. Wang. 2001. Assessment of newly developed tongue sulfide probe for detecting oral malodor. *J. Clin. Periodontol.* 28:494–496.

Morita, M., and H. L. Wang. 2001. Association between oral malodor and adult periodontitis: A review. *J. Clin. Periodontol.* 28:813–819.

Mullaby, B. H., J. A. James, W. A. Coulter, and G. H. Linden. 1995. The efficacy of a herbal-based toothpaste on the control of plaque and gingivitis. *J. Clin. Periodontol.* 22:686–689.

Nachnani, S. 2011. Oral malodor: Causes, assessment, and treatment. *Compendium* 32:22–31.

Niles, H. P., K. Rustogi, M. Pestrone, et al. 1999. Long lasting breath freshening effects of a trichlosan/coplymer/NaF toothpaste. *Proceedings of the 4th International Conference on Breath Odor*, 13. Los Angeles: Wiley.

O'Beirne, G. O., R. H. Johnson, G. Rutger Persson, and M. D. Spektor. 1996. Efficacy of a sonic toothbrush on inflammation and probing depth in adult periodontitis. *J. Periodontol.* 67:900–908.

Orchardson, R., and D. G. Gillam. 2006. Managing dentin hypersensitivity. *JADA* 137(7):990–998.

Orton, G. S., D. L. Steele, and L. T. Wolinsky. 1989. The dental professional's role in monitoring and maintenance of tissue-integrated prosthesis. *Int. J. Oral. Maxillofac. Implants* 4(4):305–310.

Page, R. C. 1997. Causes of halitosis. *Oral Care Rep.* 7(4):7–8.

Palcanis, K. G. 1996. Surgical pocket therapy. *Ann. Periodontol.* 1:589–617.

Paraskevas, S. 2005. Randomized controlled clinical trials on agents used for chemical plaque control. *Int. J. Dent. Hyg.* 3:162–78.

Philstrom, B. L., L. F. Wolff, M. B. Bakdash, E. M. Schaffer, J. R. Jensen, et al. 1987. Salt and peroxide compared with conventional oral hygiene: I. Clinical results. *J. Periodontol.* 58:291–300.

Preber, H., V. Ylipaa, J. Bergström, and H. Ryden. 1991. A comparative study of plaque removing efficiency using rotary electric and manual toothbrushes. *Swed. Dent. J.* 15:229–234.

Preti, G., L. Clark, B. J. Cowart, R. S. Feldman, L. D. Lowry, et al. 1992. Non-oral etiologies of oral malodor and altered chemosensation. *J. Periodontol.* 63:790–796.

Proskin, H. M., and A. R. Volpe. 1995. Comparison of the anticaries efficacy of dentifrices containing fluoride as sodium fluoride or sodium monofluorophosphate. *Am. J. Dent.* 8:51–58.

Ramfjord, S. P. 1987. Maintenance care for treated patients. *J. Clin. Periodontol.* 14:433–437.

Ratcliff, P. A., and P. W. Johnson. 1999. The relationship between oral malodor, gingivitis, and periodontists. A review. *J. Periodontol.* 70:485–489.

Reingewirtz, Y., O. Girault, N. Reingewirtz, B. Senger, and H. Tenenbaum. 1999. Mechanical effects and volatile sulfur compounds reducing effects of chewing gums and a control group. *Quintessence Int.* 30:319–323.

Replogle, W. H., and D. E. Beebe. 1996. Halitosis. *American Family Physician.* 53:1215–1223.

Roldán, S., D. Herrera, A. O'Connor, et al. 2005. A combined therapeutic approach to manage oral halitosis: A 3-month prospective case series. *J. Periodontol.* 76(6):1025–1033.

Rosenberg, M. J. 1996. Clinical assessment of bad breath: Current concepts. *J. Am. Dent. Assoc.* 127:475–482.

Rounds, M. C., and T. S. I. Tilliss. 1999. Personal oral hygiene: Auxiliary measures to complement toothbrushing. In eds. N. O. Harris, and F. Garcia-Godoy, *Primary preventive dentistry*, 125–154. Norwalk, CT: Appleton & Lange.

Sangnes, G. 1976. Traumatization of teeth and gingiva related to habitual tooth cleaning procedures. *J. Clin. Periodontol.* 3:94–103.

Sanz, M., and D. Herrera. 1998. Role of oral hygiene during the healing phase of periodontal therapy. In eds. N. P. Lang, R. Attström, and H. Löe, *Proceedings of the European Workshop on Mechanical Plaque Control*, 248–267. Chicago: Quintessence.

Savolainen, J. J., A. L. Suominen-Taipale, A. K. Uutela, T. P. Martelin, M. C. Niskanen, and M. L. E. Knuuttila. 2005. Sense of coherence as a determinant of toothbrushing frequency and level of oral hygiene. *J. Periodontol.* 76(6):1006–1012.

Saxer, U. P., and S. L. Yankell. 1997. Impact of improved toothbrushes on dental diseases: II. *Quintessence Int.* 28:573–593.

Schiff, T. G. 1987. The effect of a dentifrice containing soluble pyrophosphate and sodium fluoride on calculus deposits. *Clin. Prev. Dent.* 9:13–16.

Scully, C., M. El-Maaytah, S. R. Porter, and J. Greenman. 1997. Breath odor: Etiopathogenesis, assessment and management. *Eur. J. Oral Sci.* 105:287–293.

Segelnick, S. 2004. A survey of floss frequency, habit and technique in a hospital dental clinic and private periodontal practice. *NYSDJ* (May/June):28–33.

Sharma, N. C., H. J. Galustians, J. Qaqish, M. A. Cugini, and P. R. Warren. 2002. The effect of two power toothbrushes on calculus and stain. *Am. J. Dent.* 15(2):71–76.

Shellis, R. P., and R. M. Duckworth. 1994. Studies on the cariostatic mechanisms of fluoride. *Int. Dent. J.* 44(3 Suppl. 1):263–273.

Silva, M. F., M. S. Giniger, Y. P. Zhang, and W. DeVizio. 2004. The effect of a triclosan/copolymer/fluoride liquid dentifrice on interproximal enamel remineralization and fluoride uptake. *J. Am. Dent Assoc.* 135(7):1023–1029.

Silverman, G., E. Berman, C. B. Hanna, A. Salvato, P. Fratarcangelo, et al. 1996. Assessing the efficacy of three dentifrices in the treatment of dentinal hypersensitivity. *J. Am. Dent. Assoc.* 127:191–201.

Singh, S. M., M. E. Petrone, A. R. Volpe, K. N. Rustogi, and J. Norfleet. 1990. Comparison of the anticalculus effect of two soluble pyrophosphate dentifrices with and without a copolymer. *J. Clin. Dent.* 2:53–55.

Stephen, K. W. 1994. Fluoride toothpastes, rinses and tablets. *Adv. Dent. Res.* 8:185–189.

Stookey, O. K. 1994. Review of fluorosis risk of self-applied topical fluorides, dentifrices, mouthrinses and gels. *Comm. Dent. Oral Epidemiol.* 22(3):181–186.

Tammaro, S., J. L. Wennström, and G. Bergenholtz. 2000. Root-dentin sensitivity following nonsurgical periodontal treatment. *J. Clin. Periodontol.* 27:690–69.

Terézhalmy, G. T., R. D. Bartizek, and A. R. Biesbrock. 2008. Plaque-removal efficacy of four types of dental floss. *J. Periodontol.* 79(2):245–251.

Terézhalmy, G., E. Chaves, S. Bsoul, R. Baker, and T. He. 2007. Clinical evaluation of the stain removal efficacy of a novel stannous fluoride and sodium hexametaphosphate dentifrice. *Am. J. Dent.* (Feb) 20(1):53–8.

Tonzetich, J. 1997. Production and origin of oral malodor: A review of mechanisms and methods of analysis. *J. Periodontal.* 48:13–20.

Van der Weijden, G. A., M. M. Danser, A. Nijboer, M. F. Timmerman, and U. Van der Velden. 1993. The plaque-removing efficacy of an oscillating/rotation toothbrush: A short-term study. *J. Clin. Periodontol.* 20:273–278.

Van Dyke, T., S. Offenbacher, B. Pihlstrom, M. Putt, and C. Trummel. 1999. What is gingivitis? Current understanding of prevention, treatment, measurement, pathogenesis and relation to periodontitis. *J. Int. Acad. Periodontol.* 1:3–10.

Volpe, A. R., M. E. Petrone, R. Davies, and H. M. Proskin. 1995. Clinical anticaries efficacy of NaF and SMFP dentifrices: Overview and resolution of the scientific controversy. *J. Clin. Dent.* 6:1–28.

Volpe, A. R., M. E. Petrone, W. DeVizio, and R. M. Davies. 1996. A review of plaque, gingivitis, calculus and caries clinical efficacy studies with a fluoride dentifrice containing triclosan and PVM/MA copolymer. *J. Clin. Dent.* 7(Suppl):1–14.

von Troil, B., I. Needleman, and M. Sanz. 2002. A systematic review of the prevalence of root sensitivity following periodontal therapy. *J. Clin. Periodontol.* 29(Suppl. 3):173–177.

Waerhaug, J. 1981. Healing of the dentoepithelial junction following the use of dental floss. *J. Clin. Periodontol.* 8:144–150.

Watt, R. G., and V. C. Marinho. 2005. Does oral health promotion improve oral hygiene and gingival health? *Periodontology 2000* 37(1):35–47.

Westfelt, E. 1996. Rationale of mechanical plaque control. *J. Clin. Periodontol.* 23:263–267.

White, D. J., B. W. Bollmer, R. A. Baker, E. R. Cox, M. A. Perlich, et al. 1996. Quantical assessment of the clinical scaling benefits provided by phyrophosphate dentifrices with and without triclosan. *J. Clin. Dent.* 7(special issue):46–49.

Wilkins, E. M. 2012. *Clinical practice of the dental hygienist*, 11th ed. Philadelphia: Wolters Kluwer, Lippinoctt, Williams & Wilkins.

Yaegaki, K. 2000. Organoleptic measurement of oral malodor. In ed. K. Yaegaki, *Clinical guideline for halitosis*, 35–44. Tokyo: Quintessence.

Yaegaki, K., and J. M. Coil. 2000a. Examination, classification, and treatment of halitosis, clinical perspectives. *J. Can. Dent. Assoc.* 66:257–261.

Yaegaki, K., and J. M. Coil. 2000b. Genuine halitosis, pseudo-halitosis, and halitophobia: Classification, diagnosis and treatment. *Compendium.* 21:880–890.

Yaegaki, K., and T. Suetaka, 1989. The effect of zinc chloride mouthwash on the production of oral malodor, the degradation of salivary cellular elements and proteins. *J. Dent. Health.* 9:377–386.

Yankell, S. L., and U. P. Saxer. 1999. Toothbrushing and toothbrushing techniques. In eds. N. O. Harris and F. Garcia-Godoy, *Primary preventive dentistry*, 77–102. Norwalk, CT: Appleton and Lange.

Yukna, R. A., and R. L. Shaklee. 1993. Evaluation of a counter-rotational powered brush in patients in supportive periodontal therapy. *J. Periodontol.* 64:859–864.

Zambon, J. J., M. L. Mather, and Y. Gonzales. 1996. A microbiological and clinical study of the safety and efficacy of baking-soda dentifrices. *Compend. Contin. Educ. Dent. Suppl.* 17:39–44.

Zimmer, S., C. Kolbe, G. Kaiser, T. Krage, M. Ommerborn, and C. Barthel. 2006. Clinical efficacy of flossing versus use of antimicrobial rinses. *J. Periodontol.* 77:1380–1385.

21

Response to Nonsurgical Therapy

Mea A. Weinberg and Cynthia Fong

OUTLINE

EDUCATIONAL OBJECTIVES

Upon completion of this chapter, the reader should be able to:

- Discuss the rationale for periodontal debridement.
- Explain the clinical outcomes of periodontal debridement.
- Discuss the effects of nonsurgical treatment on the subgingival microbiota.
- Describe the effects of combined oral hygiene self-care with subgingival periodontal debridement on clinical attachment loss.
- Describe the healing response in gingivitis and periodontitis after periodontal debridement.
- Discuss the rationale for reevaluation of initial therapy.

GOAL: To provide an understanding of tissue healing after nonsurgical therapy.

KEY WORDS

Introduction

Because periodontal disease activity is site specific within the same mouth and differs between individuals, choice of treatment is determined on a site-by-site basis and/or on a patient-by-patient basis. The critical factor in the success of periodontal therapy is tissue response.

Nonsurgical Periodontal Therapy

The traditional emphasis of the initial phase of periodontal therapy or nonsurgical therapy is control of the supragingival microbial biofilm and disruption or removal of subgingival gram-negative microbiota, thus delaying the repopulation of pathogenic microorganisms (Magnusson, Lindhe, Yoneyama, & Liljenberg, 1984). Subgingival biofilm originates either from an apical extension of growing supragingival biofilm (Waerhaug, 1978) and/or from incomplete subgingival instrumentation. In either case, it is essential to control the supragingival microbial activity through oral hygiene self-care and subgingival biofilm removal by professional mechanical instrumentation (Cobb, 1996; Dahlen, Lindhe, Sato, Hanamura, & Okamoto, 1992; Katsanoulas, Renee, & Attström, 1992; Sbordone, Ramaglia, Gulletta, & Iacono, 1990). Subgingival debridement decreases the number of periodontal pathogens such as *Porphyromonas gingivalis* and *Prevotella intermedia* in subgingival biofilm and shifts the biofilm composition to a predominately gram-positive aerobic species associated with periodontal health.

Thus, nonsurgical therapy is based on returning the gingival tissue to a healthy, noninflamed state that can be maintained easily by the patient and the practitioner.

Terminology

The traditional therapy for removing supragingival and subgingival biofilm, its by-products and toxins, and calculus has been scaling and root planing. **Scaling** is defined as the mechanical removal of supragingival and subgingival dental biofilm, calculus, and stains (tooth-accumulated materials) from the crown and root surfaces. Thus, scaling is performed both supragingivally and subgingivally. Subgingival scaling removes the adherent biofilm and calculus attached to the root surface. Subgingival calculus is mineralized biofilm that often adheres tenaciously to root surfaces and thus is very difficult to remove. **Root planing** is defined as a "definitive treatment procedure designed to remove cementum or surface dentin that is rough, impregnated with calculus, or contaminated with toxins or microorganisms" (Ciancio, 1989). Extensive root planing is not needed to obtain healthy tissue.

Over the past few years, the term **periodontal debridement** has emerged in the literature, and it is defined as the removal of any foreign material, including dental biofilm, its by-products and toxins, calculus, and diseased or dead tissue, from the coronal tooth surfaces, root surfaces, sulcus or pocket, and periodontium (e.g., supporting bone). Thus, the difference between periodontal debridement

and scaling and root planing is that it encompasses more than just the root surfaces. It includes the pocket space, the pocket wall, and the underlying tissues (O'Hehir, 1999). Rather than total removal of cementum and the attainment of smooth root surfaces, conservation of cementum and the achievement of a good tissue healing response through control of bacterial infection are the objectives of periodontal debridement (O'Hehir, 1999). **Supragingival debridement** (also referred to as supragingival scaling) is the mechanical removal of dental biofilm and calculus from tooth surfaces above the gingival margin. **Subgingival debridement** or subgingival scaling and root planing is the mechanical removal of dental biofilm and calculus from tooth surfaces below the gingival margin. The term *deep scaling* has been used to denote subgingival scaling and root planing.

Deplaquing describes the mechanical disruption of nonattached, free-floating subgingival biofilm and its by-products from the sulcus or pocket. Deplaquing is recommended at reevaluation and maintenance appointments.

There are numerous definitions of oral **prophylaxis** in the literature. The American Dental Hygienist's Association (ADHA, 1995) reversed a change made to the prophylaxis definition published in the Current Dental Terminology (CDT)-4, which stated that prophylaxis was a scaling and/or polishing procedure to remove coronal biofilm, calculus, and stains. The change to this definition involved removal of the term */or*, thereby restoring the 1992 ADA Current Dental Terminology definition, which reads "scaling and polishing." The American Academy of Periodontology provides the most comprehensive definition of oral prophylaxis. An oral prophylaxis is the removal of biofilm, calculus, and stains from the exposed and unexposed surfaces of the teeth by scaling and polishing as a preventive measure for the control of local irritants (American Academy of Periodontology, 2003).

Polishing is performed to remove stains from the teeth and has not been shown to have any therapeutic benefits. For this reason, the American Dental Hygienist's Association's position on polishing is that it is a procedure that should be performed selectively when teeth have extrinsic stains (ADHA, 1995).

In some states, dental hygienists are permitted to perform closed gingival curettage or soft-tissue curettage. According to the American Academy of Periodontology, curettage is not an accepted procedure in periodontics. Curettage involves removal of the diseased lining of the soft-tissue pocket wall (soft-tissue debridement), including the junctional epithelium and the underlying inflamed connective tissue. The goal of gingival curettage is to reduce or eliminate periodontal inflammation. Indications for performing curettage include the presence of inflamed gingival tissues and shallow suprabony pockets. However, the benefits of soft-tissue curettage are questionable, and as a separate procedure, it has no justifiable application during active therapy for chronic periodontitis (Ciancio, 1989). Kalkwarf (1989) demonstrated that the healing effects of curettage were not any better than scaling and root planing alone.

It is noteworthy, however, that some inadvertent gingival curettage does occur as a result of scaling and root planing procedures.

Periodontal Debridement

Treatment of **inflammatory periodontal diseases** (e.g., gingivitis and periodontitis) has evolved significantly during the past decades. It was once thought that a primary goal of traditional scaling and root planing was the achievement of smooth root surfaces that were free of deposits. This intent was based on the assumption that bacteria would attach to rough surfaces (e.g., calculus and irregular root topography) and interfere with **soft-tissue healing** (Adriaens & Adriaens, 2004). It is now known that bacteria adhere to any surface, rough or smooth. Therefore, evaluation of successful periodontal debridement depends primarily on the soft-tissue response. The clinical significance of root surface roughness or smoothness is still undetermined (Jacobson, Blomlöf, & Lindskog, 1994), but the dental hygienist nevertheless, to achieve root smoothness, should strive to remove as much subgingival calculus as possible because it can affect biofilm accumulation. Oberholzer and Rateitschak (1996) concluded that striving for total root smoothness during periodontal surgery seems to be unnecessary; however, the value of a cleaned tooth surface cannot be minimized in periodontal tissue healing response.

Mechanical nonsurgical therapy consisting of oral hygiene self-care and periodontal instrumentation is intended to prevent, arrest, control, or eliminate periodontal diseases to ultimately maintain the teeth in a functional state of health (Cobb, 1996). Currently, periodontal debridement remains the foundation of nonsurgical periodontal therapy.

Combined Personal and Professional Debridement

Periodontal instrumentation is performed during the initial or preliminary phase of periodontal therapy. The beneficial effects of periodontal debridement combined with oral hygiene self-care in the treatment and prevention of periodontal diseases have been well documented. These include reduction of clinical inflammation, establishment of more beneficial microorganisms and less pathogenic microorganisms, reduction in probing depths, and a gain in attachment (American Academy of Periodontology, 1997; Kaldahl et al., 1996).

One clinical study reported that in the presence of supragingival biofilm, a subgingival microbiota containing greater than 5% spirochetes and motile rods was reestablished 4 to 8 weeks after periodontal debridement. Sites devoid of supragingival biofilm following supervised oral hygiene and mechanical instrumentation had less than 5% gram-negative bacteria (Magnusson et al., 1984). A more recent investigation studied the effects of supragingival biofilm control alone and biofilm control combined with scaling and root planing on clinical attachment loss over a 3-year period (Westfelt, Rylander, Dahlen, & Lindhe, 1998).

Results showed a reduction in bleeding scores following the combined treatment of biofilm control and scaling and root planing. Biofilm scores were reduced in both groups. Increased attachment loss of 2 mm or more was low in the combined treatment group. This study demonstrated that supragingival biofilm control is not enough to prevent further attachment loss in periodontitis patients.

Rationale and Indications for Periodontal Debridement

The purpose of periodontal debridement is to treat and resolve inflammation in the periodontal soft tissues by removing the irritants, which are the supragingival and subgingival biofilm and calculus. In conjunction with oral hygiene self-care, which also decreases supragingival biofilm accumulation, repopulation of subgingival pathogenic microbiota is delayed and shifts the composition of pocket material from a pathogenic gram-negative microbiota to gram-positive species, which are more conducive to periodontal health.

Periodontal debridement is indicated at sites showing (1) signs of gingival inflammation, (2) elevated levels of bacterial pathogens, and (3) progressive attachment or alveolar bone loss (Cobb, 1996). Various forms of instrumentation are used, including hand-activated instrumentation and power-driven instrumentation (e.g., sonic and ultrasonic instrumentation).

Outcomes of Periodontal Debridement

The ultimate long-term outcome or end point for nonsurgical periodontal debridement is preservation of the form and function of the dentition (Cobb, 1996). Determining the effects of nonsurgical periodontal treatment requires the use of measurable clinical end points. Most clinical studies, as well as private practices, measure the probing depths, gain or loss of clinical attachment (measuring the clinical attachment levels), and alveolar bone height and document bleeding on probing, visual signs of gingival inflammation, and changes in subgingival microbiota (Cobb, 1996; Suvan, 2005).

PROBING DEPTHS/CLINICAL ATTACHMENT LEVEL Root planing is contraindicated in sites that do not have periodontal pockets. A landmark clinical study showed that root planing teeth with initially shallow probing depths of less than 3 mm slightly decreased or did not alter probing depths, but loss of clinical attachment did occur (Lindhe, Socransky, Nyman, & Haffajee, 1982). A more recent study found that scaling and root planing performed with hand instruments produce a mean attachment loss of 0.76 mm, observed immediately following the procedure (Alves et al., 2004). Taking into consideration a number of clinical studies over the past years, Cobb (1996) determined that thorough debridement of moderately deep pockets (4 to 6 mm) usually results in a mean reduction in probing depth of 1.29 mm and a mean gain in clinical attachment of 0.55 mm, whereas sites with deeper probing depth (7 mm or more) showed a mean reduction in probing depth of 2.16 mm and a gain in clinical attachment of 1.29 mm. Care in selecting sites that will benefit from subgingival debridement is essential in the prevention of clinical attachment loss.

SUBGINGIVAL MICROBIOTA Periodontal debridement of pockets causes profound shifts in the composition of the subgingival microbiota (Umeda et al., 2004). After subgingival debridement, the number of gram-negative microorganisms decreases, especially spirochetes, and the number of gram-positive rods and cocci increases. However, this therapy may be ineffective in eliminating *Aggregatibacter actinomycetemcomitans* from affected subgingival sites (Cobb, 1996) because it invades soft tissue (Renvert, Wikström, Dahlen, Slots, & Egelberg, 1990).

Unfortunately, shifts in microbiotal composition are transient, and usually the pocket area becomes repopulated with subgingival microorganisms within days to months. Because the subgingival microbiota originate in supragingival areas (Waerhaug, 1978), regular and effective biofilm control and periodontal debridement are absolutely critical for long-term control of inflammatory periodontal diseases (Cobb, 1996).

BLEEDING ON PROBING Periodontal debridement has predictably reduced the levels of inflammation. A vast number of clinical studies conducted over recent years have shown that periodontal debridement has reduced bleeding in approximately 57% of sites (Cobb, 1996).

TISSUE CONSISTENCY Reduction of the fluid and cellular components of an inflammatory lesion in the lamina propria should result in an increased proportion of collagen fibers, which, when combined with reattachment of the junctional epithelium or the formation of a long junctional epithelium, will produce increased resistance to passage of the probe tip. This results in an apparent **gain in clinical attachment**.

Treatment Sequence

The treatment sequence for periodontal debridement varies depending on clinical findings and diagnosis. The first step after the dental hygiene diagnosis and treatment plan is oral hygiene self-care instructions specifically designed for the patient's needs.

Most patients undergoing subgingival debridement require topical and/or local anesthesia (Palmer & Floyd, 1995). However, the patient must not have any allergy or sensitivity to the agent used. Two types of topical anesthetics are available: amide types, such as 5% or 10% lidocaine, and ester types, such as benzocaine (varied concentrations are available, but usually it is 20%). Oraqix is a combination lidocaine/prilocaine (2.5%/2.5%) gel that is FDA approved for subgingival anesthesia. When a topical anesthetic is used, best results are obtained when a small amount is applied on a cotton-tip applicator, the tissues are dried prior to application of the agent, and the applicator is held in contact with the mucous membranes for 1 to 2 minutes. Alternatives include the use of an anesthetic patch, an anesthetic rinse, or electronic anesthesia. Topical anesthetic sprays should not be used because high doses of the agent can be absorbed into the circulatory system.

Local anesthesia is best applied by quadrant. It is recommended to treat one or two quadrants during a single visit depending on the number of teeth present as well as the degree of difficulty of the intervention. When two quadrants are treated during the same appointment, usual practice is to treat the upper and lower quadrants on either the right or the left side of the face. Both mandibular quadrants should not be treated during the same appointment to avoid patient discomfort and to prevent an inability on the part of the patient to control the mandible with both sides anesthetized.

Posttreatment care focuses on the prevention of dental biofilm formation. A long-term biofilm-free dentition is an unrealistic goal, and for this reason, periodic periodontal maintenance visits are required to monitor and identify disease recurrence (Westfelt, 1996).

Periodontal Debridement Procedures

Before debridement procedures are started, it is necessary to obtain a written informed consent from the patient. The procedure and its expected outcomes are explained to the patient. It is important for the patient to understand that the decreased probing depths primarily due to gingival shrinkage may cause gingival recession and "longer looking" teeth and that teeth may respond with hypersensitivity to cold, toothbrushing, or sweets. Such hypersensitivity is usually not permanent, but it may cause pain and discomfort that lasts for a few weeks to months.

Numerous methods to remove supra- and subgingival calculus include hand instruments, sonic scalers, ultrasonic scalers, and lasers. Although most literature reports similar healing responses after all modes of instrumentation, some research documents that the Er:YAG laser, which selectively removes calculus, may cause less damage to the cementum (Fleming & Beikler, 2011).

Subgingival Debridement

Calculus Removal. As periodontal debridement is started on a patient, the primary goal is to remove gross deposits from supragingival and subgingival tooth surfaces. The ultimate goal of subgingival debridement is to render a root surface free of biofilm, calculus, and endotoxins to enable soft-tissue healing. Complete calculus removal is essentially not attainable (Kepic, O'Leary, & Kafrawy, 1990), and total root smoothness is not necessary for adequate tissue healing. Clinical studies have shown that practitioners who spent an average of 12 to 15 minutes to complete the debridement of each tooth with hand and ultrasonic instruments fail to remove calculus from all surfaces. After debridement, about 47% of all nonfurcated surfaces and 63% of 6 mm or larger pockets showed residual calculus. Surgical access reduced the frequency of residual calculus to 20% and 38%, respectively. Teeth with furcations had a higher frequency of residual calculus, and surgical access did not provide any additional benefit (Buchanan & Robertson, 1987; Caffesse, Sweeney, & Smith, 1986; Fleischer, Mellonig, Brayer, Gray, & Barnett, 1989).

Although total elimination of causative factors is an appropriate treatment goal, reduction of dental biofilm and calculus below threshold levels appears to control the disease process and improve clinical signs of inflammation (Robertson, 1990), producing significant reductions in gingivitis, tooth loss, attachment loss, severity of disease, and probing depths (American Academy of Periodontology, 1997). Thus, if periodontal debridement can achieve elimination of inflammation and disease progression, then no further treatment is necessary. If periodontal debridement fails to achieve these objectives, then other modalities may be necessary, including more definitive debridement, use of advanced diagnostic testing, chemotherapeutics, or periodontal surgery.

Root Surface Characteristics. With the development of a gram-negative bacterial flora in the gingival crevice, events occur that eventually cause breakdown of the attachment apparatus. If elimination or disruption of the subgingival bacteria is not accomplished, rapid growth and maturation occur. During growth and after the death of subgingival gram-negative microorganisms, endotoxins or lipooligosaccharides are released from their cell walls. Endotoxins are highly toxic compounds that are capable of penetrating the junctional epithelium and entering the connective tissue, resulting in destruction of periodontal tissues. The endotoxins activate the inflammatory/immune response, which causes loss of connective tissue attachment from the root surface, apical migration of the junctional epithelium, and bone loss. A periodontal pocket forms, and the root surface (cementum) becomes contaminated when exposed to this new subgingival pocket environment. The cementum is sufficiently porous to allow superficial binding of endotoxins and colonization of dental biofilm and calculus onto the altered root surfaces. Cementum that is rough and impregnated with calculus or contaminated with toxins or microorganisms and dentin is referred to as contaminated, altered, or necrotic cementum.

Cementum Removal. The periodontal literature offers no firm conclusions about either the feasibility of or the need for removal of all contaminated cementum. In the past it was thought that the presence of cementum-bound endotoxins inhibited tissue healing after periodontal debridement.

Much investigation has been directed toward the elimination of this contaminated or necrotic cementum. *It is the consensus that endotoxins found on diseased root surfaces are weakly and superficially bound and that 99% may be removed by brushing* (Moore, Wilson, & Kieser, 1986; Nakib, Bissada, Simmelnik, & Goldstine, 1982). The primary reason for removing the superficial layer of cementum by subgingival debridement is to remove biofilm and calculus from the irregularities on the root surface. Extensive subgingival debridement for a prolonged amount of time is unnecessary (Cheetham, Wilson, & Kieser, 1988), and total removal of cementum is not the goal because the attachment of new soft tissue to the root surface is enhanced by the presence of cementum (Somerman, Archer, Shteyer, & Foster, 1987). O'Leary and Kafrawy (1983) concluded that total removal of cementum under routine clinical conditions is not a realistic objective of therapy. Smart, Wilson, Davies, and Kieser (1990), using ultrasonic instrumentation, showed that contaminated root surfaces could be rendered comparable to healthy teeth. Therefore, the key to **periodontal therapy** is the removal of biofilm and calculus to reduce the number of oral bacteria below the threshold level capable of initiating inflammation (American Academy of Periodontology, 1997). Precisely how much cementum is removed as a result of root planing is uncertain.

Therefore, it is important to attain relatively smooth root surfaces only for the purpose of reducing biofilm retention without excessive and unnecessary removal of cementum and dentin. The therapeutic goal of debridement therapy is to control bacterial infection as opposed to simply removing deposits from root surfaces.

Adverse Effects of Periodontal Debridement

Subgingival debridement may cause soft-tissue recession, making the teeth look longer and exposing the root surface to the oral environment. This may result in dentinal hypersensitivity as a result of removal of the thin outer layer of cementum and exposure of the underlying dentin. Usually, teeth are not sensitive immediately after the periodontal debridement; hypersensitivity may take about 3 to 4 days to appear. Root sensitivity occurs in approximately half of the patients following subgingival scaling and root planing (von Troil, Needleman, & Sanz, 2002). The intensity of root sensitivity increases for a few weeks after therapy, after which it decreases. In clinical practice, it may be recommended that patients should be made aware of the potential for root sensitivity prior to treatment (von Troil et al., 2002). Treatment of dentinal hypersensitivity is discussed in Chapter 20.

Limitations of Periodontal Debridement

POCKET DEPTH The effectiveness of periodontal debridement depends on the effectiveness of the mechanical removal of dental biofilm and calculus. Root debridement does not always remove all biofilm and calculus from subgingival tooth surfaces. Studies have shown that considerable amounts (54% to 57%) of calculus remain on the root surfaces of teeth with moderate or advanced pockets and that more residual calculus is found on tooth surfaces with increasing probing depths (Wylam, Mealey, Mills, Waldrop, & Moskowicz, 1993). There was no significant difference whether an anterior or a posterior tooth was debrided (Sherman et al., 1990).

Current conclusions about the effectiveness of periodontal debridement in deeper pockets are conflicting, and there is as yet no agreement on whether nonsurgical instrumentation is effective in advanced periodontal lesions (Forabosco, Galetti, Spinato, Colao, & Casolari, 1996). The most frequently lost teeth in patients receiving comprehensive periodontal treatment are the molars. Explanations for this relate to the difficulty in achieving adequate daily biofilm removal and the difficulty in properly debriding molars. Stambaugh, Dragoo, Smith, and Carasali (1981) found that the average probing depth for "efficient" removal of biofilm, calculus, and necrotic cementum was 3.73 mm. Rateitschak, Schwarz, Guggenheim, Duggelin, and Rateitschak (1992) found that surfaces where curets could reach usually were free of biofilm and calculus, but in deep pockets the curet did not reach the base of the pocket. Consequently, modified curets with longer shanks were developed to increase treatment effectiveness in deeper pockets.

FURCATIONS AND ROOT ANATOMY Access for adequate instrumentation in the furcation area is often difficult, if not impossible, given the special anatomic characteristics of multirooted teeth (Fleischer et al., 1989; Greene, 1995). Pathogenic microbiota frequently persists in furcation lesions (Loos, Claffey, & Egelberg, 1988). Narrow furcation openings make periodontal debridement a challenge. Fifty-eight percent of molars have furcation entrance diameters that are smaller than the smallest diameter of a relatively new curet, which is 0.75 mm (Bower, 1979a; Parashis, Anagnou-Vareltzides, & Demetriou, 1990).

Knowledge about the morphology of the furcation area and the variations in root form and structure is important for effective instrumentation. Root concavities, which are depressions found on the proximal root surfaces, are biofilm and calculus traps, making instrumentation extremely difficult. For instance, a deep mesial concavity is found on the maxillary first premolar. On the maxillary first molars, the mesiobuccal root has the greatest incidence of concavities, whereas both the mesio- and distobuccal roots of the mandibular first molars have concavities (Bower, 1979b; Figure 21–1 ■). Moreover, any other root also may have root concavities. Another limitation is that the smallest width of the blade of a curet is still larger than the average width of a furcation entrance, which makes it difficult to place a curet effectively into a furcation (Figure 21–2 ■).

TIME SPENT AND CLINICIAN SKILL Controversy exists over how much time should be spent on subgingival debridement. Subgingival debridement is dependent on both technique and operator skill. Because endotoxins are just weakly bound to the root surface (Moore et al., 1986), it is not necessary to spend a great deal of time debriding.

However, a considerable amount of time still should be spent in effectively removing subgingival biofilm, calculus, and necrotic cementum and being sure that the instrumentation occurs on every portio of the root surface. If this procedure is done incorrectly, root gouging may occur, resulting in the production of grooves and pits in the root surface.

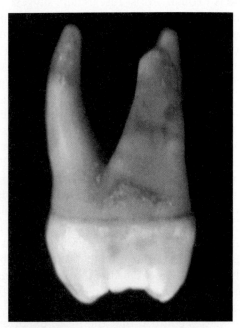

FIGURE 21–1 Root morphology. Root concavities in the maxillary molar decrease the effectiveness of debridement.

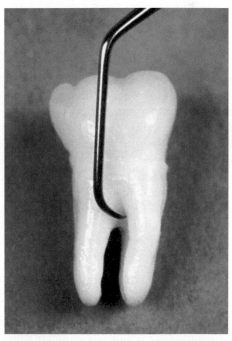

FIGURE 21–2 It is difficult to effectively scale in furcations because the narrowest width of a curet is still wider than the average width of a furcation entrance.

A clinical study (Anderson, Palmer, Bye, Smith, & Caffesse, 1996) evaluating single versus multiple episodes of subgingival instrumentation to determine effectiveness concluded that there was no significant difference between the two treatments. It was suggested that calculus remaining after one thorough episode of instrumentation is not likely to be removed by repeated instrumentation. How much time is enough? Most researchers suggest that periodontal debridement should take at least 10 minutes per tooth (Lowenguth & Greenstein, 1995). Coldiron, Yukna, Weir, and Caudill (1990) found that cementum removal was generally achieved on periodontally healthy roots with 20 strokes of a curet, but residual calculus remained. Thus, vigorous root planing is not needed and the best way to determine how much root planing should be performed is to monitor tissue healing. If the gingival tissues are still inflamed after initial therapy, then more periodontal debridement is required.

The results of a clinical study assessing periodontal debridement forces in periodontally involved molars show a broad range of forces being applied by the practitioner (Zappa, Röthlisberger, Simona, & Case, 1993). In addition, the quality of periodontal debridement done on a molar may be primarily determined by the attitude of the practitioner, who subjectively treats the tooth according to his or her habits, rather than according to the characteristics of the root surfaces being treated (Zappa et al., 1993).

Most studies confirm that the more experienced the clinician, the more calculus-free the root surfaces were in deeper pockets and in hard-to-reach areas such as furcations (Brayer, Mellonig, Dunlap, Marinak, & Carson, 1989).

Healing Response and the Outcome of Therapy

Diseased Periodontal Unit

When a periodontal probe is inserted into the pocket of a diseased and inflamed pocket, the probe penetrates the tissue apical to the junctional (pocket) epithelium, giving deeper probe readings. This occurs because the connective tissue of the gingival tissue contains less collagen and more inflammatory cells. Once the periodontium is treated, the thin junctional epithelium is closely adapted to the tooth or root surface, and collagen replaces the inflammatory cells in the connective tissue. This is responsible for the increased resistance to probing force so that the probe tip stops at a more coronal level of the junctional epithelium than when inflammation was present, resulting in shallower probing depth readings.

Healing Periodontal Unit

An expected outcome of debridement is tissue healing. Healing results in tissue repair, shrinkage of gingival tissue, and the renewal of epithelial cells in contact with tooth surfaces (Caffesse, Mota, & Morrison, 1995; Caton, Nyman, & Zander, 1980).

Generally, the same healing features of periodontal tissues are seen following debridement of any chronically inflamed site. Initially, following debridement, there is an acute inflammatory reaction due to the traumatic nature of the therapy. This inflammation subsides within 24 to 48 hours. Over the next week, there is a gradual reduction of inflammatory cells, epithelial tissue healing, and finally, connective tissue maturation with collagen deposition.

Gingivitis: Healing after Periodontal Debridement

Histologically, in gingivitis, once dental biofilm and calculus are removed, the pocket epithelium will reform into junctional epithelium and contact the adjacent tooth surface as it was in health. This happens because the basal cells of the junctional epithelium grow out and contact the tooth surface and develop into a new junctional epithelium. Reattachment of "old" junctional epithelium does not occur. Then, the apical part of the junctional epithelium moves apically until the first gingival connective tissue fibers embedded in cementum are reached. This new junctional epithelium is sometimes referred to as a "long junctional epithelium." Also, the inflammatory cells in the gingival connective tissue are replaced by collagen; these improvements result in an *apparent* "gain in clinical attachment." The formation of a new long junctional epithelium is explained in detail later.

Clinically, there is a reduction in or elimination of inflammation (e.g., bleeding) and the elimination of edema, both of which result in tissue shrinkage and occasionally gingival recession. Gingiva that is fibrotic will not shrink, as does edematous tissue. The gingiva often returns to its salmon pink color. The greatest reduction in probing depths occurs after 4 to 8 weeks (Segelnick & Weinberg, 2006) and is primarily due to (1) tissue shrinkage, which may result in gingival recession, and (2) reformation of collagen, which results in greater resistance to probing (Figure 21–3a ■). The reductions obtained in probing depths as a result of nonsurgical therapy are in the range of 1 to 2 mm.

Periodontitis: Healing after Periodontal Debridement

Histologically, in periodontitis, after the removal of dental biofilm, calculus, and necrotic cementum, some healing will occur. Healing will most likely occur by repair (e.g., long junctional epithelium) rather than regeneration, which is formation of new bone, collagen fibers, cementum, and periodontal ligament. Healing by regeneration occurs during periodontal surgery using guided tissue regeneration procedures such as barrier membranes.

The same scenario that occurs with healing of gingivitis sites also occurs with periodontitis sites. The pocket epithelium transforms back into junctional epithelium, which begins to come in contact with the root surface between the gingival connective tissue and the root (Figure 21–3b). The formation of a long junctional epithelium results in

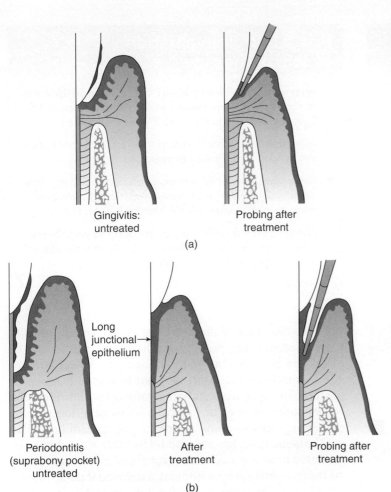

FIGURE 21–3 Healing of the gingival tissues after sub-gingival debridement. (a) In gingivitis, the tissues will heal, with approximation of the junctional epithelium to the tooth surface. (b) In periodontitis, after root planing, the tissues heal by formation of a long junctional epithelial attachment to the root surface.

closure of the pocket. This reestablishment of the junctional epithelium most likely occurs within 1 (Caton & Zander, 1979) or 2 (Waerhaug, 1978) weeks. The inflammatory cells in the gingival connective tissue are replaced by collagen, but a long junctional epithelium prevents the formation of a gingival connective tissue attachment (gingival fibers). The greatest reduction in probing depths and an *apparent* gain in clinical attachment level can be measured after 4 to 8 weeks (Segelnick & Weinberg, 2006), although true gains in clinical attachment are seen primarily after periodontal surgery, if at all (that is why the term *apparent* is used). Gains in clinical attachment level after treatment do not necessarily mean that new gingival connective tissue attachment has been achieved (Armitage, 1996). It may simply indicate that the probe is more resistant to penetration once the gingival collagen has reformed and that the probe tip, when placed into the gingival crevice, stops at a more *coronal* location of the junctional epithelium. This gives the appearance of a gain in clinical attachment when there actually may not be. A true gain in clinical attachment after periodontal treatment indicates that a new connective tissue attachment (collagen fibers inserting) to the root has occurred.

Residual or undetected calculus that instrumentation has failed to remove is often present. Despite incomplete

> ### Did You Know?
>
> It takes a lot longer for connective tissue fibers to reform than for junctional epithelium to readapt to the root surface.

calculus removal, Sherman and colleagues (1990) showed that sites still could respond favorably. Haffajee and colleagues (1997) found that periodontal debridement demonstrated clinical improvement in subjects with chronic periodontitis even though only modest changes in subgingival microbiota were seen. This suggests potential targets for therapy and indicates that radical alterations in subgingival microbiota may not be necessary.

Reevaluation of Initial Therapy

Reevaluation of initial therapy involves the assessment of treatment performed. Box 21–1 outlines different steps that should be performed on a patient during a reevaluation visit. These findings are compared with the initial clinical findings that were documented before the patient started periodontal debridement.

Box 21–1: Reevaluation Measurements

- Oral hygiene status
- Soft tissue status
- Probing depths
- Clinical attachment levels (CALs)
- Bleeding on probing
- Tooth mobility
- Furcation involvement
- Biofilm index

Box 21–2: Reevaluation of Initial Therapy

- After scaling and root planing, there is reestablishment of the junctional epithelium to the tooth surface in 1 to 2 weeks; reevaluation before 2 weeks is too early.
- After scaling and root planing, the repair of connective tissue continues for 4 to 8 weeks.
- Subgingival microbial repopulation occurs within a few months (2 months) after instrumentation of periodontal pockets in the absence of improved biofilm control.
- Longer than 2 months may be too long to wait for the reevaluation because pathogenic bacteria have already repopulated periodontal pockets.

Rapid Dental Hint

Remember that when measuring clinical attachment level, you use the cementoenamel junction (CEJ) as your reference point to take the measurement.

Tissue Response

After appropriate initial therapy, a planned **reevaluation** should assess the current state of health or disease. The treatment sequence for the reevaluation appointment consists of a medical history update, soft-tissue examination, biofilm index, determination of the presence of bleeding, oral hygiene self-care evaluation, and periodontal probing. Pretreatment findings are compared with the current status of the patient. It is important to evaluate and emphasize the patient's oral hygiene self-care techniques. Controversy exists regarding the recommended time interval between the initial therapy and the reevaluation appointment. Reprobing recommendations range from a minimum of 4 to a maximum of 8 weeks after periodontal debridement to allow for tissue healing, although waiting longer than 6 weeks may augment the healing response (Segelnick & Weinberg, 2006). However, if just a visual inspection for inflammation and tissue color is evaluated, then 1 week after debridement is sufficient. Reevaluation after regenerative periodontal surgery (e.g., bone grafts, barrier membranes) should be performed at 6 months. Key points concerning the appropriate time to perform reprobing at reevaluation are summarized in Box 21–2 (Segelnick & Weinberg, 2006).

In the absence of improved biofilm control, Magnusson et al. (1984) and Mousques, Listgarten, and Phillips (1980) observed that a subgingival microbiota containing large numbers of pathogenic spirochetes and motile rods repopulated within 4 to 8 weeks.

If results of initial therapy show improvement, but with some residual 5 mm probing depths, the patient should be placed on periodontal maintenance and reevaluated in 2 to 3 months because this is about how long it takes for bacteria to repopulate subgingivally after debridement. Reevaluation at regular intervals is essential to alert the dental hygienist to areas where biofilm control has failed and inflammation has returned. Unstable sites should be retreated or monitored closely for signs of attachment loss. At the reevaluation appointment, a decision is made regarding whether the patient qualifies for surgical intervention, continues with initial therapy, or is placed on a periodontal maintenance schedule. Factors that may influence this decision include the overall treatment plan, including restorative procedures, as well as the desires of the patient.

Reevaluation includes an examination of the gingival tissues. If inflammation persists, which is apparent clinically as bleeding on probing and redness, the cause needs to be determined. Persistent inflammation may result from incomplete debridement, patient noncompliance with home care, or a systemic disease. The desired microbial response is a change in the composition of the bacteria found within the pocket from a pathogenic gram-negative species (e.g., spirochetes, *P. gingivalis, P. intermedia*) to a more beneficial gram-positive species such as cocci or nonmotile bacteria (Mousques et al., 1980).

Ultrasonic versus Hand-Activated Instrumentation

Studies comparing hand- and power-driven scalers are difficult to assess because of the wide variety of study designs. With the advent of modified periodontal inserts, subgingival root debridement became possible. Most studies have had comparable results with hand- and power-driven scalers when considering residual biofilm and calculus. The ultimate determinant of treatment success with power-driven scalers (e.g., ultrasonics and sonics) is observation of the response of the tissues. Posttreatment evaluation consists of monitoring the soft-tissue response and determining the

Rapid Dental Hint

Shallower probing depth readings occur after debridement because healing occurs with a long junctional epithelium and/or reduction in inflammation.

critical levels of periodontal pathogenic organisms present within the gingival crevice. Thus, the outcome of scaling and root planing is similar for hand-activated instrumentation and power-driven scalers.

It has been documented that ultrasonic scalers with modified tips produced smoother roots with less damage, better access to the base of the pocket, and superior biofilm and calculus removal than hand-activated instruments and also required less time (Dragoo, 1992; Kocher & Plagmann, 1997).

Comparing manual and ultrasonic instrumentation of deep pockets (6–9 mm), it was found that both methods were equal in reducing total microbial counts and colony-forming units (Oosterwal, Matee, Mikx, van't Hof, & Renggli, 1987). Thus, the tissue healing response is similar with manual and ultrasonic instrumentation.

Lasers

All dental lasers currently used in the United States are approved by the Food and Drug Administration (FDA) as medical devices, but the ADA Council on Scientific Affairs states that clearance by the FDA may not be sufficient to scientifically demonstrate safety, efficacy, or effectiveness for marketed dental lasers in all cases (www.ada.org/1860.aspx). Each laser has a different wavelength, either the CO_2, diode, Nd:YAG, or Er:YAG (Erbium) wavelengths, which is used for different procedures. Each wavelength of laser energy is absorbed in water, pigment, or hydroxyapatite (hard tissue; Cobb, 1996). There are more than 20 cleared indications for use for dental lasers in the United States. Indications for using lasers in periodontics include sulcular and/or pocket debridement (laser curettage), reduction of subgingival bacterial loads (pocket sterilization), and scaling and root

planing. Results using the laser for these purposes are controversial. The Er:YAG wavelenths are highly absorbed in both water and hydroxyapatite, which permits it to be used for soft-tissue incision, subgingival curettage, scaling of root surfaces (removal of calculus and endotoxins), and bone reconturing during flap surgery. The CO_2 laser is best for soft-tissue surgery (e.g., soft tissue incision—frenectomy, reshaping the gingiva, soft-tissue biopsy, irradiation of aphthous ulcers, and subgingival curettage-removal of soft-tissue wall) because it is highly absorbed in water. The CO_2 laser should avoid contact with teeth.

The American Acadmey of Periodontology (2011) states that there is minimal evidence to support use of a laser for the purpose of subgingival debridement, Results are variable and conflicting when lasers are used to reduce subgingival microbial loads. However, Er:YAG lasers have shown to be effective for root debridement (removal of calculus). Cobb (1996) states that the use of lasers for the treatment of chronic periodontitis may be equivalent to scaling and root planing when it comes to reduction in probing depth and subgingival bacterial loads. But its use is not best for gain in attachment level, which is the ideal result for nonsurgical periodontal treatment.

Because the use of lasers is considered to be closed procedure (e.g, the clinician cannot see subgingival), there is much concern about damage to the root surface depending on the wavelength and power.

The intended healing response after subgingival curettage with the Er:YAG is a new attachment through regeneration of connective tissue attachment, cementum, periodontal ligament, and bone. However, healing may just be a long junctional epithelium, which has been documented to be just as good as a regenerated connective tissue attachment (Cobb, 1996; Beaumont, O'Leary, & Kafrawy 1984). Healing after laser removal of subgingival calculus is again via a long junctional epithelium.

Did You Know?

The word *laser* stands for light amplification by stimulated emission of radiation.

Dental Hygiene Application

The philosophy of periodontal therapy has changed over the past decade as a result of further understanding of the disease process. Therapy is based on up-to-date clinical and microbial studies. The decision to perform periodontal debridement as a definitive treatment should depend on the severity of periodontal disease, the inflammatory status of the gingiva, the treatment objectives of the dental hygienist,

treatment time, and the skill of the operator (Lowenguth & Greenstein, 1995).

Selection of the proper instrument involves considering the following factors: the amount of calculus, the type of tissue tone (e.g., firm or edematous, or hard and fibrotic), probing depths (or type of disease present), root morphology, and location of the calculus. Root smoothness is no longer the main criterion for periodontal instrumentation, although all detectable deposits should be removed to achieve a successful soft-tissue response. The primary goal of periodontal debridement is to make the root and the soft tissue biologically compatible (Wilson, Schoen, & Fallon, 1989). In most cases, periodontal debridement improves clinical parameters, decreasing both gingival inflammation (evidenced by less bleeding) and probing depths. Improvements in microbial parameters are transient, and the microbiota soon return to pretreatment levels. Therefore, the patient requires continuous maintenance or biofilm control. Both periodontal debridement and daily biofilm removal by the patient are equally important for the maintenance of periodontal health and will continue to be the standard of periodontal therapy. Healing after nonsurgical therapy (scaling/root planing) is clinical/histologically complete at about 3 to 6 months after final instrumentation. Clinically, there should be fewer bleeding sites, more soft-tissue recession, and a gain of clinical attachment as seen by an increased resistance of the probe.

Key Points

- Successful periodontal treatment, maintenance of periodontal health, and the regeneration of periodontal tissues depend on the removal of supra- and subgingival deposits.
- Oral hygiene self-care and periodontal debridement are indicated in the treatment of inflammatory periodontal diseases to reduce inflammation and microbial levels. The clinical end point to periodontal debridement is a good tissue healing response.
- Periodontal debridement has been shown to disrupt or alter the subgingival microbiota, thus slowing down repopulation.

- Although meticulous debridement may remove some cementum, the intentional, aggressive removal of diseased cementum does not seem to be necessary; endotoxins are loosely attached to the root surface and can be removed easily.
- The type of healing occurring after subgingival debridement is a long junctional epithelium attachment to the root surface, which is considered to be a type of repair.
- Reevaluation of initial therapy should be performed between 4 and 8 weeks after completion of scaling and root planing.

Self-Quiz

1. Which one of the following healing responses is seen in gingivitis after periodontal debridement?
   a. Formation of new bone, cementum, and periodontal ligament
   b. Formation of new cementum and periodontal ligament
   c. Reduction of inflammation
   d. Reattachment of the alveolar mucosa

2. Which one of the following healing responses is seen in periodontitis after periodontal debridement?
   a. Reattachment of the sulcular epithelium
   b. Reattachment of the desmosomes
   c. Formation of new bone, cementum, and periodontal ligament
   d. Repair with a long junctional epithelium

3. Which one of the following definitions explains an apparent gain in clinical attachment after periodontal debridement?
   a. Bone fill and formation of new cementum
   b. Improved gingival tone and reattachment of the sulcular epithelium

   c. Improved gingival tone and increased mature collagen fibers
   d. Gingival recession, bone fill, and establishment of a new periodontal ligament attachment

4. Which of the following helps determine success after periodontal debridement (reevaluation)?
   a. Amount of time spent on the procedure
   b. Number of quadrants completed
   c. Total removal of calculus
   d. Tissue response

5. Which one of the following benefits is seen after subgingival debridement?
   a. Disruption of the gram-negative microbial flora
   b. Repopulation of gram-negative anaerobic flora
   c. Removal of gram-positive facultative flora
   d. Interference with attachment of gram-positive anaerobic flora to root surfaces

Case Study

A patient has received nonsurgical periodontal therapy from the dental hygienist. The therapy included professional debridement of the periodontal pockets with related root planing where necessary. The patient is currently performing adequate home care and shows reduced plaque scores.

1. How is initial nonsurgical therapy evaluated for positive outcomes?
   a. new bone deposited in one month
   b. decreased probing depth at one week
   c. connective tissue evaluation visit in three months
   d. four to six weeks after completion of scaling and root planning

Answer: D. At four to six weeks the therapy is evaluated for fewer bleeding sites, more soft tissue recession, and gain of attachment. Assessment too early or too late will give misleading responses.

2. What technique could be utilized for professional subgingival debridement?
   a. hand instrumentation on root and furcation areas
   b. ultrasonic scalers in all areas
   c. CO_2 lasers in all areas
   d. a and b
   e. all of the above

Answer: D. Although lasers are accepted by the FDA the ADA has not offered clearance. The CO_2 lasers are used for soft tissue and the Er:YAG laser may be used for scaling and root planning.

3. What is the biological aspect that creates the decreased pocket depth after periodontal debridement?
   a. shrinkage of gingival tissue
   b. increased junctional epithelium
   c. reattachment of periodontal fibers
   d. redeposit of cementum
   e. a and b
   f. a, b, c
   g. all of the above

Answer: E. The gingival tissue reduces edema and the junctional epithelium increases resulting in increase clinical attachment. No new fibers are regenerated and the cementum does not change.

References

Adriaens, P. A., and L. M. Adriaens. 2004. Effects of nonsurgical periodontal therapy on hard and soft tissues. *Periodontology 2000* 36(1):121–145.

Alves, R.V., L. Machion, M. Z. Casati, F. H. Nociti, Jr., A.W. Sallum, and E. A. Sallum. 2004. Attachment loss after scaling and root planing with different instruments—a clinical study. *J. Clin. Periodontol.* 31:12–15.

American Academy of Periodontology. 1997. Treatment of gingivitis and periodontitis. *J. Periodontol.* 68:1246–1253.

American Academy of Periodontology. 2003. *Glossary of periodontal terms*, 4th ed. Chicago: Author.

American Academy of Periodontology. 2011. American Academy of Periodonotology Statement on the efficacy of lasers in the non-surgical treatment of inflammatory periodontal disease. American Academy of Periodontology, Chicago, IL April.

American Dental Hygienist's Association (ADHA). 1995. *A position paper on selective tooth polishing.* Chicago: Author.

Anderson, G. B., J. Palmer, F. Bye, B. Smith, and R. Caffesse. 1996. Effectiveness of subgingival scaling and root planing: Single versus multiple episodes of instrumentation. *J. Periodontol.* 67:367–373.

Armitage, G. C. 1996. Periodontal diseases: Diagnosis. *Ann. Periodontol.* 1:37–215.

Beaumont, R., T. O'Leary, and A. Kafrawy. 1984. Relative resistance of long junctional epithelial adhesions and connective tissue attachments to biofilm-induced inflammation. *J. Periodontol.* 55:213–223.

Bower, R. C. 1979a. Furcation morphology relative to periodontal treatment: Furcation entrance architecture. *J. Periodontol.* 50:23–27.

Bower, R. C. 1979b. Furcation morphology relative to periodontal treatment: Furcation root surface anatomy. *J. Periodontol.* 50:366–374.

Brayer, W. K., J. T. Mellonig, R. M. Dunlap, K. W. Marinak, and R. E. Carson. 1989. Scaling and root planing effectiveness: The effect of root surface access and operator experience. *J. Periodontol.* 60:67–72.

Buchanan, S. A., and P. S. Robertson. 1987. Calculus removal by scaling and root planing with and without surgical access. *J. Periodontol.* 58:159–163.

Caffesse, R. G., L. F. Mota, and E. D. Morrison. 1995. The rationale for periodontal therapy. *Periodontology 2000* 9:7–13.

Caffesse, R. G., P. L. Sweeney, and B. A. Smith. 1986. Scaling and root planing with and without periodontal flap surgery. *J. Clin. Periodontol.* 13:205–210.

Caton, J., S. Nyman, and H. Zander. 1980. Histometric evaluation of periodontal surgery: II. Connective tissue attachment after four regenerative procedures. *J. Clin. Periodontol.* 7:224–231.

Caton, J., and H. Zander. 1979. The attachment between tooth and gingival tissues after periodontic root planing and soft tissue curettage. *J. Periodontol.* 50:462–466.

Cheetham, W. A., M. Wilson, and J. B. Kieser. 1988. Root surface debridement: An in vitro assessment. *J. Clin. Periodontol.* 15:288–292.

Ciancio, S. G. 1989. Non-surgical periodontal treatment. In eds. M. Nevins, W. Becker, and K. Kornman, *Proceedings of the World Workshop in Clinical Periodontics*, Vol. 2, 1–22. Chicago: American Academy of Periodontology.

Cobb, C. M. 1996. Non-surgical pocket therapy: Mechanical. *Ann. Periodontol.* 1:443–490.

Coldiron, N. B., R. A. Yukna, J. Weir, and R. F. Caudill. 1990. A quantitative study of cementum removal with hand curettes. *J. Periodontol.* 61:293–299.

Dahlen, G., J. Lindhe, K. Sato, H. Hanamura, and H. Okamoto. 1992. The effect of supragingival biofilm control on the subgingival microbiota in subjects with periodontal disease. *J. Clin. Periodontol.* 19:802–809.

Dragoo, M. R. 1992. A clinical evaluation of hand and ultrasonic instruments on subgingival debridement: I. With unmodified and modified ultrasonic scalers. *Int. J. Periodont. Rest. Dent.* 12:310–323.

Fleischer, H. C., J. T. Mellonig, W. K. Brayer, J. L. Gray, and J. D. Barnett. 1989. Scaling and root planing efficacy in multirooted teeth. *J. Periodontol.* 60:402–409.

Fleming, T. F., and T. Beikler. 2011. Control of oral biofilms. *Periodontology 2000* 55:9–15.

Forabosco, A., R. Galetti, S. Spinato, P. Colao, and C. Casolari. 1996. A comparative study of a surgical method and scaling and root planing using Odontoson. *J. Clin. Periodontol.* 23:611–614.

Greene, P. R. 1995. Non-surgical periodontal therapy: Essential and adjunctive methods. *Br. Dent. J.* 179:28–34.

Haffajee, A. D., M. A. Cugini, S. Dibart, C. Smith, L. R. Kent, Jr., and S. S. Socransky. 1997. The effect of scaling and root planing on the clinical and microbiological parameters of periodontal diseases. *J. Clin. Periodontol.* 24:324–334.

Jacobson, L., J. Blomlöf, and S. Lindskog. 1994. Root surface texture after different scaling modalities. *Scand. J. Dent. Res.* 102:156–160.

Kaldahl, W. B., K. L. Kalkwarf, D. Kashinath, D. Patil, M. P. Molvar, and J. K. Dyer. 1996. Long-term evaluation of periodontal therapy: I. Response to four therapeutic modalities. *J. Periodontol.* 67:93–102.

Kalkwarf, K. L. 1989. Tissue attachment. In eds. M. Nevins, W. Becker, and K. Kornman, *Proceedings of the World Workshop in Clinical Periodontics*, Vol. 5, 1–21. Chicago: American Academy of Periodontology.

Katsanoulas, T., I. Renee, and R. Attström. 1992. The effect of supragingival biofilm control on the composition of the subgingival flora in periodontal pockets. *J. Clin. Periodontol.* 19:760–765.

Kepic, T. J., T. J. O'Leary, and A. H. Kafrawy. 1990. Total calculus removal: An attainable objective? *J. Periodontol.* 61:16–20.

Kocher, T., and H. C. Plagmann. 1997. The diamond-coated sonic scaler tip: Part II: Loss of substance and alteration of root surface texture after different scaling modalities. *Int. J. Periodontics Restorative Dent.* 17(5):484–493.

Lindhe, J., S. S. Socransky, S. Nyman, and A. Haffajee. 1982. Critical probing depth. *J. Clin. Periodontol.* 9: 323–336.

Loos, B., N. Claffey, and J. Egelberg. 1988. Clinical and microbiological effects of subgingival debridement in periodontal furcation pockets. *J. Clin. Periodontol.* 15:453–463.

Lowenguth, R. A., and G. Greenstein. 1995. Clinical and microbiological response to nonsurgical mechanical periodontal therapy. *Periodontology 2000* 9:14–22.

Magnusson, I., J. Lindhe, T. Yoneyama, and B. Liljenberg. 1984. Recolonization of a subgingival microbiota following scaling in deep pockets. *J. Clin. Periodontol.* 11:193–207.

Moore, J., M. Wilson, and J. B. Kieser. 1986. The distribution of bacterial lipopolysaccharide (endotoxins) in relation to periodontal involved root surfaces. *J. Clin. Periodontol.* 13:748–751.

Mousques, T., M. A. Listgarten, and R. W. Phillips. 1980. Effect of scaling and root planing on the composition of the human subgingival microbial flora. *J. Periodont. Res.* 15:144–151.

Nakib, N. M., N. F. Bissada, J. W. Simmelink, and S. N. Goldstine. 1982. Endotoxin penetration into root cementum of periodontally healthy and diseased human teeth. *J. Periodontol.* 53:368–378.

Oberholzer, R., and K. H. Rateitschak. 1996. Root cleaning or root smoothing: An in vivo study. *J. Clin. Periodontol.* 23:326–330.

O'Hehir, T. E. 1999. Debridement 5 scaling and root planing plus. *RDH.* 14, 62.

O'Leary, T. J., and A. D. Kafrawy. 1983. Total cementum removal: A realistic objective. *J. Periodontol.* 54:221–226.

Oosterwaal, P. J., M. I. Matee, F. H. Mikx, M. A. van't Hof, and H. H. Renggli. 1987. The effect of subgingival debridement with hand and ultrasonic instruments on the subgingival microflora. *J. Clin. Periodontol.* 14:528–533.

Palmer, R. M., and F. D. Floyd. 1995. Periodontology: A clinical approach: 3. Non-surgical treatment and maintenance. *Br. Dent. J.* 178:263–268.

Parashis, A. O., A. Anagnou-Vareltzides, and N. Demetriou. 1990. Calculus removal from multirooted teeth with and without surgical access: II. Comparison between external and furcation surfaces and effect of furcation entrance width. *J. Clin. Periodontol.* 20:294–298.

Rateitschak, P., J. Schwarz, R. Guggenheim, M. Duggelin, and K. Rateitschak. 1992. Nonsurgical periodontal treatment: Where are the limits? An SEM study. *J. Clin. Periodontol.* 19:240–244.

Renvert, S., M. Wikström, G. Dahlen, J. Slots, and J. Egelberg. 1990. Effect of subgingival debridement on the elimination of *Aggregatibacter actinomycetemcomitans* and *Bacteroides gingivalis* from periodontal pockets. *J. Clin. Periodontol.* 17:345–350.

Robertson, P. B. 1990. The residual calculus paradox. *J. Periodontol.* 61:65–66.

Sbordone, L., L. Ramaglia, E. Gulletta, and V. Iacono. 1990. Recolonization of the subgingival microbiota after scaling and root planing in human periodontitis. *J. Periodontol.* 61:579–584.

Segelnick, S., and M. A. Weinberg 2006. Reevaluation of initial therapy: When is the appropriate time? *J. Periodontol.* 77:1598–1601.

Sherman, P. R., L. H. Hutchens, Jr., L. G. Jewson, J. M. Moriarty, G. W. Greco, and W. T. McFall, Jr. 1990. The effectiveness of subgingival scaling and root planing: I. Clinical detection of residual calculus. *J. Periodontol.* 61:3–8.

Smart, G. J., M. Wilson, E. H. Davies, and J. B. Kieser. 1990. The assessment of ultrasonic root surface debridement by determination of residual endotoxins levels. *J. Clin. Periodontol.* 17:174–178.

Somerman, M. J., S. Y. Archer, A. Shteyer, and R. A. Foster. 1987. Protein production by human gingival fibroblasts is enhanced by guanidine EDTA extracts of cementum. *J. Periodont. Res.* 22:75–77.

Stambaugh, R. V., M. Dragoo, D. M. Smith, and L. Carasali. 1981. The limits of subgingival scaling. *Int. J. Periodont. Restor. Dent.* 1(5):31–41.

Suvan, J. E. 2005. Effectiveness of mechanical nonsurgical pocket therapy. *Periodontology 2000* 37(1):48–71.

Umeda, M., Y. Takeuchi, K. Noguchi, Y. Huang, G. Koshy, and I. Ishikawa. 2004. Effects of nonsurgical periodontal therapy on the microbiota. *Periodontology 2000* 36(1):98–120.

von Troil, B., I. Needleman, and M. Sanz. 2002. A systematic review of the prevalence of root sensitivity following periodontal therapy. *J. Clin. Periodontol.* 29(Suppl. 3):173–177.

Waerhaug, J. 1978. Healing of the dentoepithelial junction following subgingival biofilm control: II. As observed on extracted teeth. *J. Periodontol.* 49:119–134.

Westfelt, E. 1996. Rationale of mechanical biofilm control. *J. Clin. Periodontol.* 23:263–267.

Westfelt, E., H. Rylander, G. Dahlen, and J. Lindhe. 1998. The effect of supragingival biofilm control on the progression of advanced periodontal disease. *J. Clin. Periodontol.* 25:536–541.

Wilson, T. G., Jr., J. Schoen, and P. Fallon. 1989. Removing toothborne dental deposits: Mechanical means by the professional. In ed. T. G. Wilson, Jr., *Dental maintenance for patients with periodontal diseases*, 67–96. Chicago: Quintessence.

Wylam, J. M., B. L. Mealey, M. P. Mills, T. C. Waldrop, and D. C. Moskowicz. 1993. The clinical effectiveness of open versus closed scaling and root planing on multirooted teeth. *J. Periodontol.* 64:1023–1028.

Zappa, U., J. P. Röthlisberger, C. Simona, and D. Case. 1993. In vivo scaling and root planing forces in molars. *J. Periodontol.* 64:349–354.

Visit www.pearsonhighered.com/healthprofessionsresources to access the student resources that accompany this book. Simply select Dental Hygiene from the choice of disciplines. Find this book and you will find the complimentary study tools created for this specific title.

22

Periodontal Maintenance Therapy

Mea A. Weinberg

OUTLINE

EDUCATIONAL OBJECTIVES

Upon completion of this chapter, the reader should be able to:

- List the objectives of periodontal maintenance.
- Describe the components of periodontal maintenance.
- Describe the role of the dental hygienist in periodontal maintenance visits.
- Define the role of the dental hygienist in smoking cessation.
- Identify when retreatment is necessary.
- Explain the factors involved in patient compliance.

GOAL: To provide an overview of the role periodontal maintenance has in the long-term management of inflammatory periodontal diseases.

KEY WORDS

Introduction

Periodontal maintenance also has been referred to as periodontal recall, supportive periodontal care, and continuing care. All these terms are appropriate, but the American Academy of Periodontology (AAP) has adopted the term *periodontal maintenance*, which may be a more up-to-date and inclusive term because it is a branch of periodontal therapy.

It is known generally that after periodontal treatment is completed, patients will exhibit a decrease in biofilm control and a recurrence of gingivitis or periodontitis unless they are enrolled in a regular periodontal maintenance program (Axelsson & Lindhe, 1981). Patients must be informed of the need for periodic periodontal maintenance visits throughout their life. Because it cannot be predicted when and if gingivitis will progress into periodontitis, the disease must be monitored, and regular professional removal of dental biofilm and calculus must be accomplished.

Refractory Periodontal Diseases/ Recurrent Periodontal Diseases

Refractory periodontal disease occurs in treated periodontal patients who fail to respond to periodontal treatment including maintenance therapy. Patients may be refractory because of inadequate treatment, presence of systemic disease (e.g., diabetes mellitus), deficient immune response, or persistence of periodontal pathogens. On the other hand, *recurrent periodontal disease* occurs in patients who previously responded well to periodontal therapy but later showed signs of disease reactivation. In this situation, there was a recurrence of the disease. Recurrent disease sites also occur in patients demonstrating meticulous biofilm control and on a regular maintenance program.

Treatment for refractory periodontitis may include adjunctive use of antibiotics, or referral for medical consultation. Treatment for recurrent disease sites is based on conventional periodontal therapy (e.g., scaling/root planing, surgery, good biofilm control and maintenance).

Objectives of Periodontal Maintenance

The primary objectives of periodontal maintenance are (American Academy of Periodontology, 2003) (1) to prevent or minimize the recurrence of periodontal diseases in patients by controlling risk factors known to contribute to the disease process (e.g., dental biofilm, calculus); (2) to prevent or reduce the incidence of tooth or implant loss by monitoring the dentition and prosthetic replacements of the natural teeth; (3) to increase the probability of locating and treating other conditions or diseases found in the mouth; and (4) to preserve the health, comfort, and function of the teeth. Periodontal maintenance is also important for monitoring the overall dental health of the patient and to recognize, identify, and manage other diseases or conditions found within or related to the oral cavity (Wilson, 1996b).

Indications for Periodontal Maintenance

Periodontal maintenance is indicated for three types of patients: (1) peridontally healthy patients who have never had periodontal disease as a preventive procedure (this type of care is termed **primary prevention** and applies to a large section of the population), (2) patients who respond favorably after active periodontal therapy to prevent or minimize the recurrence and progression of periodontal disease and tooth loss (this type of care is termed **secondary prevention**), and (3) medically compromised patients or patients who maintain poor oral hygiene and are not considered candidates for periodontal surgery.

Components of the Periodontal Maintenance Visit

Patient needs at the periodontal maintenance visit vary widely and are modified on an individual basis. Regardless, standard periodontal maintenance procedures include the following steps (American Academy of Periodontology, 2003):

1. An update of medical and dental histories.
2. Extraoral and intraoral examinations.
3. Dental examination and gingival and periodontal assessment.
4. Radiographic review.
5. Oral hygiene evaluation (amount of biofilm, calculus, and stains).
6. Review of the patient's biofilm-control efficacy.
7. Removal of dental biofilm from the supragingival and subgingival areas, root debridement where indicated, teeth polishing, and adjunctive chemotherapy if necessary.

The patient's chart should be reviewed for previous periodontal treatments, including periodontal maintenance care, before any current treatment is initiated. Any medications needed before periodontal maintenance, such as antibiotic prophylaxis, can be determined before the patient is seen and acknowledged when the patient arrives at the dental office.

Two aspects emphasized and provided during periodontal maintenance are monitoring and therapy. The preceding examination steps should be performed on every patient at each periodontal maintenance visit but are subject to the judgment of the dentist and the dental hygienist. The clinical findings obtained at the periodontal maintenance visit should be compared with baseline findings. Baseline values are first established at the initial examination and again following active therapy.

Periodontal maintenance is designed to eliminate or reduce primary and secondary risk factors. The primary risk factor for inflammatory periodontal diseases is dental biofilm. Secondary factors include biofilm-retentive areas such as calculus and restorations with overhangs or defective margins. The patient removes supragingival biofilm by toothbrushing and the use of interdental aids such as floss and interproximal brushes, whereas the dental hygienist removes both supragingival and subgingival biofilm and calculus by mechanical debridement. The dentist should replace or restore defective or failed restorations. Box 22–1 provides a step-by-step list of the components of a periodontal maintenance visit.

Medical and Dental Update

The patient should be asked if there have been any medication or health changes, including hospitalizations, since the last appointment. Review current medications (prescription and over-the-counter) with the patient. Note any changes in dosage or instructions for use. A medical consultation with the patient's physician may be warranted if new illnesses are recognized or if a previous condition has changed significantly. A chief complaint should be noted, and this should be accompanied by a notation of the degree of comfort or discomfort. The patient and the dentist should sign the amended form.

Rapid Dental Hint

Remember to take a medical history at every visit.

Box 22–1: Components of a Periodontal Maintenance Visit

Examination	Remarks
Review and update medical and dental history, take blood pressure, pulse, respiration.	To determine if additional risk factors are responsible for recurrent or progressive periodontal breakdown.

Clinical examination, including
    Extra intraoral examination
    Biofilm evaluation/disclosing
    Evaluating the patient's oral hygiene technique
    Dental charting of caries, restorative care
	Changes that should be of concern during a periodontal maintenance visit include sites that have changed from nonbleeding to bleeding, sites that have increased 2 to 3 mm or more in attachment loss or probing depth, and any sites with pus or suppuration.

Periodontal charting of probing depths, gingival recession/enlargement, furcation defects, bleeding on probing, exudation, tooth mobility, fremitus	
Implant evaluation: peri-implant tissues, probing depths, bleeding on probing, stability of dental implant (mobility), examination of abutment teeth, occlusal examination	
Radiographic review	Because radiographs only show past activity (e.g., bone loss occurred approximately 6 months ago, not yesterday or today), it is important to correlate the radiographic findings with clinical probing depths and clinical attachment levels.

Treatment options
    Removal of supragingival and subgingival biofilm and
    calculus
    Selective polishing
    Oral hygiene reinstruction
	These treatment guidelines depend on the type of periodontal patient. Treatment should not be started unless the data collected are appropriately recorded.

Adjunctive therapy
    Antimicrobial therapy
    Occlusal treatment
    Counseling on control of contributing factors such as
    smoking cessation, stress reduction, and nutrition
    Restorative and prosthetic care
Reevaluation of the maintenance care interval
Scheduling of next periodontal maintenance appointment	

Counseling the patient on risk factors that contribute to periodontal diseases, such as cigarette smoking, stress, nutrition, medications (e.g., calcium channel blockers, phenytoin, cyclosporine, oral contraceptives), and systemic diseases (e.g., diabetes mellitus, AIDS), also should be done during the periodontal maintenance visit (Kerry, 1995). The patient should be informed about the availability of programs for **smoking cessation** in and outside the office.

Because many patients are on an alternating periodontal maintenance program, seeing both a general dentist and a periodontist, any communication from the last treating office should be reviewed. Any new restorative treatment should be indicated on the chart and evaluated clinically.

Extraoral/Intraoral Examination

An updated examination is performed in the head and neck area and intraoral tissues for the detection of any abnormalities, including enlarged lymph nodes or salivary glands and red, white, or pigmented lesions. If any suspicious lesions are found, the dentist should be informed for further examination or treatment.

Dental Examination

The dental examination at the periodontal maintenance visit includes caries assessment as well as documentation of the status of restorations. Restorations should be charted, noting any defective restorations or failures such as fractures or open margins of amalgams, composites, and crowns. The stability of bridges, removable partial dentures, and implants also should be noted. Documentation of tooth loss since the last charting should be recorded, including the cause. A good rule to follow is to always count the number of teeth present.

Gingival and Periodontal Assessment

GINGIVAL ASSESSMENT   Initially, a visual examination of the gingival tissues is done to determine the condition of the gingiva. The color, contour, consistency, and surface texture of the gingiva are recorded. Any mucogingival involvement should be noted. If gingival inflammation is found, the location and severity should be noted, as well as etiologic factors (e.g., dental biofilm accumulation due to poor oral hygiene self-care, medication-induced, stress, or resulting from a hormonal imbalance).

PERIODONTAL ASSESSMENT   Next, a periodontal evaluation is performed. This includes recording of probing depths, gingival recession, clinical attachment level, furcation involvement, suppuration (pus), and tooth mobility.

Gingival Recession. The position of the gingival tissues on the tooth is defined as the location of the gingival margin in relation to the cementoenamel junction (CEJ). Gingival recession that has progressed since the last appointment must be addressed and treatment options given to the patient. If the recession has remained unchanged, then monitoring is all that is needed. To treat gingival recession, the cause must be determined. Etiologic factors include inappropriate toothbrushing technique, attachment loss (disease process), and shrinkage of tissues after initial therapy. Treatment may include educating the patient on proper brushing technique or mucogingival surgery. Common patient complaints concerning gingival recession include poor aesthetics and tooth pain or hypersensitivity with air or cold application. Any dentinal hypersensitivity can be managed in most patients with desensitizing agents (e.g., potassium nitrate, sodium fluoride, or stannous fluoride).

Disease Stability: Probing Depth and Clinical Attachment Level. Monitoring of probing depths and clinical attachment levels (CALs) currently is the most reliable way to determine periodontal disease stability. It may be time consuming to determine the CAL, but it is an extremely important measurement. Probing depth recordings should be taken at six sites per tooth. If a patient's periodontal condition has deteriorated rapidly since the last periodontal maintenance visit, systemic disease such as diabetes mellitus, smoking, stress, or use of alcohol might be the cause.

Measurement of the CAL is made from the CEJ to the apical extent of the tip of the probe. Such measurements are compared with measurements obtained at the last periodontal maintenance visit. A 2 to 3 mm increase in attachment loss indicates disease progression (Haffajee, Socransky, & Goodson, 1983; Kornman, 1987), and more aggressive treatment or **retreatment** may be justified. *It should be kept in mind that even a 1 mm increase in attachment loss evident at subsequent dental appointments should be of concern.* However, a patient with a 3 mm probing depth without recession has a 3 mm CAL with no attachment loss, and this is not of great concern.

Bleeding on Probing. Probing depths should be interpreted on a patient-by-patient, site-by-site basis. For example, a 5 mm probing depth that does not bleed on probing is viewed differently from a 5 mm probing depth with bleeding on probing and suppuration. Bleeding on probing can mean two things: laceration (e.g., from too firm probe pressure) or ulceration (e.g., inflammation within the connective tissue; Armitage, 1996). Bleeding while stroking the lateral wall of the gingival crevice indicates early gingival inflammation (Van der Weijden, Timmerman, Nijbor, Reijerse, & Van der Velden, 1994). Thus, disease stability can be monitored during periodontal maintenance on the basis of bleeding on probing (Lang, Joss, & Tonetti, 1996). Bleeding sites in deep pockets seem to have an increased risk for progression of periodontitis (progressive attachment loss) in patients on periodontal maintenance care (Claffey, Nylund, Kiger, Gorrett, & Egelberg, 1990). The absence of bleeding on probing is a better indicator of gingival health than its presence is of periodontal disease (Lang et al., 1996). However, in patients who smoke, bleeding on probing may not be evident (Dietrich, 2004). One should chart the sites that bleed on probing (e.g., use a red dot over the site). Thus, sites that bleed warrant more attention during the periodontal maintenance visit and may have to be reinstrumented, whereas nonbleeding sites should be left without repeated subgingival instrumentation (Lang et al., 1996). Bleeding on probing generally is apparent 10 seconds after probing (Lang et al., 1996).

It should be emphasized that the force used while probing (probing force) varies considerably during probing depth measurements, even from tooth to tooth. Therefore, a tooth with healthy periodontium may bleed because "too much" force was used and not because of inflammation. Ideally, a probing force of 0.25 N (25 g) should be used, which clinically represents a "light probing force" (Joss, Adler, & Lang, 1994; Lang et al., 1996), or probe until slight resistance is felt. A nonmetallic probe should be used to probe around implants.

Tooth Mobility. Tooth mobility for each tooth is noted on the chart. Tooth mobility also should be measured and recorded on the chart as Grade I, II, III, or IV (Carranza & Takei, 1996). If there is increasing mobility since the last visit, the cause should be determined and appropriate treatment rendered. The presence of fremitus also should be recorded.

Radiographic Review

Radiographs show past bone destruction. It is important to monitor the patient's periodontal status with clinical probing and standardized radiographs taken at appropriate intervals to compare with previously taken radiographs. Radiographs should be taken according to the American Dental Association *Guidelines* (American Dental Association, 2004). In a recall periodontal patient with a history of bone loss and periodontal surgery, clinical judgment is used on the need for and type of radiographic images for the evaluation of periodontal disease. Imaging may consist of, but is not limited to, selected bitewing and/or periapical images of areas where periodontal disease (other than non-specific gingivitis) can be identified clinically (American Dental Association, 2004). Sites that have had bone (osseous) grafting or guided tissue regeneration can be evaluated

with radiographs at least 6 months after surgery. The need for bitewing and periapical radiographs depends on the stage and severity of the disease, risk for caries, and presence of implants. Vertical bitewing views are ideal for patients with periodontal disease because they show more of the alveolar bone than do horizontal bitewings. A radiographic evaluation is more important for monitoring of implants than probing.

Oral Hygiene Evaluation and Patient's Biofilm-Control Regimen

The next step is to evaluate gross biofilm accumulation, determine the quality of oral hygiene self-care procedures, and conduct patient education. A disclosing agent is used for patient education and as a basis for recording a biofilm index. Scoring of biofilm at a periodontal maintenance appointment may be misleading because patients frequently brush very well just before coming to such an appointment. In any event, monitoring of the biofilm level can be used to evaluate the patient's compliance with oral hygiene self-care. The patient's oral hygiene practices are reviewed by asking the patient to brush and use interdental devices while the hygienist watches. The level of patient motivation to perform daily biofilm removal must be determined. A patient may understand and show correct technique in the office but may not comply with instructions at home because of lack of interest or time constraints. It is important to recognize such patients and to spend more time explaining to them the importance of performing these tasks.

Dental Implants

Evaluation of a patient with dental implants is essentially the same as that of a patient with natural teeth. However, rather than teeth, the implants and peri-implant tissues are evaluated (Sison, 2003). If inflammation or disease is detected around an implant, the probing depth should be measured and bleeding and suppuration noted. However, it should be noted that probing depths depend on how the implant was placed. So, probing depths may not be as meaningful around implants as natural teeth. The stability of the abutment teeth and prosthesis also should be noted by recording mobility. An abutment is a tooth or implant used for support and retention of a crown or removable partial denture. The prosthesis is checked for occlusal wear. Any loosened screws should be recorded. Calculus deposits on implant surfaces are not firmly attached because the titantium surface of the implant is nonporous, which is just the opposite of natural teeth in which the cementum is porous, allowing for a firm attachment of calculus. Light, short strokes should be used to prevent trauma to the peri-implant tissues (Sison, 2003).

Because there is a correlation between implant failure and bone characteristics, it is essential to take radiographs periodically. Generally, periapical films are indicated at 6-month to 1-year intervals to determine the height of bone around an implant. The accepted standard for a stable endosseous implant 1 year after placement is vertical bone loss less than 0.2 mm per year (Albrektsson, Zarb, Worthington, & Eriksson, 1986; American Academy of Periodontology, 1989). Radiographically, an ailing, failing, or failed implant will show varying amounts of alveolar bone loss (Meffert, 1992). Mobility will occur with the failed implant.

Treatment: Recurrent Periodontal Disease versus a Well-Maintained Periodontium

Recurrent periodontal disease occurs when signs and symptoms of disease return after having subsided during active treatment. Clinical signs include bleeding on probing, increasing tooth mobility, continued soft tissue attachment loss (including deep pockets), suppuration from the pocket, and radiographic changes. Recurrent occlusal problems include increasing tooth mobility and fremitus. A good rule to follow may be that when bleeding on probing or the presence of suppuration is seen 4 to 8 weeks following the periodontal maintenance appointment, then retreatment is plausible. Another reason for retreatment includes a 1–2 mm or greater increase in probing depth or attachment loss. Specific treatment could include periodontal debridement (scaling and root planing), periodontal surgery, antimicrobial agents, occlusal adjustment, splinting, extractions, or a night guard. After the initial therapy is completed, reevaluation should be performed. If resolution does not occur after retreatment, then a systemic disease component must be considered and the patient referred to a periodontist. See AAP Guidelines for Referral (American Academy of Periodontology, 2006).

In a well-maintained patient in whom inflammation is not present (no bleeding on probing) and for whom soft tissue attachment loss or bone loss is minimal, the following treatment is recommended at a periodontal maintenance visit:

1. Point out any areas in the mouth where the patient is having difficulty with biofilm control, and correct the patient's technique, if necessary.
2. Deplaquing may be performed. In patients with little or no subgingival deposits (usually after active treatment), a deplaquing stroke can be used with a curet or ultrasonic or sonic scaler. The tip of the instrument is "floating" within the gingival sulcus, lightly touching the root surface.
3. Selective tooth polishing can be performed. Extrinsic stains may be derived from nicotine, tea, coffee, foods, and chlorhexidine oral rinse.
4. Determine the interval of the next periodontal maintenance visit.

Subgingival instrumentation, including root planing of shallow pockets, has been shown to increase soft tissue attachment loss (Lindhe, Socransky, Nyman, Haffajee, & Westfelt, 1982). Patients with dental implants should be questioned about any difficulty in oral hygiene self-care or discomfort or difficulty in chewing. Plastic periodontal probes, scalers, and curets should be used because stainless steel instruments can scratch the titanium surfaces of implants.

All patients must undergo oral hygiene reinstruction and counseling on control of contributing risk factors such as smoking. Patients should be kept informed of their current periodontal condition and treatment options. Consultation may be required with other dentists who will be providing restorative or prosthetic treatment or who will be involved in the periodontal maintenance program.

Chemotherapeutics

Chemotherapeutic agents may be beneficial in certain patients as an adjunct to standard oral hygiene procedures, but they do not replace brushing and flossing. Because chemotherapeutic agents help to prevent repopulation of potential gram-negative periodontal pathogens between periodontal maintenance appointments, medically compromised patients or those exhibiting poor oral hygiene may benefit from such agents. Because periodontitis is a subgingival malady, rinsing with an agent is ineffective. To target subgingival bacteria, oral irrigation may be helpful between periodontal maintenance visits to prevent repopulation of periodontal pathogens (Jolkovsky et al., 1990). Irrigation with water or a medicament detoxifies and removes unattached dental biofilm. Systemic antibiotics are not recommended routinely during periodontal maintenance because of the potential development of bacterial resistance, although antibiotics occasionally may be of some benefit in aggressive and refractory periodontitis cases during periodontal maintenance. Controlled-release drugs such as Arestin, PerioChip, or Atridox may be used in selected recurrent pockets of 5 mm or greater that bleed. Desensitizing agents may be applied at a periodontal maintenance visit to reduce or eliminate dentinal hypersensitivity in patients in whom gingival recession is present.

Frequency of Intervals

Periodontal maintenance intervals are determined on an individual basis according to periodontal disease severity, type of treatment performed, adequacy of oral hygiene self-care, presence of orthodontic and prosthetic appliances, systemic health, and **patient adherence** (compliance) and cooperation (American Academy of Periodontology, 1998). The premise on which a time-interval frame for periodontal maintenance has been based is the repopulation time of periodontal pathogens after the last periodontal debridement. Data suggest that periodontal maintenance intervals of 3 months or less are indicated for continued suppression of potentially pathogenic microorganisms in susceptible patients (American Academy of Periodontology, 1998).

A 12-month recall interval may be acceptable for patients with limited susceptibility to periodontitis (Rosén et al., 1999). Regardless, the periodontal maintenance interval is determined on a patient-by-patient basis. Figure 22–1 ■ is a schematic flowchart that reviews suggested time intervals for healthy and periodontal patients. Patients can return 4 to 8 weeks after periodontal debridement for further observations (Segelnick & Weinberg 2006). Any time during a periodontal maintenance program, a patient may temporarily go back into active therapy.

The time required for the periodontal maintenance visit depends on the number of teeth; disease severity; amount of biofilm, calculus, and stains; instrumentation access; presence of extensive prosthetic crowns and bridges; orthodontic appliances; depths of pockets; and patient cooperation. Although periodontal maintenance visits usually are scheduled for 1 hour, the amount of time

should be individualized (American Academy of Periodontology, 1998).

General Dentist–Periodontist Relationship

Periodontal patients can be monitored by both their general dentist and their periodontist, but they should be seen by the periodontist at least once a year for a thorough periodontal evaluation. Periodontal maintenance can be performed alternately by the general dentist and the periodontist.

Gingivitis or mild chronic periodontitis patients can receive total care, including chronic periodontal maintenance, by the general dentist. Moderate chronic periodontitis patients should alternate periodontal maintenance visits between the general dentist and the periodontist once active treatment is completed. Severe chronic periodontitis

---

At the completion of initial therapy (after reevaluation)

PERIODONTAL HEALTH (NO PREVIOUS HISTORY OF PERIODONTAL DISEASES)		GINGIVITIS
Compliant with oral hygiene self-care No extensive restorative or prosthetics No occlusal discrepancies No extensive restorative or prosthetics	No bleeding No periodontally comprised teeth Complaint with oral hygiene self-care hygiene	Generalized or localized bleeding No periodontally compromised teeth Noncomplier or irregular complier
6 months	6 months	3 months or less for the first periodontal maintenance visit; if patient responds to treatment with improvement in oral hygiene then increase interval between visits; if there is no improvement after a few periodontal maintenance visits, enroll the patient into active treatment. Risk factors including smoking and systemic diseases (e.g., diabetes mellitus, medications, hormonal imbalance) must be considered.

SLIGHT TO MODERATE PERIODONTITIS (SURGICAL AND NONSURGICAL PATIENTS)	SEVERE PERIODONTITIS (SURGICAL AND NONSURGICAL PATIENTS)
No teeth with less than 50% bone remaining Localized or no bleeding on probing Localized shallow pockets remain A controlled systemic disease that contributes to periodontal destruction Compliers with oral hygiene self-care	If many of the following factors are present: Many periodontally compromised teeth (>50% bone loss) Generalized deep pockets Occlusal problems Systemic disease (uncontrolled or poorly controlled) that predisposes to periodontal destruction (e.g., diabetes mellitus) Extensive restorative and prosthetic appliances Periodontal surgery not performed for medical, psychological, or financial reasons Noncomplier or irregular complier with oral hygiene self-care
6 months to 1 year	3 months or less depending on the number of risk factors present.

FIGURE 22–1 Schematic illustration describing suggested time intervals for periodontal maintenance.

Did You Know?

The new buzzword for compliance is *adherence*. So instead of writing *patient compliance* it is now more correct to say *patient adherence*.

patients should be seen primarily by a periodontist, with annual appointments with the general dentist for general care. Refractory periodontitis and aggressive periodontitis patients should be seen exclusively by the periodontist for all active periodontal treatment.

Patient Adherence

An essential aspect of periodontal maintenance therapy is patient adherence. Most patients do not comply with long-term behavioral changes, especially for conditions that are not life threatening. Wilson (1996a) identified three types of compliers: full compliers, irregular compliers, and noncompliers. Periodontal maintenance appointments are essential and important for all groups, but noncompliers have less-successful surgical outcomes over time. Better communication may contribute to more successful outcomes. Other methods of improving patient adherence include providing positive reinforcement and attempting to better accommodate patient needs (Wilson, 1996a). Furthermore, the severity of the periodontal problem should be stressed because the more threatening a patient perceives a disease, the higher is the adherence.

Wilson, Glover, Schoen, Baus, and Jacobs (1984) reported that of 100 treated patients who were given the opportunity for periodontal maintenance over an 8-year period in a private periodontal office, 34% never returned to the office for periodontal maintenance, and only 16% completed periodontal maintenance. Becker, Becker, and Berg (1984), in a study of 44 patients who refused to participate in periodontal maintenance, found that in the absence of periodontal maintenance, periodontal surgery was of questionable benefit in maintaining periodontal health. The patient dropout rate (43%) was highest in the first year, which, according to the authors, suggested that a patient is more likely to remain compliant in the long term if he or she is compliant with the maintenance treatment for the first year (Mendoza, Newcomb, and Nixon, 1991).

Some common reasons for patient nonadherence with office visits include the expense, the belief by patients that they no longer require treatment because they no longer have any signs of disease, fear of dental treatment (Mendoza et al., 1991; Wilson, 1996a), or lifestyle changes (e.g., job change or move).

Most longitudinal studies have shown that patients who receive therapy maintain their teeth longer than those who do not. A study by Becker and colleagues (1984) looked at patients in three categories:

1. Patients with untreated moderate to advanced periodontal disease lost an average of 0.33 teeth per year.
2. Patients who had treatment but no periodontal maintenance lost an average of 0.22 teeth per year.
3. Patients who had treatment and periodontal maintenance lost an average of 0.11 teeth per year.

Providing patients with motivational strategies may help to improve compliance. Examples of such approaches include (1) giving patients printed self-care instructions at every periodontal maintenance visit, (2) noting the next periodontal maintenance appointment on the instructions, (3) counseling patients about their condition and the benefit-to-risk ratio of having periodontal maintenance, (4) seeking out patient concerns and responding to them, and (5) sending reminders or calling patients about their next periodontal maintenance visit.

Dental Hygiene Application

Professional biofilm control, oral hygiene self-care, and periodic periodontal maintenance are and will continue to be the foundation of periodontal therapy. Following periodontal and implant therapy, regular periodontal maintenance can encourage periodontal and peri-implant health. In the majority of patients, periodontal maintenance is started after completion of active periodontal therapy, but it can be used in other phases of treatment. Periodontal maintenance evolved from a dental prophylaxis and now emphasizes treatment of areas with previous attachment loss and areas where clinical signs of inflammation are found (Wilson, 1996a). Because the timing interval for periodontal maintenance appointments is not standardized, the decision is empirical, with no real scientific basis. An interval of 3 months between periodontal maintenance visits appears to be an effective schedule to follow, but this may vary according to clinical judgment, the periodontal disease severity of the patient, and clinical findings.

A number of risk factors must be identified and monitored during periodontal maintenance. Increases in bleeding, pockets, and tooth loss will occur in high-risk patients. Clinical decisions during maintenance therapy will be influenced by the presence of risk factors, and better knowledge of these risk factors may lead to improved and more efficient risk-management efforts during periodontal maintenance (Tonetti, Muller-Campanile, & Lang, 1998).

Dental hygienists play an important role not only in the mechanical aspects of periodontal maintenance but also in promoting preventive measures and explaining the importance of periodontal maintenance. Properly motivated patients will stay on a regularly scheduled periodontal maintenance regimen.

Key Points

- Reevaluation of therapy should be performed between 4 and 8 weeks after completion of debridement.
- The desired outcome of periodontal maintenance in patients after active therapy is the maintenance of periodontal health.
- Nonadherence with regular periodontal maintenance visits may result in recurrence or progression of disease.
- Despite adequate periodontal maintenance and oral hygiene self-care, some patients may show recurrence or progression of disease, and thus active therapy should be reinstated.

Self-Quiz

1. From the following list, select the items associated with the goals of periodontal maintenance.
   a. Maintain the patient's oral status and function.
   b. Minimize inflammation and bleeding.
   c. Prevent the recurrence of disease.
   d. Prevent the patient from having surgical therapy.

2. Which one of the following assessments best determines that periodontal disease activity has occurred?
   a. Clinical attachment loss
   b. Bleeding localized to certain teeth
   c. Redness and edema of the gingival tissues
   d. Suppuration

3. From the following list, select the items associated with the presence of bleeding on probing.
   a. Laceration of the epithelium due to forceful probing
   b. Ulceration of the epithelium
   c. Inflammation
   d. Low bacterial count

4. Which one of the following procedures is appropriate if a bleeding site with a probing depth of 7 mm with furcation involvement is found during a routine periodontal maintenance visit?
   a. Reevaluate the site at the next appointment.
   b. Refer the patient to a specialist.
   c. Perform periodontal debridement.
   d. Prescribe systemic antibiotics.

5. All the following risk factors can be modified during periodontal maintenance therapy except one. Which one is the exception?
   a. Stress
   b. Smoking
   c. Interproximal biofilm accumulation
   d. Genetic susceptibility

6. Which one of the following protocols is most appropriate in a patient who shows generalized recurrence of disease at a periodontal maintenance visit?
   a. Perform periodontal surgery.
   b. Reinstate Phase I therapy.
   c. Insert tetracycline fibers into the sites.
   d. Prescribe a systemic antibiotic in conjunction with periodontal debridement.

7. From the following list, select the items associated with determining the most appropriate time interval for periodontal maintenance visits.
   a. Medical condition
   b. Level of biofilm control
   c. Number of teeth in the dentition
   d. Severity of the disease
   e. Number of medications taken

8. Which one of the following types of pockets is most appropriate for adjunctive controlled-release drug delivery?
   a. Nonbleeding, > 5 mm
   b. Nonbleeding, < 5 mm
   c. Bleeding, ≥ 5 mm
   d. Bleeding, ≤ 5 mm

9. All of the following are techniques the dental hygienist can use to improve patient adherence to periodontal therapy except one. Which one is the exception?
   a. Print self-care instructions.
   b. Counsel patients about their condition.
   c. Call the patient every week.
   d. Seek out patient concerns and respond to them.
   e. Send patients reminders about their next visit.

10. From the following list, select the items associated with objectives of periodontal maintenance.
    a. Prevent or minimize the recurrence of periodontal diseases
    b. Prevent or reduce the incidence of tooth or implant loss
    c. Increase the probability of locating and treating other conditions or diseases found in the mouth
    d. Preserve the health, comfort, and function of the teeth.
    e. Decrease attachment levels

Case Study

A periodontal practice has several patients on periodontal maintenance therapy. Some of these patients have responded favorably to therapy while others have not. Some patients adhere to the home care regimes while others continue with poor oral hygiene. The dental hygienist must review each patient profile to determine the individual care.

1. The patient who still has poor home care and bleeding pockets should be seen in which frequency interval?
   a. 3 month or less intervals
   b. 12 month intervals
   c. 6 months intervals
   d. 4–6 weeks after initial therapy

Answer: A. Intervals of three months or less allows the dental hygienist to continually suppress the potentially pathogenic microorganisms. 6 or 12 months intervals might be sufficient for a healthy patient. Maintenance intervals are established after the initial therapy is complete and evaluated at the 4–6 week interval.

2. A patient who has previously responded well to therapy and then shows signs of disease reactivation is termed
   a. refractory
   b. recurrent
   c. secondary
   d. aggressive

Answer: B. Refractory patients fail to respond to treatment including maintenance while recurrent disease occurs in patients who previously responded well to therapy. Secondary prevention is the term for care to prevent or minimize the recurrence or progression of the disease. Aggressive periodontitis is a form of rapidly progressive disease regardless of age.

3. What should the dental hygienist do for the patient who does not comply with home care or routine maintenance intervals.
   a. decrease time between maintenance interval
   b. address fear and cost issues
   c. explain risks of non-compliance
   d. all of the above

Answer: D. All of the above must be addressed. It is not just a factor of the professional debridement but also the patient involvement and commitment to the maintenance therapy.

References

Albrektsson, T., G. Zarb, P. Worthington, and A. R. Eriksson. 1986. The long-term efficacy of currently used dental implants: A review and proposed criteria of success. *Int. J. Oral Maxillofac. Implants* 1:11–25.

American Academy of Periodontology. 1989. *Proceedings of the World Workshop in Clinical Periodontics, Consensus report, Discussion section VIII: Implant therapy (VIII-11-18)*. Chicago: Author.

American Academy of Periodontology. 1998. Periodontal maintenance (PM). *J. Periodontol.* 69:502–506.

American Academy of Periodontology. 2003. Periodontal maintenance. *J. Periodontol.* 74:1395–1401.

American Academy of Periodontology. 2006. Guidelines for the management of patients with periodontal diseases. *J. Periodontol.* 77:1607–1611.

American Dental Association. 2004, November. *Guidelines for prescribing dental radiographs*. Chicago, IL. American Dental Association.

Armitage, G. C. 1996. Manual periodontal probing in supportive periodontal therapy. *Periodontology 2000* 12:33–39.

Axelsson, P., and J. Lindhe. 1981. The significance of maintenance care in the treatment of periodontal disease. *J. Clin. Periodontol.* 8:281–294.

Becker, W., B. E. Becker, and L. E. Berg. 1984. Periodontal treatment without maintenance. A retrospective study in 44 patients. *J. Periodontol.* 55:505–509.

Carranza, F. A., and H. H. Takei. 1996. Treatment of furcation involvement and combined periodontal-endodontic therapy. In eds. F. A. Carranza and M. G. Newman, *Clinical periodontology*, 640. Philadelphia: W. B. Saunders.

Claffey, N., K. Nylund, R. Kiger, S. Garrett, and J. Egelberg. 1990. Diagnostic predictability of scores of biofilm, bleeding, suppuration and probing depth for probing attachment loss. 3 1/2 years of observation following initial periodontal therapy. *J. Clin. Periodontol.* 17:108–114.

Dietrich, T. 2004. The effect of cigarette smoking on gingival bleeding. *J. Periodontol.* 75(1):16–22.

Haffajee, A. D., S. S. Socransky, and J. M. Goodson. 1983. Comparison of different data analyses for detecting changes in attachment level. *J. Clin. Periodontol.* 10:298–310.

Jolkovsky, D. L., M. Y. Waki, M. G. Newman, J. Otomo-Corgel, M. Madison, et al. 1990. Clinical and microbiological effects of subgingival and gingival marginal irrigation with chlorhexidine gluconate. *J. Periodontol.* 61:663–669.

Joss, A., R. Adler, and N. P. Lang. 1994. Bleeding on probing. A parameter for monitoring periodontal conditions in clinical practice. *J. Clin. Periodontol.* 21:402–408.

Kerry, G. J. 1995. Supportive periodontal treatment. *Periodontology 2000* 11:176–184.

Kornman, K. S. 1987. Nature of periodontal diseases: Assessment and diagnosis. *J. Periodontol. Res.* 22:192–204.

Lang, N. P., A. Joss, and M. S. Tonetti. 1996. Monitoring disease during supportive periodontal treatment by bleeding on probing. *Periodontology 2000* 12:44–48.

Lindhe, J., S. S. Socransky, S. Nyman, A. Haffajee, and E. Westfelt. 1982. "Critical probing depths" in periodontal therapy. *J. Clin. Periodontol.* 9:323–336.

Meffert, R. M. 1992. How to treat ailing and failing implants. *Implant Dent.* 1:25–33.

Mendoza, A., G., Newcomb, K. Nixon. 1991. Compliance with supportive periodontal therapy. *J Periodontol.* 62:731–736.

Rosén, B., G. Olavi, A. Baderstan, A. Rönström, G. Söderholm, and J. Egelberg. 1999. Effect of different frequencies of preventive maintenance treatment on periodontal conditions. *J. Clin. Periodontol.* 26:225–230.

Segelnick, S. L., and M. A. Weinberg. 2006. Reevaluation of initial therapy: When is the appropriate time? *J. Periodontol.* 77(9):1598–1601.

Sison, S. G. 2003, May–June. Implant maintenance and the dental hygienist. *Access* (Supplement issue):1–12.

Tonetti, M., V. Muller-Campanile, and V. Lang. 1998. Changes in the prevalence of residual pockets and tooth loss in treated periodontal patients during a supportive maintenance care program. *J. Clin. Periodontol.* 25:1008–1016.

Van der Weijden, G. A., M. F. Timmerman, A. Nijbor, E. Reijerse, and U. Van der Velden. 1994. Comparison of different approaches to assess bleeding on probing as indicators of gingivitis. *J. Periodontol.* 21:589–594.

Wilson, T. G. 1996a. Compliance and its role in periodontal therapy. *Periodontology 2000* 12:16–23.

Wilson, T. G. 1996b. Supportive periodontal treatment introduction: Definition, extent of need, therapeutic objectives, frequency and efficacy. *Periodontology 2000* 12:11–15.

Wilson, T. G., Jr., M. E. Glover, J. Schoen, C. Baus, and T. Jacobs. 1984. Compliance with maintenance therapy in a private periodontal practice. *J. Periodontol.* 55:468–473.

Visit www.pearsonhighered.com/healthprofessionsresources to access the student resources that accompany this book. Simply select Dental Hygiene from the choice of disciplines. Find this book and you will find the complimentary study tools created for this specific title.

23

Topical Drug Delivery Systems: Oral Rinses and Irrigation

Mea A. Weinberg and Deborah M. Lyle

OUTLINE

Introduction
Oral Rinses
Antiplaque/Antigingivitis Agents
Oral Irrigation
Dental Hygiene Application
Key Points
Self-Quiz
Case Study
References

EDUCATIONAL OBJECTIVES

Upon completion of this chapter, the reader should be able to:

- Describe measures, using chemical agents, taken to prevent and control the progression of periodontal diseases.
- List the different oral rinses available for the periodontal patient.
- Discuss the benefits and indications for oral irrigation.

GOAL: To provide an understanding of the fundamentals of counseling periodontal patients on the adjunctive use of chemotherapeutic agents for supragingival and subgingival plaque control.

KEY WORDS

Introduction

Topically applied **chemotherapeutic agents** have been developed based on a need for treatment of gingival bleeding and inflammation in association with gingivitis. Mouth rinsing and oral irrigation are two approaches used for supragingival application of antiseptic solutions. Oral rinses are the most common form of **topical delivery**. Oral rinses are ideal vehicles for the delivery of topical antimicrobials because of their relative simplicity of formulation and ease of use for patients.

Oral Rinses

Mouth rinses generally are divided into two classifications: therapeutic rinses, used to treat diseases such as gingival diseases, and cosmetic rinses, used to freshen the breath. Indications for using oral rinses are as follows:

- As an addition to home care regimens that have failed to achieve plaque-control goals by other means
- As an addition to periodontal instrumentation
- Where oral hygiene may be inadequate or difficult to accomplish for many people, as in the physically or mentally compromised
- Following surgical procedures, when brushing and flossing are generally not practical
- As a preprocedural rinse to reduce aerosolized bacteria in the dental office (when masked, the clinician is protected; however, after the mask is removed, aerosols remain in the dental operatory)
- For maintenance of dental implants

Topical antimicrobial agents delivered by a rinse are effective only against supragingival bacteria. Antimicrobial rinses, when used in conjunction with brushing and flossing have been reported to be an important method of reducing plaque and gingivitis (Barnett, 2006; Silverman & Wilder, 2006). No antimicrobial rinse has been shown to be effective against periodontitis because oral rinses do not reach the subgingival area. Mouth rinses may be discontinued if oral health conditions can be maintained without their use.

Antiplaque/Antigingivitis Agents

Antimicrobial agents ideally should inhibit microbial colonization on tooth surfaces and prevent the subsequent formation of plaque. They also should eliminate or suppress the pathogenicity of existing plaque. Antiseptics have a greater potential to prevent the formation of plaque than to resolve established plaque and gingivitis.

An antimicrobial agent relies on two factors for efficacy. Success depends on the amount of time the agent stays in contact with the target site and how well the agent gains access to the target site. A major requirement for the success of antimicrobial therapy is **substantivity**, which is the ability of the drug to adsorb or bind to intraoral surfaces such as teeth and soft tissues with subsequent release of the drug in its active form (Stabholz et al., 1993). Substantivity

---

> ## Did You Know?
> The total annual consumer spending on oral antiseptics/rinses is $885 million.

involves the ability of the drug to stay at the target site for longer periods of time, thus maintaining therapeutic levels. It is ideal to have a drug with high substantivity that will be bound in the oral cavity and released over a period of hours to prolong the effects. Lack of substantivity can be overcome by more frequent use of the agent, but this would likely result in noncompliance and undesirable side effects.

Classification of Oral Rinses

Topical antimicrobial oral rinses can be classified as either first- or second-generation agents. First-generation agents have antibacterial properties with low substantivity and limited therapeutic value in reducing plaque and gingivitis. Examples include phenolic compounds, quaternary ammonium compounds, peroxide, and sanguinarine. Second-generation agents have antibacterial properties in addition to substantivity. Chlorhexidine gluconate is an example of a second-generation agent and is currently the only second-generation agent proven to prevent and control gingivitis. It is available in the United States only by prescription. All first-generation mouth rinses are available over the counter (OTC) without a prescription.

In 1986, the American Dental Association (ADA) established guidelines for evaluation of the therapeutic effectiveness of products against gingivitis. For example, studies should be conducted over a minimum of 6 months, two studies with independent investigators should be conducted, and the active product should be used as part of a normal regimen and compared with a placebo or control product.

Most mouth rinses contain alcohol as a flavor enhancer and as a vehicle for the active ingredients. In the past there has been some concern about the association of alcohol in mouth rinses with oral cancer. Various studies have shown inconsistent findings. The consensus seems to agree that that there is no reason for patients to refrain from use of alcohol-containing mouth rinses (Spolarich & Gurenlian 2013). In addition, an in vitro (laboratory) setting studied the effect of acetaldehyde, a toxic compound produced by alcohol metabolism (breakdown) in the body. It was reported that acetaldehyde caused changes in gingival fibroblasts (cells involved in oral connective tissue maintenance; Poggi, Rodriguez y Baena, Rizzo, & Rota, 2003).

Bisbiguanides

Description and Mechanism of Action. Chlorhexidine gluconate (Peridex® Omni 3M, St. Paul, MN; PerioGard®, Colgate Oral Pharmaceuticals, New York, NY) is a cationic (positively charged) molecule. Originally, chlorhexidine was used in medicine as an antiseptic cream for wounds, as a preoperative skin cleanser, and as a surgical scrub. In 1970, the first study on the ability of chlorhexidine to inhibit the formation of plaque and maintain soft tissue health was released (Löe & Schiott, 1970). It was not until 1986 that chlorhexidine became available in the United States by prescription at a 0.12% concentration with an alcohol concentration of 11.6%. It has the ADA seal of acceptance for the treatment of gingivitis (Cheng, Leung, & Corbet, 2008).

After rinsing, chlorhexidine (positively charged) is attracted to and attaches onto the negatively charged bacterial cell walls, causing lysis or breakage of the cell wall, and the contents of the cells leak. Chlorhexidine enters the cell through the opening, resulting in death of the bacteria. By binding to the pellicle on the tooth surface, chlorhexidine inhibits plaque attachment. Chlorhexidine exhibits substantivity, with approximately 30% of the drug binding to oral tissues and the plaque on the teeth (Rölla, Löe, & Schiott, 1971) and showing antimicrobial activity for 8 to 12 hours afterward (Addy & Wright, 1978; Schiott et al., 1970).

In 2006 the FDA approved a nonalcoholic chlorhexidine oral rinse 0.12%. Alcohol is an inactive ingredient so the effectiveness is the same as chlorhexidine with alcohol. This product is ideal for patients susceptible to dry mouth, those who experience irritation of soft tissues (mucositis), and patients who are sensitive to alcohol.

Indications. Rinsing with chlorhexidine is indicated before, during, and after periodontal debridement to reduce plaque levels and gingival inflammation. Chlorhexidine rinses can improve wound healing and provide better plaque control after periodontal surgery when brushing and flossing is not feasible (Sanz, Newman, Anderson, & Motaska, 1987). A clinical study showed that even intermittent rinsing with chlorhexidine may provide a preventive benefit in reducing levels of bacteria but only in subjects without alveolar bone loss (Persson et al., 2007). In the office, before using dental devices that produce an aerosol, such as power-assisted instruments or air polishing, it has been shown that a preoperative rinse with chlorhexidine markedly reduces contamination of the dental office (Warrall, Knibbs, & Glenwright, 1987). Rinsing with chlorhexidine has been shown to decrease the severity of mucositis in patients receiving chemotherapy. Because peri-implantitis is similar to gingivitis, rinsing with chlorhexidine may be effective in implant plaque control (Kozlovsky et al., 2006).

Usage. It is recommended to rinse twice a day for 30 seconds. The positive charge of chlorhexidine causes it to bind to the negatively charged molecules in toothpastes such as fluorides and sodium lauryl sulfate (a detergent) and thus inactivates them. Therefore, it is best to rinse either 30 minutes before or after toothbrushing or rinse very well with water after toothbrushing. Because of this inactivation by anionic compounds, chlorhexidine is not available in toothpaste form. Chlorhexidine can be used as an irrigant, but it is usually diluted with water to reduce the incidence of staining. A recent clinical study compared the effectiveness of scaling and root planing alone or in combination

Did You Know?

Chlorhexidine 0.12% is used as an oral rinse, but chlorhexidine surgical 4.0% is used as a surgical scrub.

Rapid Dental Hint

Remind patients using chlorhexidine to brush well to help prevent calculus buildup.

with chlorhexidine in 29 patients with chronic periodontitis (Faveri et al., 2006). Results showed that scaling and root planing in combination with chlorhexidine was more effective in reducing plaque than scaling and root planing alone.

Adverse Effects. Chlorhexidine is a relatively safe drug because it is poorly absorbed from the oral membranes and systemic circulation if swallowed. The most common adverse effect is a yellow, brownish extrinsic staining of the teeth, tongue, and restorations (McCoy et al., 2008). Staining is more frequent with chlorhexidine than with other agents because of its affinity for oral surfaces. The staining may be associated with food dyes found within certain foods and beverages. This staining is not permanent and can be removed mechanically during professional prophylaxis. If the patient is compliant with oral home care, the staining is more likely on proximal tooth surfaces than facial or lingual surfaces. Other adverse effects include a temporarily impaired taste perception and increased supragingival calculus formation.

PHENOLIC COMPOUNDS Listerine® (McNeil, Titusville, NJ) is a combination of phenolic compounds or essential oils, including thymol, eucalyptol, menthol, and methyl salicylate, in an alcohol vehicle. The mechanism of action is cell wall disruption, resulting in leakage of intracellular components and lysis of the cell (Stoeken, Paraskevas, & van der Weijden, 2007). The original-formula Listerine contains 26.9% alcohol, whereas Cool Mint and Fresh Burst Listerine contain 21.6% alcohol. The newest product, Natural Citrus, also contains 21.6% alcohol.

Because of low substantivity, effectiveness is strongly related to the duration of tooth contact. Clinical studies have shown it to significantly reduce plaque development in patients with minimal plaque levels (Gordon, Lamster, & Sieger, 1985). A 6-month study comparing Listerine with a control product found that Listerine reduced plaque and gingivitis from 20% to 34%. The subjects had preexisting plaque and gingivitis, and no prophylaxis was performed at the beginning of the study (Lamster, Alfano, Seiger, & Gordon, 1983). In-office preprocedure rinsing with Listerine

---

Did You Know?

Listerine was invented in the 19th century as a powerful surgical antiseptic. It was later sold, in a distilled form, as a floor cleaner and a cure for gonorrhea. But it wasn't until the 1920s that it was advertised for chronic halitosis.

Did You Know?

Hippocrates also offered advice for bad breath. He suggested a mouthwash containing oil of anise seed, myrrh, and white wine.

---

reduced the level of bacteria in the aerosol generated during ultrasonic scaling (Fine et al., 1992).

Recommendations are to rinse for 30 seconds with 2/3 oz once in the morning and once at night. Possible adverse effects include a burning sensation and bitter taste.

QUATERNARY AMMONIUM COMPOUNDS Quaternary ammonium compounds are positively charged (cationic) compounds similar to chlorhexidine, except that after rinsing they readily bind to oral surfaces and are released more rapidly or lose their activity on binding to the surface. Substantivity is only approximately 3 hours (Roberts & Addy, 1981). An increase in bacterial cell wall permeability leads to cell lysis and decreased attachment of bacteria to tooth surfaces. Cetylpyridinium chloride is the active ingredient in Scope® Original (Procter & Gamble, Cincinnati, OH), Cepacol® (J. B. Williams, Glen Rock, NJ), and Viadent™ Advanced Care (Colgate Oral Pharmaceuticals, New York, NY). The alcohol concentration is 14% for Cepacol, 18.9% for Scope Original, and 5.5% for Viadent™ Advanced Care.

Clinical data on plaque reduction and gingivitis control have been relatively inconclusive because of the variability in results between studies. Following an initial professional prophylaxis and suspension of all oral hygiene, chlorhexidine was found to be superior to cetylpyridinium in the reduction of plaque (Renton-Harper, Addy, Moran, Doherty, & Newcombe, 1996). Cetylpyridinium chloride may have some antiplaque action but less effect on gingivitis when used as an adjunct to conventional oral home care. Lack of substantivity limits clinical efficacy. As with chlorhexidine, to obtain the maximum effect, the patient should rinse very well or wait 30 minutes after brushing with a dentifrice before using the rinse. Adverse effects are similar to those of chlorhexidine, including some staining, calculus formation, and mucosal ulceration.

A clinical study reported that in combination with toothbrushing, a mouth rinse containing 0.1% cetylpyridinium chloride or 0.06% chlorhexidine may be more effective than flossing in reducing interproximal plaque (Zimmer et al., 2006).

Rapid Dental Hint

Remember, not every patient needs to use a mouth rinse. Follow your treatment plan.

OXYGENATING AGENTS Oxygenating agents such as peroxides and perborates have been used in mouth rinse formulations primarily for acute necrotizing ulcerative gingivitis and pericoronitis. Because hydrogen peroxide liberates gaseous oxygen, it provides a cleansing action and gentle effervescence for oral wounds. Its antimicrobial effect is directed at anaerobic microorganisms that cannot live in the presence of oxygen, and it has a physical effect on plaque through the bubbling of oxygen as it is released from the peroxide (Marshall, Cancro, & Fischman, 1995). The Food and Drug Administration has approved its use as a temporary debriding agent in the oral cavity. However, antiplaque/antigingivitis claims are not well supported.

The safety of hydrogen peroxide has been disputed. Long-term use of 3% hydrogen peroxide has resulted in gingival irritation (Marshall et al., 1995; Rees & Orth, 1986) and delayed tissue healing, and it may serve as a cocarcinogen in animals (Weitzman, Weitberg, Stossel, Schwartz, & Shklar, 1986). A cocarcinogen is a compound that when administered with a low dose of a known carcinogen results in increased incidence of tumors. On the other hand, other studies found that adverse effects from exposure to 3% or less hydrogen peroxide were rare. It was concluded that exposure to less than 3% hydrogen peroxide was safe (Marshall et al., 1995). Long-term studies do not demonstrate any additional benefit over regular home care, however. Because many patients use hydrogen peroxide on a regular basis, the dental hygienist should question patients about their oral home-care practices.

POVIDONE-IODINE Povidone-iodine is antibacterial and antiseptic. Its primary use is in the prevention and treatment of surface infections. Often povidone-iodine is combined with hydrogen peroxide as a subgingival irrigant for the reduction of gram-negative microorganisms. Most studies confirm that iodine may be a beneficial adjunctive treatment for the prevention and control of gingivitis when used with optimal oral hygiene self-care procedures (Clark, Magnusson, Walker, & Marks, 1989). Iodine can stain teeth, clothing, skin, and restorations, however.

FLUORIDES Fluorides have been used in dentistry primarily for dental caries prevention by reducing demineralization and enhancing remineralization. Fluoride rinses have not been proven clinically to prevent root caries (Paine, Slots, & Rich, 1998). Its role as an antiplaque/antigingivitis agent is less well documented and shows controversial results.

Stannous fluoride (SnF_2) has been documented to exhibit antimicrobial properties in the control of gingival inflammation and bacterial repopulation. The tin molecule supposedly prevents bacterial adhesion to the tooth surface. Another indication for stannous fluoride is for dentinal hypersensitivity. Stannous fluoride is available as a dentifrice, a gel, and a concentrated oral rinse that is diluted with water. For home rinsing, available products include Gel-Kam® (available over the counter; Colgate Oral Pharmaceuticals, New York, NY) and Stanimax (0.63% SnF_2). Extrinsic tooth staining occurs with extended use. Sodium fluoride is indicated for caries prevention and has not been documented to have any antiplaque/antigingivitis action.

PREBRUSHING RINSES A prebrushing rinse (Plax®, Pfizer, New York, NY) that contains surfactants such as sodium lauryl sulfate (which functions as a detergent to help loosen and remove plaque), sodium benzoate (a preservative), and tetrasodium pyrophosphate (an anticalculus agent) is intended to be used before brushing. Studies have shown limited beneficial effects of this agent over rinsing with water alone (Grossman, 1988).

ALCOHOL-FREE MOUTH RINSES Most mouth rinses contain alcohol as a vehicle to carry other ingredients and as a flavor enhancer. The form of alcohol in the rinse is either ethanol (ethyl alcohol) or a specially denatured (SD) alcohol that is made synthetically. Alcohol can cause drying of the oral mucosal tissues, especially when the agent is used for extended periods of time. These rinses are primarily used as cosmetic rinses rather than therapeutic rinses. Indications for a nonalcoholic mouth rinse include pregnant women, former alcoholics, patients who are taking medications that would additionally dry the mouth, patients taking metronidazole (an antibiotic), and patients who prefer to avoid alcohol. Box 23–1 lists some nonalcoholic antimicrobial mouth rinses.

Oral Irrigation

Oral irrigation emerged in the early 1960s as an adjunct to brushing and flossing. It was believed that using a pulsating irrigation device did not remove supragingival plaque but research contradicts this assumption. As early as 1971, significant reductions in plaque and calculus formation were reported (Hoover & Robinson, 1971). Today numerous studies demonstrate the reduction of supragingival plaque in gingivitis patients (Sharma, Lyle, Qaqish, & Schuller, 2012; Goyal, Lyle, Qaqish, & Schuller, 2012), periodontal maintenance patients (Cutler et al., 2000), individuals in fixed orthodontics (Sharma, Lyle, Qaqish, Galustians, & Schuller, 2008), and people living with diabetes (Al-Mubarak et al., 2002). The research on daily home irrigation is extensive with over 50 clinical studies conducted at universities or independent research facilities. The research shows a significant reduction in gingival bleeding, gingival inflammation, pocket probing depth, supragingival and subgingival biofilm, and key pro-inflammatory mediators that are instrumental in bone resorption (Barnes et al., 2005; Cutler et al., 2000; Flemmig et al., 1990; Flemmig et al., 1995; Goyal et al., 2012; Jolkovsky et al., 1990; Newman et al., 1994; Rosema et al., 2011; Sharma et al., 2008; Sharma et al., 2012).

According to the American Academy of Periodontology (2005), daily oral irrigation plays an important role in the treatment of gingivitis and maintenance of periodontal patients. However, there is not much data to support that a single episode of irrigation delivered in the dental office will positively affect the benefits of scaling and root planing. There is a unique and separate body of research for professionally applied in-office irrigation and daily home irrigation, and the topics will be addressed separately in the following sections.

Daily Oral Irrigation

Irrigation was introduced as an adjunct to brushing and flossing to help clean areas that are not accessible by these traditional methods. Today, dental hygienists recommend oral irrigation based on clinical evidence, personal experience, and patient need, behavior, and/or preference. This includes patients with orthodontic appliances, implants, crowns, bridges, veneers, gingivitis, mild to moderate periodontitis, diabetes, nonflossers, and even those with good oral hygiene.

HYDROKINETIC ACTIVITY Oral irrigation devices, also known as dental water jet or water flosser, generally are power driven by either a main outlet or battery and create a pulsating stream of water or medicament (irrigant). The pulsations create two zones of hydrokinetic activity. The impact zone is the area where the irrigant comes in contact with the tooth surface, and the flushing zone is the deflection of the irrigant subgingivally and interdentally (Cobb, Rodgers, Killoy, 1988; Figure 23–1 ■). A pulsating stream of water provides better flushing than a continuous stream because it incorporates a compression and decompression phase, which allows debris and bacteria to be displaced from the pocket more efficiently. Products are available that are nonpulsating and non-power-driven, but to date, there is no evidence that they are clinically effective.

Researchers have measured the subgingival access of the irrigant delivered via a pulsating device. Eakle and colleagues (1986) found that a classic jet tip delivered an irrigant, on average, 50% into the depth of pockets. The deeper

Box 23–1: Selective Alcohol-Free Antimicrobial Mouth Rinses

- Rembrandt®
- Oral B® Antibacterial Rinse
- ProHealth Rinse
- Listermint®
- BreathRX®
- Biotene®

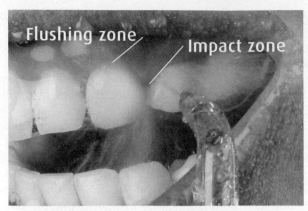

FIGURE 23-1 Impact and flushing zones caused by a pulsating oral irrigation device. (Courtesy of Water Pik, Inc., Fort Collins, CO.)

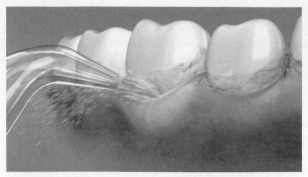

FIGURE 23-3 Classic jet tip used along the gingival margin. (Courtesy of Water Pik, Inc., Fort Collins, CO.)

the pocket the better the access with 60% of pockets over 7 mm showing delivery to 75% of the depth of the pocket. In addition, use of a classic jet tip with a Waterpik® device placed on medium pressure was found to have a positive effect on subgingival microorganisms at probing depths of up to 6 mm (Chaves et al., 1994; Cobb et al., 1988; Drisko et al., 1987). Some home irrigation devices have accessory delivery tips designed for targeted direct subgingival delivery. A Waterpik® Water Flosser using a Pik Pocket™ tip (Figure 23–2 ■) delivers an irrigant to approximately 90% of the depth of pockets ranging from 0 to 6 mm (Braun & Ciancio, 1992). The Pik Pocket® tip is designed for controlled, targeted low-pressure delivery of a medicament or water. Waterpik® irrigators come in many models and sizes with multiple tip choices (Figure 23–3 ■).

DELIVERY OF ANTIMICROBIAL AGENTS Home irrigation has been proven to reach farther into the pocket than rinsing (Braun & Ciancio, 1992; Eakle et al., 1986; Flotra, Gjermo, Rölla, & Waerhaug, 1972; Mashimo, Umemoto, Slots, Genco, & Ellison, 1980). The use of an antimicrobial agent as the irrigant has reduced clinical parameters in some studies over water irrigation. Flemmig and colleagues (1990)

demonstrated an enhanced effect on reducing gingivitis when a 0.06% solution of chlorhexidine was used as the irrigant compared with 0.12% chlorhexidine rinsing and water irrigation. Chaves et al. (1994) found that irrigating with water or 0.04% chlorhexidine showed similar reductions for bleeding, but chlorhexidine irrigant was better for reducing gingivitis scores compared to water. Both the water irrigation and chlorhexidine irrigation groups significantly reduced subgingival counts of *Prevotella intermedia* compared to 0.12% chlorhexidine rinsing. Conversely, the addition of Listerine® (Johnson & Johnson, Morris Plains, NJ) as an irrigant was as effective as placebo in reducing gingivitis and improving gingival health (Ciancio, Mather, Zambon, & Reynolds, 1989). This may be due to using only 8 ounces of Listerine® in the reservoir. However, the addition of Listerine® resulted in greater reductions in plaque and gingival bleeding and a moderate decrease in total bacteria counts, although it was not statistically significant. Subsequently, Fine and colleagues (1994) reported irrigation with Listerine® antiseptic was more effective than control in reducing plaque, bleeding on probing, redness, and putative periodontopathogens. A study that compared water irrigation with salicylic acid (aspirin) irrigation on periodontal maintenance patients found no difference between the groups but the irrigation was beneficial (Flemmig et al., 1995). Clinicians need to determine on a case-by-case basis if adding an agent to the reservoir will produce superior clinical benefits over the efficacy of using water.

INTERDENTAL EFFICACY Interdental cleaning is an important part of an oral hygiene regimen, but it has been reported that patients find flossing difficult, don't like to do it, and may demonstrate inadequate technique (Kleber & Putt, 1990; Lang, Ronis, & Farghaly, 1995;

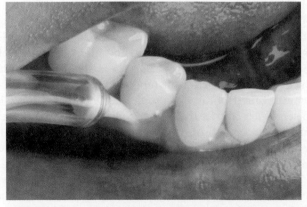

FIGURE 23-2 Pik Pocket™ tip placement below the gingival margin. (Courtesy of Water Pik, Inc., Fort Collins, CO.)

Did You Know?

The first oral irrigator was the invention of a dentist and his patient, who was an engineer, in Fort Collins, Colorado, and is the product that has been studied the most and still available today.

Tedesco, Keffer, & Fleck-Kandath, 1991). A systematic review showed there is no current evidence that adding flossing to brushing is beneficial, leading the authors to conclude that routine instruction of dental floss is not supported by research, and dental hygienists should decide on an individual basis if high-quality flossing is a goal achievable by the patient (Berchier, Slot, Haps, & Van der Weijden, 2008).

One oral irrigator (Waterpik® Ultra Water Flosser) was compared to flossing in several studies. Barnes et al. (2005) found that when paired with either a manual or power toothbrush, the irrigation group was significantly better than the brushing and flossing group in reducing gingival inflammation and bleeding. Sharma et al. (2008) evaluated the use of an oral irrigator with an orthodontic tip to brushing and flossing in a cohort of 11- to 17-year-olds with fixed orthodontic appliances. The reduction of plaque was three times better in the oral irrigation group, and the reduction of bleeding was 26% better than brushing and flossing. Other studies show a significant reduction in bleeding compared to flossing in 2 weeks, which improved at 4 weeks (Rosema et al., 2011) and was 70% more effective in reducing gingival inflammation than a powered interdental device that delivers air under pressure (Air Floss, Philips Oral Healthcare, Bethel, WA; Sharma et al., 2012).

DEVICES Waterpik® Ultra Water Flosser (Water Pik, Inc., Fort Collins, CO; Figure 23–4 ∎) is one such home irrigation device (Table 23–1 ∎). Water or a medicament is delivered to the gingival margin with a classic jet tip placed at a 90° angle to the long axis of the tooth. The jet tip is positioned at the distal of the last tooth in the arch almost touching the tooth. The tip follows the gingival margin to the next proximal area and held in place briefly. The procedure

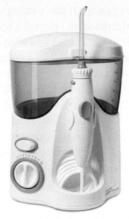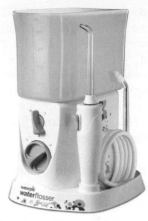

FIGURE 23–4 Waterpik® Ultra Water Flosser has 10 pressure settings and multiple tip designs. (Courtesy of Water Pik, Inc., Fort Collins, CO.)

is usually performed over a bathroom sink beginning with a low-pressure setting. Pressure may be increased as needed or according to patient comfort and gingival health. Following a pattern ensures that all areas of the facial, lingual, maxilla, and mandible are cleaned. Instructions may vary based on tip design.

Rapid Dental Hint

Tell the patient oral irrigation is easy to use and will take approximately 1 minute to irrigate their entire mouth and can be used instead of dental floss.

Table 23–1 Home Oral Irrigators

Product	Description
Waterpik® Water Flosser, Water Pik, Inc., Fort Collins, CO	Several models including countertop, cordless, traveler, kids, and combination water flosser and sonic toothbrush. Five tip designs are available; • Classic jet tip for general cleaning • Orthodontic tip • Plaque Seeker tip for crowns, bridges, implants and other dental work • Pik Pocket™ tip for targeted cleaning • Toothbrush tip
Viajet™ (Oratec Corporation, Herndon, VA)	Two standard tips for supragingival irrigation and two sulcus tips for marginal application are available. For office use: A cannula (stainless steel tube) adapter for subgingival application is also available.
Oral-B ProfessionalCare OxyJet Center, (Procter & Gamble, Cinncinati, OH)	This device is only available with the powered brush (sold as one unit). Plastic tips are available for supragingival use only, and the tips cannot be removed.

BENEFITS FOR SPECIAL NEEDS Other research has evaluated the benefits of oral irrigation on patients with special needs or situations. A study with diabetic patients (Al-Mubarak et al., 2002) found that the addition of twice daily irrigation with a specialized tip for subgingival delivery was more effective than routine oral hygiene in reducing bleeding, gingivitis, and serum levels of pro-inflammatory mediators (e.g., interleukin-1β and prostaglandin E$_2$). Implant patients can benefit from using an oral irrigator in multiple ways, such as access to areas that are inaccessible to traditional methods due to shape of restorations or bars for denture attachment. One study compared rinsing with 0.12% chlorhexidine to irrigating with 0.06% chlorhexidine with a subgingival delivery tip on implants (Felo, Shibly, Ciancio, Lauciello, & Ho, 1997; Figure 23–5 ■). The irrigation group was more effective in reducing plaque and gingivitis scores than the rinsing group. In addition, it was safe to use, and there was significantly less stain with the irrigator. Adult and adolescent orthodontic patients have been evaluated with results favoring the irrigation group for reducing gingival bleeding, gingivitis, and plaque scores using either a classic tip or a specialized orthodontic tip (Burch, Lanese, & Ngan, 1994; Sharma et al., 2008; Figure 23–6 ■). Patients with good oral hygiene have even shown improvements when adding an oral irrigator to their regimen (Chaves et al., 1994).

In-Office Irrigation

Efficacy. An alternate route of topical drug delivery is through patient or professionally applied oral irrigation. An antimicrobial agent also can be applied professionally in-office. This can be accomplished by using an air- or power-driven ultrasonic unit (piezoelectric) scaler or handheld syringe. Caution must be taken when using a handheld syringe because the delivery pressure cannot be controlled and may exceed a safe pressure for delivery into a periodontal pocket. Control is also compromised because of the inability to fulcrum and may affect the delivery to the apical aspect of the pocket. Penetration of an irrigant with an ultrasonic unit may be limited due to little lateral dispersion of agents and inaccessibility of the tip to certain areas (Nosel, Scheidt, O'Neal, & Van Dyke, 1991).

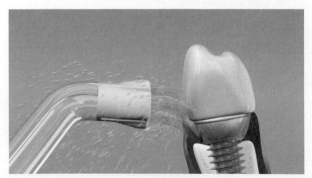

FIGURE 23–5 Plaque Seeker® tip has three tufts of bristles designed to clean around implants, crowns, bridges, and other dental work. (Courtesy of Water Pik, Inc., Fort Collins, CO.)

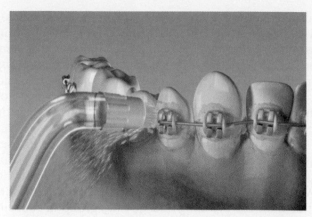

FIGURE 23–6 Orthodontic tip irrigates the gingival tissue and cleans around brackets and arch wires. (Courtesy of Water Pik, Inc., Fort Collins, CO.)

At present, a single episode of in-office irrigation has been shown only to have limited or no beneficial effects by itself, but it may be of some advantage if patients perform subgingival irrigation at home between continuing-care appointments (Jolkovsky et al., 1990). Repeated irrigations over a period of time or longer exposure to an antibiotic has shown efficacy in some patients (Christersson, Norderyd, & Puchalsky, 1993; Clark et al., 1989). The use of 2% chlorhexidine alone over a 15-week period was nearly as effective in reducing clinical parameters as periodontal debridement alone (Southard, Drisko, Killoy, Cobb, & Tira, 1989).

Studies on home oral irrigation repeatedly show statistically significant reductions in gingivitis, bleeding on probing, probing depth, and **periodontal pathogens** in gingivitis and periodontal maintenance patients with the use of oral irrigation over normal oral hygiene (Barnes et al., 2005; Flemmig et al., 1990; Goyal et al., 2012; Newman et al., 1994; Rosema et al., 2011). Subgingival calculus should be removed to prevent interference with penetration of the agent into the pocket (Pitcher, Newman, & Strahan, 1980).

Using an oral irrigation device is effective as part of an oral care routine that includes either a manual or power toothbrush (Barnes et al., 2005; Goyal et al., 2012; Rosema et al., 2011). Care must be taken when evaluating the research because not all products have been studied in clinical trials or have the same combination of pulsations and pressure. Therefore, established efficacy with one product may not be true for another. It is always advisable to check the manufacturer's website for information or copies of the clinical trials that support product claims.

Indications

Research shows that many patients may benefit from daily oral irrigation, even those with relatively good oral hygiene (Al-Mubarak et al., 2002; Chaves et al., 1994; Felo et al., 1997; Sharma et al., 2008). Oral irrigation is an ideal choice when supragingival mechanical aids (e.g., toothbrushes, floss, and interproximal brushes and devices) are not sufficient to keep the bacterial load below the threshold of disease. It is also ideal for delivering antimicrobial agents deeper into pockets and especially for those who will not floss (American Academy of Periodontology, 2005). Patients with physical challenges, orthodontic appliances, or prosthodontic replacements such as implants and crowns or those who need an adjunctive method to reduce repopulation of bacteria between periodontal maintenance appointments are also ideal candidates for home oral irrigation. Oral irrigation has the ability to reach areas that are inaccessible by other self-care aids. Subgingival irrigation may be better than rinsing in the maintenance of gingival health around dental implants (Felo et al., 1997).

Patients with plaque-induced gingivitis can benefit most from oral irrigation because the disease is in its early stage. Patients with slight and moderate chronic periodontitis also may benefit from oral irrigation. However, patients with severe chronic periodontitis and refractory periodontitis require more aggressive treatment and referral to a periodontist.

Considerations

Controlled powered-driven home irrigation devices are safe for patients to use on a daily basis. Thorough patient evaluation is always necessary prior to recommending any device or aid to a patient. It is important to match the correct

> ## Rapid Dental Hint
>
> It is important to instruct patients on the proper use of an irrigator. Many patients do not read instructions.

product with the patient's specific needs. Also, take the time to instruct patients on the proper use of their device. Oral irrigation should not be used when a periodontal abscess is present. Once the problem has been resolved, it then may be appropriate to recommend irrigation therapy.

IRRIGATION AND TOOTHBRUSHING It is well established that daily irrigation improves oral health in most patients. It is not designed as a mono-therapy and should be paired with either a manual or power toothbrush. An oral irrigator paired with a sonic toothbrush is significantly more effective than brushing with a sonic toothbrush alone. Goyal et al. (2012) found that an oral irrigator and sonic toothbrush were 70% more effective in reducing gingival bleeding, 48% better at reducing gingival inflammation, and 52% better at reducing plaque scores compared to sonic brushing alone.

Dental Hygiene Application

Antiseptics deserve continued evaluation, and their importance should not be underestimated. Currently, the most valuable application of antiplaque/antigingivitis agents is as an adjunct to conventional mechanical debridement and oral home care for short- to medium-term usage.

An important factor in the efficacy of any antiplaque/antigingivitis agent is an adequate contact time with the target site. Accordingly, the well-proven success of chlorhexidine is related to its substantivity more than to any unique action on the microbiota (bacteria). It is the function of the dental hygienist to advise patients on the role of oral rinses and dentifrices in the hygienic phase of treatment. The hygienist should use his or her knowledge of clinical studies to decide on the appropriate product for each patient.

Key Points

- Oral rinses and irrigation are types of topical delivery systems.
- Home oral irrigation can be used for interdental and subgingival cleaning, especially in patients who cannot or will not floss.

- Oral rinses are only effective supragingivally and do not have any effect on subgingival plaque.
- Home oral irrigation may be useful between maintenance appointments to reduce bacterial reinfection (repopulation).

Self-Quiz

1. Which one of the following substances can cause extrinsic tooth staining?
   a. Cetylpyridinium
   b. Alcohol
   c. Phenols
   d. Chlorhexidine

2. From the list provided, select the indications for the use of mouth rinses in periodontics
   a. Limited manual dexterity
   b. Gingivitis
   c. Periodontitis before periodontal debridement
   d. Peri-implantitis

3. Which one of the following antimicrobial agents possesses high substantivity to the oral soft tissues?
   a. Cetylpyridinium
   b. Alcohol
   c. Chlorhexidine
   d. Erythromycin
   e. Tetracycline

4. Which of the following dosing is correct for chlorhexidine rinse?
   a. Rinse only in the morning before brushing for 1 minute.
   b. Gargle in the night before bedtime for 1 minute.
   c. Gargle in the morning for 30 seconds.
   d. Rinse twice a day for 30 seconds.

5. Which one of the following antimicrobial mouth rinses contains the highest concentration of alcohol?
   a. Listerine
   b. PerioGard
   c. Scope
   d. Viadent Advanced Care

Case Study

A 55 year old male has many restorations and a 3 unit bridge with #30 as a pontic. The patient is not on any medications that cause xerostomia and has functional ability to brush and floss. The patient however does not routinely floss and brushes only once a day. There is localized papillary gingivitis in the molar of all quadrants. There are 4 mm pockets on #3 mesial and distal and # 15 mesial. The dental hygienist wishes to consider additional modalities to remove the biofilm from the interproximal and subgingival areas.

1. The use of a daily home irrigator with water would have what effect?
   a. disrupts biofilm under pontic
   b. dries gingival tissue
   c. replaces tooth brushing
   d. dislodges all subgingival biofilm

Answer: A. The daily home irrigators have been shown effective to remove interdental plaque. The water has no effect on the tissue. It is an adjunct to brushing and may replace flossing. Depending upon the patient's ability and depth of pocket it may or may not remove all subgingival biofilm.

2. If an antimicrobial mouthwash was to be recommended which one(s) meet this criteria?
   a. Chlorhexidine
   b. Listerine
   c. Scope
   d. all of the above

Answer: D. Although all products contain active ingredients to be antimicrobial not all will be as effective to one another. The dental hygienist is advised to monitor the gingival and the tissue response.

3. If an antimicrobial is added to a home irrigation device what could be the expected result?
   a. twice as effective as water alone
   b. some studies have shown effectiveness
   c. the dental hygienist should confirm evidence
   d. use of any product at half strength is advised

Answer: C. Although some studies have shown effectiveness, the dental hygienist should use evidence-based literature to make a final decision.

References

Addy, M., and R. Wright. 1978. Comparison of the in vivo and in vitro antibacterial properties of povidone-iodine and chlorhexidine gluconate mouth rinses. *J. Clin. Periodontol.* 5:198–205.

Al-Mubarak, S., Ciancio, S., Aljada, A., et al. 2002. Comparative evaluation of adjunctive oral irrigation in diabetics. *J. Clin. Periodontol.* 29:295–300.

American Academy of Periodontology. 2005. The role of supra- and subgingival irrigation in the treatment of periodontal diseases. *J. Periodontol.* 76:2015–2027.

Barnes, C. M., C. M. Russell., R. A. Reinhardt, et al. 2005. Comparison of irrigation to floss as an adjunct to tooth brushing: Effect on bleeding, gingivitis, and supragingival plaque. *J. Clin. Dent.* 16:71–77.

Barnett, M. L. 2006. The rationale for the daily use of an antimicrobial mouthrinse. *JADA* 137(11 supplement):16S–21S.

Berchier, C. E., D. E. Slot, S. Haps, and G. A. Van der Weijden. 2008. The efficacy of dental floss in addition to a toothbrush on plaque and parameters of gingival inflammation: A systematic review. *Int. J. Dent. Hygiene* 6:265–279.

Braun, R., and S. Ciancio. 1992. Subgingival delivery by an oral irrigation device. *J. Periodontol.* 63:469–472.

Burch, J. G., R. Lanese, and P. Ngan. 1994. A two-month study of the effects of oral irrigation and automatic toothbrush use in an adult orthodontic population with fixed appliances. *Am. J. Orthod. Dentofacial Orthop.* 106:121–126.

Chaves, E. S., K. S. Kornman, and M. A. Manwell, et al. 1994. Mechanism of irrigation effects on gingivitis. *J. Periodontol.* 65(11):1016–1021.

Cheng, H. R. W., W. K. Leung, and Corbet E. F. 2008. Non-surgical periodontal therapy with adjunctive chlorhexidine use in adults with Down syndrome: A prospective case series. *J. Periodontol.* 79(2):379–385.

Christersson, L. A., O. M. Norderyd, and C. S. Puchalsky, 1993. Topical application of tetracycline HCl in human periodontitis. *J. Clin. Periodontol.* 20:80–95.

Ciancio, S. G., M. L. Mather, J. J. Zambon, and H. S. Reynolds. 1989. Effect of a chemotherapeutic agent delivered by an oral irrigation device on plaque, gingivitis, and subgingival microflora. *J. Periodontol.* 60:310–315.

Clark, W. B., I. Magnusson, C. B. Walker, and R. G. Marks. 1989. Efficacy of Perimed antibacterial system on established gingivitis I. Clinical results. *J. Clin. Periodontol.* 16:630–635.

Cobb, C. M., R. L. Rodgers, and W. J. Killoy. 1988. Ultrastructural examination of human periodontal pockets following the use of an oral irrigation device in vivo. *J. Periodontol.* 59:155–163.

Cutler, C. W., T. W. Stanford, C. Abraham, et al. 2000. Clinical benefits of oral irrigation for periodontitis are related to reduction of pro-inflammatory cytokine levels and plaque. *J. Clin. Periodontol.* 27:134–143.

Drisko, C. L., C. L. White, W. J. Killoy, et al. 1987. Comparison of dark-field microscopy and a flagella stain for monitoring the effect of a Water Pik on bacterial motility. *J. Periodontol.* 58:381–386.

Eakle, W. S., C. Ford, and R. L. Boyd. 1986. Depth of penetration in periodontal pockets with oral irrigation. *J. Clin. Periodontol.* 13:39–44.

Faveri, M., L. C. Gursky, M. Feres, J. A. Shibli, S. L. Salvador, and L. C. de Figueiredo. 2006. Scaling and randomized, placebo-controlled clinical trial. *J. Clin. Periodontol.* 33:819–828.

Felo, A., O. Shibly, S. G. Ciancio, F. R. Lauciello, and A. Ho. 1997. Effects of subgingival chlorhexidine irrigation on peri-implant maintenance. *Am. J. Dent.* 10:107–110.

Fine, D. H., C. Mendieta, M. L. Barnett, D. Furgang, R. Meyers, et al. 1992. Efficacy of preprocedural rinsing with an antiseptic in reducing viable bacteria in dental aerosols. *J. Periodontol.* 63:821–824.

Fine, J. B., D. S. Harper, J. M. Gordon, C. A. Hovliaras, and C. H. Charles. 1994. Short-term microbiological and clinical effects of subgingival irrigation with an antimicrobial mouthrinse. *J. Periodontol.* 65:30–36.

Flemmig, T. F., B. Epp, Z. Funkenhauser, et al. 1995. Adjunctive supragingival irrigation with acetylsalicylic acid in periodontal supportive therapy. *J. Clin. Periodontol.* 22:427–433.

Flemmig, T. F., M. G. Newman, F. M. Doherty, E. Grossman, A. H. Mechkel, and M. B. Bakdash. 1990. Supragingival irrigation with 0.06% chlorhexidine in naturally occurring gingivitis: I. Six-month clinical observations. *J. Periodontol.* 61:112–117.

Flotra, L., P. Gjermo, G. Rölla, and J. Waerhaug. 1972. A 4-month study on the effect of chlorhexidine mouth rinses on 50 soldiers. *Can. J. Dent. Res.* 80:10–16.

Gordon, J. M., I. B. Lamster, and M. C. Sieger. 1985. Efficacy of Listerine antiseptic in inhibiting the development of plaque and gingivitis. *J. Clin. Periodontol.* 12:697–704.

Goyal, C. R., D. M. Lyle, J. G. Qaqish, and R. Schuller. 2012. The addition of a water flosser to power tooth brushing: Effect on bleeding, gingivitis, and plaque. *J. Clin. Dent.* 23:57–63.

Grossman, E. 1988. Effectiveness of a prebrushing mouthrinse under single-trial and home-use conditions. *Clin. Prev. Dent.* 10:3–9.

Hoover, D. R., and H. B. G. Robinson. 1971. The comparative effectiveness of a pulsating oral irrigator as an adjunct in maintaining oral health. *J. Periodontol.* 42:37–39.

Jolkovsky, D. L., M. Y. Waki, M. G. Newman, et al. 1990. Clinical and microbiological effects of subgingival and gingival marginal irrigation with chlorhexidine gluconate. *J. Periodontol.* 61:663–669.

Klebler, C. J., and M. S. Putt. 1990. Formation of flossing habit using a floss-holding device. *J. Dent. Hyg.* 64:140–143.

Kozlovsky, A., Z. Artzi, O. Moses, et al. 2006. Interaction of chlorhexidine with smooth and rough types of titanium surfaces. *J. Periodontol.* 77(7):1194–1200.

Lamster, I. B., M. C. Alfano, M. C. Seiger, and J. M. Gordon. 1983. The effect of Listerine antiseptic on existing plaque and gingivitis. *J. Clin. Prev. Dent.* 5:12–16.

Lang, W. P., D. L. Ronis, and M. M. Farghaly. 1995. Preventive behaviors as correlates of periodontal health status. *J. Public Health Dent.* 55:10–17.

Löe, H., and C. R. Schiott. 1970. The effect of mouthrinses and topical application of chlorhexidine on the development of dental plaque and gingivitis in man. *J. Periodont. Res.* 5:79–83.

Marshall, M. V., L. P. O. Cancro, and S. F. Fischman. 1995. Hydrogen peroxide: A review of its use in dentistry. *J. Periodontol.* 66:786–796.

Mashimo, P. A., T. Umemoto, J. Slots, R. J. Genco, and S. A. Ellison. 1980. Pathogenicity testing of Macaca arctoides subgingival plaque following chlorhexidine treatment. *J. Periodontol.* 51:190–199.

McCoy, L. C., C. J. Wehler, S. E. Rich, et al. 2008. Adverse events associated with chlorhexidine use. *JADA* 1239:178–183.

Newman, M., M. Cattabriga, D. Etienne, T. Flemmig, M. Sanz, et al. 1994. Effectiveness of adjunctive irrigation in early periodontitis: Multicenter evaluation. *J. Periodontol.* 65:224–229.

Nosel, G., M. Scheidt, R. O'Neal, and T. Van Dyke. 1991. The penetration of lavage solution into the periodontal pocket during ultrasonic instrumentation. *J. Periodontol.* 62:554–557.

Paine, M., J. Slots, and S. Rich. 1998. Fluoride use in periodontal therapy: A review of the literature. *J. Am. Dent. Assoc.* 129:69–77.

Persson, G. R., J. Yeates, R. E. Persson, et al. 2007. The impact of a low-frequency chlorhexidine rinsing schedule on the subgingival microbiota (the TEETH clinical trial). *J. Periodontol.* 78(9):1751–1758.

Pitcher, G. R., H. N. Newman, and J. D. Strahan. 1980. Access to subgingival plaque by disclosing agents using mouth rinsing and direct irrigation. *J. Clin. Periodontol.* 7:300–308.

Poggi, P., R. Rodriguez y Baena, S. Rizzo, and M. T. Rota. 2003. Mouth rinses with alcohol: Cytotoxic effects on human gingival fibroblasts in vitro. *J. Periodontol.* 74:623–629.

Rees, T. D., and C. E. Orth. 1986. Oral ulcerations with use of hydrogen peroxide. *J. Periodontol.* 57:689–692.

Renton-Harper, P., M. Addy, J. Moran, R. M. Doherty, and R. G. Newcombe. 1996. A comparison of chlorhexidine, cetylpyridinium chloride, triclosan, and C3LG mouth rinse products for plaque inhibition. *J. Periodontol.* 67:486–489.

Roberts, W. R., and M. Addy. 1981. Comparison of in vitro and in vivo antibacterial properties of antiseptic mouth rinses containing chlorhexidine, alexidine, CPC and hexetidine: Relevance to mode of action. *J. Clin. Periodontol.* 8:295–310.

Rölla, G., H. Löe, and R. C. Schiott. 1971. Retention of chlorhexidine in the human oral cavity. *Arch. Oral Biol.* 16:1109–1116.

Rosema, N. A. M., N. L. Hennequin-Hoenderdos, C. E. Berchier, et al. 2011. The effect of different interdental cleaning devices on gingival bleeding. *J. Int. Acad. Periodontol.* 13:2–10.

Sanz, M., M. G. Newman, L. Anderson, and W. Motaska. 1987. A comparison of the effect of a 0.12% chlorhexidine gluconate mouth rinse and placebo on postperiodontal surgical therapy. *J. Dent. Res.* 66:280 (Abstract).

Schiott, C. R., H. Löe, S. B. Jensen, M. Kilian, R. M. Davies, and L. Glavid. 1970. The effect of chlorhexidine mouth rinses on the human oral flora. *J. Periodont. Res.* 5:84–89.

Sharma, N. C., D. M. Lyle, J. G. Qaqish, J. Galustians, and R. Schuller. 2008. Effect of a dental water jet with orthodontic tip on plaque and bleeding in adolescent patients with fixed orthodontic appliances. *Am. J. Ortho. Dentofacial Orthop.* 133:565–571.

Sharma, N. C., D. M. Lyle, J. G. Qaqish, and R. Schuller. 2012. Comparison of two power interdental cleaning devices on the reduction of gingivitis. *J. Clin. Dent.* 23:22–26.

Silverman, S., and R. Wilder. 2006. Antimicrobial mouthrinse as part of a comprehensive oral care regimen. *JADA* 137(11 supplement):22S–26S.

Southard, S. R., C. L. Drisko, W. J. Killoy, C. M. Cobb, and D. E. Tira. 1989. The effect of 2 percent chlorhexidine digluconate irrigation on clinical parameters and the level of *Bacteroides gingivalis* in periodontal pockets. *J. Periodontol.* 60:302–309.

Spolarich, A. E., and J. R. Gurenlian. 2013. Dispel the myths. *Dimensions of Dental Hygiene*, 11(4):20–22, 24.

Stabholz, A., J. Kettering, R. Aprecio, G. Zimmerman, P. J. Baker, and U. M. E. Wikesjo. 1993. Antimicrobial properties of human dentin impregnated with tetracycline HCl or chlorhexidine: An in vitro study. *J. Clin. Periodontol.* 20:557–562.

Stoeken, J. E., S. Paraskevas, and G. A. van der Weijden. 2007. The long-term effect of a mouthrinse containing essential oils on dental plaque and gingivitis: A systematic review. *J. Periodontol.* 78(7):1218–1228.

Tedesco, L. A., M. A. Keffer, and C. Fleck-Kandath. 1991. Self-efficacy, reasoned action, and oral health behavior reports: a social cognitive approach to compliance. *J. Behav. Med.* 14:341–355.

Warrall, S. F., P. J. Knibbs, and H. D. Glenwright. 1987. Methods of reducing contamination of the atmosphere from use of an air polisher. *Br. Dent. J.* 163:118–119.

Weitzman, S. A., A. B. Weitberg, T. P. Stossel, J. Schwartz, and G. Shklar. 1986. Effects of hydrogen peroxide on oral carcinogenesis in hamsters. *J. Periodontol.* 57:685–688.

Zimmer, S., C. Kolbe, G. Kaiser, T. Drage, M. Ommerborn, and C. Barthel. 2006. Clinical efficacy of flossing versus use of antimicrobial rinses. *J. Periodontol.* 77(8):1380–1385.

Visit www.pearsonhighered.com/healthprofessionsresources to access the student resources that accompany this book. Simply select Dental Hygiene from the choice of disciplines. Find this book and you will find the complimentary study tools created for this specific title.

Systemic and Local Drug Delivery Systems: Systemic Antibiotics, Local Drug Devices, and Enzyme Suppression Therapy

Mea A. Weinberg

OUTLINE

EDUCATIONAL OBJECTIVES

Upon completion of this chapter, the reader should be able to:

- Discuss the rationale for the use of antimicrobials in the treatment of the inflammatory periodontal diseases.
- List and discuss the various types of drug delivery systems.
- Describe the different types of controlled-release devices.
- Discuss enzyme suppression therapy.

GOAL: To provide an understanding of current concepts about the adjunctive use of chemical agents in the prevention and treatment of the inflammatory periodontal diseases.

KEY WORDS

adjunctive *335*

antibiotic resistance *334*

chemotherapeutic agents *334*

controlled-release delivery
    devices *335*

periodontal pathogens *334*

substantivity *338*

systemic drug delivery *335*

Introduction

The foundation for the treatment of periodontal diseases is mechanical debridement. However, in some patients the adjunctive use of antibiotics, antimicrobial agents, or an enzyme suppression drug (e.g., doxycycline 20 mg) is justified. The newest approach in the treatment of inflammatory periodontal diseases is enzyme suppression therapy. Instead of targeting bacteria, enzyme suppression therapy targets the enzyme collagenase, which causes destruction of collagen.

The purpose of chemotherapy is to aid the host defenses (body) in controlling and eliminating bacteria that have overwhelmed the host. These chemotherapeutic agents can be administered to the patient via oral rinses, irrigation, systemically in a pill or capsule, in a controlled-release device placed subgingivally in a pocket, or in dentifrices (e.g., triclosan). The use of chemotherapeutic agents and enzyme suppression therapy is based on the type of periodontal disease the patient has and the nature of the offending bacteria.

Selected Drug Information Resources

It is important for the dental hygienist to be aware of the generic names and trade names of drugs. The generic name is the official name of the drug as determined by the United States Adopted Names Council. The trade name of a drug is the registered property of a specific manufacturer and is protected for 17 years so that the manufacturer has the exclusive rights for that specific drug.

Numerous drug references on the Internet, on personal digital assistants (PDAs), and in books are available. Selected resources include the following:

- *The Physicians' Desk Reference* (PDR® Medical Economics Company, Inc., Montvale, NJ). This is published once a year and is essentially a conglomerate of the patient package inserts that the manufacturers supply for each drug.
- *Delmar's Dental Drug Reference* (Delmar Thompson™ Learning, Albany, NY).
- *Mosby's Dental Drug Reference* (Mosby-Year Book, Inc., St. Louis, MO).
- *Drug Information Handbook for Dentistry* (Lexi-Comp, Inc., Hudson, OH).
- *ADA Guide to Dental Therapeutics* (ADA, Chicago).

Rationale for Use of Antibiotics

Although periodontal debridement and periodontal surgery are currently the foundation for controlling inflammatory periodontal diseases, several factors can substantiate

---

Did You Know?

Cochrane Reviews (www.cochrane.org/cochrane-reviews) compares a variety of antimicrobials for efficacy.

---

the adjunctive use of chemical or **chemotherapeutic agents** (e.g., antiseptic mouth rinses and antibiotics; American Academy of Periodontology, 2004; Beikler, Prior, Ehmke, & Flemmig, 2004; Haffajee, Socransky, & Gunsolley, 2003; Kaner et al., 2007; Seymour, 2008). An antiseptic is a substance that prevents or inhibits the growth of microorganisms or kills microbes on contact. An antibiotic is a substance that is synthesized by microorganisms that prevents or inhibits the growth of bacteria by either stopping multiplication or killing the bacteria.

Instrumentation often leaves behind significant numbers of periodontal pathogens. Repopulation of these pathogens can occur within 60 days of periodontal debridement (Sbordone, Ramaglia, Gulletta, & Iacono, 1990). In addition, certain **periodontal pathogens**, such as *Aggregatibacter actinomycetemcomitans* and *Porphyromonas gingivalis*, invade the junctional epithelium and connective tissue and elude removal by periodontal debridement (de Graaf, van Winkelhoff, & Goené, 1989; Renvert, Wikström, Dablén, Slots, & Egelberg, 1990). Other periodontal pathogens, such as *Tannerella forsythensis*, *Prevotella intermedia*, and *Peptostreptococcus micros*, live in nonperiodontal sites such as the tongue, tonsils, saliva, and buccal mucosa (Asikainen, Alaluusua, & Saxén, 1991). These sites are a source for reinfection and must be considered in the overall treatment process. Other factors influencing the use of chemical plaque-control agents include the manual dexterity of the patient.

A number of chemical agents have been studied clinically and shown to be successful in the further suppression of dental plaque in certain types of periodontal diseases when used in conjunction with periodontal debridement and surgery. The role of antimicrobial agents as part of the periodontal treatment plan in certain patients has gained significant importance in recent years since the acknowledgment that periodontal diseases are infectious diseases with specific bacteria as the cause (Loesche, 1976). Based on the specific plaque hypothesis, treatment is geared toward the elimination or reduction of specific bacteria (e.g., *A. actinomycetemcomitans, P. gingivalis, P. intermedia*, and spirochetes). Thus, antimicrobial agents can be instituted as a supplement, not a replacement, during nonsurgical and surgical therapy. Because there are also beneficial bacteria living in the mouth, it is not desirable nor a goal to eliminate all intraoral bacteria. Unfortunately, systemic antibiotics used indiscriminately can result in **antibiotic resistance**, in which an antibiotic is ineffective against certain bacteria. This is becoming a worldwide problem.

Delivery Systems

Currently, two systems are available for the delivery of chemotherapeutic agents: local and systemic systems. Topical and controlled (sustained)-release (American Academy Periodontology, 2000) drug devices are types of local delivery systems. Each delivery system has advantages and limitations (Table 24–1).

Topical application delivers the agent or drug to an exposed surface such as the teeth and gingiva. The most common route for the supragingival topical delivery of antimicrobial agents is by a mouth rinse, a dentifrice, or an oral irrigator. Subgingival topical delivery of antimicrobial agents is by oral irrigation or the use of controlled-release devices.

Controlled-release delivery devices are placed directly into the periodontal pocket and are designed to release a drug slowly over 24 hours for prolonged drug action. Antimicrobials are delivered into the periodontal pocket by fibers, gels, chips, powder, ointments, acrylic strips, or collagen films.

Systemic drug delivery involves taking a tablet or a capsule orally with subsequent distribution of the agent through the circulation to the subgingival pocket area.

Choice of the delivery system is based on the target site. For instance, if gingivitis were being treated, oral rinses or irrigation would be chosen for supragingival plaque control. If, on the other hand, a certain type of periodontitis is being treated, the target site is the base of the periodontal pocket. Because oral rinses do not reach subgingivally, the delivery system of choice would be either oral irrigation or systemic or controlled-release delivery.

Dental Plaque as a Biofilm

As mentioned earlier, dental plaque exists as a biofilm. A plaque or oral biofilm is defined as matrix-enclosed bacterial populations adherent to each other and/or to surfaces or interfaces (Costerton et al., 1994). Plaque biofilms are of varying thicknesses, and to penetrate the biofilm, antibiotic concentrations must be several times greater than that needed to kill bacteria in a test tube (laboratory conditions; Kleinfelder, Müller, & Lange, 1999). Subgingival biofilms cannot be removed by toothbrushing, flossing, or the use of antimicrobial agents. It is necessary to physically remove the biofilm by instrumentation, and then the antimicrobial agent can be administered. For this reason, administration of antimicrobial agents should never be the sole treatment and always should be an adjunct to periodontal debridement and/or periodontal surgery. The biofilm structure also may account for the rapid rebound or repopulation of the pathogenic bacteria, which occurs frequently after the use of antimicrobial agents (Page, Offenbacher, Schroeder, Seymour, & Kornman, 1997).

Drug Actions

When considering the use of chemotherapeutic agents, the dental hygienist should be aware of the pharmacokinetics and pharmacodynamics of each drug. Pharmacokinetics involves knowledge of the drug's absorption, distribution, metabolism, and excretion. Pharmacodynamics relates to the drug's mechanism of action. In addition, any adverse effects (Seymour & Rudralingham, 2008), drug–drug interactions, and drug–food interactions should be noted, and the patient should be informed.

Systemic Drug Delivery

Indications

Systemic drug delivery through oral administration has several advantages and disadvantages (see Table 24–1 ■; Seymour & Hogg, 2008; Walker & Karpinia, 2002). Antibiotics generally are unnecessary and inappropriate for reducing plaque levels and treating gingivitis, with the exception of necrotizing periodontal diseases.

Systemic antibiotics are useful as adjuncts in periodontal treatment for patients with aggressive periodontitis, all types of refractory periodontitis, and immunodeficiency diseases. Patients with refractory periodontal diseases usually harbor persistent subgingival pathogens that are likely to be resistant to conventional treatment. In localized aggressive periodontitis patients, *A. actinomycetemcomitans* invades the gingival connective tissue and thus evades removal by mechanical instrumentation. Antibiotics will benefit patients with a periodontal abscess when there are systemic signs such as fever or lymphadenopathy. A recent study reported that there may be no benefit in using antibiotics for the sole purpose of preventing postsurgical infections (Powell, Mealey, Deas, McDonnell, & Moritz, 2005). Bacterial invasion (spirochetes) of periodontal tissues seen in nectrotizing gingivitis (NUG) also evades mechanical removal with instruments.

SELECTION **Adjunctive** systemic antibiotics may be used during initial and/or surgical therapy. In patients with refractory or recurrent periodontitis it may be advantageous to perform microbiologic testing to determine the presence of specific bacteria. Reevaluation with microbiologic testing 1 to 3 months after antimicrobial therapy may be done to verify elimination or suppression of the pathogens. However, the expense of this procedure may preclude its generalized use. Long-term use (1 to 2 months or longer) of systemic antibiotics is considered to be without foundation.

Proper selection and dosing of the appropriate antibiotic are necessary to avoid untoward reactions and antibiotic resistance. Many categories of antibiotics are available, and several are indicated in periodontal infections (Box 24–1). The dental hygienist must be familiar with both the generic and brand or trade names of each drug.

Good oral hygiene is still mandatory and will foster a positive clinical response when patients are prescribed systemic antibiotics. As mentioned earlier, periodontal debridement must be performed before the administration of any antimicrobial agent. This will remove the biofilm that protects subgingival microorganisms, except in cases where the bacteria have invaded the soft tissue. Systemic antibiotics are given in certain situations and should be used as a supplement or adjunct to conventional periodontal debridement and oral hygiene self-care. Antibiotics should never be given as the only treatment regimen. Antibiotics are classified as being either bacteriostatic, which means they suppress the multiplication

Table 24–1 Main Features of Drug Delivery Systems

Delivery System	Target Site	Adequate Concentration at Target Site	Stays at Target Site Long Enough	Reaches the GCF	Advantages
Systemic: tablets, capsules	Periodontal pocket; epithelium and connective tissue; nonperiodontal sites (e.g., saliva, tongue, buccal mucosa, tonsils)	Fair concentrations reached due to some dilution by the time it reaches pocket area; frequent dosing is necessary to maintain therapeutic levels	No	Yes	Reaches all intraoral sites where bacterial reservoirs are found
Topical: oral rinses	Supragingival	Adequate concentrations, but therapeutic level dramatically declines by being washed out by saliva	No	No	No systemic adverse effects; no antibiotic resistance develops
Topical: dentifrices	Supragingival	Adequate concentrations, but therapeutic level dramatically declines by being washed out by saliva	No	No	No systemic adverse effects; high patient compliance
Topical: subgingival irrigation	Periodontal pocket	Adequate concentrations, but therapeutic level dramatically declines by being washed out by GCF	No	No	No systemic adverse effects
Controlled-release: powder, gel, chip	Periodontal Pocket	Adequate concentrations; therapeutic levels are relatively constant for several days	Yes	Yes	Maintains therapeutic levels in the GCF for several days; no systemic adverse effects; concentrates in pocket without dilution through entire body; possible development of bacterial resistance to the antibiotic (more studies needed)

of the bacteria, or bactericidal, which means they kill the bacteria.

Adverse Drug Events

Heightened public interest in adverse drug events has motivated the government to require pharmaceutical companies to provide adverse drug reaction (ADR) information (Smith, 1999). The requirement is to provide information on the percentage of adverse drug reactions caused by antibiotics in both hospital and nonhospital settings.

ADRs can range from mild reactions that disappear when the antibiotic is discontinued to severe reactions that are life threatening, are disabling, or result in hospitalization (Smith, 1999). Table 24–2 ■ lists common adverse effects associated with antimicrobial agents.

Box 24–1: Classification of Systemic Antibiotics Used in Periodontics

Tetracyclines

- Tetracycline HCl
- Doxycycline hyclate
- Minocycline HCl

Penicillins (Beta-lactams)

- Penicillin VK
- Amoxicillin trihydrate
- Amoxicillin
- + clavulanic acid

Nitroimadazoles

- Metronidazole

Azalides (derivative of erythromycin)

- Azithromycin dihydrate

Lincomycins

- Clindamycin HCl

Fluoroquinolones

- Ciprofloxacin HCl

Systemic Antibiotics

TETRACYCLINES Tetracyclines as a group are bacteriostatic, inhibiting bacterial growth and multiplication by inhibiting protein synthesis. Two semisynthetic analogues of tetracycline, doxycycline hyclate and minocycline HCl, are broad-spectrum antibiotics, affecting both gram-positive and gram-negative microorganisms. Doxycycline and minocycline have been used in the treatment of *Aggregatibacter actinomycetemcomitans* infections in localized aggressive periodontitis and refractory periodontitis. Mandell, Tripodi, Savitt, Goodson, and Socransky (1986) reported that although surgery and treatment with tetracycline were superior in localized aggressive periodontitis patients, it appeared that there was a possibility of reinfection with or incomplete elimination of *A. actinomycetemcomitans*.

Anticollagenase Feature. Tetracyclines have both antibacterial and nonantibacterial properties. Besides affecting bacterial growth, they also affect the host response by inhibiting the production and secretion of collagenase by cells in the body such as polymorphonuclear leukocytes (PMNs; Golub, Ramamurthy, McNamara, Greenwald, & Rifkin, 1984). Collagenase is an enzyme responsible for the destruction of collagen, which makes up the connective tissue of the periodontium. Tetracyclines also were found to inhibit bone resorption by affecting osteoclast function (Rifkin, Vernillo, & Golub, 1993). This anticollagenase property does not depend on the drug's antibacterial actions.

Table 24–2 Classification of Adverse Effects of Systemic Antimicrobial Agents

Adverse Effect	Features
Hypersensitivity reactions	Involves allergic reactions to the antibiotic (e.g., rashes).
Gastrointestinal disturbances	Very common; includes nausea, vomiting, and diarrhea. Pseudomembranous colitis is the most severe gastrointestinal complication that requires immediate discontinuation of the antibiotic. Although initially believed to be a complication associated primarily with clindamycin, most oral and injectable antibiotics may produce this side effect.
Hepatotoxicity	Liver disease can occur with commonly administered antibiotics such as erythromycin, amoxicillin-clavulanic acid, and quinolones.
Photosensitivity reactions	Occurs with fluoroquinolones and tetracyclines (less with minocycline). Seen as an exaggerated sunburn. Patients should not be exposed to sun when taking these antibiotics.
Fungal infection	Fungal infections can occur especially with use of broad-spectrum antibiotics, which destroy bacteria, allowing fungi (*Candida albicans*) to overgrow, which may produce gastrointestinal irritation, stomatitis, and vaginal infection. Acidophilus (available in a soft gel tablet) or yogurt taken in conjunction with the antibiotic (except tetracycline) will replace some of the bacteria, thereby possibly preventing a fungal infection.

Did You Know?

Doxycycline is unique because it is the only antibiotic that also has nonantibiotic properties when prescribed at sub-antimicrobial doses.

Rapid Dental Hint

Doxycycline should be taken with plenty of water in an upright or sitting position. Patients should not lie down for a few hours after taking it.

Concentration in Gingival Crevicular Fluid. Another property of tetracyclines is their ability to concentrate in the gingival crevicular fluid (GCF) at two to four times blood levels following multiple doses (Gordon, Walker, Murphy, Goodson, & Socransky, 1981). Doxycycline (Pascale et al., 1986) and minocycline also concentrate in higher levels in the GCF than in serum. Tetracyclines exhibit higher **substantivity** than other antibiotics (Baker, Evans, Coburn, & Genco, 1983; Stabholz et al., 1993), which allows binding to root surfaces with a slow release into the GCF. The binding of tetracyclines to calcium ions in the GCF enhances their substantivity. These properties allow the drug to maintain high therapeutic levels in the GCF. It is advantageous for a drug to concentrate in high levels in the GCF because the GCF bathes the subgingival pocket area where the periodontal pathogens live.

Adverse Effects, Drug–Drug Interactions, and Drug–Food Interactions. Common adverse effects of tetracyclines include esophageal ulcers (Segelnick & Weinberg, 2008), nausea, vomiting, and diarrhea. Gastrointestinal (stomach) upset is much less with the semisynthetic drugs because they are more highly absorbed from the gastrointestinal tract. Instructions to the patient on how to take tetraycyclines is important to avoid these adverse effects. Taking doxycycline (or any tetracycline) with plenty of water and in an upright position will help avoid the development of esophageal ulcers (Segelnick & Weinberg, 2008). Tetracyclines stain newly formed teeth during enamel deposition and should not be used during the last half of pregnancy or in children up to 8 years of age. A complex is formed with calcium orthophosphate that produces a yellow-gray fluorescent discoloration. Photosensitivity is another adverse effect, resulting in exaggerated sunburn when patients are exposed to the sun.

Tetracyclines, except doxycycline and minocycline, should not be taken concomitantly with dairy products because tetracycline binds to calcium, inhibiting its absorption. Tetracycline should be taken on an empty stomach (1 hour before or 2 hours after meals) because food delays its absorption. Doxycycline and minocycline can be taken without regard to meals. Absorption of all tetracyclines into the bloodstream is delayed with antacids. Tetracyclines, as well as other antibiotics, interfere with the metabolism of oral contraceptives. Estrogens, a component in oral contraceptives, must be metabolized (broken down) to its active form in the stomach by bacteria. Most antibiotics kill or stop the growth of these bacteria, inhibiting estrogen breakdown. Patients must use other forms of birth control if they are taking antibiotics concomitantly. Tetracyclines or any other bacteriostatic drug should not be given together with bactericidal antibiotics such as penicillin, metronidazole, or ciprofloxacin that would interfere with the bactericidal action of that drug. For a bactericidal drug to work, the bacteria need to be multiplying.

PENICILLINS (BETA-LACTAMS) Penicillins as a group are bactericidal, and their mechanism of action is to inhibit bacterial cell wall synthesis. Penicillin VK has limited activity against gram-negative periodontal pathogens. It is indicated primarily in certain acute periodontal infections such as abscesses. Amoxicillin, a broad-spectrum penicillin, is used frequently in periodontics. Some bacteria produce enzymes called beta-lactamases that inactivate the penicillin molecule. To overcome this vulnerability, a beta-lactamase inhibitor such as clavulanic acid is combined with amoxicillin (Augmentin).

Adverse Effects, Drug–Drug Interactions, and Drug–Food Interactions. Approximately 5% to 10% of individuals are allergic to penicillin. It is best to take this antibiotic with food to decrease gastrointestinal upset. Severe gastrointestinal upset (e.g., nausea, vomiting, and diarrhea) occurs as a result of the acid component. Food does not interfere with absorption of amoxicillin into the bloodstream. Penicillins should not be taken together with bacteriostatic antibiotics because for a bactericidal antibiotic to work, the bacteria need to be multiplying, and this would be inhibited if a bacteriostatic antibiotic were administered concomitantly with penicillin.

CEPHALOSPORINS Cephalosporins are not considered to be the drug of choice for most types of dental infections, including periodontal diseases. These antibiotics do not provide an advantage over amoxicillin or penicillin.

Nitroimadazoles

Mechanism of Action and Indications. Metronidazole is specifically effective against obligate or strict anaerobic (live in a pure nonoxygen environment) microorganisms. Metronidazole penetrates well into the GCF, but not as high as the tetracyclines. Metronidazole is bactericidal, and its mechanism of action is to inhibit bacterial DNA synthesis.

Metronidazole is indicated in the treatment of NUG. Metronidazole is also indicated when barrier membranes are used during guided tissue regeneration surgery. *P. gingivalis*, a strict anaerobe, is the primary bacteria that colonize on porous membrane material. It has been reported in both professional journals and in the lay press that periodontal debridement in conjunction with metronidazole may reduce the need for periodontal surgery (Loesche, Giordano, Soehren, & Kaciroti, 1996), but this remains controversial. Metronidazole in combination with amoxicillin or Augmentin may be effective against refactory and aggressive forms of periodontitis associated with *Aggregatibacter actinomycetemcomitans* and *P. gingivalis* infection. However, a recent study of 21 patients with moderate, untreated periodontal diseases evaluated the benefits of amoxicillin and amoxicillin plus clavulanic acid after initial therapy. Patients received periodontal debridement twice during the study. After the second debridement, patients were assigned randomly to either the group that received the drug combination or the placebo group. Results indicated no added benefit when amoxicillin and Augmentin were taken after initial therapy (Winkel et al., 1999).

Adverse Effects and Drug–Drug Interactions. Antibiotic resistance to metronidazole is rare, but there are numerous adverse effects. Gastrointestinal upset is seen frequently, especially nausea. A metallic taste in the mouth has been reported, as well as darkened urine. Consumption of alcohol beverages, including use of alcohol-containing mouth rinses, while taking metronidazole results in a disulfiram-like reaction. Disulfiram is a drug given to wean alcoholics off alcohol by acting to deter further ingestion of alcohol. It works by inhibition of the enzyme aldehyde dehydrogenase, causing a buildup of acetaldehyde, a toxic by-product of ethanol metabolism (Garey & Rodvold, 1999). Within 5 to 10 minutes after metronidazole is taken with alcohol, serious non-life-threatening adverse effects occur, including headache, flushing, nausea, vomiting, and cramps. The reaction usually lasts for up to 1 hour; however, it may continue for a few days after discontinuation of the medication (Walker, 1996). Alcohol should not be consumed during metronidazole therapy and for at least 3 days after discontinuing the drug. Metronidazole is contraindicated in patients taking anticoagulants (e.g., warfarin), lithium (a drug used for manic depression), and cimetadine (an antiulcer drug).

MACROLIDES Erythromycin, a macrolide antibiotic, is not used in the treatment of periodontal diseases because it is primarily effective against gram-positive microorganisms and does not penetrate gram-negative bacterial cells. Erythromycin also does not penetrate the GCF to effective levels. Erythromycins are bacteriostatic and inhibit bacterial protein synthesis. Adverse effects include severe gastrointestinal disturbances, including nausea, vomiting, and diarrhea.

Second-Generation Drugs: Azalides. The newer second-generation erythromycins, referred to as azilides, have a broader spectrum of action with fewer adverse effects. Azithromycin dihydrate shows promising results in periodontics. Azithromycin has several unique features. It concentrates in phagocytes such as PMNs and macrophages, which contribute to its distribution into inflamed

periodontal tissues (gingival connective tissue) in greater amounts than in plasma (Dastoor et al., 2007; Malizia, Tejada, Ghelardi, Senesi, & Gabriele, 1997). In addition, a postantibiotic effect is seen, whereby high antibiotic levels remain after the drug is discontinued (Malizia et al., 1997).

Adverse Effects, Drug–Drug Interactions, and Drug–Food Interactions. All erythromycins, except for azithromycin, should not be taken with cholesterol-lowering "statin" drugs (such as lovastatin and simvastatin) because erythromycin and clarithromycin inhibit the metabolism of these drugs, resulting in high blood levels. Concurrent use of erythromycins and theophylline (an antiasthma drug) increases blood levels of theophylline. Capsules of azithromycin should be taken on an empty stomach, but tablets can be taken with food.

LINCOMYCINS Clindamycin HCl penetrates well into the GCF and is active against most periodontal pathogens, except *A. actinomycetemcomitans* and *Eikenella corrodens*, and is especially useful in treating refractory periodontitis. Clindamycin HCl inhibits bacterial protein synthesis and is bacteriostatic. Although the development of pseudomembranous colitis has been associated with the use of clindamycin, it can occur with any antibiotic. Suppression of normal intestinal bacteria allows the overgrowth of *Clostridium difficile*, which produces a toxin that causes severe watery diarrhea and fever. The antibiotic should be discontinued as soon as such signs appear. Clindamycin can be taken with food.

QUINOLONES Quinolones are bactericidal because they inhibit bacterial DNA replication. Quinolones (e.g, ciprofloxacin, levofloxacin) are not actually antibiotics, however, because they are totally synthetic. Antibiotics are chemical substances produced by bacteria; some antibiotics can be semisynthetic, which means that they are a mixture of natural and synthetic substances. Nevertheless, they are frequently referred to as broad-spectrum antimicrobials with good activity against facultative gram-negative anaerobes. Adverse effects include dizziness, convulsions, headache, hallucinations, and joint and cartilage damage.

Did You Know?

Any antibiotic can cause pseduomembranous colitis, not just clindamycin.

Did You Know?

Quinolones (e.g., Cipro, Levaquin) should not be taken by athletes because it can cause joint and cartilage damage.

Ciprofloxacin should not be given to children younger than 18 years of age because of its effect on cell growth. Ciprofloxacin should not be administered with theophylline or caffeine because it inhibits metabolism, resulting in increased blood levels. Dairy products and antacids delay absorption. Food does not slow absorption.

Antibiotic Resistance

Bacterial resistance to antibiotics raises serious questions for healthcare providers. The danger is that an antibiotic will not be effective if administered later for a truly life-threatening bacterial infection because the bacteria have become resistant to that antibiotic. Thus, antibiotic resistance can lead to an increase in the incidence of disease. Patients often stop their antibiotic treatment prematurely, believing that if they feel better, it is not necessary to take the full course. Patients also self-medicate with leftover antibiotics from a previous infection. Patients may request antibiotics or other medications because they believe they will be beneficial. Many practitioners comply with such patient requests without evaluating the situation clinically, and many practitioners simply overprescribe antibiotics.

Therefore, it is extremely important to use antibiotics and antimicrobials conservatively, only when indicated, and with the narrowest possible spectrum of activity. Prolonged or repetitive courses of antibiotic treatment should be avoided. Antibiotics are an adjunct to periodontal debridment.

Local Delivery: Controlled (Sustained)-Release Drug Delivery

The development of site-specific, controlled (sustained)-release delivery systems has provided a further option for antimicrobial therapy by allowing therapeutic levels of a drug to be maintained in the periodontal pocket for prolonged periods of time (Bonito, Lux, & Lohr, 2005). The decision to use local drug delivery during active treatment or maintenance is based on clinical findings, clinical response to therapy, desired clinical outcomes, and the patient's dental and medical history (Greenstein, 2006). If the drug is released from the device past 24 hours, it is called a controlled-release device; if the drug is released within 24 hours, it is called a sustained-release device. Many devices are available in the United States and Europe that incorporate an antimicrobial agent into a specific material (a polymer) that is placed into the periodontal pocket. The active ingredient is then released from the material, which subsequently exerts its antibacterial activity on subgingival bacteria over several days. Then the material is

absorbed (dissolves). Once the material is absorbed, healing between the tooth and the gingival can occur. The concentration of antimicrobials administered in a controlled (sustained)-release device does not enter the bloodstream and thus does not trigger adverse effects. Types of materials used to incorporate antimicrobial drugs include fibers, gels, chips, collagen film, and acrylic strips. Controlled (sustained)-release drug therapy is used as an adjunct to periodontal debridement and should not replace conventional mechanical therapy. It is necessary to disrupt subgingival biofilms to improve the drug's action on the bacteria. In fact, the American Academy of Periodontology reported in the 2003 Annals that it would be premature to conclude that insertion of sustained-release antimicrobial systems is as effective as scaling and root planing in all populations of patients (Hanes & Purvis, 2003). They are indicated for use in *localized* recurrent pockets of 5 mm or greater that continue to bleed on probing. *The indication for use of controlled-release drug devices is localized (< 30% of sites) chronic periodontitis.* Controlled-drug delivery is intended for localized sites because it would be impossible to use it on every tooth in the mouth. *The intended results with controlled-release drug devices are gains in clinical attachment level, reductions in probing depths, and reductions in bleeding on probing.*

The first controlled-release device approved in the United States in the early 1990s was Actisite, which was an ethylene vinyl acetate flexible fiber impregnated with 12.7 mg of tetracycline HCl. It was placed subgingivally into the periodontal pocket, where the tetracycline is released slowly over 7 to 10 days. It is no longer available.

Currently in the United States, PerioChip, Atridox, and Arestin are available commercially. Other controlled-release systems are available in Europe that have not been approved for use in the United States.

Absorbable Controlled (Sustained)-Release Devices

CHLORHEXIDINE GLUCONATE CHIP The PerioChip (Dexcel Pharma) is a gelatin maxtrix (bovine origin) containing 2.5 mg of chlorhexidine gluconate. This product received Food and Drug Administration (FDA) approval in June 1998. PerioChip is indicated for use as an adjunct to instrumentation in maintenance patients with pockets 5 mm or larger that bleed recurrently on probing (Jeffcoat et al., 1998; Paolantonio et al., 2008). A recent clinical study comparing the efficacy of periodontal debridement alone with that of periodontal debridement plus PerioChip revealed statistically significant reductions in probing depth and gains in clinical attachment in the periodontal debridement plus PerioChip group. However, the magnitude of these changes was small (0.3 mm), so the results are not clinically significant (Jeffcoat et al., 1998). In this study, mechanical debridement was limited to only 1 hour in patients with moderately advanced peridontitis (5 to 8 mm pockets), which does not seem realistic.

After periodontal debridement, the chip is placed into the periodontal pocket. In contact with subgingival fluids it becomes sticky and binds to the epithelium lining the pocket, so no periodontal dressing is indicated. Its antibacterial action occurs when chlorhexidine is released over 7 to 10 days, after which the chip resorbs and does not have to be removed. Up to eight chips can be inserted into pockets in one visit. Another round of treatment can be done at 3 months.

DOXYCYCLINE HYCLATE GEL Atridox is composed of 10% (42.5 mg) doxycycline hyclate in a gel formulation that is biodegradable and subsequently will resorb. The ingredients are available in two syringes (powder and liquid) that are mixed together and injected into the pocket around the entire tooth. The gel form allows for ease of flow, readily subgingival root morphology. When the gel comes in contact with gingival fluid in the pocket, it solidifies to a wax-like substance.

Atridox is indicated as an adjunct to scaling and root planing procedures in patients with chronic periodontitis (Novak et al., 2008). Local anesthesia is not required. Results of therapy are to promote attachment level gain, to reduce pocket depths, and to reduce bleeding on probing. Atridox may also be used in patients who refuse to have periodontal debridement or periodontal surgery and who are medically, physically, or emotionally compromised.

A randomized, controlled clinical study (Garrett, Johnson, & Stoller, 1998) comparing Atridox alone (all patients had a history of periodontal debridement at least 2 months before the study) and periodontal debridement alone reported that Atridox produced clinical results comparable with periodontal debridement alone. Both groups showed a statistically significant reduction in pocket depths (an average of 1.3 mm) and gains in attachment level (average of 0.8 mm).

Levels of doxycycline in the pocket (GCF) peaked at 2 hours after placement into the pocket, and effective drug levels were maintained at 28 days (Stoller, Johnson, Trapnell, Harrold, & Garrett, 1998). However, within a few days levels of doxycycline have peaked.

MINOCYCLINE HYDROCHOLORIDE MICROSPHERES The most recently FDA-approved sustained-release device is Arestin. Arestin microspheres (OraPharm) are a sustained-release product containing the antibiotic minocycline hydrochloride. Minocycline is a type of tetracycline but it is longer acting and has a broader spectrum of antibiotic activity. Each cartridge of Arestin contains 1 mg of minocycline

(Figure 24–1 ■). Arestin is indicated as an adjunct to scaling and root planing procedures for the reduction of pocket depth in patients with chronic localized periodontitis.

Results

Most studies have shown that scaling and root planing (in pockets ≥ 5 mm) followed by the application of controlled-release local delivery antimicrobial agents resulted in a reduction in pocket depths (0.25–0.5 mm) at 9 months compared to scaling and root planing alone (American Academy of Periodontology, 2006). However, even if the results were statistically significant, the additional improvement in probing depth was not clinically significant because there was a similar reduction achieved by scaling and root planing alone (American Academy of Periodontology, 2006).

Many periodontal pathogens, including *Porphyromonas gingivalis*, *Prevotella intermedia*, *Fusobacterium nucleatum*, *Eikenella corrodens*, and *Aggregatibacter actinomycetemcomitans*, are susceptible to minocycline.

Other Products

Some controlled-release products are available in other countries. Elyzol (Dumex, Copenhagen, Denmark) is a 25% metronidazole gel that is injected into the pocket. Periocline (Sunstar Corp., Osaka, Japan) and Dentomycin (Cyanamid International, Wayne, NJ) are 2% minocycline gels.

Precautions/Contraindications

Subgingival placement of devices containing antibiotics or antimicrobials is not recommended in an acutely abscessed periodontal pocket. Any antibiotic product should be used with caution in patients with a history of predisposition to oral candidasis because antibiotics suppress the growth of or kill bacteria, which allows for the growth of other microorganisms such as fungi.

The use of tetraycycline and its analogs, doxycycline and minocycline, should not be used during tooth development, which includes the last half of pregnancy, infancy, and childhood up to the age of 8 years.

Rapid Dental Hint

The patient does not need to be anesthetized when applying Atridox or Arestin.

Rapid Dental Hint

It is important to remove biofilms with debridement before antibiotics/antimicrobials are administered because biofilms act as a barrier to the penetration of the drug.

Did You Know?

These controlled-release medicaments are used for localized chronic periodontitis sites.

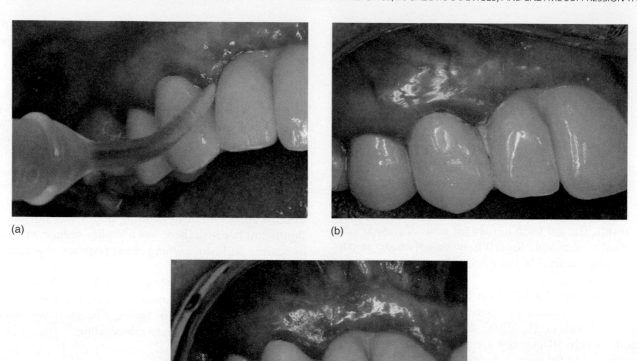

(a)

(b)

(c)

FIGURE 24–1 Arestin being administered into a pocket. Arestin is a powder containing minocycline.

Enzyme-Suppression Therapy

Although bacteria are the culprits in initiating inflammatory periodontal diseases, the inflammatory mediators, including cytokines and prostaglandins produced by the host (body) cells in response to the bacteria, are partly responsible for periodontal tissue breakdown. When produced in excess, inflammatory mediators induce destruction of healthy periodontal tissues. For example, prostaglandins facilitate bone resorption by stimulating the activity of osteoclasts.

Matrix Metalloproteinases

Host cells, including PMNs and fibroblasts, also respond to bacterial products by synthesizing and secreting matrix metalloproteinases (MMPs) in the host connective tissue. The MMPs are a family of enzymes that work together to break down connective tissue proteins, including collagen. MMPs that cause the breakdown of the periodontium include collagenase and gelatinase.

In healthy oral tissues, as part of the normal turnover of connective tissue, fibroblasts synthesize and secrete collagenase, which removes "old" collagen while new collagen is laid down. However, in the presence of disease (bacterial infection), PMNs produce collagenase in excessive amounts, which destroys periodontal tissues (collagen). Thus, the third approach to therapy is to inhibit the collagenase synthesized and released by PMNs. Antibiotics are aimed at reducing or eliminating the periodontal pathogens but do not target the enzyme-producing PMNs.

Subantimicrobial-Dose Doxycycline (SDD)

Golub and colleagues (1984) found that tetracyclines, especially doxycycline, have anticollagenase properties and inhibit collagenase activity. This group of investigators discovered that by using only 20-mg tablets of doxycycline, instead of the customary 50- or 100-mg tablets, collagenase would be inhibited. At these subantimicrobial doses, doxycycline only has anticollagenase activity and no antibacterial action. Doxycycline 20 mg is indicated as an adjunct to periodontal debridement to promote attachment level gain and to reduce pocket depths in patients with chronic periodontitis. A recent study reported that adjunctive subantimicrobial doxycycline in chronic periodontitis reduced gingival crevicular fluid (GCF) collagenase inducers levels and clinical periodontal parameters more than the placebo (Emingil, Atilla, Sorsa, & Tervahartiala, 2008). It is intended to improve the clinical outcome of periodontal debridement. This drug should be taken twice daily. Efficacy beyond 9 months of continuous dosing and safety beyond 12 months of continuous dosing have not been established.

Rapid Dental Hint

Because doxycycline 20 mg is still doxycycline, the same precautions and contraindications as with tetracyclines must be followed with doxycycline 20 mg.

A recent clinical study (Preshaw et al., 2008) reported that a modified-release subantimicrobial dose doxycycline (40 mg) that is taken once daily rather than twice with the 20-mg formulation resulted in significantly greater clinical benefits than scaling and root planing alone in periodontitis patients.

In a large-scale clinical study, patients received debridement and either doxycycline 20 mg or a placebo twice a day for 9 months. The results of the study showed that after 3 months of daily use, reductions in probing depth and improvements in attachment levels were statistically greater with SDD and debridement than with placebo and debridement (Ciancio & Ashley, 1998). Reductions in probing depth from baseline were up to 38% greater with SDD in tooth sites with mild to moderate periodontitis (probing depths of 4 to 6 mm) and severe periodontitis (probing depths of 7 mm or more). Improvements in attachment from baseline were up to 54% greater with the SDD than with placebo in severely diseased sites. Although treatment differences in the per-patient mean change in probing depth and clinical attachment level were statistically significant, these differences were relatively small. However, the frequency of probing depth reduction of 2 mm or more was greater in the doxycycline group than in the placebo group.

Antimicrobial Treatment of Inflammatory Conditions of Dental Implants

Peri-implantitis is a general term defined as an inflammatory process that affects the peri-implant bone around a dental implant. An ailing implant is also referred to as peri-implant mucositis, where only the gingiva around the implant is inflamed; there is no bone loss on the radiograph. A failing implant is referred to as peri-implantitis, where there is bone loss on the radiograph. A failed implant is an implant that is mobile, and the only treatment is removal. There is much controversy regarding the treatment of peri-implant mucositis and failing implants. In cases of peri-implant mucositis where there is only gingival inflammation around the implant, oral hygiene instructions, nonsurgical periodontal debridement, and if necessary an antimicrobial rinse such as chlorhexidine gluconate is recommended. Systemic antibiotics have no advantage in treating peri-implant mucositis (Hallström, Persson, Lindgren, Olofsson, & Renvert, 2012). The use of repeated local drug delivery such as minocycline microspheres has been documented to improve probing depths in patients with peri-implantitis (Renvert, Lessem, Dahlen, Renvert, & Lindahl, 2008). In addition, if the probing depths are greater than 5 mm and there is bone loss of less than 2 mm, then systemic antibiotics or local drug delivery is recommended. If bone loss is greater than 2 mm and there is bleeding on probing with probing depths greater than 5 mm, then regenerative periodontal surgery using some type of bone material with a membrane is encouraging (Froum, Froum, & Rosen, 2012).

Dental Hygiene Application

The multifaceted approach to treating periodontal diseases uses mechanical instrumentation, which reduces the bacterial load, and locally and systemically administered antibiotics and host-modulating pharmacotherapies as treatment adjuncts.

Treatment of patients with gingivitis or chronic periodontitis is related to reducing the number of bacteria to a level conducive to health (Loesche, 1976). This may involve periodontal debridement, periodontal surgery, and oral rinses and oral irrigation. Frequently, patients are overtreated using systemic antibiotics, which can lead to the development of bacteria that become resistant to antibiotics. Systemic antibiotics are contraindicated in patients with gingivitis or chronic periodontitis.

Antibiotic resistance of bacteria has enormous clinical and societal implications. In essence, when bacteria become resistant to an antibiotic, that antibiotic becomes ineffective. Although the prudent use of antibiotics will continue to be a valuable treatment option for certain forms of periodontal disease, the abuse and misuse of antibiotics must be addressed and monitored to prevent antibiotic resistance.

Systemic antibiotics are indicated in about 20% of patients with periodontitis (Loesche, 1976), where specific bacteria including *A. actinomycetemcomitans, P. gingivalis, P. intermedia*, and spirochetes (Loesche, 1976; Slots, 1986) have invaded the soft tissues. Treatment including systemic antibiotics is needed to eliminate the bacteria in the tissues because periodontal debridment is ineffective. Examples include patients with localized aggressive periodontitis, necrotizing periodontal diseases, and refractory forms of periodontal diseases. In addition, patients with a compromised immune system, such as AIDS patients, can benefit from the use of antimicrobial agents.

The controlled (sustained) drug devices may be useful in the adjunctive treatment of chronic periodontitis. The clinician's decision to use local antimicrobial agents remains the matter of individual clinical judgment. Even though scaling and root planing disrupts the subgingival biofilms that cause periodontitis, the placement of sustained-release antimicrobial devices subgingivally may help in slowing the rapid return of the biofilm and thus may slow the progression of disease.

As advances are made in the development of new antimicrobial and antibiotic agents, the oral healthcare team will continue to play an integral part in ensuring that these agents are used appropriately. No data are available to support the long-term effectiveness of the newly approved controlled-release devices. Although many studies on site-specific drug therapy and submicrobial-dose doxycycline report statistically significant reductions in probing depths and improvements in attachment levels, the clinical benefit may not be significant. Further clinical studies are needed to determine clinical significance.

Antimicrobial therapy is indicated for teeth as well as dental implants. Almost the same theory for the selection of the appropriate agent is used. For instance, periodontal therapy including oral hygiene instructions, mechanical periodontal debridement, and polishing are indicated for gingivitis as well as peri-implant mucositis when probing depths are less than 3 mm with bleeding on probing and the presence of plaque. When probing depths are 4–5 mm with bleeding on probing without bone loss, then the addition of an antimicrobial rinse and irrigation (referred to as antiseptic cleaning) may be warranted. When there is bone loss around the implant, then a systemic or locally delivered antibiotic may be necessary.

Key Points

- Systemic antibiotics are indicated in certain inflammatory periodontal diseases, such as localized or generalized aggressive periodontitis, and refractory forms of periodontal diseases.
- Systemic antibiotics are not indicated for chronic periodontitis.
- Controlled-release drug devices that slowly release antimicrobial agents are used in site-specific (recurrent) areas in chronic localized periodontitis.

- Enzyme-suppression therapy involves the inhibition of collagenase that is synthesized and released by neutrophils.
- Dental practitioners should contribute to limiting antibiotic use to prevent drug resistance.
- Treating peri-mucositis may require the use of an antimicrobial rinse and irrigation.
- Treating a failing implant with mild bone loss may require the use of systemic or locally delivered antibiotics.

Self-Quiz

1. From the following list, select the items associated with site-specific chemotherapy.
   a. Reduction in probing depth
   b. Gain in clinical attachment
   c. Reduction in bleeding
   d. Formation of alveolar bone
   e. Reattachment of the junctional epithelium
   f. Reformation of parallel inserting periodontal ligament fibers

2. Which one of the following procedures most effectively removes supra/subgingival dental biofilms?
   a. Oral irrigation
   b. Systemic antibiotics
   c. Periodontal debridement
   d. Controlled-release drugs

3. From the following list, select the items associated with treatment of peri-implant mucositis.
   a. oral hygiene instructions
   b. surgical periodontal debridement
   c. nonsurgical periodontal debridement
   d. polishing
   e. chlorhexidine rinse
   f. metronidazole
   g. Arestin
   h. Atridox

4. Which of the following agents is the active ingredient in Arestin?
   a. Tetracycline HCl
   b. Minocycline HCl
   c. Doxycycline hyclate
   d. Chlorhexidine gluconate

5. From the following list, select the items associated with high substantivity to the root surface and oral mucosal tissues.
   a. Cetylpyridinium
   b. Sanguinarine
   c. Tetracycline
   d. Erythromycin
   e. Chlorhexidine

6. All the following are ways a dental practitioner can contribute to limiting antibiotic resistance except one. Which one is the exception?
   a. Prescribe drugs at the first sign of purulent exudate.
   b. Avoid prolonged course of the medication.
   c. Instruct the patient on proper use.
   d. Prescribe an antibiotic with the narrowest possible spectrum of activity.

7. From the following list, select the items associated with tetracycline.
   a. Substantivity
   b. Antifungal
   c. Antibacterial
   d. Anticollagenase
   e. Antibiotic
   f. Doxycycline
   g. Cannot take with milk

8. Which one of the following indications is for site-specific drug delivery?
   a. Probing depths of less than 4 mm
   b. Pockets with suppuration and bleeding
   c. Nonresponding bleeding sites with probing depths of 5 mm or more
   d. Sites with bone loss, suppuration, bleeding, and probing depths of less than 5 mm

9. Which of the following is an adverse effect that may occur when taking antibiotics?
   a. Bacterial resistance
   b. Mucosa inflammation
   c. Bone degeneration
   d. Tissue mucositis

10. Which of the following drugs is used in chronic periodontitis to suppress the production and secretion of host cell collagenase?
    a. Minocycline
    b. Doxycycline
    c. Tetracycline
    d. Metronidazole
    e. Penicillin V

Case Study

A 45-year-old male has chronic periodontitis with some horizontal bone loss between #3 and 4, 14 and 15 and vertical bone loss on distal #30. The pocketing on these teeth is 4–5 mm. Tooth #18 is a single implant. The tissue around the implant is edematous and bleeds occasionally. There is no bone loss in the implant area. The dental hygienist is considering other adjunctive therapy to assist in the maintenance for this patient.

1. Which delivery system would be appropriate for the chronic periodontitis?
   a. systemic antibiotic
   b. oral rinse
   c. controlled-release
   d. topical

Answer: C. Systemic antibiotics are contra-indicated for gingivitis or chronic periodontics. Oral rinse will not reach subgingival areas. Topical delivery will not reach subgingival areas. The controlled-release is placed in the pocket and may help slow the return of the biofilm.

2. What would be the correct adjunct or system for the implantitis?
   a. Chlorhexidine
   b. systemic antibiotics
   c. subgingival controlled-release
   d. Metronidazole

Answer: A. The peri-implant mucositis is treated with chlorhexidine or antimicrobial oral rinses. Systemic antibiotics are not indicated. The peri-implant mucositis is not indicated for local controlled release as it is only the gingival around the implant that is inflamed.

3. What effect does enzyme-suppression therapy have on the subgingival biofilm?
   a. targets collagenase not bacteria
   b. used when have antibiotic resistant bacteria
   c. replaces periodontal debridement
   d. eliminates *Aggregatibacter Actinomycetemcomitans*

Answer: A. Enzyme suppression therapy inhibits the collagenase synthesized and released by PMN's. The therapy does not affect the bacteria. Adjunctive therapy does not replace scaling and root planning or other modalities of disrupting the biofilm.

References

American Academy of Periodontology. 2000. The role of controlled drug delivery for periodontitis. Position paper. *J. Periodontol.* 71:125–140.

American Academy of Periodontology. 2004. Systemic antibiotics in periodontics. *J. Periodontol.* 75:1553–1565.

American Academy of Periodontology. 2006. American Academy of Periodontology Statement on Local Delivery of Sustained or Controlled Release Antimicrobials as Adjunctive Therapy in the Treatment of Periodontitis.

Asikainen, S., S. Alaluusua, and L. Saxén. 1991. Recovery of *A. actinomycetemcomitans* from teeth, tongue, and saliva. *J. Periodontol.* 62:203–206.

Baker, P., T. Evans, R. Coburn, and R. Genco. 1983. Tetracycline and its derivatives strongly bind to and are released from the tooth surface in active form. *J. Periodontol.* 54:580–585.

Beikler, T., K. Prior, B. Ehmke, and T. F. Flemmig. 2004. Specific antibiotics in the treatment of periodontitis—a proposed strategy. *J. Periodontol.* 75:169–175.

Bonito, A. J., L. Lux, and K. N. Lohr. 2005. Impact of local adjuncts to scaling and root planing in periodontal disease therapy: A systematic review. *J. Periodontol.* 76(8):1227–1236.

Ciancio, S. G., and R. Ashley. 1998. Safety and efficacy of subantimicrobial-dose doxycycline therapy in patients with adult periodontitis. *Adv. Dent. Res.* 12:27–31.

Costerton, J. W., Z. Lewandowski, D. DeBeer, D. Caldwell, D. Korber, and G. James. 1994. Biofilms, the customized microniche. *J. Bacteriol.* 176:2137–2142.

Dastoor, S. F., S. Travan, R. F. Neiva, et al. 2007. Effect of adjunctive systemic azithromycin with periodontal surgery in the treatment of chronic periodontitis in smokers: A pilot study. *J. Periodontol.* 78:1887–1896.

de Graaf, J., A. J. van Winkelhoff, and R. J. Goené. 1989. The role of *Actinobacillus actinomycetemcomitans* in periodontal disease. *Infection* 17:269–271.

Emingil, G., G. Atilla, T. Sorsa, and T. Tervahartiala. 2008. The effect of adjunctive subantimicrobial dose doxycycline therapy on GCF levels in chronic periodontitis. *J. Periodontol.* 79(3):469–576.

Froum, S. J., S. H. Froum, and P. S. Rosen. 2012. Successful management of peri-implantitis with a regenerative approach: A consecutive series of 51 treated implants with 3- to 7.5-year follow-up. *Int. J. Periodoontics Restorative Dent.* 32(1):11–20.

Garey, K. W., and K. A. Rodvold. 1999. Disulfiram reactions and anti-infective agents. *Infect. Med.* 16(11):741–744.

Garrett, S., L. Johnson, and N. Stoller. 1998. The influence of subgingival calculus levels on outcomes following treatment of periodontitis with subgingivally delivered doxycycline or periodontal debridement. *J. Dent. Res.* 77:923 (Abstract 2336).

Golub, L. M., N. S. Ramamurthy, T. F. McNamara, R. A. Greenwald, and B. R. Rifkin. 1984. Tetracyclines inhibit tissue collagenase activity: A new mechanism in the treatment of periodontal diseases. *J. Periodont. Res.* 19:651–655.

Gordon, J. M., C. B. Walker, J. C. Murphy, J. M. Goodson, and S. S. Socransky. 1981. Tetracycline: Levels achievable in gingival crevice fluid and in vitro effect on subgingival organisms: 1. Concentrations in crevicular fluid after repeated doses. *J. Periodontol.* 52:609–612.

Greenstein, G. 2006. Local drug delivery in the treatment of periodontal diseases: Assessing the clinical significance of the results. *J. Periodontol.* 77(4):565–578.

Haffajee, A. D., S. S. Socransky, and J. C. Gunsolley. 2003. Systemic anti-infective periodontal therapy. A systematic review. *Ann. Periodontol.* 8(1):115–181.

Hallström, H., G. R. Persson, S. Lindgren, M. Olofsson, and S. Renvert. 2012. Systemic antibiotics and debridement of peri-implant mucositis. A randomized clinical trail. *J. Clin. Periodontol.* 39:674–581.

Hanes, P. J., and J. P. Purvis. 2003. Local anti-infective therapy: Pharmacological agents. A systematic review. *Ann. Periodontol.* 8:79–98.

Hersh, E. V., and P. A. Moore. 2008. Adverse drug interactions in dentistry. *Periodontology 2000* 46(1):109–142.

Jeffcoat, M. K., K. S. Bray, S. G. Ciancio, A. R. Dentino, D. H. Fine, et al. 1998. Adjunctive use of a subgingival controlled-release chlorhexidine chip reduces probing depth and improves attachment level compared with periodontal debridement alone. *J. Periodontol.* 69:989–997.

Kaner, D., C. Christan, T. Dietrich, et al. 2007. Timing affects the clinical outcome of adjunctive systemic antibiotic therapy for generalized aggressive periodontitis. *J. Periodontol.* 78:1201–1208.

Kleinfelder, J., R. Müller, and D. Lange. 1999. Antibiotic susceptibility of putative periodontal pathogens in advanced periodontitis patients. *J. Clin. Periodontol.* 26:347–352.

Loesche, W. 1976. Chemotherapy of dental plaque infections. *Oral Sci. Rev.* 9:65–107.

Loesche, W. J., J. Giordano, S. Soehren, and N. Kaciroti. 1996. The nonsurgical treatment of patients with periodontal disease. *Oral Surg. Oral Med. Oral Pathol.* 81:533–543.

Malizia, T., M. R. Tejada, E. Ghelardi, S. Senesi, and M. Gabriele. 1997. Periodontal tissue disposition of azithromycin. *J. Periodontol.* 68:1206–1209.

Mandell, R. L., L. S. Tripodi, E. Savitt, J. M. Goodson, and S. S. Socransky. 1986. The effect of treatment on *Actinobacillus actinomycetemcomitans* in local juvenile periodontitis. *J. Periodontol.* 57:94–97.

Novak, M. J., D. R. Dawson, I. Magnusson, et al. 2008. Combining host modulation and topical antimicrobial therapy in the management of moderate to severe periodontitis: A randomized multicenter trial. *J. Periodontol.* 79(1):33–41.

Page, R. C., S. Offenbacher, H. E. Schroeder, G. J. Seymour, and K. S. Kornman. 1997. Advances in the pathogenesis of periodontitis: Summary of developments, clinical implications and future directions. *Periodontology 2000* 14:216–248.

Paolantonio, M., M. D'Angelo, R. F. Grassi, et al. 2008. Clinical and microbiologic effects of subgingival controlled-release delivery of chlorhexidine chip in the treatment of periodontitis: A multicenter study. *J. Periodontol.* 79(2):271–282.

Pascale, D., J. Gordon, I. Lamster, P. Mann, M. Seiger, and W. Arndt. 1986. Concentration of doxycycline in human gingival fluid. *J. Clin. Periodontol.* 13:841–844.

Powell, C. A., B. L. Mealey, D. E. Deas, H. T. McDonnell, and A. J. Moritz. 2005. Post-surgical infections: Prevalence associated with various periodontal surgical procedures. *J. Periodontol.* 76: 329–333.

Preshaw, P. M., M. J. Novak, J. Mellonig, et al. 2008. Modified-release subantimicrobial dose doxycycline enhances scaling and root planing in subjects with periodontal disease. *J. Periodontol.* 79:440–452.

Renvert, S., J. Lessem, G. Dahlén, H. Renvert, and C. Lindahl. 2008. Therapy using a local drug delivery system in the treatment of peri-implantitis: A randomized clinical trail. *J. Periodontol.* 79:836–844.

Renvert, S., M. Wikström, G. Dahlén, J. Slots, and J. Egelberg. 1990. On the inability of root debridement and periodontal surgery to eliminate *Actinobacillus actinomycemtemcomitans* from periodontal pockets. *J. Clin. Periodontol.* 17:351–355.

Rifkin, B. R., A. T. Vernillo, and L. M. Golub. 1993. Blocking periodontal disease progression by inhibiting tissue destructive enzymes: A potential therapeutic role of tetracyclines and their chemically modified analogs. *J. Periodontol.* 64:819–827.

Sbordone L., L. Ramaglia, E. Gulletta, and V. Iacono. 1990. Recolonization of the subgingival microflora after scaling and root planing in human periodontis. *J. Periodontol.* 61(9): 579–584

Segelnick, S., and M. A. Weinberg. 2008. Recognizing doxycycline-induced esophageal ulcers in dental practice: A case report and review. *JADA* 139:581–585.

Seymour, R. A. 2008. Pharmacology and therapeutics in dentistry. *Periodontology 2000* 46(1):7–8.

Seymour, R. A., and S. D. Hogg. 2008. Antibiotics and chemoprophylaxis. *Periodontology 2000* 46(1):80–108.

Seymour, R. A., and M. R. Rudralingham. 2008. Oral and dental adverse drug reactions. *Periodontology 2000* 46(1):9–26.

Slots, J. 1986. Bacterial specificity in adult periodontitis: A summary of recent work. *J. Clin. Periodontol.* 13:912–917.

Smith, C. 1999, May. Adverse effects of antibiotics. *U.S. Pharmacist.* 46–60.

Stabholz, A., J. Kettering, R. Aprecio, G. Zimmerman, P. J. Baker, and U. M. E. Wikesjo. 1993. Antimicrobial properties of human dentin impregnated with tetracycline HCl or chlorhexidine: An in vitro study. *J. Clin. Periodontol.* 20:557–562.

Stoller, N., L. Johnson, S. Trapnell, C. Harrold, and S. Garrett. 1998. The pharmacokinetic profile of a biodegradable controlled-release delivery system containing doxycycline compared to systemically delivered doxycycline in gingival crevicular fluid, saliva, and serum. *J. Periodontol.* 69:1085–1091.

Walker, C. B. 1996. Selected antimicrobial agents: Mechanism of action, side effects and drug interactions. *Periodontology 2000* 10:12–28.

Walker, C., and K. Karpinia 2002. Rationale for use of antibiotics in periodontics. *J. Periodontol.* 73(10):1188–1196.

Winkel, E., A. van Winkelhoff, D. Barendregt, G. van der Weijden, M. Timmerman, and U. van der Velden. 1999. Clinical and microbiological effects of initial periodontal therapy in conjunction with amoxicillin and clavulanic acid in patient with adult periodontitis. *J. Clin. Periodontol.* 26:461–468.

Visit www.pearsonhighered.com/healthprofessionsresources to access the student resources that accompany this book. Simply select Dental Hygiene from the choice of disciplines. Find this book and you will find the complimentary study tools created for this specific title.

Principles of Periodontal Surgery: Gingivectomy, Osseous Resection, and Periodontal Plastic Surgery

Mea A. Weinberg

OUTLINE

EDUCATIONAL OBJECTIVES

Upon completion of this chapter, the reader should be able to:

- Discuss the rationale for periodontal surgical therapy.
- Describe the indications and contraindications for periodontal surgical therapy.
- Compare and contrast the different surgical treatment modalities.
- Demonstrate postoperative care following periodontal surgery.
- Identify and explain the management of postoperative complications.
- Discuss surgical wound healing and how soon after surgery a reevaluation can be performed.

GOAL: To provide an understanding of the basic indications and principles of periodontal surgery and postoperative care.

KEY WORDS

Introduction

The term *surgery* is a generic word to describe the branch of medical science concerned with the treatment of diseases or injuries by manual or operative means. Periodontal debridement (scaling and root planing) meets this definition, but it is not considered surgery. The term **periodontal surgery**, as used in the dental literature, is applied only to surgical procedures used to treat periodontal diseases or to modify the morphology of soft tissues and bone.

Different surgical procedures have been used to treat gingivitis and periodontitis, as well as to gain access to the underlying root surface and supporting bone.

Objectives, Indications, and Contraindications of Periodontal Surgery

Over the past several years, subgingival scaling and root planing techniques and local and systemic antibiotic periodontal therapy have improved dramatically. Nevertheless, periodontal surgery remains a valid option for many patients. It is imperative for the dental hygienist to have a thorough knowledge of various basic periodontal surgical procedures as well as a clear understanding of the indications and contraindications of these procedures. This is particularly important on consideration of the limitations of scaling and root planning. Egelberg (1995) reviewed these limitations, which include the fact that complete removal of subgingival calculus may not be predictably attainable after subgingival root planning. This was demonstrated in one study in which pockets with initial probing depths of ≥ 5 mm showed inadequately debrided root 65% of the time (Greenstein, 2000).

The primary objectives of periodontal surgery include the following (Palcanis, 1996):

- Reduction in the pocket depth, which allows the patient and the dental practitioner access for plaque control.
- In patients with very deep pockets and bone loss, to gain access to the root and underlying bone to achieve more effective removal of calculus and subgingival bacterial biofilm to maintain periodontal attachment levels and perhaps even gain "new attachment." New attachment is defined as the union of connective tissue with a root surface that has been deprived previously of its original attachment apparatus (American Academy of Periodontology, 2001).
- To regenerate periodontal tissues lost due to the disease.
- To arrest disease progression.
- To create an oral environment that is maintainable by both the patient and the dental team.

After the surgical procedures have been performed, the therapeutic end points of clinical success are measured by the attainment of stable or improved clinical attachment levels, minimal inflammation (bleeding on probing), and reduced and stable probing depths (Palcanis, 1996).

Indications for periodontal surgery include the following:

- Pocket elimination/reduction on teeth with gingival/periodontal pockets
- Correction of mucogingival defects (e.g., for root coverage, increasing the zone of keratinized/attached gingiva, augmentation of alveolar ridges)
- To improve aesthetics—that is, aesthetic crown lengthening
- Creation of a favorable restorative environment such as lengthening of the clinical crown
- Placement of dental implants
- Incision and drainage of a gingival or periodontal abscess
- Regeneration of the attachment apparatus that was destroyed as a result of periodontal disease

Periodontal surgical therapy is contraindicated or at least delayed for the following reasons:

- Systemic diseases that cannot be controlled by medications or otherwise, such as diabetes mellitus, cardiovascular conditions (e.g., hypertension).
- Systemic diseases that are associated with excessive bleeding, such as leukemia, hemophilia, and renal (kidney) dialysis (consult with the patient's physician).
- Patients taking anticoagulation medication (warfarin, heparin), which could result in extensive and difficult to control bleeding. This may not be a contraindication, but precautions must be followed due to the possible extensive bleeding.
- Patients who are unable to undergo periodontal surgery.
- Patients taking intravenous bisphosphonates are not candidates for periodontal surgery; contact physician.
- For patients taking oral bisphosphonates, use professional and clinical judgment; contact physician.
- Patients who are noncompliant with plaque control or periodontal maintenance appointments.
- Concern for cosmetic outcome (e.g., postsurgical gingival shrinkage), especially in anterior areas.
- Treating teeth that have hopeless prognoses.

Did You Know?

John M. Riggs originated a surgical technique for the treatment of pyorrhea alveolaris (periodontal disease) and contributed it to the *Pennsylvania Journal of Dental Science* in 1876. He was referred to as the "Father of Periodontal Surgery."

Preoperative Preparation

Preoperative management involving patient preparation for surgery includes removal of soft and hard deposits, reinforcement of oral hygiene self-care, selective occlusal adjustment, and selective adjunctive antimicrobial or antibiotic agents. It is important to complete initial therapy because this may eliminate the need for surgery or at least reduce or eliminate gingival inflammation, which will increase the manageability of the tissues during surgery and allow for better healing. Evaluation for surgery is done at a minimum of 4 to 6 weeks after completion of the initial phase of therapy. At this time, a soft tissue examination will determine the tissue healing or response to the initial therapy. An evaluation of the patient's oral hygiene status also is made. If there is residual calculus, additional sessions of periodontal debridement may be necessary. A complete periodontal charting is done, including identification and cause of bleeding sites and sites with clinical attachment loss (Carranza, 1996).

Requirements for Periodontal Surgery

Specific requirements must be met before surgery is performed. Any uncontrolled or poorly controlled systemic disease (i.e., diabetes) should be addressed by referring the patient to his or her physician prior to surgery. Elimination of plaque-retentive restorations should be performed before surgery (e.g., overhanging margins of restorations or overcontoured restorations; Flores-de-Jacoby & Mengel, 1995). Any carious lesions should be repaired and hopeless teeth extracted. Necessary endodontic treatment should be performed prior to periodontal therapy. The hygienist and dentist should recommend a smoking cessation program to the patient prior to surgery. Smoking seems to alter the inflammatory response during healing. Risk factors such as smoking have been shown to delay wound healing after surgery (Boström, Linder, & Bergström, 1998; Persson, Mand, Martin, & Page, 2003; Preber & Bergström, 1990), and this may need to be addressed with the patient.

Types of Periodontal Surgery

There are many types of surgical procedures, and selection of the appropriate surgery depends on the pattern of bone loss (e.g., horizontal versus vertical or a combination of both) and the presence of mucogingival involvement. Periodontal surgery usually is done in quadrants or sextants, depending on the number of teeth involved and the decision of the surgeon. Most important, the practitioner and the patient should be aware of the limitations of periodontal surgery (Box 25–1).

Lang and Löe (1993) proposed a convenient classification of periodontal surgical procedures. It includes five categories:

1. Procedures for supragingival pocket reduction or elimination (gingivectomy)
2. Procedures for gaining access to root surfaces for debridement (periodontal flap surgery)

Box 25–1: Limitations of Periodontal Surgery

- Periodontal surgery does not compensate for the patient's poor plaque control.
- Some adverse effects from surgery include gingival recession, which may compromise aesthetics to some degree.
- It will not routinely produce miraculous and complete regeneration of all lost periodontal tissues.

3. Procedures for treatment of osseous defects (flap surgery with osseous reduction)
4. Procedures for correcting mucogingival defects (periodontal plastic surgery)
5. Procedures for regeneration of lost periodontium (periodontal regeneration)

Healing Following Periodontal Surgery

There are four types of **healing responses** of periodontal tissues that can occur after periodontal treatment (Carranza, 1996). Repair is the healing of periodontal tissues with tissues that do not replicate the original lost periodontium. After periodontal debridement and periodontal surgery, instead of the gingival connective tissue attaching to the tooth, the junctional epithelium reforms on the root surface by migrating along the root surface, forming a long junctional epithelium attachment. Another example of repair is scar formation, in which the new tissue formed is considered epithelium and connective tissue but does not replicate the original tissue that was lost or damaged. Reattachment is the reunion of epithelial or connective tissue to a root surface that was not damaged by periodontal disease. This would occur after an incision or injury or where a surgical flap has to be extended to a tooth with a healthy periodontium for better access. New attachment is the union of connective tissue or epithelium with a root surface that was deprived of its original attachment apparatus. Regeneration is the reformation of the periodontal tissues that were destroyed by periodontal disease with the formation of new cementum, periodontal ligament, and bone. This is the ideal treatment result and is the goal of various surgical procedures. However, it is not always attained. Rather, a partial regeneration or new attachment is more often obtained. Epithelium is the first tissue to move or migrate into the wound area. Epithelium migrates up to 0.5 mm a day, which is faster than connective tissue or bone cells. This can interfere with the formation of a new attachment or regeneration. General postoperative instructions are given in Box 25–2.

Box 25–2: General Postoperative Instructions

Discomfort	Usually, minimal discomfort is expected, especially after the anesthesia wears off. If you have been given a prescription, fill it and take the medication as directed. Aspirin should not be used. If discomfort persists, call the office.
Swelling	If swelling occurs, it will peak 48 to 72 hours after the surgery. You may use an ice pack on the outside of your face, 20 minutes on and 20 minutes off, for the next 2 hours. If swelling occurs after the first day, a moistened heated towel may be used on the area. If excessive swelling occurs, call the office.
Bleeding	There may be occasional blood stains in the saliva for the first 4 or 5 hours. This is not unusual; do not be alarmed. If bleeding continues, do not rinse to stop bleeding. Apply firm pressure using a moistened gauze pad or fresh tea bag for 20 minutes, without interruption. Repeat as necessary. If the bleeding does not stop, call the office.
Physical activity	It is recommended that you rest and limit your activities for the rest of the day. Avoid excessive exertion (jogging, swimming, tennis, etc.) for the next week.
Eating	Limit your diet to soft foods on the day of the surgery. Do not drink hot liquids (tea, coffee, soup) for 24 hours following surgery. Do not chew on the area where the surgery was performed. Avoid alcoholic beverages for 1 week following the surgery.
Sutures	If sutures were used, avoid that area. They will be removed approximately 7 to 14 days following surgery.
Dressing	To help minimize irritation, a periodontal dressing may be placed around the surgical area. It will harden within about 2 hours and should not be removed. It is of no concern if a few pieces of the dressing break off. However, if the dressing seems to be loose or has come off, contact the office for instructions.
Smoking	Do not smoke. Smoking may negatively affect the healing process, which may result in a poor outcome.
Home care	The most important element required for good healing is meticulous oral hygiene. If a dressing is placed, avoid pressing down on it. Use a soft or ultrasoft toothbrush to carefully clean the occlusal surface and the surface of the dressing. If no dressing was placed, gently use a soft or ultrasoft toothbrush to cleanse the area. Do not floss the surgical site. Brush and floss the untreated areas as usual. Do not rinse on the day of the surgery. On the second day, use the prescribed mouth rinse as directed.
Medications	In some cases, analgesics and/or antibiotics will be prescribed. Use prescribed medications as directed.

Procedures for Pocket Reduction/Elimination

Gingivectomy/Gingivoplasty

DEFINITION **Gingivectomy** is the excision or removal of the soft tissue walls (gingiva) to eliminate a pocket. Gingivoplasty, on the other hand, refers to surgical reshaping or recontouring of the oral surface of the gingiva without removing any portion of the gingiva that is attached to the tooth.

INDICATIONS The main objectives of gingivectomy/gingivoplasty procedures are to reduce or eliminate suprabony periodontal pockets that are associated with horizontal patterns of bone loss and to eliminate pseudopockets (gingival enlargement) induced by certain medications, such as phenytoin, cyclosporine, valproic acid, and nifedipine (Bosco, Bonfante, Luize, Bosco, & Garcia, 2006). Enlarged gingiva and interdental papillae seen in mouth breathers also can be treated with these techniques. Oftentimes, localized or generalized gingival enlargement is seen during pregnancy, which may or may not resolve postpartum. Surgery in these cases, unless the gingival overgrowth becomes infected or interferes with chewing, is delayed until a reevaluation is made postpartum. Frequently, the gingival enlargement will recur, and gingivectomy procedures may have to be repeated. Less frequently, lengthening of the clinical crown can be achieved using gingivectomy.

CONTRAINDICATIONS Contraindications for gingivectomy include lack of attached gingiva and the presence of infrabony pockets associated with vertical bone loss.

TECHNIQUE After the patient receives local anesthesia, the gingivectomy is begun by marking the base of the pockets with a periodontal probe or other instrument. Incisions are made with a surgical blade angled at 45 degrees to the gingiva slightly coronal to the base of the pocket (Figure 25–1 ■). Incisions are not made into the sulcus, but rather on the outer epithelium, with the blade directed in an occlusal or incisal direction rather than apically. Root debridement is performed followed by gingivoplasty to reestablish a physiologic gingiva. After hemostasis is obtained (bleeding is controlled), the area

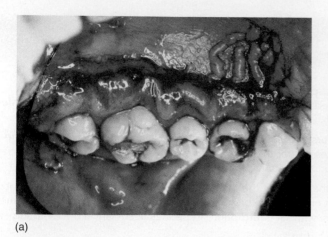

(a)

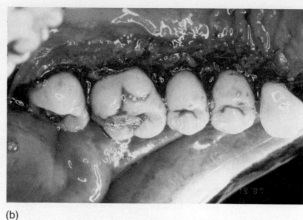

(b)

FIGURE 25–1 (a) Clinical picture of a gingivectomy procedure. A 38-year-old patient with pseudopockets (gingival enlargement) due to phenytoin therapy. The incision is made apical to the bleeding points, which demarcate the base of the pocket. (b) After the incision is made, the tissue is removed, exposing the underlying bleeding connective tissue.

is dried, and a periodontal dressing is placed. The patient is given postoperative instructions. Postoperative instructions to the patient for this procedure are given in Table 25–1 ■. This includes care of the surgical wound, oral hygiene measures taken during initial healing, and reporting adverse signs and symptoms. The patient then returns in 7 to 10 days for a postoperative visit.

HEALING Epithelialization of the wound surface starts within a few days of surgery and usually takes 7 to 14 days, depending on the size of the wound. Soft tissue healing is completed within 4 to 5 weeks, although clinically it may appear healed within 2 weeks. Clinically, it is important to avoid probing the area until the connective tissue has healed.

Table 25–1 Surgical Care Procedures

Surgical Procedure	Postoperative Care	Reevaluation Procedures
Gingivectomy	1. Instruct patient not to brush the area where the periodontal dressing is located.	1. Periodontal probing should not be done until a minimum of 6 weeks after surgery.
	2. The area will heal by secondary intention; the wound is open and exposed because there is no flap and no sutures. This area is similar to a scraped knee or pizza burn on the palate. It will be sore.	2. Final prosthetic restorations should not be completed until 6 weeks or more after surgery.
	3. Avoid smoking, if possible.	
	4. At postoperative visit, carefully remove the dressing, irrigate with sterile water or saline, and wipe off the white film (this consists of dead epithelial cells).	
	5. Reapply dressing if needed.	3. Supragingival scaling can be done after 1 week, but subgingival periodontal debridement should not be performed until 6 weeks after surgery.
	6. After the first postoperative visit, the patient may start to brush the teeth around the surgical site gently with a roll technique. Bleeding will occur but will gradually lessen. The patient should continue to brush even if light bleeding is seen.	

Surgical Procedure	Postoperative Care	Reevaluation Procedures
Flap surgery (with or without osseous resection)	1. Instruct patient not to brush the area where the periodontal dressing is located. 2. Apply ice pack. 3. At postoperative visit, carefully remove the dressing and sutures, irrigate with sterile water or saline, and wipe off the white film (this consists of dead epithelial cells). 4. Reapply dressing if needed; patient may start to brush surgical site gently with a roll technique. Bleeding will occur but will gradually lessen. The patient should continue to brush even if bleeding is seen. 5. Avoid smoking, if possible.	1. Periodontal probing should not be done until a minimum of 3 months after surgery. 2. Final prosthetic restorations should not be completed until a minimum of 3 months after surgery. 3. Supragingival scaling can be done after 1 week, but subgingival periodontal debridement should not be performed until 3 months after surgery.
Mucogingival surgery (soft-tissue grafts)	1. Instruct patient not to brush the area where the periodontal dressing is located. 2. At postoperative visit, carefully remove the dressing and sutures at the donor site, irrigate with sterile water or saline, and wipe off the white film (this consists of dead epithelial cells). 3. Avoid smoking. 4. Reapply dressing if needed; patient may start to brush surgical site gently with a roll technique. Advise the patient not to hit the gums with the toothbrush. The patient should discontinue brushing if bleeding is seen and only rinse the area with warm water.	1. Gingival grafts with root coverage would be reevaluated a minimum of 6 months after surgery. 2. Gingival grafts without root coverage can be reevaluated a minimum of 2 months after surgery.

Did You Know?

The use of lasers in periodontal therapy is FDA approved only for sulcular debridement and not for surgery. Lasers deliver wavelengths. Using a laser instead of a scalpel is intended to increase coagulation (blood clotting) allowing for a dry surgical field and better visualization. (See American Academy of Periodontology, 2006.)

Periodontal Flap Surgery

A flap is defined as that loosened portion of the gingiva, alveolar mucosa, and/or periosteum that is separated from the underlying structures except at its base, from which the flap receives its blood supply. Flaps are the most commonly used periodontal surgical procedure. Flap procedures are designed to gain access to the underlying bone and root surface for the purpose of debridement, bone recontouring, or regeneration. Generally, a flap is made by an incision with a surgical blade or knife into the pocket (intracrevicular) or slightly subgingival to the gingival margin (internal bevel incision). The amount of attached gingiva present and the depth of the pockets primarily determine the type of incision made. The flap is then reflected away from the tooth with an instrument called a periosteal elevator to expose the underlying tooth and root surface.

FLAP CLASSIFICATION Flaps are classified on the basis of tissue components included in the flap and the positioning of the flap at the end of the procedure. In a full-thickness or mucoperiosteal flap, the gingiva, alveolar mucosa, and periosteum are reflected from the root and the underlying bone surfaces (Figure 25–2a ■). A partial- or split-thickness

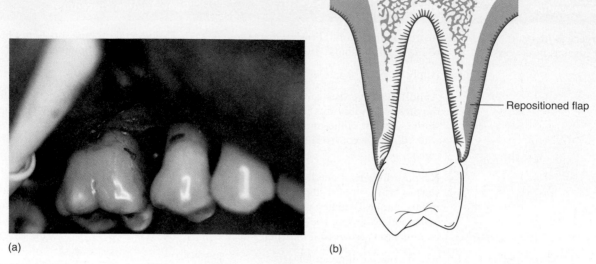

(a)

(b)

Repositioned flap

FIGURE 25–2 (a) Full-thickness flap consists of the full thickness of mucosa and underlying connective tissue (periosteum) exposing the underlying bone. (b) Replaced flap postoperative.

flap is one in which the periosteum and some connective tissue are left attached to the bone and are not included in the flap (Figure 25–3 ■). Partial-thickness flaps are used when the bone is thin and exposure to the environment is not desirable because this would increase the chances of bone resorption. It is controversial if a partial-thickness flap results in less bone resorption. When the bone needs to be visualized, a full-thickness flap is required.

Based on the final positioning of the flap at the end of the surgical procedure, flaps are classified as replaced (e.g., modified Widman), apically positioned, coronally (Gürgan, Oruç, & Akkaya, 2004), and laterally positioned.

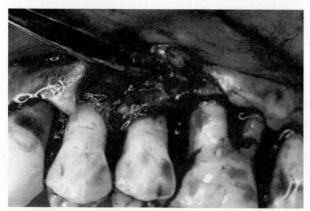

FIGURE 25–3 Split- or partial-thickness flap consists of the mucosa and submucosa but not the periosteum. Periosteum is left on the bone.

The most frequently used periodontal flap procedures are the modified Widman flap and apically positioned flap.

MODIFIED WIDMAN FLAP Ramfjord and Nissle (1974) described the modified Widman flap (MWF) as a flap for better visualization of the area.

Objective. The specific objective of the MWF is to gain access to root surfaces for improved periodontal debridement and a reduction in inflammation and pocket depths.

Indications. The procedure is indicated for deep pockets, infrabony pockets, and where aesthetics is important, such as in the anterior region. An advantage of this procedure is direct visualization with debridement of deep pockets. Widman flap procedures also allow complete removal of pocket epithelium, and because the flaps can be placed in close approximation, healing takes place by primary intention. Healing of wounds occurs by primary, secondary, or tertiary intention. Primary intention occurs where the wound heals by fibrous adhesion (edges of flap approximate each other) without the formation of granulation tissue. A gingivectomy wound heals by secondary intention where the wound is left open. Healing by tertiary intention is usually used in surgical wounds complicated by infection whereby they must heal by contraction of the wound edges.

Contraindications. The MWF is contraindicated if there are bony defects that need to be recontoured or regenerated.

Technique. After adequate anesthesia is obtained, incisions are made through the crest of the gingiva approximately 1 mm from the margin (Figures 25–4 ■, 25–5 ■). This is called an inverse bevel incision. This incision is scalloped and extended as far interproximally as possible to preserve the interdental papillae. Gingival tissues are then reflected only far enough to allow the surgeon direct vision of the root surfaces and the crest of bone. After complete debridement of plaque, calculus, and diseased tissue from the root surfaces and bony defects, the flaps are readapted to cover the crest of bone; flaps are replaced to their original position before the surgery. In some cases, bone recontouring is required for better flap adaptation. Interrupted interproximal sutures are then placed, and the surgical area is covered with a periodontal dressing. The patient receives postoperative instructions (Table 25–1). The dressing and sutures are removed after 1 week, and the patient is placed on a chlorhexidine mouth rinse.

Healing. Following traditional **flap surgery**, the debrided root surface becomes repopulated with epithelial cells that form a long junctional epithelium along the root surface with no new connective tissue attachment (gingival fibers inserting into the cementum; Figure 25–2b).

APICALLY POSITIONED FLAP An apically positioned flap is a full-thickness or split-thickness flap made with an internal bevel incision that following suturing is apically positioned at or near the level of the alveolar crest.

Objective. The main objective is to surgically reduce or eliminate deep pockets by apically positioning the gingival complex while retaining the entire width of gingiva.

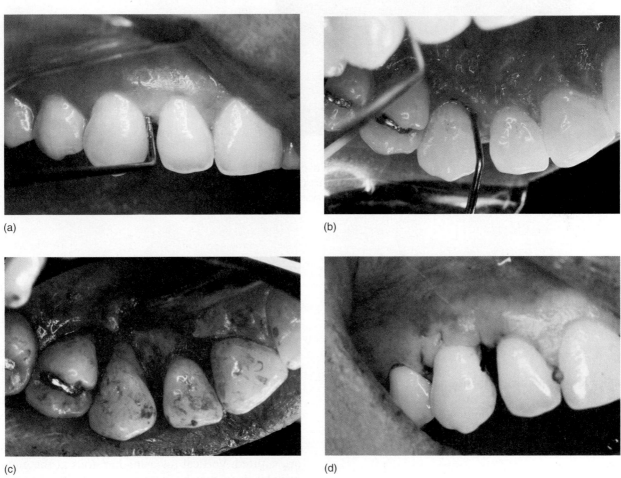

(a)   (b)

(c)   (d)

FIGURE 25–4 Preoperative measurements on the maxillary canine: (a) 7 mm pocket on the mesiofacial and (b) 5 mm pocket depth on the mesiopalatal. (c) Buccal and palatal flaps allowed access to the underlying root and bone for root and defect debridement. (d) Flaps are replaced to their original position and sutured.

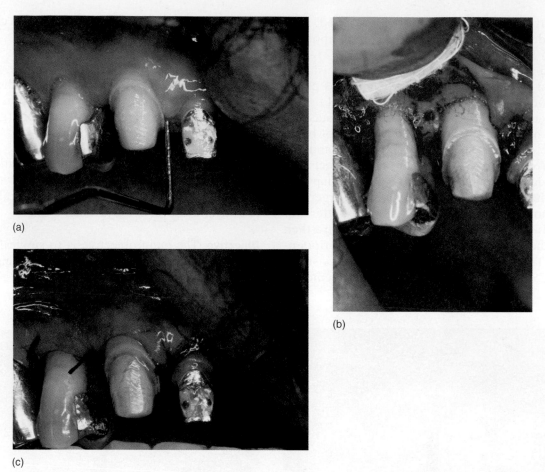

(a)

(b)

(c)

FIGURE 25–5 (a) Preoperative: Note amalgam overhang on the mesial of the premolar. The canine and lateral incisor were being prepared for crowns. (b) Intrasulcular incisions were placed, and full-thickness flaps were reflected. The amalgam was recontoured. (c) The flaps were replaced and sutured to the original position.

Indications. This procedure is used to (1) eliminate moderate or deep pockets by positioning the gingival tissue apically, (2) lengthen the clinical crown for restorative/prosthetic procedures, and (3) increase the zone of attached gingiva.

Contraindications. The apically positioned flap is contraindicated where aesthetics is a concern, such as in the anterior region, where root exposure would be unaesthetic. This type of surgery is also contraindicated in patients at high risk for root caries. It is also contraindicated in areas of advanced bone loss.

Technique. (Figures 25–6 ■, 25–7 ■) The apically positioned flap can be used on buccal surfaces of both mandibular and maxillary arches as well as on the mandibular lingual

surface. The palatal gingiva cannot be displaced or moved because it is composed entirely of keratinized gingiva without alveolar mucosa, which is what gives the flap its flexibility.

After obtaining adequate local anesthesia, a reverse (internal) bevel incision is made from the gingival margin to the crest of bone. The location of the initial incision in relation to the gingival margin depends on the width and thickness of the attached gingiva, as well as the depth of the pocket. The incision is scalloped interproximally to obtain optimal coverage of alveolar bone when the flaps are sutured. Vertical releasing incisions at the ends of the initial incision may be placed for flexibility and easier positioning of the flap apically. Next, a split-thickness flap is raised (coronally, a full-thickness flap is necessary if bone is to be contoured), and the incised gingival tissue collar is

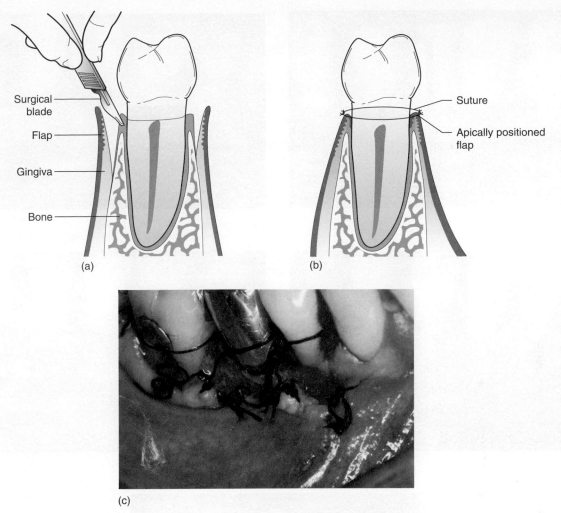

Surgical blade
Flap
Gingiva
Bone
(a)

Suture
Apically positioned flap
(b)

(c)

FIGURE 25–6 The apically positioned flap procedure. (a) An inverse bevel incision is made slightly apical to the free gingival margin, and the flap is reflected from the alveolar process. (b) The flap is positioned apically, and it is sutured. This procedure attempts to help eliminate or reduce the soft-tissue pocket depth. Apically positioned flap eliminates deep pockets and increases the zone of attached gingiva. (c) In this case, the split-thickness flap is sutured apically, exposing the tissue and bone, which when healed allows for an increased width of attached gingiva. (Courtesy of Dr. James B. Fine, Columbia University College of Dental Medicine)

removed with a curet. Using power-driven scalers and hand instruments, diseased tissue is removed, and root and bony defect debridement is performed.

If bony defects are present, the bone can be recontoured. Bone recontouring is done with a high-speed handpiece and/or hand chisels to establish a harmonious relationship between the gingiva and the bone. The flap is then positioned apically to cover the bone and is sutured. A **periodontal dressing** can be applied.

Healing. The attachment or closure of the soft tissue to the root surface in the apically positioned flap is by a long junctional epithelium, with no new connective tissue attachment. Complete healing occurs within 30 to 35 days. **Postoperative care** procedures are reviewed in Table 25–1 (Figure 25–2b).

Rapid Dental Hint

When removing the periodontal dressing, sometimes the sutures get embedded. Do not pull on the dressing. Carefully hold the dressing and see where the suture is buried and then cut the suture with scissors.

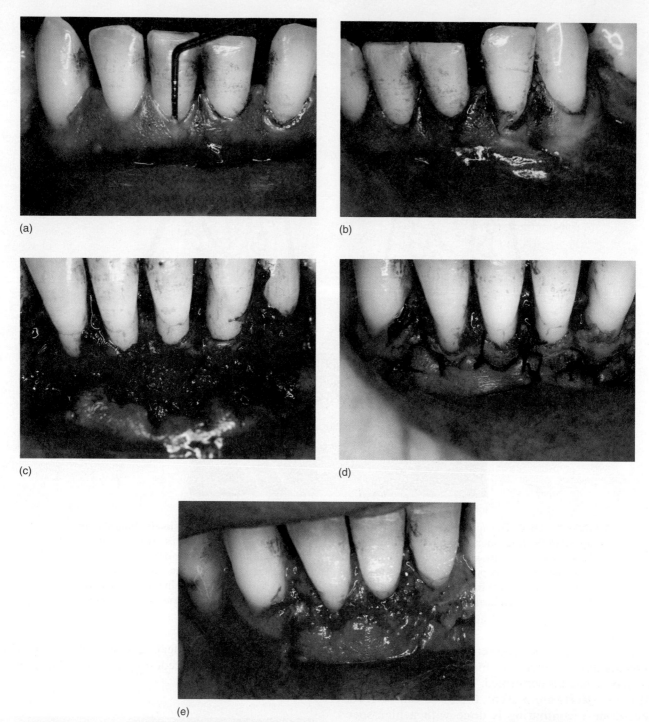

FIGURE 25–7 The apically positioned flap procedure. (a) Preoperative: Note mucogingival defects (no attached gingiva) on the anterior teeth. (b) An inverse bevel incision was made. (c) Split-thickness flap was reflected. (d) Apically positioned flap was sutured. (e) One week postop: Note that the position of the flap allows for the underlying tissue to be exposed. This allows for new keratinized gingiva to granulate in.

Procedures for Treating Osseous Defects

Periodontal Flap Surgery with Osseous Resection

Periodontitis is a disease that involves loss of connective tissue attachment and loss of alveolar bone. This loss creates osseous defects and deformities leading to an uneven gingival architecture, which makes it difficult for the patient and the dental hygienist to maintain a healthy dentition. Osseous surgery is periodontal surgery involving modification of the bone supporting the teeth to eliminate pockets and obtain optimal physiologic gingival contours. The elimination or modification of bone defects can be either by resection or recontouring, which is removing bone, or by adding bone, which is termed periodontal regeneration (Figure 25–8 ■). Whether to perform osseous resection or periodontal regeneration depends on the type of osseous defect. This is reviewed in the following paragraph. Periodontal regeneration is discussed in Chapter 26.

CLASSIFICATION OF OSSEOUS DEFECTS The surgical approach (e.g., resection or regeneration) depends on the pattern of bone loss. There are two types of bone loss: horizontal and vertical.

In a suprabony pocket, the base of the pocket is coronal to the alveolar crest, and the pattern of bone destruction is horizontal, where the bone height is reduced evenly between two adjacent teeth, creating flat interproximal bone or a horizontal pattern of bone loss (Figure 25–9 ■). On the other hand, in infrabony pockets, the base of the osseous defect is apical to the crest of the alveolar bone. The pattern of bone destruction is vertical (angular), where the bone is "scooped out" along the side of the root.

Intraosseous or infrabony (vertical) defects are classified according to the number of remaining osseous walls

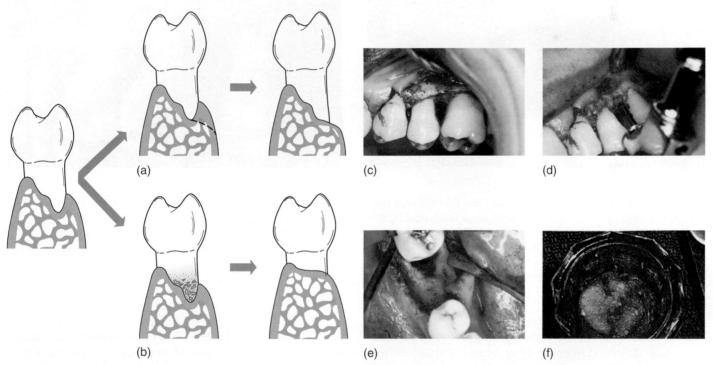

(a)

(b)

(c)

(d)

(e)

(f)

FIGURE 25–8 A periodontal bony defect is treated either by (a) reshaping or recontouring the bone (top diagram) or (b) filling in the defect (bottom diagram) with bone or a bone substitute (regeneration). (c) Flap reflected showing a two-wall bony defect in between the premolar and molar. (d) A high-speed round bur is used to do osseous recontouring to eliminate the defect. (e) This three-wall bony defect (the buccal, lingual, and mesial walls remain) on the mesial surface of the molar is best treated with a regenerative procedure. (f) Bone in the dappen dish is used to place into the infrabony defect.

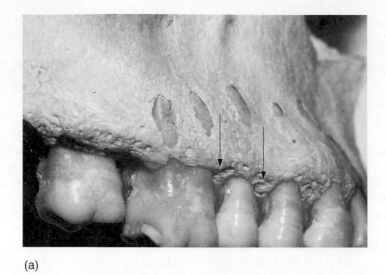

(a)

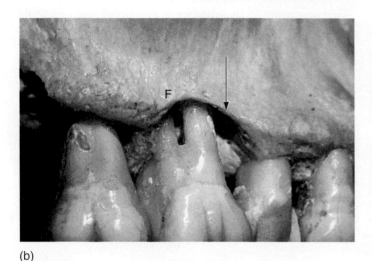

(b)

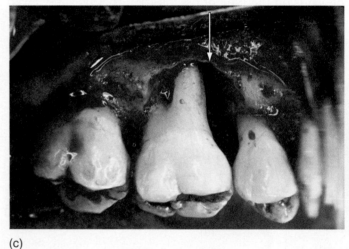

(c)

FIGURE 25–9 (a) Horizontal pattern of bone loss between the premolars and second premolar and first molar. Interproximal bone (arrows) is destroyed on both sides of adjacent teeth equally. (b) *Left side:* Dry skull specimen showing furcation involvement (F) and vertical pattern of bone loss on the mesial aspect of the first molar. Note that the interproximal bone is not flat as with horizontal bone loss. (c) *Right side:* After the gingiva has been reflected from the tooth and bone, a vertical defect is seen on the mesial aspect of the first molar.

and by their predominant morphology: one-, two-, and three-wall defects (Figure 25–10 ■). Most infrabony defects are a combination of one–two- or two–three-wall morphology. Most infrabony defects are interproximal, but they can be located on the direct facial or lingual surface. A crater is a specific type of two-wall defect in which the remaining osseous walls are the facial and lingual walls. A hemiseptal defect is a type of one-wall defect in which the remaining wall is usually the facial or lingual. A circumferential defect is a three-wall defect that wraps around the line angle of the tooth to involve the lingual or facial surface. Only by probing through the soft tissue pocket (bone sounding), but more precisely by surgical entry, can a determination of the type of infrabony defect be made.

OSTECTOMY AND OSTEOPLASTY Ostectomy and osteoplasty are the two types of osseous recontouring during osseous surgery (Figure 25–11 ■). Ostectomy is the removal of supporting bone or bone that is in contact with the root, and osteoplasty is the reshaping or recontouring of nonsupporting bone or bone that is not in contact with the root (e.g., bony ledges) to achieve physiologic contours.

Objectives. The objectives of osseous resective surgery are to create optimal physiologic contours that reduce bony ledges or irregular contours to permit primary flap closure and to eliminate infrabony pockets by eliminating the bony walls of the defect.

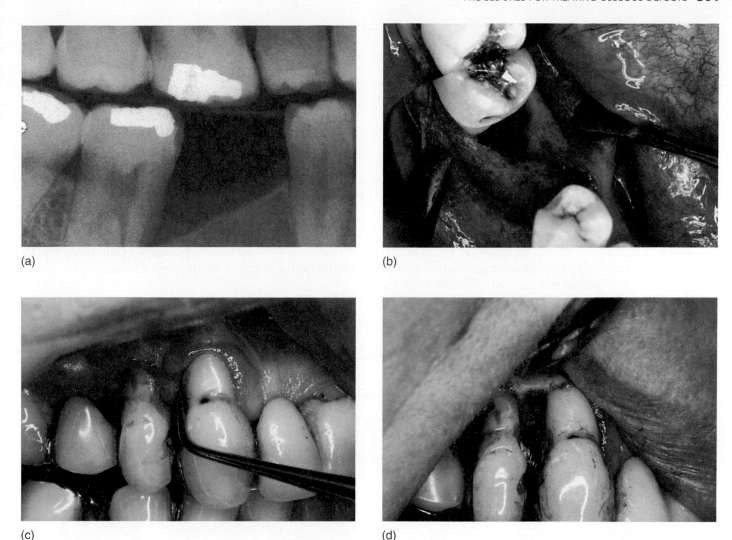

FIGURE 25–10 (a) X-ray of three-wall defect; surgical entry. Note that the distal bony wall against the molar is destroyed. Thus, three walls remain: buccal, lingual, and mesial. (b) Surgical entry of a three-wall defect—the buccal, lingual, and distal walls remain. (c) Probing distal of canine. (d) Surgical entry shows a deep three-wall bony defect.

Indications. Indications for osseous resective surgery include the following: (1) to permit optimal flap adaptation by removing bony ledges or exostosis, (2) to eliminate shallow infrabony pockets (1 to 2 mm deep), (3) to open furcations for easier maintenance, and (4) to lengthen crowns for restorative procedures (e.g., crowns).

Contraindications. Osseous resective surgery is contraindicated in the following situations: (1) patients with advanced periodontitis (teeth in these patients already have compromised bone support; additional resection of tooth-supporting structures would be contraindicated); (2) aesthetics (removal of bone in aesthetic areas, especially the anterior maxillary area, will result in an aesthetically unacceptable appearance); (3) isolated deep vertical

defects (attempts to reduce or eliminate such defects would result in removing too much supporting bone from the adjacent tooth); and (4) the existence of local anatomic factors, such as the external oblique ridge, maxillary sinus, and flat palate limits achieving the intended results from osseous resection.

Technique. (Figure 25–12 ■) The patient receives local anesthesia. The flap is reflected from the root and bone. When the flaps are elevated, the alveolar crest and marginal bone are inspected. If the marginal bone is thick with ledges, osteoplasty is performed with burs on a high-speed handpiece with copious irrigation. If infrabony defects are present, ostectomy is performed with burs and hand instruments to flatten the interproximal bone. A question

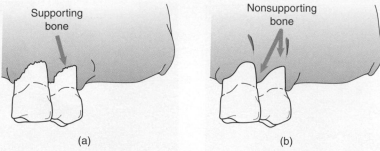

FIGURE 25–11 (a) Ostectomy removes bone attached to the tooth, which is called supporting bone. (b) Osteoplasty is the reshaping of the nonsupporting bone.

arises of how much bone should be removed. The answer is enough bone is removed to eliminate or significantly reduce the depth of the defect but not enough to compromise the tooth or adjacent teeth. These procedures will create a harmonious environment for the alveolar process and the overlying gingiva. The apically positioned flap is the technique of choice when pocket elimination is anticipated. If desired,

periodontal dressing may be placed over the surgical area. Postoperative instructions are given (Table 25–1).

Healing. The soft tissue attachment to the root surface is by a long junctional epithelium. Healing also results in gingival recession with root exposure. Healing is complete by 2 to 3 months.

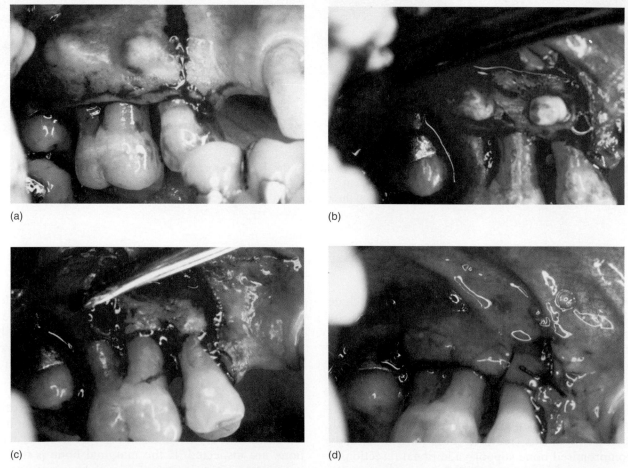

FIGURE 25–12 (a) A horizontal and vertical releasing incision is made on the facial surface. (b) A full-thickness flap is reflected away from the bone. There is a furcation involvement on the first molar. Note the two bony protuberances called exostoses (singular: exostosis) on the facial surface. A two-wall bony crater exists between the premolar and molar. (c) Osteoplasty removed the exostoses, resulting in a thin, smooth, bony surface. Ostectomy removed the bony crater. (d) An apically positioned flap. The flap is moved in an apical position to the crest of bone to eliminate the depth of the pocket.

Crown-Lengthening Procedures

Crown lengthening or crown extension is a surgical procedure designed to expose more tooth structure for restorative purposes (e.g., placement of a crown or other restoration; Deas et al., 2004). Indications for crown lengthening are as follows: (1) a tooth that is fractured close to the gingival margin and/or alveolar crest and (2) subgingival caries.

Before surgery is performed, the concept of the biologic width must be considered. Biologic width is the soft-tissue dimension that is occupied by the junctional epithelium and the gingival connective tissue attachment (gingival fibers). The average length of the junctional epithelium is 0.97 mm, and the average length of the gingival fibers is 1.07 mm, making the dimension of the biologic width approximately 2.04 mm. Thus, the biologic width is the soft tissue attachment from the base of the sulcus to the crest of alveolar bone. There must be enough length of root surface to allow for these two attachments. This distance is necessary for gingival health. The margin of a crown or other restoration should not be placed within this space. When a margin is placed less than 2 mm from the alveolar crest, it causes gingival inflammation and damage to the attachment apparatus. Bone resorption will then take place to reestablish this biologic width. Thus, if a tooth is fractured, a radiograph will indicate how close the most coronal part of the remaining tooth structure is to the alveolar bone. Osseous resective surgery may be indicated to create more exposed tooth structure and allow for reestablishment of soft tissue attachments and proper placement of restorative margins (Perez, Smukler, & Nunn, 2007; Figure 25–13 ■).

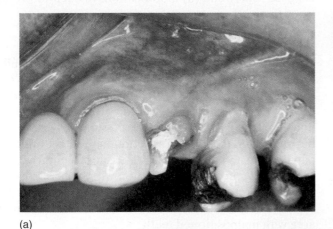

(a)

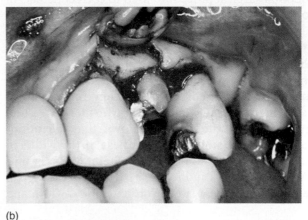

(b)

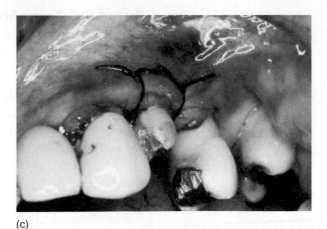

(c)

FIGURE 25–13 (a) The premolar fractured due to caries. (b) Flap is elevated, and surgical removal of bone was necessary to lengthen the crown so a crown could be placed without impinging on the biologic width. (c) The flap was positioned apically and sutured.

Root Resection

In patients with substantial furcation involvements (class III or IV) with extensive bone loss around the roots of molar teeth and defective, decayed, or resorbed roots, root resection or hemisection may be indicated. Root resection or amputation is defined as the removal of a root while leaving the crown on a multirooted tooth (Figure 25–14 ■). Root resection is usually done on maxillary molars. Hemisection is the surgical sectioning and removal of one root and the crown portion and is usually done on mandibular molars that have a furcation involvement with severe bone loss around the root. If a molar is adequately stable with sufficient bony support but displays a class III or IV furcation involvement, a bisection or bicuspidization procedure can be done. This involves the sectioning or cutting of the molar in half, creating two separate teeth. Endodontics (root canal therapy) must be done before any of these procedures. The long-term survival of resected teeth is not predictable (Blomlof, Jansson, Ehnevid, & Lindskog, 1997).

Periodontal Plastic Surgery

The mucogingival relationship is important in sustaining the health of the gingival attachment. Mucogingival surgery is a periodontal surgical procedure used to correct defects in the morphology, position, and/or amount of gingiva.

Indications

Historically, the use of **mucogingival surgical** procedures was limited to treatment of gingival recession. A certain amount of attached gingiva was considered necessary to maintain gingival health and prevent further recession. However, several studies have shown that periodontal health can be maintained regardless of the width of attached gingiva (Salkin, Freedman, Stein, & Bassiouny, 1987; Wennström & Lindhe, 1983). Therefore, gingival augmentation is used in sites with inadequate width and

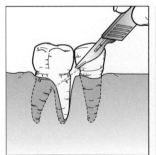
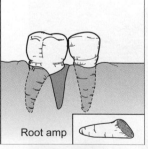

Root resection
presurgical defect
(a)

Root resection
affected root removed
(b)

Root amp

FIGURE 25–14 Root resection: Surgical blade used to reflect the flap; buccal furcation involvement with bone loss of the mesiobuccal root of the mandibular first molar allows for the surgical resection of the mesiobuccal root.

thickness of attached gingiva that exhibit persistent inflammation (bleeding) or progressive recession and sites with inadequate dimensions of gingiva that have subgingival restorations or orthodontics. In sites where crown margins are to be placed subgingivally, recession with exposure of the crown margins may occur when there is inadequate gingival dimensions. Other indications for mucogingival procedures include (1) elimination of frenum and muscle pull at or near the gingival margin (Figure 25–15 ■), (2) areas in which the base of a periodontal pocket extends to or beyond the mucogingival junction, (3) deepening of the buccal vestibule, (4) aesthetic reasons (e.g., to cover exposed roots), and (5) modifications of edentulous ridges prior to prosthetic reconstruction.

Classification of Gingival Recession

The original classification of gingival recession by Sullivan and Atkins (1985) was later expanded by Miller (1985; Figure 25–16 ■). The Miller classification includes: I: soft-tissue recession not extending to the mucogingival junction; II: isolated soft-tissue recession that extends to or beyond the mucogingival junction with intact interdental papillae and no bone loss; III: sof-tissue recession extending beyond the mucogingival junction with bone or soft-tissue loss in the interdental area; and IV: extensive soft-tissue recession and bone loss or soft-tissue loss in the interdental area with malpositioned teeth.

Types of Soft-Tissue Grafts

Mucogingival defects are corrected using different types of soft-tissue grafts. In addition, guided tissue regeneration procedures also may be used for this purpose.

PEDICLE GRAFT OR LATERALLY POSITIONED FLAP The pedicle graft, as the name implies, is used to move gingiva from an adjacent tooth or edentulous area to a prepared recipient site on another tooth with an inadequate amount

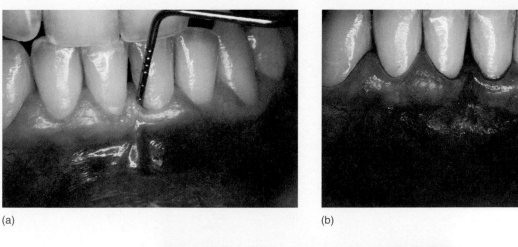

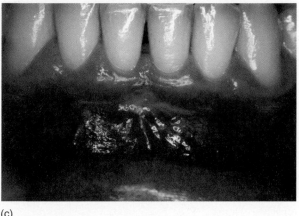

(a)

(b)

(c)

FIGURE 25–15 Frenectomy: (a) Note the lack of attached gingiva on the central incisors and the high frenum attachment that was pulling on the gingival margin. (b) A frenectomy using a split-thickness flap was performed. The frenectomy cuts the frenum, allowing it to relocate further apically. (c) One month postoperative.

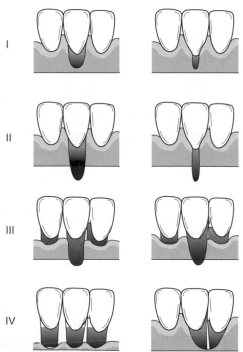

I

II

III

IV

FIGURE 25–16 P. D. Miller's classification of gingival recession.

of attached gingiva. The pedicle graft is "freed" on three aspects but retains its attachment (blood supply) from its base. This procedure requires sufficient width and thickness of gingiva to be present in the donor site. There should be no underlying bone dehiscence or fenestration. The pedicle graft is best used for single-site recession for root coverage and augmentation (increasing the amount) of attached gingiva.

Technique. A V-shaped incision is made around the recipient site (Figure 25–17 ■). Incised tissue is removed, and root planing of the root surface is performed. A full- or split-thickness flap is elevated on the tooth away from the defect and rotated to cover the defect. The flap is sutured, and pressure is applied (this is done with all soft-tissue grafts) for about 4 to 5 minutes, ensuring that no blood clot has formed under the graft. A periodontal dressing to protect the flap can be placed. If a periodontal dressing is not used, the patient should not brush the area. Postoperative instructions are given to the patient (see Table 25–1), and the patient returns 1 to 2 weeks later. At the first postoperative visit, the sutures and the dressing are removed, and the area either may be left uncovered or may be redressed for an additional week.

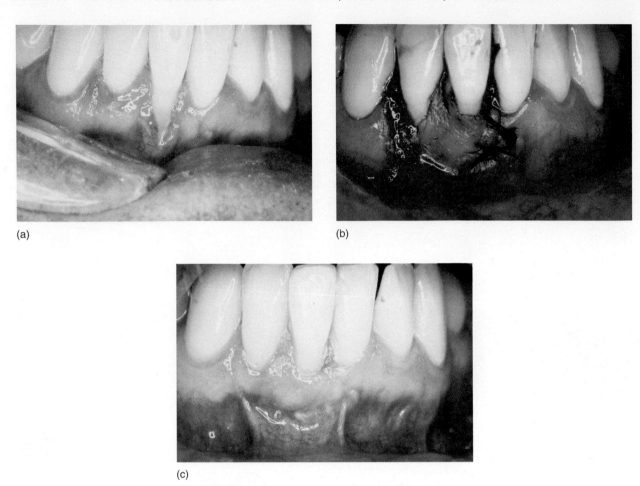

(a)

(b)

(c)

FIGURE 25–17 (a) Lateral incisor with severe gingival recession with root exposure. (b) A laterally positioned flap was used to move gingiva from the right central incisor to the left central incisor. An anchor suture is around the lateral incisor. (c) Two months healing shows good root coverage and increased width of attached gingiva.

Healing. Usually, clinical healing occurs in about 1 month. However, complete maturation can take up to 1 year.

DOUBLE PAPILLAE FLAP The double papillae flap is a modification of the laterally positioned flap. The papillae from each side of the tooth with the defect are reflected and rotated over the midfacial aspect of the recipient tooth and sutured.

FREE GINGIVAL SOFT-TISSUE GRAFT Unlike a pedicle graft, a free gingival graft (FGG) has a donor site located away from the grafted site. Thus, the blood supply is not attached to the graft but depends on the recipient bed. The most common site for donor tissue is the palate, but in many cases, edentulous areas also can be used. Free gingival grafts are more predictable for augmentation of attached gingiva than for root coverage because significant shrinkage of the graft occurs during healing. Thicker free gingival grafts can be used for root coverage because there is less tissue shrinkage. Often, after a frenectomy a free gingival graft is placed at the site to prevent frenum reattachment.

Technique. After local anesthesia is administered on the palate and the recipient area, split-thickness flaps are reflected at the recipient site (Figure 25–18 ■). A piece of gingiva about 1.5 mm thick is obtained from an intraoral area. Although the most common donor site is the hard palate, edentulous areas also can be used. The donor tissue (graft) is placed on the recipient bed, and the graft is sutured in place, usually with absorbable sutures, making sure that it does not move, because this will interfere with the establishment of a blood supply from the recipient bed and the graft may fail. A periodontal dressing may be applied. Postoperative instructions are given, and the patient returns in 1 week (see Table 25–1). Smoking is strictly prohibited because soft-tissue grafts are more likely to fail if the patient smokes. This was demonstrated by Miller (1987), where he found a 100% correlation between failure to obtain root coverage and heavy smoking. A major disadvantage of free gingival grafts is the poor color match between the graft and the existing gingiva.

Healing. The graft will swell initially, then shrinkage occurs (Figure 25–18d). The graft receives blood and nutrients

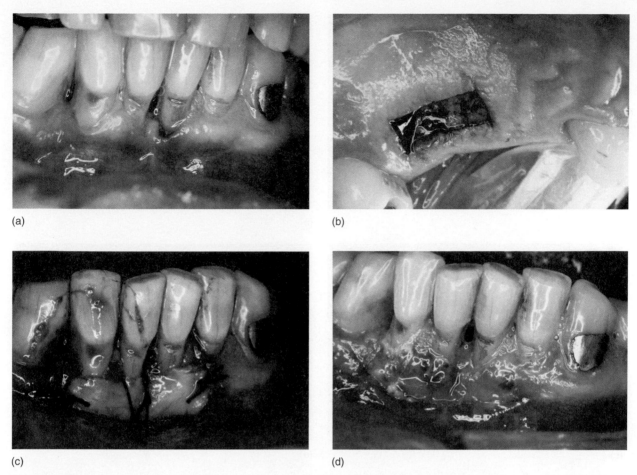

(a)

(b)

(c)

(d)

FIGURE 25–18 (a) Mandibular central and right lateral incisors have no attached gingiva (Miller classification III). (b) A free gingival graft was harvested from the palate and (c) sutured into place at the recipient site. (d) Posttreatment healing of the grafted site. Increased width of attached gingiva was achieved. Note that root coverage was not obtained using this type of grafting procedure.

from the underlying connective tissue. Complete healing with keratinization occurs in about 1 month.

SUBEPITHELIAL CONNECTIVE TISSUE GRAFT The subepithelial connective tissue graft (SCTG) is the procedure of choice for root coverage of single or multiple teeth. The subepithelial connective tissue graft was first described by Langer and Calagna (1982) as having several advantages over the other grafts: (1) There is no open wound on the palate as in a free gingival graft, (2) the graft has a better blood supply coming from both the underlying connective tissue and the overlaying flap, and (3) better aesthetics and tissue and color blend are seen. A recent meta-analysis of randomized controlled clinical trials concluded that SCTGs have the best predictability for complete root coverage (Chambrone, Pannuti, Tu, & Chambrone, 2012).

Indications. The subepithelial connective tissue graft may be used for both single and multiple adjacent teeth with gingival recession and root exposure (Chambrone & Chambrone, 2006). It is limited by the amount of donor tissue able to be harvested.

Rapid Dental Hint

The free gingival graft donor site will heal by secondary intention (open wound). It may be painful.

Technique. After local anesthesia is obtained, a split-thickness flap is raised at the recipient site using a surgical blade (Figures 25–19 ■, 25–20 ■). A flap is raised at the donor site on the palate, and connective tissue is harvested while leaving the epithelium on the outside of the flap. This palatal flap is sutured into place. The connective tissue is placed on the recipient site and sutured in place with absorbable sutures. A periodontal dressing may be applied. Postoperative instructions are given to the patient, and the patient returns in 1 to 2 weeks (see Table 25–1). At 1 to 2 weeks, the dressing and sutures are removed, and the area is either left uncovered or redressed for another week.

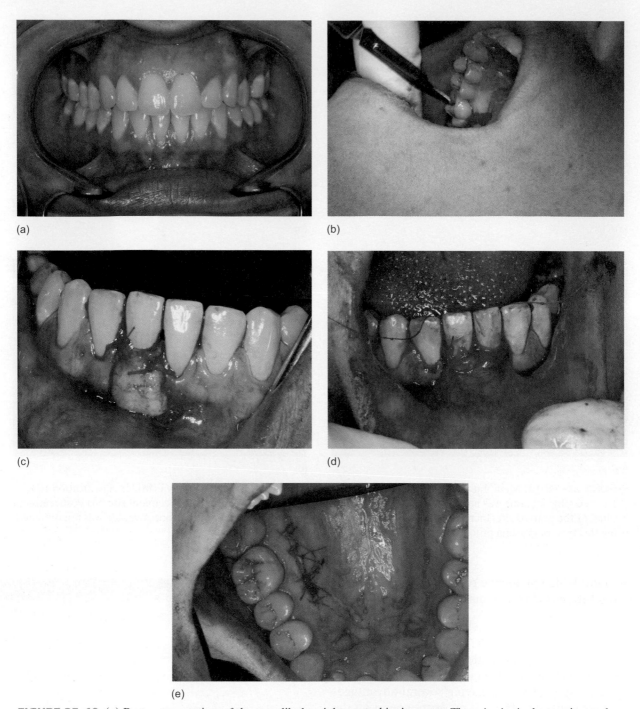

FIGURE 25–19 (a) Pretreatment view of the mandibular right central incisor area. There is gingival recession and exposed root surfaces (Miller classification II). A connective tissue graft was selected to cover the root surfaces. (b) The subepithelial connective tissue graft was harvested from the palate. Incisions were made, and the epithelium was reflected. Note the vascular connective tissue underlying the epithelium. (c and d) The graft was sutured to the recipient site and the flap sutured. (e) Flap at donor site is sutured. (Courtesy of Dr. Jesse Sorrentino, New York University College of Dentistry.)

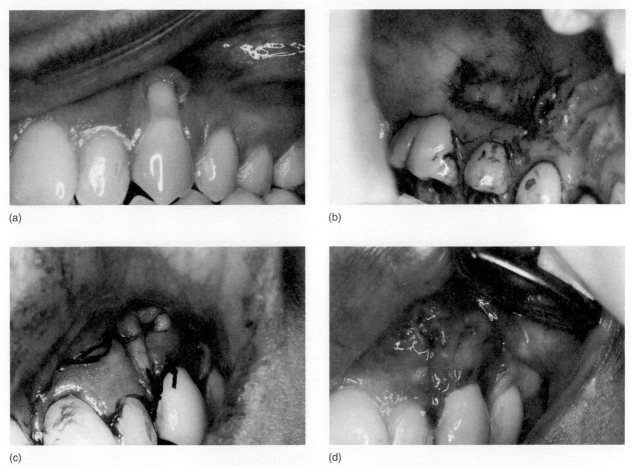

(a)

(b)

(c)

(d)

FIGURE 25–20 (a) Pretreatment view of the maxillary canine. Miller classification II. Gingival recession occurs beyond the mucogingival junction. The patient complained that the area was sensitive to cold and was not aesthetic. (b) Incisions made on the palate to obtain subepithelial connective tissue. This is the donor site. (c) The connective tissue graft is sutured in placed and then covered by the flap. (d) Healing at 2 weeks. (Courtesy of Dr. James B. Fine, Columbia University College of Dental Medicine.)

Healing. Healing occurs through a double blood supply. Both the connective tissue from the recipient site and the overlying flap aid in healing of the soft-tissue graft. Complete healing occurs in approximately 1 month (Figure 25–20d).

GUIDED TISSUE REGENERATION FOR ROOT COVERAGE
Guided tissue regeneration (GTR) will be discussed further in Chapter 26. Essentially, GTR involves the use of a barrier membrane that is designed to prevent the gingival tissue from establishing contact with the root surface, creating a space for the formation of a new attachment and new bone rather than a long junctional epithelial attachment. This concept was intended originally for the treatment of class II buccal furcation defects and certain infrabony defects. A newer application is for the treatment of gingival recession and for root coverage (Pini Prato et al., 1992).

Alloderm® is a biomaterial that is processed from human tissue. The process removes all epidermal and dermal cells (acellular dermal matrix), while preserving the remaining biological dermal matrix. All cells are removed to remove the risk of rejection or inflammation. This material is indicated for recession defects and for periodontal sites that have little to no attached gingiva where the goal is to increase the amount of keratinized/attached gingiva and to obtain root coverage (Gapski, Parks, & Wang, 2005; Tal, Moses, Zohar, Meir, & Nemcovsky, 2002).

AlloDerm is used in a similar way that a tissue graft from the patient's mouth (e.g., free gingival graft or connective tissue graft) is used, except there is no harvesting of donor tissue (e.g., palatal tissue) and thus less pain is involved. At the time of surgery, AlloDerm is rehydrated in sterile saline before it is sutured in place on the recipient bed. AlloDerm acts like a scaffold to support regeneration of the patient's own tissue. Six to 8 months postsurgery, AlloDerm becomes integrated into the patient's own soft tissue. A surgical case using AlloDerm is presented in Figure 25–21 ■.

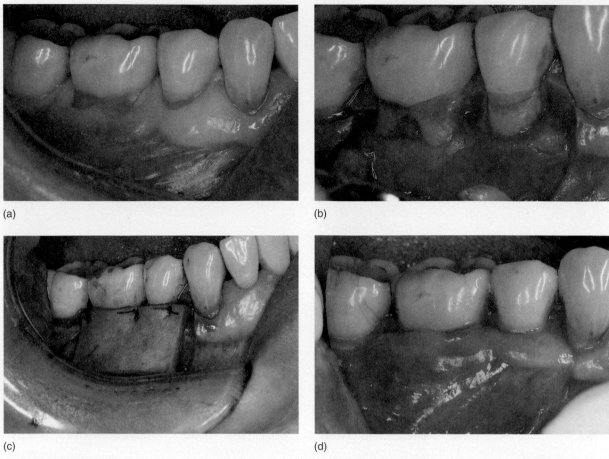

(a)   (b)

(c)   (d)

FIGURE 25–21 (a) Preoperative view of the mandibular right quadrant. Note the gingival recession (Miller Classification I). (b) Flap reflected exposing underlying bone. (c) Placement of AlloDerm at recipient site. Flap sutured in place, covering the AlloDerm. (d) Three weeks postop. Note the root coverage obtained.

A clinical study showed that treatment with a coronally positioned graft plus AlloDerm significantly increased gingival thickness when compared with a coronally positioned flap alone. Coverage of a recession defect was significantly improved with the use AlloDerm (Woodyard et al., 2004).

Technique. After local anesthesia is obtained, a full-thickness flap is raised at the recipient site. Root planing is completed on the root surface. A barrier membrane is placed over the recession and bone and sutured. The flap is positioned coronally covering both the membrane and the enamel. If the membrane is resorbable, it is not removed and will resorb in about 6 to 8 weeks after surgery. The flap sutures are removed after 2 to 4 weeks. Patients should not brush the area for at least 6 weeks and are recommended to rinse with chlorhexidine gluconate.

Sutures

Sutures are used to co-apt or closely adapt a flap to a tooth surface until the wound has healed sufficiently to withstand normal functional stresses. Closure of the wound provides good hemostasis and covers exposed bone. Suture material is broadly classified as absorbable or nonabsorbable and synthetic or nonsynthetic. Absorbable sutures are absorbed by the healing tissues by the breakdown process of hydrolysis (a process by which water gradually penetrates the suture filaments, causing the breakdown of the suture's polymer chain) or proteolysis (a process by which the suture filaments are absorbed by protein [salivary] enzymes and then digested by body enzymes). Nonabsorbable sutures do not get absorbed and remain in the tissues until removed (Table 25–2 ■).

Absorbable Sutures

Surgical gut is a natural material from the intestines of sheep or cows and is absorbable. Surgical gut is not too strong and is hard to handle, getting knotted easily. Chromic gut is plain gut that has been treated with chromic salts, which makes it more resistant to absorption. Through proteolysis, enzymes in saliva will absorb surgical gut sutures within 7 to 10 days and chromic gut in about 14 days. However, depending on the patient's saliva, sutures may still be seen up to 2 to 4 weeks later.

The other type of absorbable suture is synthetic. These sutures are easier to handle, the knot will not loosen easily,

Table 25–2 Suture Materials Used in Periodontics

Material	Synthetic/Nonsynthetic	Product Name
Nonabsorbable Sutures		
Silk	Nonsynthetic (natural)	PERMA-HAND Black Silk
Nylon	Synthetic	Ethilon
Polyester	Synthetic	Ethibond Green polyester
e-PTFE (expanded polytetrafluoroethylene)	Synthetic	Gore-Tex
Absorbable Sutures		
Plain gut	Natural	Plain gut
Chromic gut	Natural	Chromic gut
PGA (Polyglycolic acid)	Synthetic	Absorbex
PGA-FA (FA refers to fast absorption)	Synthetic	PGA-FA
Poliglecaprone 25	Synthetic	Monocryl
Polygalactin 910	Synthetic	Vicryl

and they cause less tissue irritation and inflammation than surgical gut because of the more reliable, constant rate of absorption through hydrolysis. Resorption of sutures begins between 10 and 15 days and is usually completed in 28 to 70 days.

Nonabsorbable Sutures

Silk, a type of nonabsorbable natural suture, is the most frequently used suture material because of its ease in handling and superior visibility. Silk sutures can elicit tissue inflammation, so they should be removed not later than 10 days after surgery. If sutures need to be left in place for several weeks, absorbable sutures are recommended.

Rapid Dental Hint

It is important to obtain hemostasis (stoppage of bleeding) before suturing.

Needles

Needle and suture material come in various sizes. Needles also are classified according to their shape and curvature. Needles are available in a 1/4-, 3/8-, 1/2-, and 5/8-inch circle, with 3/8- or 1/2-inch being used most commonly in periodontal surgery. Suture size is classified numerically. An increase in the number indicates a decrease in the diameter of the suture. Thus 4-0 and 3-0 sutures are used most often in periodontal flap surgery. The 6-0 and 5-0 sutures are smaller and are used in more delicate mucogingival surgical procedures such as soft-tissue grafts (Hutchens, 1995).

Suturing Techniques

Suturing technique varies among surgeons. Basically, there are different ways to tie the suture. The most common and simplest suture is the interrupted suture, which is tied with a square or surgeon's knot (Figure 25–22 ■). After the needle engages the buccal and lingual gingiva, it should be tied on the buccal rather than the lingual so that it is easier to remove, and the sutures are in a more protected area. When tying a suture, leave about a 2 mm end. Other types of sutures include continuous sutures,

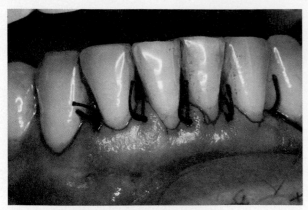

FIGURE 25–22 Interrupted (simple loop) sutures (interproximal) using 4-0 silk.

mattress sutures, and sling sutures (Figure 25–23 ■). Mattress technique is usually used in areas where tension-free flap closure cannot be accomplished (Silverstein, 1999). Mattress suturing techniques generally are used to resist muscle pull and to adapt the tissue flaps tightly to the underlying structures (e.g., bone graft, tissue graft, alveolar ridge, regenerative membrane, or dental implant; Silverstein and Kurtzman, 2005). Continuous sutures can

Did You Know?

Natural materials doctors used in ancient times were flax, hair, grass, cotton, silk, pig bristles, and animal gut.

Rapid Dental Hint

Remember to knot the suture from the buccal because it is easier to see and remove later.

Did You Know?

Suture manufacturing comes under the control of the Food and Drug Administration (FDA) because sutures are classified as medical devices.

be used to attach two surgical flap edges or to secure multiple interproximal papillae of one flap independent of the other flap (Silverstein and Kurtzman, 2005). The disadvantage of using continuous sutures is that there is only one knot, and if the knot or loop breaks, the entire surgical site will be compromised.

The number of sutures placed should be documented in the chart. When the patient returns for the postoperative visit, count the number of sutures before removing them. This will verify that all sutures were removed. Sutures should be removed by gently holding the knot with collage pliers in your nondominant hand while using scissors to cut the suture by the knot. The suture is then gently pulled through the tissue to remove it.

Periodontal Dressing

In today's clinical practice, periodontal dressings are of the noneugenol type that does not cause irritation or burning to the tissue or bone. The primary purpose of using a periodontal dressing over a surgical area is for patient comfort. Periodontal dressings also protect the wound area after surgery. Some practitioners prefer not to use a dressing because the dressing creates an anaerobic (nonoxygen) area under itself that favors the growth of pathogenic microorganisms. However, this theory has not been proven.

The most widely used noneugenol dressing is a COE-pak® (GC America, Inc., Alsip, IL). It is supplied in two tubes: the accelerator tube and the base tube. Equal amounts of dressing from each tube are mixed for 30 to 45 seconds. In the hard and fast set, the working time is about 5 to 8 minutes; in the regular set, it is 10 to 15 minutes.

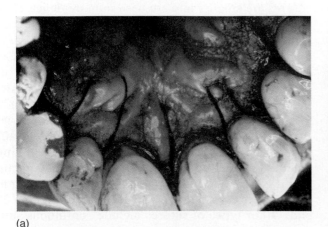
(a)

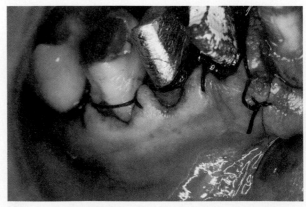
(b)

FIGURE 25–23 (a) Horizontal mattress suture using 4-0 silk. (b) Continuous suture using one knot.

The material is then formed into a strip. Hemostasis should be achieved before the dressing is applied, and the area should be dried. The end of the facial strip is wrapped around the distal aspect of the last tooth and meets with the lingual strip. Finger pressure is applied interproximally to wedge the dressing into place. A dressing placed on a surgical site should not overextend onto the gingiva, vestibule, or occlusal surfaces (Figure 25–24 ■). Any excess dressing should be trimmed with a curet.

A light-cured periodontal dressing is available (Barricaid™, Dentsply International, Inc., Milford, DE). It is transparent and is used frequently on anterior areas where aesthetics are a concern. The material is first applied to the area (which does not necessarily have to be completely dry) and then is light-cured.

Surgical and Postoperative Care

The dental hygienist plays an important role in the postoperative care of patients.

Surgical Complications

Syncope is defined as a temporary loss of consciousness caused by a loss of blood flow to the brain. Patients have been known to faint before, during, or after surgical procedures. If a patient faints, treatment should be stopped and the patient positioned with the head lower than the body. The patient's vital signs, including blood pressure, respiration, and pulse, should be monitored. Oxygen can be administered if necessary. Causes for patient syncope include fear or anxiety about the procedure, the sight of blood, pain, or low blood sugar.

Rapid Dental Hint

Sometimes putting petrolatum (Vaseline) on your fingers will help prevent the dressing from sticking.

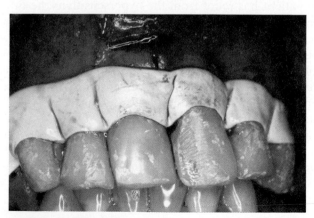

FIGURE 25–24 Placement of a periodontal dressing. The packing should not interfere with occlusion or impinge on the gingiva.

Immediately after the administration of a local anesthetic containing epinephrine, patients may complain of a fast heartbeat or begin to shake or shiver. This is caused by the inadvertent injection of the anesthetic solution into a vein rather than a nerve. Keep the patient calm by reassuring that this will pass very soon and in most cases the patient will be fine. To prevent this situation, it is essential to aspirate while injecting.

During periodontal surgery, bleeding will occur because blood vessels are severed and the diseased tissue is vascular. Small blood vessels will be severed or broken when making incisions. However, it is important not to sever certain arteries such as the greater palatine artery in the maxillary palatal area. Once the diseased tissue is removed and the flaps are raised, bleeding should diminish. Excessive bleeding is controlled by finding the source of the bleeding and applying pressure by administering a vasoconstrictor (e.g., lidocaine 2% with 1:50,000 epinephrine) or by tying the offending artery.

It is important to avoid unnecessary or excessive hemorrhaging or bleeding. The patient's medical history should be evaluated carefully and updated to help avoid these situations. For example, a patient may be taking aspirin every day or even several times a week as a preventive measure for stroke. Aspirin (acetylsalicylic acid) binds to platelets and inhibits the formation of prostaglandins, resulting in a prolonged bleeding time that lasts for approximately 7 days, until new platelets are formed. A similar situation occurs with nonsteroidal anti-inflammatory drugs such as ibuprofen. It is best to consult with such a patient's physician before performing surgery for patients taking these drugs.

Postoperative Complications

After periodontal surgery, the patient is given a number of written suggestions and instructions. These instructions must be reviewed carefully with the patient before he or she is allowed to leave the office. An example of postoperative patient instructions is given in Table 25–1. During the first postoperative week, the patient may experience swelling, pain, and sensitivity; these are usually mild and transient. Swelling generally can be controlled by the use of ice packs for the first day. An ice pack should be applied extraorally 20 minutes on and 20 minutes off for the first day. If swelling continues, the patient should switch to warm packs. Swelling can be due to soft-tissue inflammation from the surgical procedure or an infection. If swelling continues, advise the patient to return to the office. Pain is usually due to swelling. If there is severe pain, the patient should return to the office. The patient may be given systemic antibiotics and analgesics (pain medication). The dental hygienist should confirm that the patient is taking the appropriate medications as prescribed. The patient should be asked if he or she is taking any over-the-counter medications, vitamins, or herbal remedies.

The patient may complain of seeing blood in the mouth for a few hours after the surgery. Most of the time this is residual blood in the saliva probably remaining on the tongue after surgery. If there is frank bleeding coming from the surgical site, the patient should apply pressure to the site and return to the office as soon as possible. Rinsing should not be done because it will prevent a blood clot from forming.

Oral Hygiene Instructions

Maintenance of the surgical area is important, and the dental hygienist must instruct the client on proper care (see Table 25–1). It has been demonstrated that regardless of the type of surgery performed (i.e., gingivectomy, MWF, or osseous recontouring), all will fail and probing depths recur if plaque control is not meticulously controlled following surgery (Nyman, Lindhe, & Rosling, 1977). Vigorous toothbrushing and flossing should not be done until healing is complete, yet it must be stressed to patients that removal of dental plaque is important for healing. The period of time the patient refrains from toothbrushing varies with each surgeon. While a periodontal dressing is in place, the patient should not brush that area. Rinsing with chlorhexidine gluconate is recommended. After the dressing and sutures are removed, patients are instructed to brush gently with a roll technique. Gradually, as healing occurs, regular brushing can be resumed. After surgery, the interdental papillae are usually absent or blunted, creating large gingival embrasures. Plaque removal in these areas is best accomplished with an interdental brush (single-tuft brush). Also, plaque removal on teeth with Class III/IV furcation involvement is best with a single-tuft brush. If no large interdental spaces develop after surgery, the patient can continue to use dental floss or a small interdental brush.

Postoperative Visit Management

The dental hygienist may be called on to attend to a patient at the first postoperative visit. Box 25–2 describes various reevaluation procedures that may be performed at this visit. At the 7- to 10-day postoperative visit, the dressing and sutures are removed. After the dressing is carefully removed, the number of sutures are counted and compared with the number of documented sutures placed at the time of the surgery. Frequently, parts of or all of the periodontal dressing may have come off during the week. When the dressing is removed, care must be taken not to pull the sutures. If the sutures are being pulled by the dressing, cut the interfering sutures before the dressing is further removed. Once the dressing is removed, a white layer can be seen on the tissue surface. This represents dead epithelial cells. A moistened (with water, saline, or chlorhexidine) cotton-tipped applicator is used to carefully cleanse the area. Following suture removal, the area is again thoroughly irrigated with water or saline. Only supragingival debridement should be performed; subgingival debridement should be postponed

until complete healing has occurred. The decision to apply another dressing to the area depends on the amount of discomfort the patient is experiencing and the rate of healing.

Effects of Surgical Procedures

As a consequence of surgery, several problems may arise. Patients should be informed about these adverse side effects before surgery. All patients also should sign an informed consent form.

Tooth Mobility

Tooth mobility may increase immediately after surgery and may not return to preoperative levels for as long as 6 months. The patient should be told that this is a normal consequence of surgery. Increased tooth mobility is due to the extension of inflammation into the periodontal ligament and to the surgical manipulation. The occlusion should be checked to verify that there is no occlusal trauma. Any occlusal interferences should be eliminated. Check for fremitus to help determine occlusal interferences.

Gingival Recession: Dentinal Hypersensitivity and Root Caries

Gingival recession with longer clinical crowns may occur after surgery. With exposure of the root surface, the patient may experience dentinal hypersensitivity and can develop root caries due to demineralization.

Maintaining adequate plaque control can reduce both the sensitivity and risk for root caries. For immediate hypersensitivity relief, an in-office application of DentinBloc® (Colgate Oral Pharmaceuticals, New York) or Seal and Protect® (Dentsply, Pa) is done. Other in-office desensitizing products are available, including chemical agents (oxalates, fluorides), sealants, and bonding agents. Reducing plaque accumulation is important for reducing hypersensitivity.

It is also helpful for the patient to use at home a dentifrice containing potassium nitrate (Sensodyne®). Unfortunately, the use of dentifrices is controversial, and they may take several weeks to have a positive effect. Once the patient has relief from the hypersensitivity, he or she can start to use the regular dentifrice but should return to the desensitizing dentifrice if the sensitivity returns. An over-the-counter 0.4% stannous fluoride gel (Gel-Kam®, Colgate Oral Pharmaceuticals) that is applied to the toothbrush may reduce dentinal hypersensitivity and prevent demineralization of the exposed root surfaces. A 0.63% stannous fluoride oral rinse (Gel-Kam® Oral Care Rinse, Colgate Oral Pharmaceuticals) is available by prescription for patient use at home. Adverse effects of stannous fluoride include staining of the dentin and stinging of the soft tissue.

Dental Hygiene Application

The range of treatment alternatives for periodontitis is wide. The type of treatment depends on a number of factors, including the patient's level of plaque control, the type of gingival or periodontal pocket, and the type of periodontal defect. Careful assessment and planning of a case are important in the overall surgical treatment.

Key Points

- Periodontal flap surgery is indicated for increasing access to the underlying root and bone in deeper periodontal pockets.
- The patient must be able to maintain excellent plaque control before periodontal surgery is performed.
- The therapeutic clinical end point of success for surgical pocket therapy is an oral environment that is easily maintainable by the patient and the clinician; there should be minimal inflammation (bleeding) and minimal probing depths.

- Cigarette smoking adversely affects the outcome of surgery.

Self-Quiz

1. All of the following factors are indications for periodontal surgery except one:
   a. Maintain teeth with a hopeless prognosis
   b. Pocket elimination
   c. Arrest disease progression
   d. Gain access to underlying bone

2. Which one of the following healing responses is usually seen after periodontal flap surgery?
   a. New bone, cementum, and periodontal ligament
   b. New bone and cementum
   c. Long junctional epithelium
   d. Connective tissue attachment

3. Which one of the following surgical procedures is indicated for gingival enlargement in a patient who is taking phenytoin?
   a. Mucogingival
   b. Gingivectomy
   c. Periodontal flap
   d. Excisional new attachment

4. When placing sutures, the knot is usually tied on the palatal surface because this is a protected area.
   a. Both the statement and the reason are correct and related.
   b. Both the statement and the reason are correct but not related.
   c. The statement is correct, but the reason is not.
   d. The statement is not correct, but the reason is correct.
   e. Neither the statement nor the reason is correct.

5. After periodontal surgery, which one of the following hygiene aids is best recommended to clean exposed furcations?
   a. Dental floss
   b. Manual toothbrush
   c. Powered toothbrush
   d. Single-tuft brush

6. Which one of the following surgical procedures is best recommended for augmenting the amount of attached gingiva and covering exposed root surfaces before a patient undergoes orthodontic treatment?
   a. Gingivectomy
   b. Connective tissue graft
   c. Modified Widman flap
   d. Crown lengthening

7. Which one of the following immediate measures should be advised to a patient who calls the office 2 days after periodontal surgery and states that he or she has bleeding from the surgical site?
   a. Rinse with warm saltwater
   b. Lie down on a couch
   c. Remove the packing
   d. Apply pressure

8. Which of the following is the primary objective of periodontal flap surgery?
   a. Gain access to the bone and root surface
   b. Augment the amount of free gingiva
   c. Provide easy-to-maintain areas
   d. Allow for healing by regeneration

9. A patient has experienced some root sensitivity in the area of flap surgery. Which one of the following recommendations can the dental hygienist make to alleviate the pain?
   a. Floss the area
   b. Rinse with a nonfluoride mouth rinse
   c. Rinse and brush with a baking soda solution
   d. Meticulous plaque control

10. All the following are adverse effects the patient should be informed about before periodontal surgery is performed except one. Which one is the exception?
   a. Dentinal hypersensitivity
   b. Gingival recession
   c. Tooth mobility
   d. Root caries
   e. Open bite

Case Study

A 45-year-old male has treatment planned for periodontal surgery to reduce the pocket depths and recontour the bony defects. He smokes a pack of cigarettes a day, has poor home care, and generalized chronic periodontitis. He is scheduled for an initial series of dental hygiene visits including one postoperative the surgery.

1. What factor is a consideration for this patient in preoperative preparation?
   a. noncompliant with plaque control
   b. smoking may delay healing
   c. calculus may not have been totally removed in scaling
   d. A and B
   e. all of the above

Answer: E. All are considerations for a better prognosis. The surgery may access the root to remove the remaining calculus. Smoking is a consideration in healing and the patient should be advised to quit. Poor home care may permit repopulation of bacteria.

2. What postoperative instruction might be given?
   a. rinse with warm salt water twice daily
   b. do not drink hot liquids for 12 hours
   c. apply pressure to stop bleeding
   d. brush and floss all areas as normal

Answer: C. Apply pressure to stop bleeding and call the office if continues. Do not rinse until second day and then with prescribed mouthrinse. Do not floss site until directed. Do not drink hot liquids for 48 hours.

3. After surgery the gingival margin is more apical and some recession has occurred to expose the cementum. What might the dental hygienist consider in a treatment?
   a. surgery needs to be redone for grafting
   b. desensitizing dentifrice
   c. splint for stability
   d. periodontal dressing for additional week.

Answer: B. The exposed cementum may be sensitive and desensitizing office treatment, toothpaste, or rinses may be provided. Periodontal dressing is placed immediately after surgery if needed for wound protection. Recession is an expected result in some surgeries. Splints relate to mobility which was not indicated in the data.

References

American Academy of Periodontology. 2001. *Glossary of periodontal terms*, 4th ed. Chicago: Author.

American Academy of Periodontology. 2006. Position paper: Lasers in periodontics: A review of the literature. *J. Periodontol.* 77:545–564.

Blomlof, L., L. Jansson, H. Ehnevid, and S. Lindskog. 1997. Prognosis and mortality of root-resected molars. *Int. J. Periodontics Restorative Dent.* 17(2):190–201.

Bosco, A. F., S. Bonfante, D. S. Luize, G. M. D. Bosco, and V. G. Garcia. 2006. Periodontal plastic surgery associated with treatment for the removal of gingival overgrowth. *J. Periodontol.* 77(5):922–928.

Boström, L., L. E. Linder, and J. Bergström. 1998. Influence of smoking on the outcome of periodontal surgery: A 5-year follow-up. *J. Clin. Periodontol.* 25:194–201.

Carranza, F. A., Jr. 1996. The surgical phase of therapy. In eds. F. A. Carranza, Jr., and M. G. Newman, *Clinical Periodontology* 565–569, 584–587. Philadelphia: W. B. Saunders.

Chambrone, L., C. M. Pannuti, Y. Tu, and L. A. Chambrone. 2012. Evidence-based periodontal plastic surgery: II. An individual data meta-analysis for evaluating factors in achieving complete root coverage. *J. Periodontol.* 83:477–490.

Chambrone, L. A., and L. Chambrone. 2006. Subepithelial connective tissue grafts in the treatment of multiple recession-type defects. *J. Periodontol.* 77(5):909–916.

Deas, D. E., A. J. Moritz, H. T. McDonnell, et al. 2004. Osseous surgery for crown lengthening: A 6-month clinical study. *J. Periodontol.* 75(9):1288–1294.

Egelberg, J. 1995. Effectiveness of subgingival scaling and root planning. In *Periodontics the scientic way. Synopses of human clinical studies*, 2nd ed., 71–90. Malmo, Sweden: OdontosSience.

Flores-de-Jacoby, L., and R. Mengel. 1995. Conventional surgical procedures. *Periodontology 2000*. 9:38–54.

Gapski, R., C. A. Parks, and H. L. Wang. 2005. Acellular dermal matrix for mucogingival surgery: A meta-analysis. *J. Periodontol.* 76(11):1814–1822.

Greenstein, G. 2000. Nonsurgical periodontal therapy in 2000. A literature review. *J. Am. Dent. Assoc.* 131:1580–1592.

Gürgan, C. A., A. M. Oruç, and M. Akkaya. 2004. Alterations in location of the mucogingival junction 5 years after coronally positioned flap surgery. *J. Periodontol.* 75(6):893–901.

Hutchens, J. L., Jr. 1995. Periodontal suturing: A review of needles, material, and techniques. *Postgrad. Dent.* 2(4):3–14.

Lang, N. P., and H. Löe. 1993. Clinical management of periodontal diseases. *Periodontology 2000* 2:128–139.

Langer, B., and L. Calagna. 1982. The subepithelial connective tissue graft: A new approach to the enhancement of anterior cosmetics. *Int. J. Periodont. Rest. Dent.* 2:22–23.

Miller, P. D. 1985. A classification of marginal tissue recession. *Int. J. Periodont. Rest. Dent.* 5:15–37.

Miller, P. D. 1987. Root coverage with free gingival grafts. Factors associated with incomplete coverage. *J. Periodontol.* 58:674–681.

Nyman, S., J. Lindhe, and B. Rosling. 1977. Periodontal surgery in plaque infected dentitions. *J. Clin. Periodontol.* 4:240–249.

Palcanis, K. G. 1996. Surgical pocket therapy. *Ann. Periodontol.* 1:589–617.

Perez, J. R., H. Smukler, and M. E. Nunn. 2007. Clinical evaluation of the supraosseous gingivae before and after crown lengthening. *J. Periodontol.* 78(6):1023–1030.

Persson, G. R., L. A. Mand, J. Martin, and R. Page. 2003. Assessing periodontal disease risk. *J. Am. Dent. Assoc.* 134(5):575–582.

Pini Prato, G., C. Clauser, P. Cortellini, C. Tinti, G. Vincenzi, and U. Pagliaro. 1992. Guided tissue regeneration versus mucogingival surgery in the treatment of human buccal gingival recession. *J. Periodontol.* 63:919–928.

Preber, H., and J. Bergström. 1990. Effect of cigarette smoking on periodontal healing following surgical therapy. *J. Clin. Periodontol.* 17:324–328.

Ramfjord, S. P., and R. R. Nissle. 1974. The modified Widman flap. *J. Periodontol.* 45:601–607.

Salkin, L. M., A. L. Freedman, M. D. Stein, and N. A. Bassiouny. 1987. A longitudinal study of untreated mucogingival defects. *J. Periodontol.* 58:164–166.

Silverstein, L. H. 1999. *Principles of dental suturing: The complete guide to surgical closure*. Mahwah, NJ: Montage Media.

Silverstein, L. H., and G. M. Kurtzman. 2005. A review of dental suturing for optimal soft-tissue management. *Compendium* 2(3):163–169.

Sullivan, H. C., and J. H. Atkins. 1968. Free autogenous gingival grafts: I. Principles of successful grafting. *Periodontics* l6:121–129.

Tal, H., O. Moses, R. Zohar, H. Meir, and C. Nemcovsky. 2002. Root coverage of advanced gingival recession: A comparative study between acellular dermal matrix allograft and subepithelial connective tissue grafts. *J. Periodontol.* 73:1405–1411.

Wennström, J. L., and J. Lindhe. 1983. Role of attached gingiva for maintenance of periodontal health. *J. Clin. Periodontol.* 10:206–221.

Woodyard, J. G., H. Greenwell, M. Hill, C. Drisko, J. M. Iasella, and J. Scheetz. 2004. The clinical effects of acellular dermal matrix on gingival thickness and root coverage compared to coronally positioned flap alone. *J. Periodontol.* 75:44–56.

26

Principles of Periodontal Surgery: Periodontal Regeneration

Stuart J. Froum

OUTLINE

Introduction
Periodontal Regenerative Surgery
Biologics and Growth Factors
Bone Grafts and Bone Substitutes:
  Surgical Procedure
Guided Tissue Regeneration
Regenerative Surgery: Postoperative
  Care
Root Surface Treatment
Risk Factors for Regenerative
  Therapy
Dental Hygiene Application
Key Points
Self-Quiz
Case Study
References

EDUCATIONAL OBJECTIVES

Upon completion of this chapter, the reader should be able to:

- Describe the process of periodontal regeneration, including the type and origin of cells involved in the regenerative process.
- Describe the different bone grafts and bone substitutes that are used in periodontal regeneration.
- Discuss the role of enamel matrix protein derivatives and growth factors in regeneration of bony defects.
- Compare and contrast the different clinical procedures used to attain periodontal regeneration.

GOAL: To provide an understanding of the basic principles of periodontal surgical regeneration.

KEY WORDS

Introduction

The goals of periodontal therapy have long included arresting the disease process, preventing disease recurrence, and providing for the regeneration of periodontium lost as a result of the disease. Over the past four decades, great strides have been made in the field of periodontal regeneration. **Periodontal regeneration** is defined as healing after periodontal surgery that results in the reconstruction of lost tissues, including supporting alveolar bone, cementum, and a functionally oriented periodontal ligament (American Academy of Periodontology, 2001). Guided bone regeneration is defined as healing after periodontal surgery that results in the formation of only new bone and includes use of a barrier membrane. This procedure is usually performed to increase the height or width of bone before implant placement and is discussed in Chapter 27. This chapter provides a review of the various regenerative therapies and materials currently in use today (Box 26–1). Future directions in this ever-changing field also will be discussed. Techniques currently in use include open flap debridement, the use of bone grafts and bone substitutes, guided tissue regeneration, combination techniques, root surface treatment, and the use of biomimetics and growth factors.

Periodontal Regenerative Surgery

Objectives

Once inflammation of the gingiva is resolved with initial therapy (e.g., periodontal debridement and oral hygiene self-care instruction), the periodontitis component still must be treated. Periodontitis is characterized by apical migration of the junctional epithelium resulting in periodontal pocket formation, loss of clinical attachment (connective tissue fibers attached to the tooth surface), and alveolar bone loss. **Periodontal tissue regeneration** involves surgery using bone grafts, bone substitute materials, and/or barrier membranes, and modulators of tissue healing are aimed at regenerating the periodontal attachment apparatus lost due to periodontitis (Froum, Gomez, & Breault, 2001).

The primary goal of regenerating lost attachment is the preservation of the natural tooth . Secondary goals of using such bone-replacement materials as bone grafts and bone substitutes in infrabony defects include the following: (1) a reduction in probing depths, (2) a gain in clinical attachment level (this refers to a reduction in probing depth caused by decreased penetration of the probe at the base of the pocket), (3) filling of the osseous defects with new bone, and (4) regeneration of new supporting alveolar bone, new cementum, and a functionally oriented periodontal ligament (Brunsvold & Mellonig, 1993; Laurell, Bose, Graziani, Tonetti, & Berglundh, 2006; Schallhorn, 1977). The latter can only be determined by histologic examination of the healed periodontal tissues.

Regenerative surgery significantly differs from osseous resective procedures, in which the osseous (bony) walls are removed surgically to eliminate the intraosseous component of the defect. Often, the morphology of the defect requires the removal of too much bone to obtain complete elimination of the defect (parabolic interdental bone), which would further compromise the affected tooth. Periodontal regenerative surgery involves "adding" bone (bone fill) into the intraosseous defect instead of its removal. Certain bony defects are more amenable to regeneration than others (Table 26–1 ■). The type of periodontal defects that respond best to the use of bone grafts include three-wall, two-wall, and combination-type intraosseous defects. This is because the remaining bony walls contain and hold the bone graft in the defect. The depth and width of these infrabony type defects influence the amount of bone and connective tissue attachment gain. For example, an infrabony defect that is deep and narrow will most likely achieve better regeneration than a defect that is deep and wide (Tonetti, Pini Prato, & Cortellini, 1993). Moreover, the additional surrounding bony walls provide more surface area on which bone can form. Horizontal patterns of

Box 26–1: Procedures Used to Enhance Periodontal Regeneration

- Bone and bone substitute grafting to fill the periodontal defect

- Prevention or retardation of junctional epithelial down growth and selective cell repopulation: Guided tissue regeneration (GTR)

- Guided bone regeneration (GBR)

- Acid conditioning of the root surface

- Application of enamel matrix protein derivatives

- Growth factor application to promote specific cell proliferation

Rapid Dental Hint

To diagnosis an infrabony defect, the clinician must probe the area and evaluate the radiographs.

Rapid Dental Hint

Remember that an "infrabony" defect is the generic term used for a vertical defect in the alveolar bone, whereas an "intrabony" defect is a special type of three-wall defect with cancellous bone between the cortical lining and the cortical plate.

Table 26–1 Bony Defects: Response to Regeneration

Defects That Heal Best after Regeneration	Defects with a Lower Chance for Regeneration
Three-wall infrabony defect	One-wall infrabony defect
Class II buccal furcation involvement on mandibular molars	Class III furcation involvement
Deeper bony defects (deeper than 3 mm)	Shallower bony defects

Rapid Dental Hint

Class II buccal furcation defects and three-wall vertical bony defects are most amenable to regenerative procedures.

bone loss, loss of buccal or lingual plates of bone, and furcation defects cannot be treated predictably with bone graft and bone substitute materials alone. Furcation defects are more predictably treated with GTR. Class II buccal furcation defects on the mandibular molars are most predictable types of furcation defects for periodontal regeneration.

The following are different types of regenerative techniques.

Surgery: Open Flap Debridement

As a surgical technique, open flap debridement (OFD), in which a flap is reflected and the roots and pocket area are debrided without the addition of any bone or bone substitute material, has been used primarily as a control for comparison in assessing other treatment. In most histologic

studies, open flap debridement resulted in repair rather than regeneration of periodontal tissues. A greater recurrence of probing depth over time has been shown with open flap debridement alone (Smith, Ammons, & van Belle, 1980) when compared with traditional osseous resective procedures. A review of the literature shows that OFD results in an average clinical attachment level gain of 1.5 mm and average bone fill of 1.1 mm (Stahl, Froum, & Kushner, 1982).

Surgery: Bone Grafts and Bone Substitutes

Bone grafts and their substitutes are classified into four categories: **autografts**, **allografts**, **alloplasts**, and **xenografts**. **Bone grafts** refer to naturally occurring autografts and allografts (Hanes, 2007). Despite the benefits of autografts and allografts, the limitations of each have necessitated the pursuit of alternatives. Many of these alternatives, or **bone substitutes** (also referred to as bone replacement materials), can be synthetic (manufactured, not naturally occurring) materials (alloplasts), including natural and synthetic polymers and ceramics or natural and recombinant growth factors (Reynolds, Aichelmann-Reidy, & Branch-Mays, 2010; Christgau et al., 2006) or materials processed from the bone of other species (xenografts). Table 26–2 ■ describes the different types of bone graft materials.

Table 26–2 Types of Bone Grafts/Bone Replacement Materials

Name	Features
Autografts	Bone harvested from one part of the body and grafted to another part of the same patient's body. The bone can be obtained from an intraoral site such as the maxillary tuberosity area, edentulous area, chin, ramus, healing extraction site, or mandibular torus during implant placement or an extraoral site (e.g., tibia, femur). Osteogenic
Allografts	Bone material obtained from other individuals of the same species but genetically different. Donors include human cadavers. Allografts are obtained from bone banks. The main forms of bone allografts used in clinical practice are demineralized freeze-dried bone (DFDBA) and freeze-dried bone (FDBA). Osteoinductive
Alloplasts	Made of biocompatible, inorganic, inert materials including synthetic hydroxyapatite, calcium sulfate, bioactive glass, and tricalcium phosphate. Osteoconductive
Xenografts	A type of natural bone substitute derived from a genetically different species (e.g., bovine). Osteoinductive

AUTOGRAFTS (AUTOGENOUS GRAFTS) Autogenous bone is living bone derived directly from the patient's own body. This has shown the best potential of any of the bone fill material for periodontal regeneration and bone fill. This bone is often mixed with the patient's blood. However, when a sufficient amount of bone is not available intraorally, or if the patient does not want bone obtained from extraoral sites such as the hip, other materials must be considered. Autogenous bone has long been considered to be the gold standard of grafting materials in terms of stimulating new bone formation.

A bone blend is a mixture of cancellous and cortical bone. When cortical bone is mixed with the patient's blood, it becomes an osseous coagulum.

ALLOGRAFTS (ALLOGENEIC GRAFTS) Allografts such as demineralized freeze-dried bone (DFDBA) obtained from human cadavers have demonstrated bone-forming properties. Bone allografts are obtained from bone banks. The issue of safety (e.g., nontransmission of hepatitis, HIV, and other known diseases) when using allografts has been well established, thus minimizing this factor as a concern (Marx & Carlson, 1993; Mellonig, Preuett, & Moyer, 1992). Controlled clinical studies have shown greater bone fill in sites treated with DFDBA than in nongrafted controls, with DFDBA reporting a mean bone fill of 2.6 mm (65% defect fill) compared with 1.3 mm (30% defect fill) in nongrafted controls (Mellonig, 1984). A recent review of the literature concluded that both autogenous bone and DFDBA support the formation of a new attachment apparatus (Reynolds, Aichelmann-Reidy, Branch-Mays, & Gunsolley, 2003).

ALLOPLASTS (ALLOPLASTIC GRAFTS) Alloplastic bone substitutes are manufactured synthetic materials. They are classified as implant material. Alloplasts (implants) are differentiated from grafts, which are defined as "any tissue or organ used for implantation or transplantation" (Hallmon, Carranza, Drisko, Rapley, & Robinson, 1996). Advantages of alloplasts include zero risk of disease transmission as compared with allografts and no additional surgical sites required in the mouth or body to harvest bone (as with autografts). However, alloplasts are not as effective in forming bone as are graft materials. Alloplasts are inert (nonliving) materials acting as a bone "filler" in the defect, and when effective, they act as a scaffold for bone to form around them (osteoconductive).

A number of alloplastic materials have been introduced in an attempt to create a readily available material for bone fill of infrabony periodontal defects. Synthetic alloplasts may be divided into ceramic and nonceramic categories. These may be further divided into absorbable and nonabsorbable materials. Absorbable materials will absorb or dissolve (it may take years) and be replaced with new bone, whereas nonabsorbable grafts may never absorb. Ceramic alloplasts are materials that include calcium phosphate such as hydroxyapatite and tricalcium phosphate. The most commonly used ceramic materials are nonporous hydroxyapatite, porous hydroxyapatite, and tricalcium phosphate. Frequently, these materials result in a repair that evidences a long junctional epithelium to the root surface and/or adhesion of connective tissue fibers oriented parallel to the root (Yukna, 1993).

Bioactive glass is another type of alloplast. In a clinical study of the treatment of infrabony periodontal defects, a bioactive glass showed significant clinical superiority in gain of clinical attachment and defect fill compared with sites that were treated with open flap debridement alone (Froum, Weinberg, & Tarnow 1998). Bioactive glass particles contain silicon dioxide, sodium oxide, calcium oxide, and phosphorus pentoxide. Advantages of this material include the ability to bond to both hard and soft tissue (Hench, 1988), its cohesiveness (Hench & West, 1996), and its ability to inhibit the apical migration of junctional epithelium (Fetner, Martigan, & Low, 1994). One human histological study showed the clinical improvement to be a repair rather than a regenerative response (Nevins et al., 2000).

Although many of these materials serve as scaffolds or fillers that allow bone from the surrounding area to grow over and into them, to date alloplasts have failed to demonstrate human histologic evidence of new cementum and a functionally oriented periodontal ligament. From a clinical standpoint, these materials appear to be biocompatible, nontoxic, nonallergenic, noncarcinogenic, and noninflammatory.

XENOGRAFTS (XENOGENEIC GRAFTS) Heterografts or xenografts are taken from a donor of another species. Bio-Oss (Osteohealth Co., Shirley, NY) and Osteograf/N (CeraMed Dental, Lakewood, CO) are types of natural bone mineral obtained from the cow (bovine). This bone is anorganic and deproteinated. A histological study showed that Bio-Oss used in periodontal osseous defects has the potential to

Rapid Dental Hint

Bone grafts and substitutes are indicated for infrabony (vertical) defects and not for sites with horizontal bone loss.

Rapid Dental Hint

Bone grafting materials act as scaffolds and provide a framework for attachment and proliferation of osteoblasts or bone forming cells.

regenerate lost periodontal support (Camelo et al., 1998). The safety of these materials has also been demonstrated in regard to causing mad cow disease.

Properties of Bone Grafts and Bone Substitutes

Bone grafts and bone replacement materials are divided into their properties of osteogenesis, osteoinduction, and osteoconduction. Osteogenic bone contains bone cells called osteoblasts that make new bone and obtain a bone fill in the defect. Autogenous bone (e.g., bone from the host—intraoral or extraoral) is an example of osteogenic bone, and it is considered the gold standard that bone alternatives must meet. Autogenous bone directly lays down new bone during wound healing after it is placed in the periodontal defect. This is ideal; however, there are many limitations to autogenous bone, including limited amounts obtained and donor site morbidity.

Osteoinductive agents are bone grafts and bone graft substitutes, generally proteins, which induce the transformation of immature stem cells into bone-producing osteoblasts, which make new bone through growth factors that are found only in living bone (Fox, 1997). This bone does not contain osteoblasts as autogenous bone. Examples of osteoinductive agents include demineralized freeze-dried bone (DFDBA) from cadavers, bone morphogenic proteins (BMPs), and growth factors (platelet derived growth factor).

This differs from alloplastic grafts, which, when placed into a periodontal defect, at best function as osteoconductive material. In these situations, the alloplastic graft acts as a scaffold or framework to allow bone cells from the surrounding bone in the defect to lay down bone against its surface. In addition, the porous surface of the graft material provides for bone in growth from bone adjacent to the bone material. Such osteoconductive materials require the presence of existing bone, and the more bone there is (greater number of bony walls in an intraosseous defect), the greater is the chance of a successful bone fill (Reyonlds et al., 2010; Fox, 1997). These materials are not osteoinductive and do not produce new bone. The size and shape of the bone substitute particles influence their osteoconductive capacity. Eventually, the particles of material are either replaced by bone growing over them or incorporated into the new bone.

Biologics and Growth Factors

Biologics is a rapidly developing field that is generating new clinical studies. Wound healing is a complex, well-orchestrated sequence of events. In studying the dynamics of cell-to-cell and cell-to-tissue interaction, scientists discovered the presence of growth factors. Attempts have been made to use these factors to enhance wound healing (repair and regeneration).

Growth factors are naturally occurring proteins that mediate or regulate cellular events such as cell proliferation. Growth factors are found only in living tissue in cells such as bone, platelets, and macrophages. The most widely studied growth factor has been platelet-derived growth factor (PDGF). Platelet derived growth factor is a potent wound healing growth factor and stimulates the proliferation and recruitment of periodontal ligament cells and bone cells. The incorporation of PDGF in bone allograft (product is available as GEM21—Osteohealth, NY) may induce periodontal regeneration during wound healing when placed in a periodontal defect (Lynch, Wisner-Lynch, Nevins, & Nevins, 2006; McGuire & Scheyer, 2006).

Platelet-rich plasma (PRP) in the form of autologous platelet concentration (APC), which is enriched with growth factors, is used to promote periodontal bone formation and accelerate healing during periodontal and implant surgery (Nevins et al., 2012). This concept is used not only in periodontics and implantology but also in medicine and orthopedics to fixate bone grafts and to enhance bone growth. APC growth factors are produced from the body's own blood and are incorporated into bone and soft tissue grafts to stabilize the graft material. To obtain APC, about 1.5 ounces of blood is taken from the patient in the dental office just before surgery. The blood is centrifuged, which spins and separates the red blood cells from the plasma. The plasma is again centrifuged to concentrate the autologous platelets. This procedure takes less than 30 minutes. The APC is usually applied topically to the wound site or to bone grafts and soft tissue grafts to stabilize the graft material. Platelet-rich plasma containing growth factors PDGF, insulin-like growth factors (IGFs), and transforming growth factors (TGFs) and fibrin can also be added to maxillary sinus graft material for sinus augmentation (to increase bone height before implants can be placed; Froum, Wallace, Tarnow, & Cho, 2002).

Other proteins called bone morphogenic proteins (BMPs) are normally found in bone and can induce new bone formation. Recently, a bone graft material composed of recombinant (genetically manufactured) BMP-2 and a bovine collagen sponge (available as Infuse Bone Graft—Medtronic, TN) has been used in periodontal defects to stimulate bone formation in the bony defect.

There are still questions about the concentration of growth factors when they are used by themselves or in combination with other factors. The variability of growth factor responses locally and systemically is still unknown (Nevins, Hanratty, & Lynch, 2007).

Another material referred to as enamel matrix proteins (amelogenins) are retrieved from the developing teeth in pigs (porcine). This product, Emdogain (Straumann, Switzerland, Chicago), is used in periodontal regenerative techniques. Clinical studies have shown improved clinical results and gain in clinical attachment and bone fill in sites treated with Emdogain versus open flap debridement (Froum, Weinberg, Rosenberg, & Tarnow, 2001). Multicenter studies have been performed with this material and verify the safety of multiple uses in the same patient (no allergies or immunologic problems; Froum et al., 2004). After flap reflection and debridement, EDTA (ethylenediaminetetraacetic acid) is applied to the root surface to remove the smear layer. This is then washed off with sterile water or saline. Emdogain is applied to the root surface, which promotes attachment of certain cells that will eventually encourage the formation of cellular cementum and bone. Emdogain is available in a premixed, one-vial preparation. After flap reflection and debridement of the infrabony defect, Emdogain is syringed onto the root surface and the flap is sutured.

Bone Grafts and Bone Substitutes: Surgical Procedure

For bone grafting, intracrevicular incisions are made, and a gingival flap is reflected. The root surface and osseous defect are debrided to remove all granulomatous (diseased) tissue (Table 26–3 ■). A combination of power-driven and hand

Table 26–3 Common Bone Grafts and Bone Substitutes

For Periodontal Defects	Composition	Supplied	Company
Puros	Cadaver (allograft)	Cancellous particles, cortical particles, corticocancellous block	Zimmer Dental, Carlsbad, CA
MinerOss	Cadaver (allograft)	Cortical and cancellous chips	Biohorizons Alabama
Bio-Oss	Bovine (xenograft)	Particles	Geistlich Biomaterials, Switzerland
Osteo-graf	Hydroxyapatite (alloplast)	Particles	Dentsply, York, PA/Friadent/Ceramed
SynthoGraft	Pure phase beta-tricalcium phosphate (alloplast)	Particles	Synthograft, Boston
Perioglas, Biogran	Bioactive glass (calcium, phosphorus, sodium, silicon) (alloplast)	Particles	NovaBone Products, Jacksonville, FL; Implant Innovations Inc. ("3i"), a Biomet Company, Warsaw, IN
Capset	Calcium sulfate (plaster of Paris) (alloplast)	Particles	LifeCore Biomedicals, Chaska, MN
DFDBA (demineralized freeze dried bone)	Cadaver (allograft)	Particles	many
Demineralized and mineralized cortical bone	Cadaver (allograft)	Particles	many
Regenafil	Cadaver (allograft)	Powder/fluid	Exactech Inc., FL
OrthoBlast II	Demineralized bone matrix (DBM) and cancellous bone in a reverse phase medium (allograft)	Putty and paste	Isotis Orthobiologics, Irvine, CA
Dynablast	Demineralized bone matrix with cancellous bone (allograft)	Putty and paste	Keystone Dental, MA

(continued)

Table 26–3 Common Bone Grafts and Bone Substitutes (continued)

For Periodontal Defects	Composition	Supplied	Company
GEM 21S	Bioactive protein (highly purified recombinant human platelet derived growth factor, rhPDGF-BB) and a biocompatible osteoconductive matrix (beta-tricalcium phosphate, β-TCP)	Particles and liquid	Osteohealth, New York
PepGen P-15	Synthetic P-15 peptide, bovine hydroxyapatite	Flow, particles, putty	Dentsply/Friadent/CeraMed
Emdogain	Enamel matrix derivative; porcine	Gel	Straumann, Andover, MA

For Ridge Augmentation—Implant	Composition	Supplied	Company
Infuse	Recombinant human bone morphogenic protein 2 (rhBMP)	Apply to an absorbable collagen sponge carrier	Medtronic, TN
DFDBA, FDBA (bone allografts)	Cadaver	Block	many
Bio-Oss Cortical Block	Bovine	Block	Geistlich Biomaterials, Switzerland
Regenaform	Cadaver	Thermoplastic/moldable	Exactech, FL

instruments is commonly used to ensure that all calculus and plaque as well as altered cementum are removed from the root surface (Brunsvold & Mellonig, 1993). The defect is filled and packed with bone or a bone replacement material. The flap is replaced and sutured in an attempt to fully cover the material (Figures 26–1 ■, 26–2 ■, 26–3 ■). Often a barrier membrane is placed covering and protecting the bone material and aiding the process of periodontal regeneration (Lindfors, Tervonen, Sandor, & Ylikontiola, 2010). A periodontal dressing may be placed if desired. The patient returns 7 to 14 days later for suture removal, light debridement, and oral hygiene instruction during the first postoperative visit.

Guided Tissue Regeneration

Cells Involved in Regeneration

The periodontal unit can be divided into five tissue components: the gingival epithelium, the gingival connective tissue, the periodontal ligament (PDL), the supporting alveolar bone, and cementum. In 1976 it was theorized that the type of tissue that predominates in the healing wound after periodontal surgery determines whether the response is either repair (e.g., long junctional epithelial attachment or connective tissue adherence) or regeneration (e.g., new bone, new cementum, and new periodontal ligament; Melcher, 1976; Zeichner-David, 2006).

Rapid Dental Hint

Many bone materials are either mixed with the patient's blood or sterile saline before being placed in the defect. Some products such as Emdogain are already premixed.

Did You Know?

Hydroxyapatite for bone grafting comes from coral from the ocean.

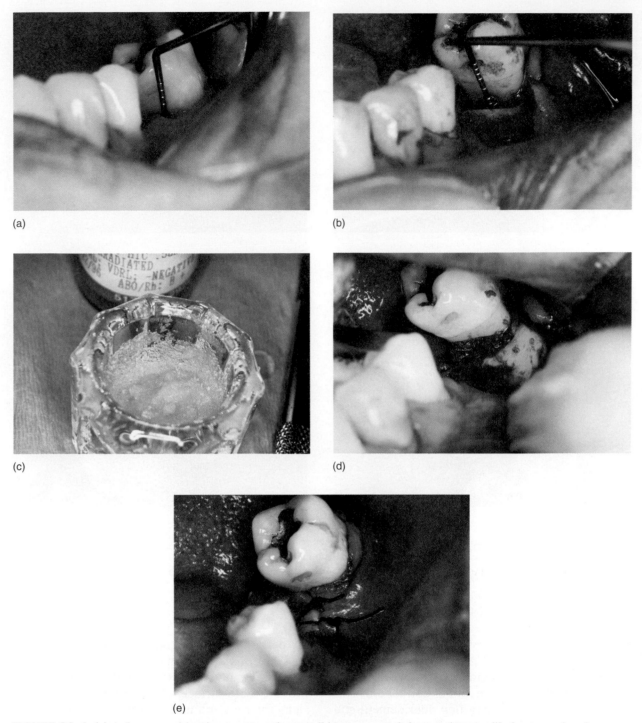

(a)

(b)

(c)

(d)

(e)

FIGURE 26–1 (a) A 6-mm combination one-two-three-wall intraosseous defect on the mandibular second molar.
(b) After flaps are reflected and the roots and defect thoroughly debrided, demineralized freeze-dried bone autograft
(DFDBA) (c, d) was placed into the defect and the flap sutured to cover the bone (e).

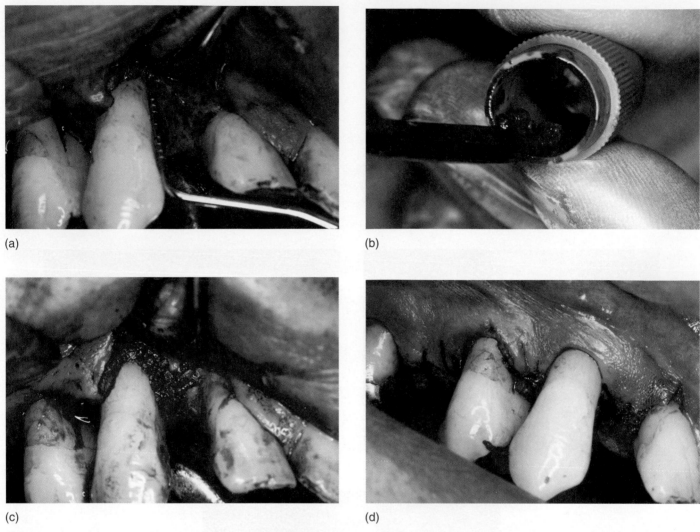

FIGURE 26–2 (a) A 9-mm intraosseous periodontal defect is present on the mesial aspect of the maxillary cuspid. (b) Following reflection of a periodontal flap and defect and root debridement, a bone blend is mixed consisting of autogenous bone and the patient's blood and (c) placed into the defect. (d) The replaced flap is sutured with silk sutures to cover the graft material.

Epithelium is the fastest growing tissue, migrating at a rate of 0.5 to 1.0 mm per day. A periodontal wound in which unimpeded epithelial migration is allowed to occur results in repair with a long junctional epithelium. This type of healing occurs after open flap debridement and osseous resective surgical procedures. Regeneration does not occur when either gingival (junctional) epithelium or gingival connective tissues (e.g., tissue inside the flap) contact the root surface during healing. For regeneration to occur, cells capable of forming new cementum, PDL, and supporting alveolar bone must migrate into the periodontal osseous defect and produce these tissues. It is believed that these cells come from the PDL (osteoblasts, fibroblasts, and cementoblasts) and/or alveolar bone remaining around the tooth (Melcher, McCulloch, Cheong, Nemeth, & Shiga, 1987). For these cells to migrate into

the periodontal defect, apical epithelial migration must be delayed, and the gingival connective tissue from the gingival flap must be excluded. If the flap makes contact with the tooth surface, a long junctional epithelium forms along the root and may prevent the necessary regenerative cells from gaining access to the periodontal defect. This concept led to the theory of selective cell repopulation or **guided tissue regeneration** (GTR; Gottlow, Nyman, Karring, & Wennström, 1986; Nyman, Gottlow, Karring, & Lindhe, 1982).

This concept has been the basis for clinical techniques using barrier membranes inserted between the gingival flap and the root surface. The membrane maintains a "space" between the tooth and the flap. This procedure is designed to retard apical migration of the junctional epithelium and exclude the gingival connective tissue cells

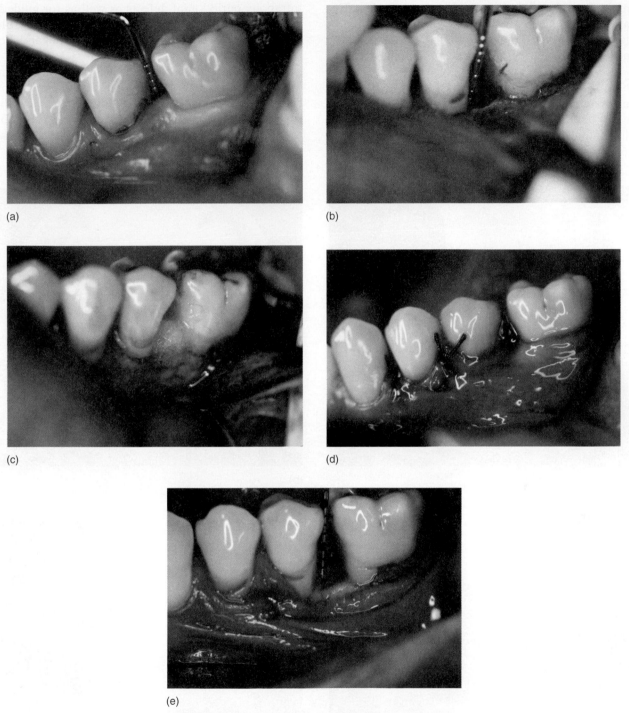

FIGURE 26–3 (a) Probing between the mandibular second premolar and first molar. (b) Probing of the deep defect after flap reflection. (c) After thorough tooth and root debridement, Perioglas® was placed into the defect, and the flaps were sutured with silk sutures to cover the graft material. (d) Flap sutured with interrupted sutures. (e) Reentry of the site 6 months later shows that the bony defect has been filled in with new bone (also there is slight crestal resorption). The interproximal bone is flat, not cratered. Compare with Figure 26–3b.

from making contact with the root surface and defect. This then allows cells originating from the PDL space and/or alveolar bone cells to migrate coronally into the defect to form new bone, cementum, and attachment (Figure 26–4 ■).

Surgical Procedure

Barrier membranes have been used in the treatment of Grade II buccal furcation defects in both maxillary and mandibular molars and in two- and three-wall interproximal

infrabony periodontal defects as well as for guided bone regeneration (GBR) applications. Optimal results are obtained in patients who are healthy nonsmokers who demonstrate good oral home care.

Clinically, GTR techniques are performed by making intrasulcular incisions and full-thickness flap reflection. Following debridement of the periodontal defect and the root surface, a membrane barrier is placed on the tooth to cover the periodontal bony defect (Figures 26–5 ■, 26–6 ■). The

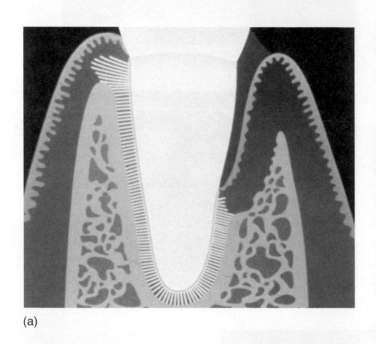

(a)

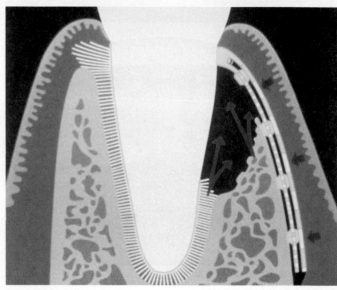

(b)

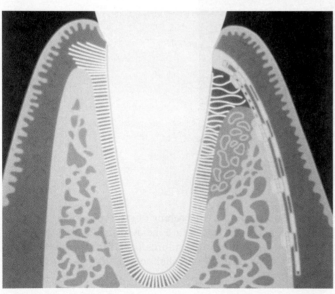

(c)

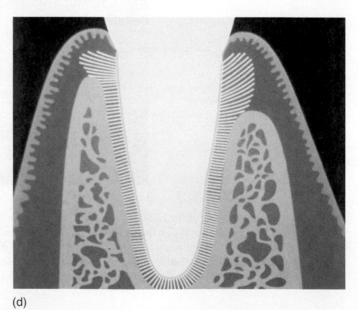

(d)

FIGURE 26–4 Schematic illustration of a guided tissue regeneration procedure. (a) The periodontal defect with the junctional epithelium on the root surface. (b) After a flap is raised and the defect debrided, a barrier membrane is placed over the defect to create a space for the defect to heal. The periodontal ligament and bone cells attempt to migrate coronally (arrows) into the defect to produce new cementum, periodontal ligament, and supporting alveolar bone. The flap is then sutured over the membrane covering it. (c) Healing by regeneration. (d) The result of therapy after healing.

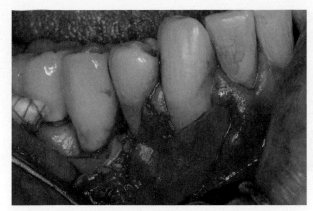

FIGURE 26–5 Bone + membrane: infrabony defect on the canine. Flaps are reflected and surgical debridement performed until the defect is visualized. Bio-Oss is placed into the defect and BioGide placed on top of the bone graft. Then the flaps are sutured to cover both the bone and membrane.

membrane is situated between the inner flap and the tooth and bone. The flap is sutured so that the membrane is fully covered and not exposed to the oral cavity. Frequently, a bone graft is first placed into the periodontal defect to prevent the membrane from collapsing into the defect and to aid in regeneration.

Types of Barrier Membranes

NONABSORBABLE MEMBRANES Membranes are classified as nonabsorbable or absorbable. Nonabsorbable membranes were the first to be used and studied clinically. Because the body does not absorb (degrade) a nonabsorbable membrane, it has to be removed. A second surgical procedure, therefore, is performed a minimum of 6 to 8 weeks later to remove the barrier. The most commonly used nonabsorbable barrier membrane is expanded polytetrafluoroethylene (e-PTFE). Examples of an e-PTFE membrane are Gore-Tex® and Gore-Tex® Regenerative Membrane Titanium Reinforced, in which the titanium enhances the space creating ability of the membrane (Gore Associates, Flagstaff, AZ). Similar nonabsorbable barriers are TefGen-FD™ and TefGen-RE™ (Lifecore Biomedical, Chaska, MN), which are less porous than Gore-Tex® and thus may limit the amount of connective tissue in growth.

Most studies using nonabsorbable membranes in infrabony defects showed positive results. Over the past two decades, studies of infrabony defects in humans treated with e-PTFE barriers showed definitive clinical gains in new attachment, with three-wall defects having the greatest improvement (Gottlow et al., 1986). A 12-month study of one-, two-, and three-wall infrabony defects treated with e-PTFE barriers showed a 93% fill

of three-wall defects, an 82% fill of two-wall defects, and a 39% fill of one-wall defects (Cortellini, Pini Prato, & Tonetti, 1993a, 1993b).

ABSORBABLE MEMBRANES Absorbable membranes appeared half a decade after nonabsorbable membranes. These membranes have various compositions, including collagen (Bornstein, Bosshardt, & Buser, 2007). Absorbable membranes offer a distinct advantage over nonabsorbable barriers in that there is no need for a second surgery to retrieve the membrane. Macrophages, a type of phagocyte, are always involved in the degradation process. The barrier must remain in place a minimum of 3 to 4 weeks (Minabe, 1991) for proper wound healing. Several membranes are available commercially (Table 26–4 ■).

The general consensus seems to be that furcation closure in a horizontal dimension is better with absorbable membranes (Garrett, 1996). The clinician must choose the appropriate barrier for the appropriate defect. Although nonabsorbable barriers do not have breakdown products that can interfere with tissue healing, the need for a second procedure to remove the membrane is a distinct disadvantage to wound healing.

The membrane should be covered completely by the flap to prevent bacterial colonization on the outer part of the membrane. Membrane exposure may lead to early infection and poor results. Unfortunately, membrane exposure to the oral cavity occurs with both barrier types. Tissue management when membrane exposure occurs with nonabsorbable barriers may be a problem. Bacteria from the oral cavity may contaminate the exposed membrane by attaching to it. If complete flap closure is not possible, absorbable membranes may be the best choice.

Although GTR using nonabsorbable and absorbable membranes has revolutionized clinical practice, the technique is not as yet predictable for class II, class III, and horizontal bone defects. More research in regeneration of furcation and interproximal defects is needed.

Barrier membranes need to be secured around the tooth to hold them in place and prevent them from moving. Either sutures or bone tacks can be used to attach and immobilize the membrane. A mallet is used to secure the tacks in place. The bone tacks are either stainless steel or titanium. Most are nonabsorbable, thus a second surgery is needed to remove the tacks. Osteo-Pin (Osteohealth, Shirley, NY) is a bioabsorbable fixation pin that does not need to be removed.

Several bacteria, including *A. actinomycetemcomitans* and *P. gingivalis*, have been shown to attach to bioabsorbable membranes, which could cause a bacterial infection. In addition, these bacteria produce and release proteolytic bacterial enzymes that may take part in the degradation of collagen barrier membranes such as Bio-Gide and Biomend (Sela, Kohavi, Krausz, Steinberg, & Rosen, 2003).

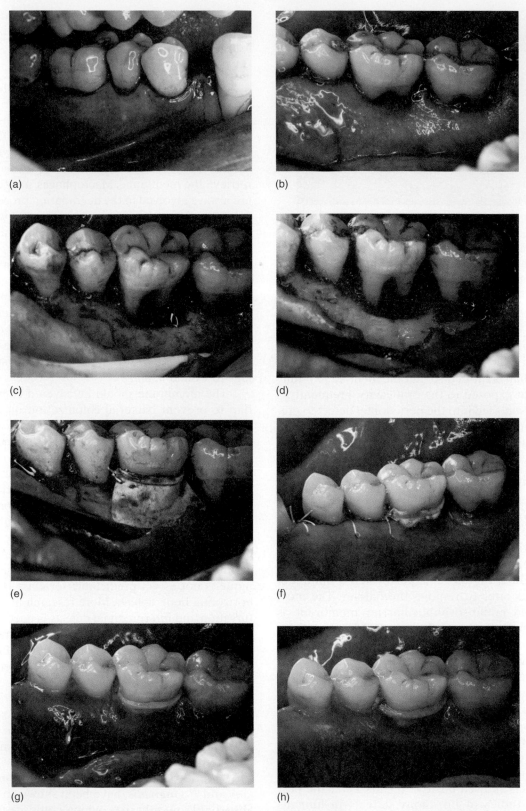

FIGURE 26–6 Mandibular right quadrant: initial incisions on the buccal (a) and lingual (b). (c) Full-thickness flap is reflected showing circumferential bony defects (bone destruction from the interproximal to the lingual surface) and furcation involvement. (d) After debridement, the bony defects are grafted with DFDBA (demineralized freeze-dried bone), and (e) an absorbable membrane is sutured over the defect. (f) The flaps are sutured. (g) One week postoperative; sutures removed and (h) 4 weeks postoperative with the membrane still in place. (Courtesy of Dr. James B. Fine, Columbia University College of Dental Medicine.)

Table 26–4 Absorbable Barrier Membranes

Material	Product	Manufacturer
Synthetic: Polyglycolic acid, polylactic acid, and trimethylene carbonate	Gore OsseoQuest	W. L. Gore, Flagstaff, AZ; distributed by Nobel Biocare, Yorba Linda, CA
	Gore Resolut XT	W. L. Gore
Synthetic: Polyglycolic acid and trimethylene carbonate	Gore Resolut Adapt	W. L. Gore, Flagstaff, AZ; distributed by Nobel Biocare, Yorba Linda, CA
	Gore Resolut Adapt LT	
Synthetic: PLA (poly-DL-lactide)	Epi-Guide	Curasan Inc., NC
	Atrisorb FreeFlow	Tolmar, Fort Collins, CO
	Atrisorb-D FreeFlow (with 4% doxycycline)	Tolmar
Natural: Collagen (bovine)	BioMend	Zimmer Dental, Carlsbad, CA
(bovine)	BioMend Extend	Zimmer Dental
(porcine)	BioGide	Geistlich, Switzerland; distributed by Osteohealth Company, Shirley, NY
(bovine)	OsseoGuard	Biomet 3i, Warsaw, IN
(porcine)	Ossix Plus	OraPharma, Warminster, PA

Rapid Dental Hint

Do not probe or do subgingival scaling for at least 6 months in areas that have a bone graft or barrier membrane placed either around a tooth or implant.

Regenerative Surgery: Postoperative Care

The patient's oral home care is of utmost importance for a desirable outcome. The dental hygienist should provide the patient with thorough home care instructions. Guidelines for postoperative care are outlined in Table 26–5 ■ (Becker & Becker, 1993; Garret & Bogle, 1993; Yukna, 1993). An antimicrobial mouth rinse such as chlorhexidine gluconate may be prescribed. The patient may be prescribed an antibiotic before and after the surgery to prevent infection. The first postoperative visit is within 7 to 14 days.

Professional maintenance and plaque control have been repeatedly shown to correlate with successful clinical results of regenerative therapies including open flap debridement (Froum et al., 1982; Nyman, Lindhe, & Rosling, 1977; Rosling, Nyman, & Lindhe, 1976), bone grafting (Rosen, Reynolds, & Bowers, 2000), and guided tissue regeneration (Cortellini, Pini Prato, & Tonetti, 1994). The hygienist thus plays a key role in the short- and long-term success of regenerative therapy.

Complications can occur during the healing period after GTR surgery. Some complications (Becker & Becker, 1993) are outlined in Table 26–6 ■.

Root Surface Treatment

Animal studies have shown that the root surface becomes contaminated by bacteria, bacterial by-products, and endotoxins that will prevent connective tissue attachment and regeneration (Garrett, 1977). The classic method of scaling and root planing, although effective in removing endotoxins from the root (Smart, Wilson, Davies, & Kieser, 1990), in most cases will not result in new connective tissue attachment, but rather a long junctional epithelium. Use of an acid solution such as citric acid or tetracycline HCl has been studied to determine if a new connective tissue attachment results. The proposed purposes of using acidic solutions on contaminated root surfaces are to detoxify the root and expose collagen fibers for a connective tissue attachment. However, two recent reviews of periodontal regeneration studies with and without the use of citric acid root conditioning showed no clinical advantage to its use (Garrett, 1996; Mariotti, 2003).

Table 26–5 Periodontal Regenerative Surgery: Postoperative Care

Surgical Procedure	Postoperative Home Care	In-Office Reevaluation Procedures
Bone grafting	• If a periodontal dressing is placed, instruct the patient not to brush the area. Instruct the patient to rinse with 0.12% chlorhexidine gluconate twice a day. • Following suture removal the patient may start to brush (soft or ultrasoft brush) surgical site gently with a circular technique. Bleeding may occur but will gradually lessen, and the patient should continue to brush. • If an antibiotic was prescribed, instruct the patient to continue until all medication is finished.	• At the postoperative visit (7 to 14 days), carefully remove the dressing (cut sutures if embedded in dressing), wipe off the white film (this consists of dead epithelial cells); and irrigate the area with sterile water or saline. • Reapply dressing if needed (especially if sutures and dressing are removed before 10 days). • Periodontal probing should not be done prior to 6 months after surgery. • Final prosthetic restorations should not be completed until 6 months or more after surgery. • Initial appointments for professional plaque removal should be every 2 to 3 weeks for the first month, then every month for four visits, followed by every 3 months (alternate with visits to the general dentist).
Guided tissue regeneration	• A periodontal dressing is usually not placed. Instruct the patient not to floss or brush around the surgical area for 6 weeks after the surgery. However, a soft or ultrasoft toothbrush may be used for coronal brushing of the surgical area. • Rinse with 0.12% chlorhexidine gluconate twice a day, and use cotton swabs saturated with chlorhexidine around the surgical area. • Instruct the patient to continue to take the prescribed antibiotic until finished.	• At the first postoperative visit (1 to 2 weeks), the surgical area is inspected and flap sutures are removed. • The patient should be seen regularly for the first 6 weeks (every week or twice a week) for supragingival scaling and tooth polishing with sterile water. • At 2 weeks the patient can carefully brush with a soft toothbrush. • Between 4 and 6 weeks, the membrane-attached sutures are removed. • Absorbable membranes: wait for membrane resorption. Instruct patient to resume normal toothbrushing and interdental cleaning at week 6. • For nonabsorbable membranes: At 8 to 12 weeks, an incision is made to remove the nonabsorbable membrane. • Periodontal probing and deep scaling instrumentation should not be done prior to 6 months after surgery. • Final prosthestic restorations should not be completed prior to 6 months after surgery.

Sources: Becker & Becker, 1993; Garrett & Bogle, 1993; Yukna, 1993.

Table 26–6 Complications after Periodontal Regenerative Surgery

Complication	Procedures to Follow
Membrane becomes uncovered	Instruct the patient to call the office. Most often the membrane will become exposed within a few weeks after surgery. If there is no infection, instruct patient to keep optimal oral hygiene. Monitor the area. Instruct the patient not to disrupt the membrane. Bacteria associated with exposed membranes include *A. actinomycetemcomitans* and *P. gingivalis*. Aggressive antimicrobial therapy may be necessary, including chlorhexidine mouth rinses and antibiotics such as metronidazole alone or combined with amoxicillin.
Gingival recession at the surgical site	If recession occurs, it will usually happen within 1 to 3 weeks after surgery. Because increased plaque accumulation may result, optimal plaque control is stressed.
Pus	If an infection develops, it is most likely at the fourth and fifth postoperative visit. Remove the membrane and place the patient on an antibiotic. If the patient is already on an antibiotic, change to another antibiotic in a different classification.

Risk Factors for Regenerative Therapy

The same contraindications for any surgical periodontal therapy apply to regenerative therapies. These include any acute or chronic uncontrolled systemic diseases that put the patient at risk (e.g., diabetes mellitus), inadequate plaque control, and smoking (especially more than one pack per day). Smoking has been shown to have a negative influence on the results of regenerative therapy. Using GTR therapy, smokers had less than 50% gain in attachment levels compared to results in nonsmokers (Tonetti, Pino Prato, & Cortellini, 1996). Of the failures with GTR, the majority (80%) occurred in smokers (Rosenberg, Dent, & Cutles, 1984).

Dental Hygiene Application

Today, the role of periodontics in dentistry focuses not only on arresting the progression of inflammatory periodontal diseases, but also on the regeneration of periodontal structures (cementum, PDL, supporting alveolar bone) that were destroyed by disease. Periodontal regenerative therapy uses bone replacement materials and guided tissue regeneration (GTR) techniques. The use of growth factors (e.g., bone morphogenic proteins, platelet-derived growth factor, and tissue modifiers) holds great promise. These factors most likely will be the next addition to periodontal regenerative techniques.

Key Points

- Periodontal regeneration is defined as healing after periodontal surgery that results in the reproduction of cementum, PDL, and supporting alveolar bone that was lost or destroyed by periodontal diseases.
- Ideally, after periodontal surgery, healing by regeneration is preferred over repair.
- Periodontal regenerative techniques include the use of bone grafts, synthetic bone substitutes, guided tissue regeneration (GTR), and a combination of these.
- Bone-replacement materials may contribute to new bone formation or serve as a filler material for bone formation that starts from the adjacent bone and grows into the defect.
- GTR is used to delay apical migration of the junctional epithelium and exclude gingival connective tissue (inner flap) from the surgical site. The goal is to allow periodontal regenerative cells to repopulate the wound first.
- A barrier membrane is placed over the osseous defect and root to create a space for the migration of cells from the PDL and alveolar bone to repopulate the wound.

Self-Quiz

1. For each substance listed, select the correct type of bone graft, bone graft substitute, biologic, or growth factors from the list provided.

Substance	Type of bone graft, bone graft substitute, or growth factor
1. Demineralized freeze-dried bone	a. Allograft
2. Bone from the tuberosity	b. Autograft
3. Enamel matrix proteins	c. Alloplast
4. Bovine bone (Bio-Oss)	d. Xenograft
5. Platelet rich plasma (PRP)	e. Growth factors
6. Bioactive glass	f. Amelogenin

2. Cells coming from which one of the following structures is required for successful periodontal regeneration?
   a. Periodontal ligament
   b. Alveolar bone
   c. Gingival connective tissue
   d. Gingival epithelial

3. Guided tissue regeneration (GTR) focuses on the isolation or exclusion of what type of tissue cells?
   a. Junctional epithelial and gingival connective tissue
   b. Alveolar bone and sulcular epithelium
   c. Connective tissue and alveolar bone
   d. Alveolar bone and junctional epithelial

4. Which one of the following types of material is BioMend membrane?
   a. Polytetrafluoroethylene (e-PTFE)
   b. Poly-DL-lactide (PLA)
   c. Polylactic acid/polyglycolate (PLA/PGA)
   d. Bovine collagen

5. After surgical placement of a barrier membrane around an intraosseous defect, it is important to cover the membrane with the flap because
   a. brushing the area is easier.
   b. bacterial colonization can be prevented.
   c. aesthetics are enhanced.
   d. tooth mobility is reduced to pretreatment levels.

6. Which one of the following defects heals best when treated with bone grafts or bone substitutes?
   a. One-wall
   b. Two-wall
   c. Three-wall
   d. Class III furcations
   e. Horizontal bone loss

7. All the following are objectives of using bone grafts or bone-replacement materials in the treatment of infrabony defects except one. Which one is the exception?
   a. Reduction in probing depth
   b. Reduction of bleeding
   c. Gain in clinical attachment
   d. Fill of the defect
   e. Regeneration of the attachment apparatus

8. For each barrier membrane listed, select the correct material from the list provided.

Membrane	Material
1. BioMend	a. synthetic: polygycolic acid
2. BioGuide	b. natural: bovine collagen
3. Gore Resolut XT	c. natural: porcine collagen

9. All the following complications may be seen after placement of barrier membranes except one. Which one is the least likely?
   a. Suppuration
   b. Gingival overgrowth
   c. Soft-tissue recession
   d. Membrane exposure

10. From the following list, select the items associated with postoperative instructions after a regenerative procedure using a barrier membrane.
    a. Floss the surgical area.
    b. Rinse the area frequently with diluted saltwater.
    c. Use an antimicrobial mouthrinse.
    d. Take antibiotics as prescribed.

Case Study

A 55-year-old female has treatment planned for a dental implant for tooth #30. At the time of extraction for #30 it was determined to use guided bone regeneration. The dental hygiene visit prior to extraction included periodontal debridement and oral hygiene self-care instruction.

1. What is the goal of guided bone regeneration?
   a. replaces horizontal bone loss prior to implant placement
   b. restore cementum for attachment
   c. creates long junctional epithelium
   d. forms new bone with barrier membrane

Answer: D. New bond is formed and the epithelium is blocked by the membrane. The cementum is not affected. Walled bony defects are more conducive to retaining the membrane.

2. After the tooth had been extracted and the membrane placed, what do the dental hygiene intervention(s) include?
   a. probing depths recorded at 6 week evaluation
   b. chlorhexidine and thorough home care
   c. subgingival scaling at 4 months
   d. normal brushing at 2 weeks after suture removal

Answer: B. Rinsing and home care are extremely important. Office visits may be weekly at first and resume normal routines at 6 weeks. Probing and subgingival scaling does not occur until 6 months.

3. What role could use of growth factors have for this patient?
   a. used as autogenous bone
   b. stimulates new periodontal ligament cells
   c. contains osteoblasts for new bone formation
   d. used as osteoconductive agent as a framework

Answer: B. The growth factors have been shown to enhance wound repair and regeneration. They are osteoinductive or osteoconductive agents that do not contain osteoblasts.

References

American Academy of Periodontology. 2001. Tissue banking of bone allografts used in periodontal regeneration. *J. Periodontol.* 72:834–838.

Becker, W., and B. E. Becker. 1993. Clinical applications of guided tissue regeneration: Surgical considerations. *Periodontology 2000.* 1:46–53.

Bornstein, M. M., D. Bosshardt, and D. Buser. 2007, October. Effect of two different bioabsorbable collagen membranes on guided bone regeneration: A comparative histomorphometric study in the dog mandible. *J. Periodontol.* 78(10):1943–1953.

Brunsvold, M. A., and J. T. Mellonig. 1993. Bone grafts and periodontal regeneration. *Periodontology 2000* 1:80–91.

Camelo, M., M. L. Nevins, R. K. Schenk, M. Simion, G. Rasperini, et al. 1998. Clinical, radiographic, and histological evaluation of human periodontal defects treated with Bio-Oss and Bio-Guide. *Int. J. Periodontics Restorative Dent.* 18:321–331.

Christgau, M., D. Moder, K. A. Hiller, A. Dada, G. Schmitz, and G. Schmalz. 2006. Growth factors and cytokines in autologous platelet concentrate and their correlation to periodontal regeneration outcomes. *J. Clin. Periodontol.* 33:837–845.

Cortellini, P., G. Pini Prato, and M. S. Tonetti. 1993a. Periodontal regeneration in human intrabony defects: I. Clinical measures. *J. Periodontol.* 64:254–260.

Cortellini, P., G. Pini Prato, and M. S. Tonetti. 1993b. Periodontal regeneration in human intrabony defects: II. Reentry procedures and bone measurements. *J. Periodontol.* 64:261–268.

Cortellini, P., G. Pini Prato, and M. Tonetti. 1994. Periodontal regeneration of human infrabony defects (V). Effect of oral hygiene on long-term stability. *J. Clin. Periodontol.* 21:606–610.

Fetner, A. E., M. S. Martigan, and S. B. Low. 1994. Periodontal repair using Perioglas® in nonhuman primates: Clinical and histologic observations. *Compend. Contin. Ed. Dent.* 15:932–939.

Fox, J. S. 1997. Bone grafting materials for dental applications: A practical guide. *Compend. Contin. Ed. Dent.* 18:1013–1038.

Froum S. J., M. Coran, B. Thaller, L. Kushner, I. W. Scopp, and S. S. Stahl. 1982. Periodontal healing following open flap debridement. *J. Periodontol.* 53:8–14.

Froum S. J., C. Gomez, and M. R. Breault. 2001. Current concepts of periodontal regeneration. *NYSDJ* 68(9):14–22.

Froum, S. J., S. S. Wallace, D. P. Tarnow, and S. C. Cho. 2002. Effect of platelet-rich plasma on bone growth and osseiointegration in human maxillary sinus grafts: Three bilateral case reports. *Int. J. Periodontics Restorative Dent.* 22:45–53.

Froum, S. J., M. A. Weinberg, J. Novak, J. Mailhot, J. Mellonig, et al. 2004. A multicenter study evaluating the sensitization potential of enamel matrix derivative after treatment of two infrabony defects. *J. Periodontol.* 75:1001–1008.

Froum, S. J., M. A. Weinberg, E. Rosenberg, and D. Tarnow. 2001. A comparative study utilizing open flap debridement with and without enamel matrix derivative in the treatment of periodontal intrabony defects: A 12-month re-entry study. *J. Periodontol.* 72:25–34.

Froum, S. J., M. A. Weinberg, and D. Tarnow. 1998. Comparison of bioactive glass synthetic bone graft particles and open debridement in the treatment of human periodontal defects: A clinical study. *J. Periodontol.* 69:698–709.

Garrett, S. 1977. Root planing: A perspective. *J. Periodontol.* 48:553–557.

Garrett, S. 1996. Periodontal regeneration around natural teeth. *Ann. Periodontol.* 1:621–666.

Garrett, S., and G. Bogle. 1993. Periodontal regeneration: A review of flap management. *Periodontology 2000* 1:100–108.

Gottlow, J., S. Nyman, T. Karring, and J. Wennström. 1986. New attachment formation in the human periodontium by guided tissue regeneration: Case reports. *J. Clin. Periodontol.* 13:604–616.

Hallmon, W. W., F. A. Carranza, Jr., C. L. Drisko, J. W. Rapley, and P. Robinson. 1996. Surgical therapy. In *Periodontal literature review*, 167–194. Chicago: American Academy of Periodontology.

Hanes, P. J. 2007, November. Bone replacement grafts for the treatment of periodontal intrabony defects. *Oral Maxillofac. Surg. Clin. North Am.* 19(4):499–512, vi.

Hench, L. L. 1988. Bioactive ceramics. *Ann. N.Y. Acad. Sci.* 523:54–71.

Hench, L. L., and J. K. West. 1996. Biological application of bioactive glasses. *Life Chem. Rep.* 13:187–241.

Laurell, L., M. Bose, F. Graziani, M. Tonetti, and T. Berglundh. 2006. The structure of periodontal tissues formed following guided tissue regeneration therapy of intra-bony defects in the monkey. *J. Clin. Periodontol.* 33:596–603.

Lindfors, L. T., E. A. Tervonen, G. K. Sandor, and L. P. Ylikontiola. 2010. Guided bone regeneration using a titanium-reinforced ePTFE membrane and particulate autogenous bone: The effect of smoking and membrane exposure. *Oral Surg. Oral Med. Oral Pathol. Oral Radiol. Endod.* 109:825–830.

Lynch, S., L. Wisner-Lynch, M. Nevins, and M. L. Nevins. 2006. A new era in periodontal and periimplant regeneration: Use of growth factor enhanced matrices incorporating rhPDGF. *Compend. Contin. Educ. Dent.* 27(12):672–679.

Mariotti, A. 2003. Efficacy of chemical root surface modifiers in the treatment of periodontal disease. A systematic review. *Ann. Periodontol.* 8:205–226.

Marx, R. E., and E. R. Carlson. 1993. Tissue banking safety: Caveats and precaution for the oral and maxillofacial surgeon. *J. Oral Maxillofac. Surg.* 51:1372–1379.

McGuire, M. K., and E. T. Scheyer. 2006. Comparison of recombinant human platelet-derived growth factor-BB plus beta tricalcium phosphate and a collagen membrane to subepithelial connective tissue grafting for the treatment of recession defects: A case series. *Int. J. Periodont. Restor. Dent.* 26(2):127–133.

Melcher, A. H. 1976. On the repair potential of the periodontal tissues. *J. Periodontol.* 47:256–260.

Melcher, A. H., C. A. G. McCulloch, T. Cheong, E. Nemeth, and A. Shiga. 1987. Cells from bone synthesize cementum-like and bone-like tissues in vitro and may migrate into periodontal ligament in vivo. *J. Periodontol. Res.* 22:246–247.

Mellonig, J. T. 1984. Decalcified freeze-dried bone allograft as an implant material in human periodontal defects. *Int. J. Periodont. Restor. Dent.* 4(6):41–55.

Mellonig, J. T., A. B. Preuett, and M. P. Moyer. 1992. HIV inactivation in a bone allograft. *J. Periodontol.* 63:979–983.

Minabe, M. 1991. A critical review of the biologic rationale for guided tissue regeneration. *J. Periodontol.* 62:171–179.

Nevins, M., M. L. Nevins, N. Karimbux, et al. 2012. The combination of purified recombinant human platelet-derived growth factor-BB and equine particulate bone graft for periodontal regeneration. *J. Periodontol.* 83:565–573.

Nevins, M., J. Hanratty, and S. E. Lynch. 2007, October. Clinical results using recombinant human platelet-derived growth factor and mineralized freeze-dried bone allograft in periodontal defects. *Int. J. Periodont. Restor. Dent.* 27(5):421–427.

Nevins, M. L., M. Camelo, M. Nevins, C. J. King, R. J. Oringer, et al. 2000. Human histologic evaluation of bioactive ceramic in the treatment of periodontal osseous defects. *Int. J. Periodont. Restor. Dent.* 20:459–467.

Nyman, S., J. Gottlow, T. Karring, and J. Lindhe. 1982. The regenerative potential of the periodontal ligament: An experimental study in the monkey. *J. Clin. Periodontol.* 9:257–265.

Nyman, S., J. Lindhe, and B., Rosling. 1977. Periodontal surgery in plaque-infected dentitions. *J. Clin. Periodontol.* 4:240–249.

Reynolds, M. A., M. E. Aichelmann-Reidy, and G. L. Branch-Mays. 2010. Regeneration of periodontal tissue: bone replacement grafts. *Dent. Clin. North Am.* 54:55–71.

Reynolds, M. A., M. E. Aichelmann-Reidy, G. L. Branch-Mays, and J. C. Gunsolley. 2003. The efficacy of bone replacement grafts in the treatment of periodontal osseous defects. A systematic review. *Ann. Periodontol.* 8:227–265.

Rosen, P. S., M. A. Reynolds, and G. M. Bowers. 2000. The treatment of intrabony defects with bone grafts. *Periodontology 2000.* 22:88–103.

Rosenberg, E. S., H. D. Dent, and S. H. Cutles. 1994. The effect of cigarette smoking on the long-term success of guided tissue regeneration: A preliminary study. *Ann. Royal Aust. Coll. Dent. Surg.* 112:89–93.

Rosling, B., S. Nyman, and J. Lindhe. 1976. The effect of systematic plaque control on bone regeneration in infrabony pockets. *J. Clin. Periodontol.* 3:38–53.

Schallhorn, R. G. 1977. Present status of osseous grafting procedures. *J. Periodontol.* 48:570–576.

Sela, M. N., D. Kohavi, E. Krausz, D. Steinberg, and G. Rosen. 2003. Enzymatic degradation of collagen-guided tissue. Regeneration membranes by periodontal bacteria. *Clin. Oral Impl. Res.* 4, 263–268.

Smart, G. J., M. Wilson, E. H. Davies, and J. B. Kieser. 1990. The assessment of ultrasonic root surface debridement by determination of residual endotoxin levels. *J. Clin. Periodontol.* 17:174–178.

Smith, D., W. Ammons, and G. van Belle. 1980. A longitudinal study of periodontal status comparing osseous recontouring with flap curettage: II. Results after 6 months. *J. Periodontol.* 51:367–375.

Stahl, S. S., S. J. Froum, and L. Kushner. 1982. Periodontal healing following open debridement flap procedures. II. Histologic observations. *J. Periodontol.* 53(1):15–21.

Tonetti, M., G. Pini Prato, and P. Cortellini. 1993. Periodontal regeneration of human infrabony defects. IV. Determinants of the healing response. *J. Periodontol.* 64:934–940.

Tonetti M., G. Pini Prato, and P. Cortellini. 1996. Factors affecting the healing response of intrabony defects following guided tissue regeneration and access flap surgery. *J. Clin. Periodontol.* 23:548–556.

Yukna, R. 1993. Synthetic bone grafts in periodontics. *Periodontology 2000* 1:93–99.

Zeichner-David, M. 2006. Regeneration of periodontal tissues: Cementogenesis revisited. *Periodontology 2000* 41(1):196–217.

27

Implantology

Pinelopi Xenoudi and Raymond A. Yukna

OUTLINE

EDUCATIONAL OBJECTIVES

Upon completion of this chapter, the reader should be able to:

- Define the role of the dental hygienist in the management of patients with dental implants.
- Explain the various types of dental implants currently in use.
- Discuss the general sequence of implant placement, uncovering, and restoration.
- Compare the tissues around natural teeth and dental implants.
- Discuss the steps in evaluating tissue conditions around dental implants.
- Describe proper instrument selection and therapeutic steps for in-office maintenance procedures.
- Choose appropriate home-care techniques for patients with dental implants.

GOAL: To provide an understanding of dental implants and the establishment of proper implant evaluation procedures and maintenance.

KEY WORDS

Introduction

The dental hygienist plays a critical role in implant dentistry, providing valuable information on treatment and maintenance. The dental hygienist should know the types of implants used in his or her dental office. It is usually beneficial to have before and after pictures of patients who have undergone implant procedures in the office to show prospective patients potential end results.

A potential implant patient must be well educated about the entire procedure, especially the need for follow-up care. Although most implants now have a success rate of over 90%, they still require maintenance and routine care for long-term survival.

Age, Systemic, and Social Factors

The age of the patient has not shown to have an effect on the success or failure of implants (Dao, Anderson, & Zarb, 1993).

Implant therapy may not be an option for patients with certain systemic diseases or adverse risk factors. Systemic diseases such as reduced immune defense (HIV/AIDS) and uncontrolled diabetes mellitus can cause an increased susceptibility to infection and interfere with wound healing. Similarly, social risk factors such as smoking, excessive alcohol intake, drug abuse, and stress have been shown to be associated with an increased frequency of implant infections, including failure (Bain, 1996). Consultation with a patient's physician is required if a patient has disturbances of blood coagulation (including anticoagulation therapy), is on long-term steroids, or has a cancer that requires chemotherapy (Belser et al., 1996). An alternate method of replacing missing teeth should be pursued for such patients, such as fixed partial dentures, removable partial dentures, or complete dentures.

Patients taking intravenous bisphosphonates for cancer, osteoporosis, multiple myeloma, or other medical condition are not candidates for implant surgery. Implant surgery is a precipitating factor associated with ONJ whereby there is *poor or delayed wound healing* in patients taking bisphosphonates.

According to the most current *JADA* report (Edwards, Hellstein, & Jacobson, 2008), patients taking oral bisphosphonates can have implant surgery, but the patient may be at increased risk of developing osteonecrosis of the jaw when extensive implant placement is necessary or bone augmentation surgery can be performed (Cartsos, Zhu, & Zavras 2008; Fugazzotto, Lightfoot, Jaffin, & Kumar, 2007; Grant, Amenedo, Freeman, & Kraut, 2008; Marx, 2007; Marx, Cillo, & Ulloa, 2007; Marx, Sawatari, Fortin, & Broumand, 2005). Thus, patients on long-term oral bisphosphonates should still be treated with caution (Wang, Weber, & McCauley, 2007).

Components of Dental Implants

The components of a **dental implant** include the following (Figure 27–1 ■):

1. The implant body or fixture is the part that is surgically placed into the bone.
2. The abutment (or metal post) is the part that is attached to the implant body and will be fitted with a restoration that can be placed on top of it.
3. The superstructure is the prosthetic replacement (e.g., crown or denture) that is either screwed or cemented to the abutment.

Types of Dental Implants

Several types of implants have been used to replace teeth or support prostheses over the centuries. A few types have been developed that provide the predictable success rates that clinicians and patients expect (Albrektsson & Sennerby, 1991; Brånemark, Zarb, & Albrektsson, 1985).

Implant success and survival rates are affected by the anatomic region of the jaw, the quality of bone, and the length and width of the implant (Cochran, 1996). Minimal criteria for a successful implant should include absence of clinical mobility, absence of persistent and/or irreversible signs and symptoms of pain or infections, no peri-implant radiolucency, no irreversible mechanical failures (e.g., implant fractures), support and/or retention of functional restoration(s), and lack of progressive bone loss beyond physiologic remodeling (0.2 mm per year after the first year of loading [occlusal function]). There are five types of implants: endosseous, subperiosteal, transosteal, transitional, and endodontic.

Endosseous Implants

Endosseous means "within the bone." **Endosseous implants** have several different shapes, including blade, cylinder, and screw types, with each manufacturer having its own designs. These are the most commonly used implants, and they are placed in edentulous areas of the maxilla or mandible (endosseous). Blade-type implants were popular in the 1960s and 1970s and were associated with a fibrous type of attachment to bone (connective tissue found between the implant and bone). They have been replaced generally by root-form implants, which are associated with a direct bony attachment called osseointegration (see Figures 27–1b and 27–1c).

Did You Know?

The oldest evidence of the use of dental implants dates back to 550 B.C. in Turkey.

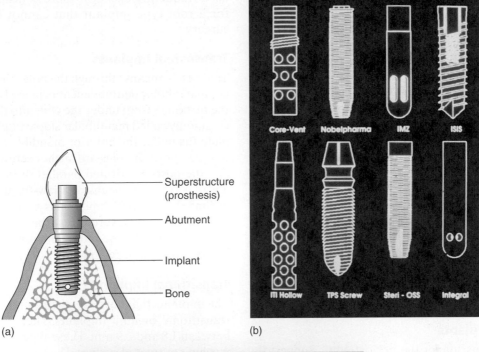

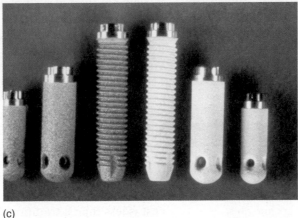

FIGURE 27–1 (a) Parts of a dental implant. Osseointegration occurs with direct anchorage of bone to the implant. Diagrammatic (b) and clinical (c) examples of different types of root-form dental implants showing different shapes, surfaces, and coatings.

Rapid Dental Hint

There are many types of dental implant systems available. These systems are based on their shapes and the relation to the patient's bone.

OSSEOINTEGRATION **Osseointegration** is a term introduced by Brånemark and coworkers in 1969 to describe the direct contact of a load-carrying dental implant (inert metal) with bone without any intervening connective tissue. Thus, the implant becomes an integral part of the bone and is,

in effect, ankylosed, as seen at the light microscopic level (Brånemark et al., 1969). Osseointegration has revolutionized implant dentistry and made it the mainstream form of therapy it is today.

Osseointegrated description has been expanded by the same group of investigators to characterize the long-term success of an osseointegrated implant. Success rates have been reported to be greater than 90% in both fully edentulous and partially edentulous patients. Such success requires full occlusal function without pain and, most important, after an initial marginal bone height loss in the first year of 1 to 2 mm at the bone crest, a crestal bone height loss of no more than 0.1 to 0.2 mm per year. Inflammation of the gingiva around the implant neck is acceptable as long as it is contoured and does not affect the bone or jeopardize long-term implant success rates (Smith & Zarb, 1989).

The implant fixture that initially showed long-term success was made of machined pure titanium with a screw shape. The titanium surface oxidizes into a thin nonreactive titanium oxide layer to which bone adheres, at least at the light-microscopic level. This type of bone-implant interface is called osseointegration. Although almost all dental implants today are titanium based (pure titanium or titanium alloy), some are coated, sprayed, or otherwise treated to create a rough surface, thus producing more surface area for the bone to contact or adhere to (see Figures 26–1b, 26–1c). The coatings used are usually acid-etched and sprayed, a titanium plasma spray, titanium beads, grit blasted-acid etched, or calcium-phosphate ceramics (hydroxyapatite and others). Some research has shown that the initial bone bonding to hydroxyapatite may be greater and stronger than the bonding to titanium (Weinlander, 1991). Endosseous implants are the predominant type (> 90%) used in current practice (Figure 27–2a ■).

Subperiosteal Implants

Subperiosteal means "under the periosteum." Subperiosteal implants are individually designed cast-metal frames that fit intimately over the bone and under the periosteum and gingiva. Resting on the bone for support, the frame may or may not be fixed by screws to the bone. Posts protrude through the gingiva as anchors for the replacement

Did You Know?

Swedish Professor Per-Ingvar Brånemark discovered that titanium can be successfully fused into bone when osteoblasts grow on and into the rough surface of the implanted titantium; hence the discovery of Brånemark implants.

teeth (Figure 27–2b). Currently, this type of implant is not used frequently except if there is insufficient bone mass for a root-type implant that cannot be corrected with surgery.

Transosteal Implants

Transosteal means "through the bone." Transosteal implants are mandibular denture anchors placed all the way through the mandible from under the chin into the mouth. They are commonly called mandibular staple implants. A curved, flat plate fits under the anterior mandible and usually has five to seven pins. The pins are anchor screws to hold the plate, and the posts are drilled parallel through the mandibular alveolar ridge by means of a jaw-fixation jig with parallel drilling sleeves. This implant has a good success record and is used for very severely resorbed mandibles. However, complications may be more common, and there is greater risk of tissue damage and infection.

Transitional Implants

The implants that have less than 3 mm diameter are called transitional or mini implants. Their diameter can range between 1.8 and 2.9 mm. These types of implants can have machine or treated surface. The last decade they have been used for orthodontic anchorage and also for prosthetic rehabilitation. It is the consensus that they are best used as an alternative to provisional restorations (Heberer, Hildebrand, & Nelson, 2011; Froum, Emtiaz, Bloom, Scolnick, & Tarnow, 1998; Petrugaro & Windmiller, 2001) even though success rates over 90% have been reported for long-term prosthesis (Balaji, Mohamed, & Kathiresan, 2010; Bulard & Vance, 2005). Their main advantages are that they provide retention, stability, and support of the prosthesis; better chewing and phonetics for the patient; and protection of an augmentation site as well as a vertical stop. They have a very easy surgical protocol, and their cost is less than a traditional dental implant (de Almeida, Filho, & Goiatto, 2011).

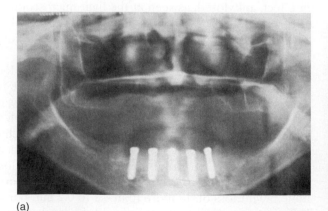

(a)

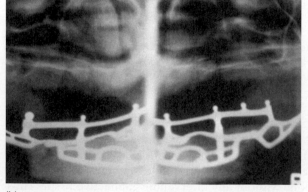

(b)

FIGURE 27–2 (a) Panoramic radiograph of root-form dental implants in mandible. (b) Panoramic radiograph of supraperiosteal dental implants on mandible.

Endodontic Implants

Endodontic implants are placed "in and through the tooth." They are also called endodontic stabilizers because they consist of a long, wide post inserted into the prepared root canal space that purposely extends at least a centimeter beyond the apex. The rationale is that this extension will stabilize the tooth and improve its usefulness as an abutment. However, this type of implant is not used commonly in the United States and has a poor prognosis because of the potential for root fracture, mechanical retention problems, and root resorption.

Surgical Procedure

Surgical protocol for implant placement varies from two-stage surgery, to single-stage surgery, and to single-stage surgery with immediate or early loading.

Dental hygienists should be familiar with the basics of dental implant therapy, including the surgical procedures. Although dental implant treatment may sound extensive, involved, and painful, most patients receive their dental implants in an outpatient setting and have few postoperative problems such as bleeding, infection, or pain. The general stages of dental implant treatment are outlined in Figure 27–3 ■.

The patient should be aware that several preoperative steps usually are necessary before the actual implant surgery. The restorative dentist (and the surgeon) should do a full workup on the patient. This includes mounted study casts, a wax-up of the planned restoration, fabrication of a radiographic and surgical guide stent, and appropriate pretreatment radiographs such as periapicals, panoramic, and computed or linear tomography for a three-dimensional view of the bone. These steps are needed to ensure accurate planning of implant number, diameter, length, and location based on the restorative needs of the patient, bone quantity and quality, and anatomic structures.

Bone quantity and quality of the maxilla and mandible is also important for implant success. Bone quantity refers to the available bone at the future implant site. Bone quantity factors that must be evaluated are the bone width (distance between facial and lingual cortical plates of bone; a minimum of 5 mm is recommended), height (measured

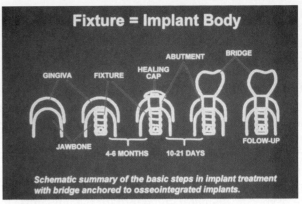

FIGURE 27–3 Diagram of sequence of dental implant placement using two-stage technique. The body of the implant (fixture) is surgically placed in the bone under the gingiva, allowed to heal for several months, uncovered so that a healing post can be connected to the implant, and the restoration completed.

from the crest of the edentulous ridge to an anatomical structure such as the maxillary sinus or mandibular canal), and length (mesiodistal distance in an edentulous site or the distance between two adjacent implants; recommended distance between two implants is 3 mm). Determination of bone quality is based on bone density (Table 27–1 ■), which reflects the strength of the bone (Lekholm & Zarb, 1985). Types I, II, and III bone offer good strength, whereas type IV bone has poor strength because this type of bone has a thin cortical plate and low trabecular density.

Implant placement can be done as a two-stage or single-stage procedure in which the implant body is placed in the bone and following a healing period is surgically exposed

Did You Know?

Cortical bone allows for a greater implant-bone contact and implant fixation than cancellous bone because cortical bone has an 80% to 90% volume density of bone matrix versus 20% to 25% for cancellous bone.

Table 27–1 Quality of Bone for Implant Placement

Type of Bone	Quality of Bone
I	Homogenous cortical (compact) bone
II	Core of dense trabecular (cancellous) bone with a thick layer of compact bone surrounding it
III	Thin layer of cortical bone surrounding dense trabecular bone of favorable strength
IV	Thin layer of cortical bone surrounding a core of low-density trabecular bone

to prepare the implant for a restoration. In the single-stage procedure the implant body is placed in bone with a portion of the implant body (collar) or abutment (post) left exposed until the time of restoration some time later.

Two-Stage Surgical Procedure

FIRST-STAGE SURGERY Once the patient is made comfortable and the areas of implant placement are anesthetized, the surgical guide stent is positioned and the specific implant locations marked. An incision is made through the crest of the gingiva, and flaps are reflected to expose the bone. A specific sequence of drills/burs is used to create a hole of specific diameter and depth for the implant(s) to be used. The drilling is done at relatively slow speed with copious irrigation to keep the bone cool and minimize trauma to the potential bone-healing cells. The root-form implant is then threaded or gently tapped into position so that its top is flush with the top of the bone. A cover screw is placed on top of the implant to seal the screw hole for cleanliness. The gingiva is then sutured to cover the implant(s) (Figure 27–4 ■). The implant surgeon may prescribe analgesics and antibiotics as needed. Sutures are left in place for

approximately 7 to 14 days. Although most patients would like to have a temporary tooth replacement in the implant area immediately, pressure on top of the implant should be avoided. A fixed temporary restoration relieved over the implant sites often can be placed in the partially edentulous implant patient.

The implants are allowed to heal undisturbed for 3 to 6 months so osseointegration occurs before second-stage uncovering surgery is performed. The time period needed for osseointegration varies depending on the bone quality or density and therefore is shortest for the mandibular anterior area, which is composed of dense cortical bone (3 to 4 months), and longest for the maxillary posterior area, which is composed of more fragile cancellous bone (5 to 6 months). However, recent advances in implant surfaces have allowed manufacturers to claim implants can be loaded as early as 2 months after placement (Avila, Galindo, & Rios, 2007).

SECOND-STAGE SURGERY Second-stage or uncovering surgery is performed to expose the top of the implant to create a permanent opening and replace the cover screw with a

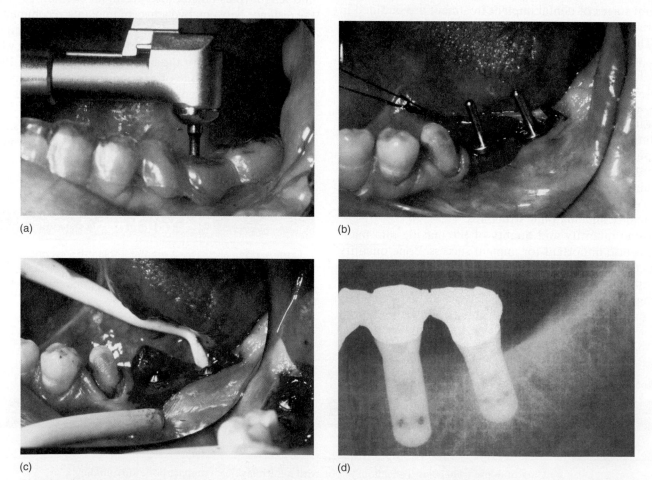

(a)

(b)

(c)

(d)

FIGURE 27–4 Clinical case illustrating implant placement. (a) Initial drill hole (osteotomy) using surgical guide stent. (b) Test pins placed to verify position and angulation of the planned implants. (c) Two implants placed into properly drilled holes to be level with bone crest. (d) Five-year follow-up radiograph illustrating fixed-bridge design for good oral hygiene and maintenance of bone level.

temporary healing abutment or post that screws into the implant fixture and protrudes through the gingival tissue into the oral cavity. This surgery is usually performed using local anesthesia. After a small incision is made over the implants, the cover screw is removed, and the healing abutment is placed. The gingiva is then sutured tightly around the protruding abutment. After 2 to 3 weeks of soft-tissue healing, the restoration process continues. Impressions of the implant(s) are taken, and crowns are fabricated to cement or screw onto the implant abutments. A removable prosthesis can also be attached to the abutment, which allows the patient to remove and clean the tooth.

Single-Stage Surgical Procedure

Some implant systems avoid the second-stage surgery with one-stage implants. Single-stage implants are left exposed but not loaded at the time of surgery. This single-stage surgery still requires a 3- to 6-month healing time, but rather than performing a second surgery, the cover screw or healing abutment is removed and the final restoration (crown) is placed.

SINGLE-STAGE SURGICAL PROCEDURE WITH EARLY/IMMEDIATE LOADING Implants placed with primary stability can be put into function immediately as long as the forces are controlled and below the critical movement threshold. If primary stability cannot be achieved, then delayed (extended time for healing) loading is required. This procedure allows the attachment of a temporary prosthesis at the time of implant placement rather than waiting months until healing is complete. Early loading of implants with a dental prosthesis occurs at another visit after the surgery, whereas immediate loading of implants with dental prosthesis/tooth occurs at the same visit as the surgery (Assad, Hassan, Shawky, & Badawy, 2007; Esposito et al., 2007).

Single-Tooth Replacements

Single-tooth replacement with dental implants is a treatment option for anterior or posterior teeth. Single missing anterior and posterior teeth are generally caused by trauma/injury, congenitally missing, extensive caries, or failed endodontic procedures. In the past, the primary concern with single-tooth placements in the anterior maxilla was with aesthetics and having the single dental implant closely resemble adjacent natural teeth (Figure 27–5 ■). Advancements in clinical application, concepts, and technology have developed into single-tooth replacements with a high rate of success.

Immediate Implant Placement in Extraction Sockets

Implants can also be placed at the same visit that a natural tooth is extracted. Immediately following extraction of a tooth, the implant is placed into the socket. Loading can be performed at a future time or in the same visit. There are a number of considerations for success, including adequate availability of bone, primary stability of the implant, and absence of infection. Drawbacks to this type of surgery include protracted healing time, excessive pain and swelling, and a large ridge defect if the implant fails and has to be removed (Froum, 2005; Froum et al., 2007; Wagenberg & Froum, 2006).

Dental Implant Site Preservation and Development

A tooth that is going to be extracted and later used as an implant site requires intact cortical plates of bone after the extraction for optimal aesthetics and implant function. Atraumatic extraction and socket preservation techniques have been introduced to minimize bone resorption after tooth extraction (John, De Poi, & Blanchard, 2007). However, sometimes this is not possible, and the socket needs to be grafted with bone and membrane to preserve the alveolar plates. An implant is usually placed about 6 months after socket bone grafting (Figure 27–6 ■).

Although the surgical procedures just outlined are basic and apply to patients with good bone quantity, quality, and form, additional procedures often must be used to build up the bone or gingival tissues to allow proper implant placement and restoration. These other procedures may include such therapy as guided bone regeneration (with bone grafts and membranes), soft tissue grafts, sinus bone grafts (sinus lift), distraction osteogenesis, or combinations of these. These additional procedures may extend the total treatment time until the final restoration can be delivered.

Guided bone regeneration (GBR) is a surgical procedure performed to increase the amount of alveolar bone available for the proper placement of a dental implant (Esposito, Grusovin, Coulthard, & Worthington, 2006). The terms *guided tissue regeneration* and *guided bone regeneration* are often used interchangeably in literature, but they are really two different terms—however, based on the same basic principles. Guided bone regeneration describes the

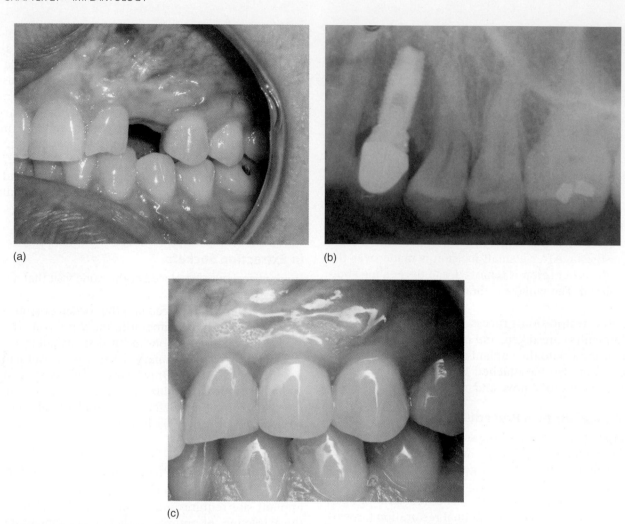

(a)

(b)

(c)

FIGURE 27–5 (a) Preoperative clinical view of a missing maxillary canine. (b) Radiograph of implant placement to replace maxillary canine. (c) Final clinical view of single tooth implant. (Courtesy of Dr. Stuart J. Froum, New York, New York.)

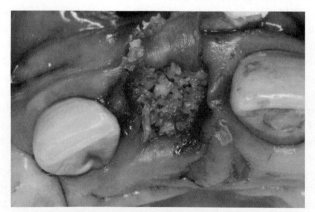

FIGURE 27–6 Extraction + graft: The maxillary central incisor was extracted and a bone graft placed in the extraction socket to preserve the bony walls for a future implant.

formation of only bone, not any other tissue (McAllister & Haghighat, 2007), whereas guided tissue regeneration involves the formation of bone, cementum, and periodontal ligament around teeth. Guided bone regeneration surgery is indicated when there is a volume, height, or width deficiency of the residual ridge that prohibits implantation or optimal implant installation for aesthetic and functional needs (Keith & Salama, 2007; Kfir, Kfir, Eliav, & Kaluski, 2007; Migani & Esposito, 2007). Bone grafting and use of an absorbable (or nonabsorbable) membrane, which is placed over the bone defect site, is used to stimulate the patient's osteoblasts (bone-producing cells) to develop additional alveolar bone mass. This procedure is done about 6 months prior to placement of dental implants; however, it can be done in conjunction with dental implant placement surgery.

Sinus grafts are needed to increase the height of the posterior alveolus (Figure 27–7 ■). Surgery is performed

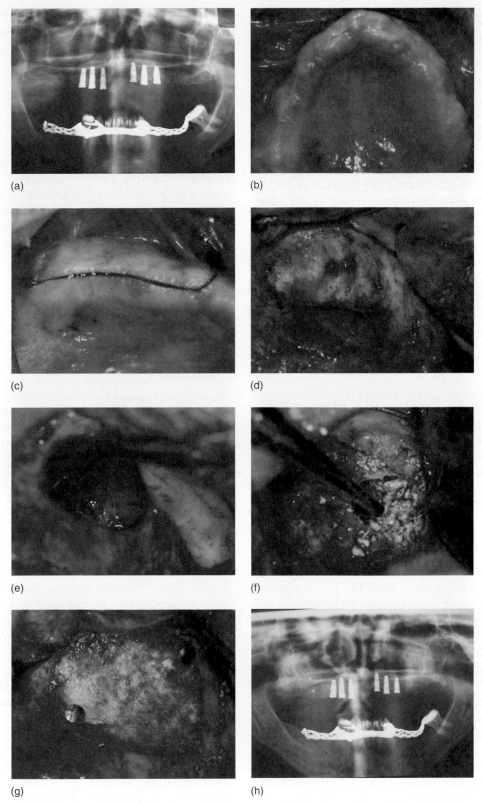

FIGURE 27–7 Sinus lift procedure: (a, b) Preoperative X-ray and clinical slide of the maxillary right side. This procedure is performed to increase the amount of bone in the maxilla for implant placement. (c) Surgical incision made on the edentulous ridge. (d) Soft tissue in anterior maxilla has been reflected back to expose the bone. An outline of the maxillary sinus area has been made. (e) Osteotomy in bone. Bone flap created by osteotomy has been pushed inward with maxillary sinus membrane (referred to as the Schneiderian membrane), creating space that is packed with bone graft material as shown in (f). (g) A membrane is placed over the bone material with bone tacks that hold the membrane in place to prevent movement. These tacks must be removed after healing has occurred. (h) Postoperative X-ray showing increased alveolar ridge height (right). Now implants can be placed.

Rapid Dental Hint

GTR (guided tissue regeneration) is regeneration of tissue around a tooth. GBR (guided bone regeneration) is regeneration of bone on a deficient alveolar ridge.

to expose and elevate the maxillary sinus membrane from the floor of the sinus, and bone graft material is placed into this area. Onlay bone block grafts (bone is placed on the alveolar ridge) are required to augment thin ridges (buccal/lingual dimension; Fugazzotto & Vlassis, 2007; Wallace et al., 2005).

Distraction osteogenesis is a surgical procedure used to increase the bone height of the alveolar ridges by cutting the bone into two pieces, which are gradually separated by 1 mm a day to form new bone between the cut pieces of bone. This allows for the displacement of bone into the deficient site. This procedure does not require placement of bone grafts. Figure 27–8 ■ reviews a case involving distraction osteogenesis.

Implant patients and dental office personnel must realize the stages and timeline involved in dental implant therapy. Generally, it takes 9 to 12 months to arrive at the point of delivery of the desired restoration. Longer times are necessary if implant sites require bone grafts or guided tissue (bone) regeneration procedures prior to implant placement. After the final restoration is placed, patients must commit to long-term professional maintenance and optimal oral hygiene self-care.

Prostheses

The original Brånemark implant system in the 1980s was initially recommended for edentulous (no teeth) patients and used "hybrid" prostheses supported by implants in the anterior area of the maxilla or mandible with the abutments visible when the lips are retracted. The function was good, but the appearance of these hybrid prostheses was not highly acceptable, and alternative, more aesthetic restorations were needed. Completely edentulous mouths may be treated with fixed prostheses or overdentures, whereas partially edentulous mouths may be treated with fixed partial prostheses and single-tooth replacements.

Implant-supported overdentures are recommended in edentulous (completely without teeth) patients to provide more stability to the denture and may help stop alveolar ridge resorption. Usually, two mandibular implants are placed in the canine area and a denture is fabricated to attach to the implants (Figure 27–9 ■).

If the patient is not totally edentulous, fixed dentures (bridges) attached to multiple implants may be a treatment option. Although some studies showed that splinting of implants to natural teeth resulted in intrusion of the natural tooth (Sheets & Earthman, 1993), a recent long-term study showed no higher risk for implant or prosthetic failure for implants splinted to teeth compared to implants splinted only to implants.

Implants versus Teeth

There are obvious differences between implants and teeth in structure and components (Table 27–2 ■). Implants are not prone to caries, endodontic (pulpal) problems, or root sensitivity, as are teeth. However, implants depend on proper restoration and occlusion, good oral hygiene, and regular maintenance, just as teeth do. Having a healthy soft tissue barrier is very important. Superstructures should be designed to help facilitate this. It has been shown that plaque accumulation and excessive occlusal forces are primary causes for implant failures (Meffert, Langer, & Frutz, 1992).

Anatomy

IMPLANT–TISSUE INTERFACE Natural teeth are surrounded by the periodontium: alveolar and supporting bone, cementum, periodontal ligament, and gingiva. Dental implants are surrounded by peri-implant tissues, including osseointegrated bone surrounding the fixture. There is no periodontal ligament. The abutment, like the crown of a natural tooth, is surrounded by gingiva. After surgery, the gingiva heals around the abutment. During the healing process, a new free gingival margin forms, including a gingival sulcus.

On natural teeth, the junctional epithelium provides a seal at the base of the sulcus against the invasion of bacterial substances. If the seal is disrupted and/or the gingival fibers are destroyed, the junctional epithelium migrates in an apical direction onto the root surface, and connective tissue fibers are destroyed, forming a periodontal pocket. The evidence supports the fact that a junctional epithelium, referred to as a **perimucosal seal**, adheres to implant component surfaces and has similar biologic features to the epithelial–tooth interface of a natural tooth.

On the other hand, the implant–connective tissue interface shows marked differences when compared with the connective tissue in teeth. There is a lack of cementum, and no connective tissue fibers insert into the implant surface. Connective tissue fibers subjacent to the epithelium on implants have been shown to be either parallel or circular in orientation to the implant surface, but they do not insert directly into the implant surface. These circular fibers are likely the first line of defense against bacteria. The arrangement of fibers is sometimes called a pursestring arrangement, and it helps to keep the soft tissues tightly adapted to the implant (Listgarten, Lang, Schroeder, & Schroeder, 1991).

KERATINIZED GINGIVA There are conflicting reports concerning the need for keratinized tissue around implants. However, multiple factors may influence the

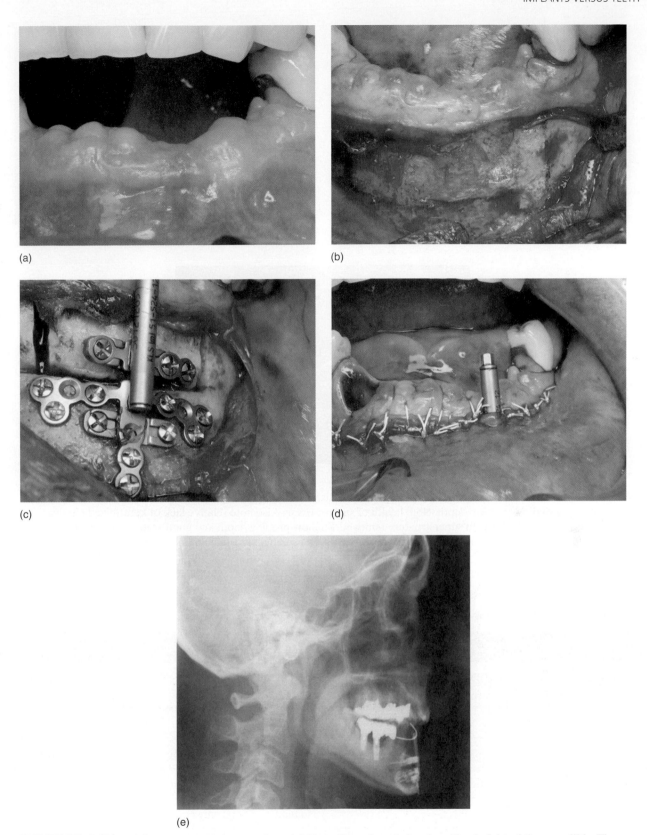

(a)

(b)

(c)

(d)

(e)

FIGURE 27–8 Distraction osteogenesis procedure. (a) Note the reduced alveolar ridge height of the mandible. The mandibular bone height must be lengthened to place dental implants. (b) Surgical procedure starts with raising a flap and exposure of the cortical bone. The area is outlined where the distraction device will be placed. This device is used to transmit controlled torque for elongation of the device thereby affecting distraction osteogenesis. (c) This device for lengthening bone by distraction osteogenesis (separating bone pieces) comprises a telescoping screw assembly. (d) The flap is repositioned to cover the device and sutured. The lead screw is exposed and is left in place until bone healing occurs. (e) Final case complete. (Courtesy of Dr. Stuart J. Froum, New York, New York.)

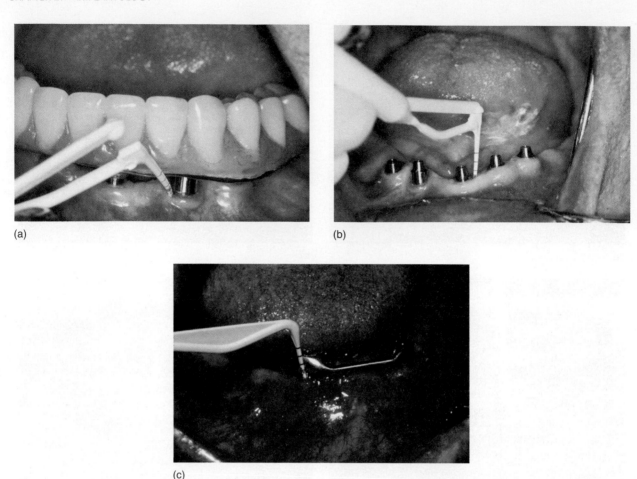

(a)

(b)

(c)

FIGURE 27–9 Periodontal probing around implants and tissue health. (a) Plastic probe with pressure-limiting mechanisms showing shallow probing depth. Note health of surface tissue. Also note relative lack of keratinized gingiva. (b) Probing access is easier with superstructure removed. Shallow probing depth and good zone of keratinized gingiva. (c) Inflamed tissue with deeper probing depth and bleeding on probing indicating an unhealthy implant site.

Table 27–2 Biologic Environment

Natural Tooth	Dental Implant
Perpendicular connective tissue (PDL) attachment inserting into cementum	No PDL; parallel connective tissue fibers because there is no cementum for attachment
Cementum	No cementum
Greater blood supply at neck	Less blood supply at neck due to scar formation during healing
Plaque—more confined inflammation	Plaque—more widespread inflammation
Transseptal/supracrestal fibers	No limiting fibers; only circular or parallel
Aggressive or slow bone loss in suprabony or infrabony patterns	Earlier, faster bone loss—circumferential around the implant
Inflammation not found in bone marrow	Inflammation into bone marrow
May show slight mobility	Any mobility means implant failure

desirability for the presence of keratinized tissue (Bahat, 1996; Greenstein & Cavallaro, 2011; Nemcovsky & Ofer, 2002). The type of tissue around an implant is essential to create the ideal emergence profile and an aesthetic illusion of a natural tooth (Kois, 2001). The type of tissue that surrounds a dental implant dictates the long-term health of the implant and its ability to withstand peri-implantitis (Nemcovsky & Ofer, 2002).

Blood Supply

Implants have less blood supply near their neck with more of a scar tissue appearance. Lack of a periodontal ligament limits the blood supply to the area to only the periosteal vessels (blood vessels covering the surface of bone) and bone marrow spaces.

Inflammatory Lesion

Dental plaque has been shown to grow faster on titanium than on enamel (Quirynen, Van Steenberghe, Jacobs, Schotte, & Darius, 1991). When plaque accumulation occurs, it results in more widespread inflammation around implants than the confined nature of the inflammatory lesion seen around teeth (Ericsson, Berglund, Marinello, Liljenberg, & Lindhe, 1992; Lekholm, 1986). This is due primarily to a lack of limiting attached connective tissue fibers such as the transseptal and supracrestal fiber groups that are present on teeth. Similarly, natural teeth tend to exhibit slow bone loss, and the inflammation does not usually extend into the bone marrow to any great degree. Infected implants, however, tend to have earlier and more rapid bone loss that extends into the adjacent bone marrow, creating a low-grade osteomyelitis.

Bacteriology

Neither dental implants nor natural teeth are immune to plaque accumulation. Regular, effective plaque control is imperative for soft tissue health and a good long-term prognosis with both.

Several studies have investigated the amount, rate, and contents of plaque deposits on implants as compared with teeth. Virtually all these studies show that there are no differences in the amount of plaque or the type of bacteria that accumulate on teeth or various implant surfaces. The types of pathogens found on both teeth and implants are similar (Newman & Flemmig, 1988; Box 27–1). Peri-implantitis (inflammation of the soft tissues around the implant) and marginal bone loss have been associated with the presence of these pathogens in both partially and fully edentulous patients.

For both implants and teeth, smooth surfaces inhibit and roughened surfaces encourage plaque accumulation. Therefore, in-office maintenance procedures should not roughen the surface of implant components (or teeth). Care should be taken not to locally damage the implant surface with metal ultrasonic or manual instruments. Plastic instruments should be used instead.

In summation, the major difference between implants and teeth, therefore, is the mechanism by which they are attached to the jawbone. Teeth are connected to the bone by means of a connective tissue sling, the periodontal ligament, which is a dynamic, responsive, adjustable attachment mechanism. Implants, by design, become osseointegrated or ankylosed without the cushioning effect of a periodontal ligament. Teeth can move as a result of occlusal or orthodontic forces. Implants do not have any physiologic movement.

Implant Maintenance Program

Periodontal maintenance procedures (continuing care) provided by the dental hygienist for implant patients include assessment of the entire oral cavity as well as the implant sites. A thorough assessment of plaque and calculus accumulation, as well as evaluation of soft and hard tissues, should be a part of the protocol for each maintenance visit. Box 27–2 reviews these assessment procedures.

The goal for maintenance therapy is to continually monitor the stable condition created by active treatment. Recall appointments should take place at three-month intervals, and the frequency should be increased if that interval is not adequate to maintain oral health.

Some clinicians assumed that patients with a history of tooth loss caused by periodontal disease presented a

Box 27–1: Pathogens Associated with Peri-Implantitis

Porphyromonas gingivalis	*Fusobacterium nucleatum*
Campylobacter recta	*Eikenella corrodens*
Tannerella forsythensis	*Eubacterium* species
Prevotella intermedia	*Selemonas* species
Peptostreptococcus micros	Spirochetes
Aggregatibacter actinomycetemcomitans	

Box 27–2: Assessment of Dental Implants and Maintenance Procedures (In-Office)

1. Review medical history.
2. Head and neck examination, oral cancer screening.
3. Take radiographs every 3 months for first year after implant restoration is placed; then yearly to check for bone loss. Place radiographs in sequential mounts.
4. Remove superstructure if necessary and possible.
5. Clean superstructure.
6. Check tissues for surface inflammation.
7. Check for plaque and review oral hygiene practices.
8. Record probing depths using a plastic or nylon periodontal probe.
9. Record bleeding on probing.
10. Clean implant abutments using special nonmetallic instruments.
11. Irrigate with antimicrobial solution if indicated.
12. Replace superstructure, if removed.
13. Have occlusion checked.
14. Review dental hygiene again with superstructure in place.
15. Reschedule for 3- or 4-month recall, depending on evaluation of tissue and oral hygiene.

Box 27–3: Periodontal Criteria for Success with Dental Implants

- No mobility
- Frequent inspection and debridement
- Shallow, stable pockets
- No bleeding on probing
- Effective oral hygiene
- Patient ability/accessibility
- Keratinized gingiva
- Accurate, secure fit of parts
- No trauma from occlusion
- Change in dental behavior pattern
- Maintenance of biocompatible interface

potentially higher risk for implant failure. However, several publications disproved this assumption demonstrating successful osseointegration in patients with different types of periodontal disease (Ellegaard, Baelum, & Karring, 1997; Mengel, Stelzel, Hasse, & Flores-de-Jacoby, 1996; Nevins & Langer, 1995). However, because the same periodontal microbiota colonizes teeth and implants placed in patients with periodontally compromised teeth, it is essential that optimum oral hygiene and plaque control be maintained prior to and following implant placement.

Clinical Parameters of Evaluation

SOFT TISSUE EVALUATION The clinical similarities between the natural dentition and dental implants have led to the use of similar parameters for evaluation of the periodontium and peri-implant tissues (Box 27–3). Clinical similarities provide a means of monitoring and observing peri-implant health status and the effectiveness of treatment. Evaluation of the soft tissue surrounding dental implants is very similar to that of natural tooth structure. A basic assessment begins with the color, contour, and consistency (texture) of the surrounding soft tissue. The presence of erythema, edema, and suppuration, which are the traditional signs of inflammation, should be noted. Thorough documentation of the changes in the soft tissue is important because change may signify current disease activity.

Probing Depth. Probing depth also can be used to assess the health of peri-implant tissues. However, the use of periodontal probes for evaluation of the peri-implant condition is highly controversial (Brägger, 1994). Some clinicians feel that probing depth is not an important clinical parameter in the success of an implant (Smith & Zarb, 1989). Concern has been expressed that probing for pockets around an implant may create a pathway for bacteria to attack the peri-implant seal. The probe may carry microorganisms from an infected site and seed a noninfected site. Also, different probing forces allow the probe to penetrate into the connective tissue/bone region easily because of the lack of a connective tissue attachment. Gentle probing is recommended around implants if the practitioner suspects pathology.

If probing is performed, four measurements around the circumference of the implant should be recorded. As with natural teeth, minimal probing depth (< 4 mm) is preferable (Balshi, 1986; Orton, Steele, & Wolinsky, 1987). Changes in probing depth over a period of time around an implant may be more important as an indicator of disease activity than a single probe depth measurement (Balshi, 1986). The use of a plastic or nylon periodontal probe is recommended to prevent scratching of the titanium components. With some abutment and superstructure designs, accurate probing may be difficult because the probe is prevented from reaching the base of the sulcus; thus the probing depth may be underestimated. A more accurate measurement may be obtained by removing the superstructure, which would allow probe insertion parallel to the long axis of the implant. However, more important than the actual probing depth is detecting early changes in the depth of the pocket. Early detection provides an opportunity for therapeutic intervention before irreversible changes have occurred. Probing level has been demonstrated to correlate highly with the marginal bone level (Quirynen et al., 1991; Figure 27–9).

Bleeding on Probing. Controversy also can be found in the literature regarding the use of bleeding on probing as a clinical assessment parameter for implants. As with natural teeth, bleeding on probing can be a significant clinical finding. Despite the apparent healthy look of surface tissues and even shallow probing depths, bleeding on probing is an indication that there is underlying disease (Lekholm, 1986). Any bleeding site (especially if the same site bleeds from visit to visit) should be inspected closely for the presence of irritants, and appropriate therapy should be instituted. However, some researchers find that bleeding may be related to probing force and wounding of the tissue rather than actual inflammation (Esposito, Hirsch, Lekholm, & Thomsen, 1998) and should not be used as an indicator of healthy or diseased peri-implant tissue.

KERATINIZED GINGIVA As mentioned earlier, the presence of keratinized gingiva adjacent to implants is associated with improved tissue health. As with natural teeth, keratinization improves the strength and stability of the epithelium and promotes long-term implant success. An inadequate zone of keratinized gingiva may lead to increased recession, tissue soreness with toothbrushing or eating, and the ability of metallic components to be seen through mucosal tissues.

Hard Tissue Evaluation

RADIOGRAPHIC PROCEDURES Implant bone levels are best determined by regular accurate radiographic evaluations. Panoramic radiographs commonly are taken for baseline data following abutment placement; however, individual periapical or vertical bitewing radiographs should be taken using the paralleling technique with a gridded film (film with millimeter markings). Such radiographs are preferable for determining bone height and density. Marginal bone height should be measured both mesially and distally and recorded in relation to a landmark on the implant system. For dental implant success, 0.2 mm or less of bone loss annually along the implant surface is acceptable (Albrektsson, Zarb, Worthington, & Eriksson, 1986). For proper continued evaluation, radiographic examinations are recommended after prosthetic connection, at 6 and 12 months and subsequently at 1- to 3-year intervals.

Mobility

It is recommended that the prosthesis be removed at least once a year to test for implant and abutment mobility. Because the truly osseointegrated implant has no periodontal ligament, there should be zero mobility around healthy implants. Mobility of an implant after an appropriate healing period is a sign of implant failure, indicating lack of osseointegraton. Radiographic examinations together with implant mobility tests seem to be the most reliable parameters in the prognostic assessment of osseointegrated implants (Esposito et al., 1998).

Mobility of the superstructure can be evaluated by wedging a curet between the prosthesis and the abutment head or by traditional mobility detection. If the abutment is loose, the screws may need to be examined and possibly tightened.

Identifying the Problem Implant

Although endosseous root-form dental implants are quite successful, with most studies showing greater than 90% long-term success with a variety of systems, some do develop problems. Identification of these problems when they first begin is important for effective management. The two primary reasons for ailing and failing implants are bacterial infection and mechanical trauma.

Criteria for Success

The periodontal criteria for success are similar for dental implants and natural teeth (Box 27–3). The basis of success is frequent inspection and debridement. As with natural teeth, shallow and stable probing depths are desirable at each visit. In addition, there should be no bleeding on probing at any evaluation site. An adequate zone of keratinized gingiva may be advantageous to protect the soft tissue interface (Brånemark et al., 1985). The main difference in success criteria involves mobility. Although unchanging mobility within physiologic limits is acceptable with natural teeth, any implant mobility is unacceptable.

Restoratively, the prosthesis must fit accurately and securely. There should be no trauma from occlusion (excessive occlusal force on the implant), especially in lateral excursions. Moreover, there should be no mobility of the superstructure and especially of the implant itself. Radiographically, no radiolucency should be present around the implant, and less than 0.2 mm of bone loss per year should be present.

Perhaps the most important factor in success is to effect a change in the patient's dental behavior pattern. If this occurs, and the preceding technical aspects are achieved, then a biocompatible interface between the implant and the host tissues can be maintained for a long time. These criteria are summarized in Box 27–3 (Smith & Zarb, 1989).

Overloading of Implants

Mechanical failures of both the implant components and prosthetic superstructures have been associated with occlusal overload and ill-fitting restorative frameworks. Because implants do not have a periodontal ligament, occlusal forces placed on the implant are transmitted directly to alveolar bone instead of the periodontal ligament. Thus, excessive occlusal force (overloading) generated either from improper placement/angle of implant, prosthesis design, and/or parafunctional activity may cause loosening and/or fracture of the screws through bending overload (Akça & Iplikçioğlu, 2001). Marginal bone loss around implants also has been associated with implant overload.

Rapid Dental Hint

There should be at least 1.5 to 2 mm of interproximal bone between an implant and a natural tooth.

Stages of Peri-Implant Disease

Plaque-induced inflammation occurs in a similar fashion around dental implants as around natural teeth. The pathogenesis is very similar for both entities, but there are several differences, as noted earlier in this chapter. **Peri-implant diseases** keep classified as peri-implant mucositis and peri-implantitis.

Peri-implant mucositis is similar to gingivitis; it is a reversible inflammatory reaction with bleeding on probing. There may be slight increased probing depths, but the perimucosal seal is intact.

Peri-implantitis has many of the same clinical manifestations and stages as periodontitis and is characterized by rapid loss of bone that can occur without any classic signs of pain or mobility. Peri-implantitis is an aggressive lesion. It can be graded from slight to severe, and its treatment parallels that of the stages of periodontitis (Figures 27–10 ■, 27–11 ■, 27–12 ■). Slight problems are treated with improved oral hygiene and nonsurgical local therapy (controlled-release antibiotics, mouth rinses; Ciancio, Lauciello, Shibly, Vitello, & Mather, 1995). Moderate problems usually require systemic antibiotics (Mombelli & Lang, 1992) or flap access surgery. Severe problems require flap surgery for access, with the likelihood of regenerative therapy, including bone-replacement grafts and guided tissue regeneration barriers. The latter has not been shown to be as effective with implants as with natural teeth. The best results in severe cases of peri-implantitis are obtained when the implant has the plaque removed and can be reburied to recapture the lost osseointegration. Sometimes, the problem is so advanced that the implant must be removed.

In 2004 the ITI group published a consensus on clinical procedures regarding implant survival and complications (Lang et al., 2004). They proposed the protocol shown in Figure 27-13 ■.

Superstructure Removal

On some occasions, the prosthetic superstructure supported by an implant must be removed for better access for maintenance of the implant abutment posts. Some superstructures are removable prostheses anyway, and the patient is familiar with their removal and replacement. Others (increasingly common) are fixed prostheses (screw-retained or cemented) and must be removed by dental office personnel.

Because the hygienist may be asked to remove a superstructure, he or she must be familiar with the removal and replacement process (Box 27-4).

Removing the superstructure generally entails unscrewing it from the abutments. This must be done in a systematic way. For example, a patient may have crowns and bridges from tooth 2 to tooth 15 with six implants under this superstructure. The hygienist should have six containers, small cups, or dappen dishes, with markings on them to correspond to the jaw location of the implants. When the screw from implant 2 is removed, it should be placed in the container marked 2. When the screw from implant 6 is removed, it should be placed in the container marked 6, and so on. The hygienist will want to back the screws off a little at a time, alternating among them, much in the way a tire is removed and replaced on a car. Unscrewing one side, for example, implant screws 2, 4, and 6 all the way, and not unscrewing implant screws 11, 13, and 15, may cause the integrity of the implants and superstructure to be compromised. When removing screws, the hygienist should employ a throat pack (gauze) to block and prevent any loose screws or abutments from being accidentally swallowed by the patient. Once the superstructure is removed, better access is available to evaluate the soft tissue and gingiva and provide maintenance therapy to the individual implants. The superstructure itself should be thoroughly inspected and

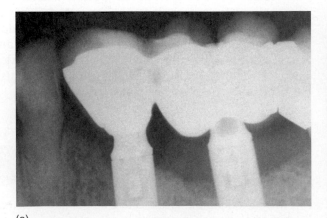

(a)

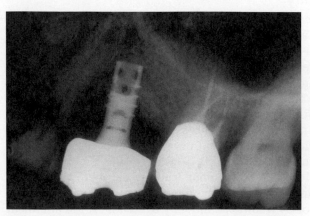

(b)

FIGURE 27–10 Radiographic evidence of bone loss around dental implants, indicating peri-implantitis.

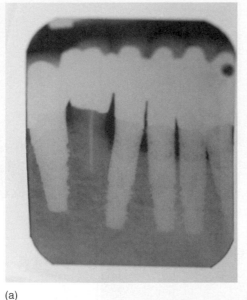
(a)

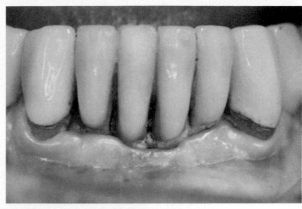
(b)

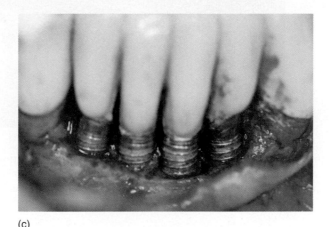
(c)

FIGURE 27–11 (a) X-ray showing implants with peri-implantitis. There is bone loss around the threads of the implant. (b) Clinical characteristics of these implants. Note the presence of gingival inflammation and swelling. (c) Surgical site with flap reflected showing bone loss around the implants.

Did You Know?

The peri-implant sulcus and the surfaces of endosseous dental implants acquire the patient's indigenous periodontal microflora.

Rapid Dental Hint

It is very important for patients to be on a regular recall schedule for maintenance, including plaque control, of the implant-supported prostheses.

cleaned. The hygienist must be aware that the inside of the screw holes always must be kept free of debris or pumice, or the screws may not fit, and the superstructure may not seat properly.

When replacing the superstructure, begin with one implant, and slightly tighten the screw. Then move to the next implant, and so on, just like replacing a tire on a car. Once all the screws are in position and slightly tightened, the hygienist can begin to tighten them down fully. Because peri-implant bone loss may result from occlusal overload, always make sure the occlusion is checked once the superstructure is in place.

Appropriate Instruments for Implants

Deposits that accumulate on supra- and subgingival surfaces of dental implant components should be removed. Normally, calculus on these surfaces is not as tenacious as on natural teeth because the deposits do not penetrate or interlock with the implant component surfaces (Lang, Mombelli, & Attström, 2003).

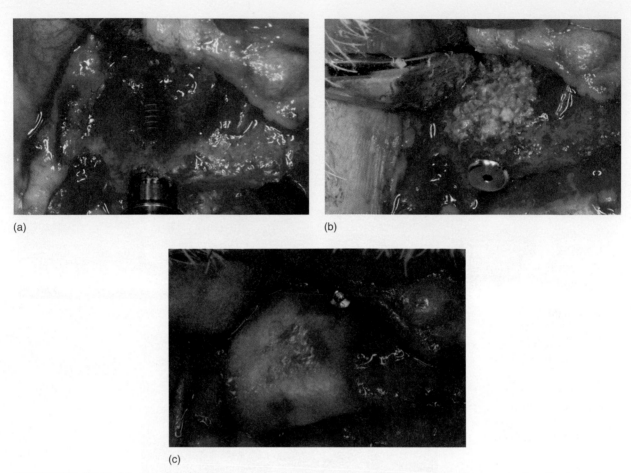

(a)

(b)

(c)

FIGURE 27–12 Peri-implantitis: (a) Surgical exposure of an implant. Bone resorption has occurred on the buccal aspect. Note the dehiscence with exposure of the threads of the implant. (b) Placement of Bio-Oss bone graft in the bony defect and (c) a barrier membrane attached to the bone with bone tacks. (Courtesy of Dr. Stuart J. Froum, New York, New York.)

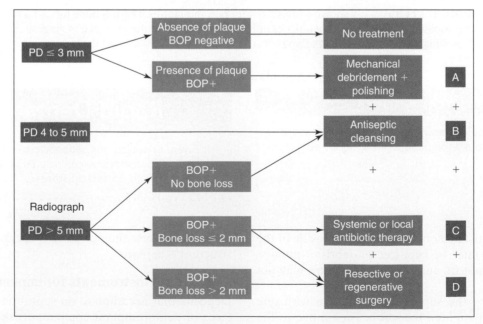

FIGURE 27–13 According to the CIST decision tree (Cumulative Interceptive Supportive Therapy) in part A, implants with probing depths 5 mm are first viewed by radiography. Those that have bleeding on probing, but no bone loss are treated the same as the latter. Those with > 5 mm with bleeding on probing and bone loss 5 mm PD, BOP and > 2 mm bone loss receive the same as the latter, followed by either resective or regenerative surgery (D).

Box 27–4: Removal and Replacement of Superstructure

1. Review radiographs and familiarize yourself with the implant location(s).
2. Note location of each implant under superstructure.
3. Have appropriately sized screws and instruments for removal and replacements available.
4. Remove any temporary filling material that may be in the screw hole area.
5. Have small containers, dappen dishes, or envelopes available. When removing the screws use a throat pack.
6. Once screws are removed, place in containers labeled as to location.
7. If removing extensive restorations, loosen screws a little at a time. Then return to each screw and loosen fully.
8. Remove superstructure and examine underside for debris.
9. Clean appropriately, keeping the integrity of the interface with the abutments and the screw holes free of debris.
10. Clean around implant abutments.
11. Replace superstructure.
12. Using correct screws, screw into place using same sequential technique as was used when removing superstructure.
13. Place temporary filling material over screws if indicated.
14. Check occlusion.

The nature of the surface of implant components must be considered when deciding which instruments to use during office procedures. Most implant components are titanium, a very tough but easily scratchable metal. Stainless steel and carbon steel instruments used directly on titanium can cause marring and scratching of the surface, resulting in roughness, which can increase plaque adherence. Curets made of **nonmetallic materials**, such as plastic, graphite, Teflon®, or nylon, are recommended, and these are available from several manufacturers (Figures 27–14 ■, 27–15 ■). Cleaning around the tissue surface of the prosthesis and implant abutments also can be performed with gauze or tufted floss.

Air-powder abrasive units are effective, but they should not be used directly on implant components for any length of time. The use of ultrasonic- and sonic-powered scalers with metal tips is also contraindicated with implants. Specific plastic or nylon sleeves placed over the tip are available that allow cleaning of implants without scratching (Figure 27–16 ■).

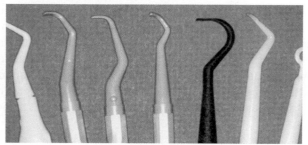

FIGURE 27–14 Several types of nonmetallic scalers and curets for use on dental implant components.

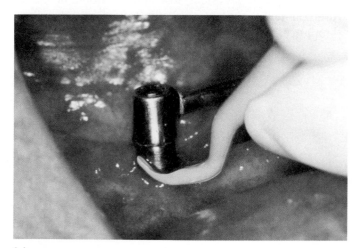

(a)

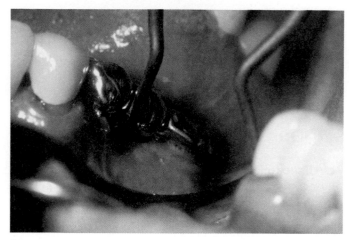

(b)

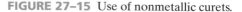

FIGURE 27–15 Use of nonmetallic curets.

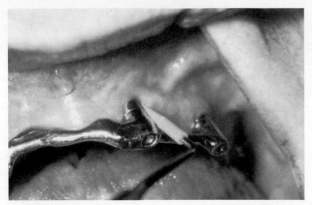

FIGURE 27–16 Nylon or plastic sleeve for ultrasonic or sonic instruments to prevent scratching of implant components.

In-Office Irrigation

The purpose of in-office irrigation is to attempt to irrigate to the base of the pocket. Plastic rather than metal irrigation tips or needles should be used when irrigating around implants, and care should be taken not to become too aggressive in forcing the tip into the pocket. Using an irrigation device with an antimicrobial solution at every maintenance visit is considered to be of some benefit by certain practitioners. Irrigation can be used if pathologic changes are present (Meffert et al., 1992). However, this information is anecdotal, and there are not enough controlled clinical studies to support implant irrigation.

Dental Hygiene Application

Implant therapy is a rapidly growing part of dental care. With the growing number of implants being placed, the dental team will have an important role in helping attain and preserve the oral health of these patients. Patient education regarding the scope of implant procedures, recommendations for daily home-care regimens, periodic maintenance visits, and regular evaluations are all part of the role of the dental hygienist. The hygienist probably will spend the most time with the patient and can help contribute substantially to the success of dental implant treatment. The dental hygienist has a significant role not only in implant maintenance but also in patient motivation and education. It is important to keep in mind that implant therapy is not for everyone. For this reason, it is crucial that the dental hygienist be informed about implant types, the sequence of therapy, and the social and systemic factors that influence implant success.

Key Points

- Controversy exists regarding the use of periodontal probes around healthy implants.
- Progressive bone loss is a pathologic sign that can lead to implant failure.
- The implant should not be mobile; mobility indicates lack of osseointegration and implant failure.
- Different prosthetic designs are used for final implant restorations.
- Implant placement can be done as a single- or second-stage procedure.
- Metal (e.g., stainless steel) instruments should never be used on dental implants; use only Teflon®, wood, nylon, graphite, rubber, or plastic instruments.

Self-Quiz

1. All the following systemic conditions are precautions or contraindications to implant placement except one. Which one is the exception?
   a. Uncontrolled diabetes mellitus
   b. Controlled hypertension
   c. Smoking
   d. AIDS

2. Which one of the following types of dental implants is used most commonly today to support prostheses?
   a. Submucosal
   b. Subperiosteal
   c. Endosseous
   d. Transosteal

3. Which one of the following similarities is common between dental implants and natural teeth?
   a. Bone interface
   b. Microbial flora
   c. Connective tissue attachment
   d. Probing depths topography

4. The presence of keratized gingiva is important around implants because it may improve tissue health.
   a. Both the statement and the reason are correct and related.
   b. Both the statement and the reason are correct but not related.
   c. The statement is correct, but the reason is not.
   d. The statement is not correct, but the reason is correct.

5. In which one of the following drugs a patient is taking is implant placement a contraindication?
   a. IV bisphosphonate
   b. Aspirin
   c. Acetaminophen
   d. Vitamin D

6. All the following types of instruments are used to clean implant abutments except one. Which one is the exception?
   a. Teflon®
   b. Stainless steel
   c. Nylon
   d. Wood

7. Which one of the following factors is the major criterion for success of an implant?
   a. Inflammation
   b. Mobility
   c. Bleeding
   d. Bone level

8. Which one of the following parameters is most reliable in the assessment of the prognosis for osseointegrated implants?
   a. Color and contour of the gingiva
   b. Bleeding on probing and mobility
   c. Radiographic changes and mobility
   d. Periodontal probing and color of the gingiva

9. Which one of the following signs indicates implant failure?
   a. Deep probing depths
   b. Edematous tissue
   c. Bleeding
   d. Mobility

10. Oral irrigation should be used routinely around dental implants because there is no periodontal ligament attachment to an implant, allowing for easy access of the irrigant to the implant surface.
    a. Both the statement and the reason are correct and related.
    b. Both the statement and the reason are correct but not related.
    c. The statement is correct, but the reason is not.
    d. The statement is not correct, but the reason is correct.
    e. Neither the statement nor the reason is correct.

Case Study

A 55-year-old male has had an implant placed for tooth #30 for five years. He routinely comes for his preventive visits. Over the last year the dental hygienist has noticed that there is some gingival inflammation around his mandibular molars, including the tissue around the implant. Currently there is one thread showing on the implant. There is no mobility on the implant. The dental hygienist is preparing for this preventive visit.

1. Which instrument will not be used in this visit for the implant tooth?
   a. Plastic curet
   b. Teflon curet
   c. Carbon steel curet
   d. Graphite curet

Answer: C. Carbon or stainless steel instruments should not be used as they might mar or scratch the surface of the implant and increase biofilm adherence. Implant curets may be plastic, Teflon, or graphite.

2. What criteria will be an indicator for clinical health of the implant?
   a. No mobility
   b. Wide zone of keratinized tissue
   c. Firm transeptal fibers
   d. 2 mm sulcus

Answer: A. Mobility is an identified indication of implant failure. There are conflicting reports of need for keratinzed tissue around implants. There are no transeptal fibers, only circular or parallel fibers. Probing is controversial and does not have established guidelines; however, change in depth is more critical.

3. Bacterial biofilm on the implant has which characteristic?
   a. Contains same colonies as biofilm on natural teeth
   b. Grows faster on titanium than enamel
   c. Invades bone faster with more bone loss than natural teeth
   d. A and B
   e. All of the above

Answer: E. All are characteristics of implant biofilm. Optimal oral hygiene is essential to implant success.

References

Akça, K., and H. Iplikçioğlu. 2001. Finite element stress analysis of the influence of staggered versus straight placement of dental implants. *Int. J. Oral Maxillofac. Implants.* 16:722–730.

Albrektsson, T., and L. Sennerby. 1991. State of the art in oral implants. *J. Clin. Periodontal.* 16:474–481.

Albrektsson, T., G. Zarb, P. Worthington, and A. R. Eriksson. 1986. The long-term efficacy of currently used dental implants: A review and proposed criteria of success. *Int. J. Oral Maxillofac. Implants* 1:11–25.

Assad, A. S., S. A. Hassan, Y. M. Shawky, and M. M. Badawy. 2007, June. Clinical and radiographic evaluation of implant-retained mandibular overdentures with immediate loading. *Implant Dent.* 16(2):212–223.

Avila, G., P. Galindo, and H. Rios. 2007. Immediate implant loading: Current status from available literature. *Implant Dent.* 16(3):235–245.

Bahat, O. 1996. Interrelations of soft and hard tissues for osseointegrated implants. *Compend. Contin. Educ. Dent.* 12:1161–1170.

Bain, C. A. 1996. Smoking and implant failure: Benefits of a smoking cessation protocol. *Int. J. Oral Maxillofac. Implants* 11:756–759.

Balaji A., J. B. Mohamed, and R. Kathiresan. 2010. A pilot study of mini implants as a treatment option for prosthetic rehabilitation of ridges with sub-optimal bone volume. *J. Maxillofac. Oral Surg.* 9(4):334–338.

Balshi, T. J. 1986. Hygiene maintenance procedures for patients treated with the tissue integrated prosthesis (osseointegration). *Quintessence Int.* 17:95–102.

Belser, U., R. Mericske-Stern, D. Buser, J. P. Bernard, D. Hess, and J. P. Martinet. 1996. Preoperative diagnosis and treatment planning. In eds. A. Schroeder, F. Sutter, D. Buser, and G. Krekeler, *Oral implantology*, 231–255. New York: Thieme Medical.

Brägger, U. 1994. Maintenance, monitoring, therapy of implant failures. In eds. N. P. Lang and T. Karring, *Proceedings of the 1st European Workshop on Periodontology.* Chicago: Quintessence.

Brånemark, P. I., U. Breine, R. Adell, O. Hansson, J. Lindström, and A. Ohlsson. 1969. Intraosseous anchorage of dental prosthesis. *Scand. J. Plast. Reconstr. Surg.* 3:81–100.

Brånemark, P. I., G. Zarb, and T. Albrektsson. 1985. *Tissue-integrated prosthesis osseointegration in clinical dentistry.* Chicago: Quintessence.

Bulard R. A., and J. B. Vance. 2005. Multi-clinic evaluation using mini-dental implants for long-term denture stabilization: A preliminary biometric evaluation. *Compend. Contin. Educ. Dent.* 26(12):892–897.

Cartsos, V. M., S. Zhu, and A. Zavras. 2008. Bisphosphonate use and the risk of adverse jaw outcomes. *JADA* 139(1):23–30.

Ciancio, S. G., C. Lauciello, O. Shibly, M. Vitello, and M. Mather. 1995. The effect of an antiseptic mouthrinse on implant maintenance: Plaque and peri-implant gingival tissues. *J. Peridontol.* 66:962–965.

Cochran, D. 1996. Implant therapy. *I. Ann. Periodontol.* 1:707–820.

Dao, T. T., J. D. Anderson, and G. A. Zarb. 1993. Is osteoporosis a risk factor for osseointegration of dental implants? *Int. J. Oral Maxillofac. Implants.* 8:137–144.

de Almeida E. O., H. G. Filho, and M. C. Goiatto. 2011. The use of transitional implants to support provisional prostheses during the healing phase: A literature review. *Quintessence Int.* 42(1):19–24.

Edwards, B. J., J. W. Hellstein, and P. L. Jacobson. 2008. Updated recommendations for managing the care of patients receiving oral bisphosphonate therapy: An advisory statement from the American Dental Association Council on Scientific Affairs. *J. Am. Dent. Assoc.* 139:1674–1677.

Ellegaard, B., V. Baelum, and T. Karring. 1997. Implant therapy in periodontally compromised patients. *Clin. Oral Implants Res.* 8:180–188.

Ericsson, I., N. T. Berglund, C. Marinello, B. Liljenberg, and J. Lindhe. 1992. Long-standing plaque and gingivitis at implants and teeth in the dog. *Clin. Oral Implant Res.* 3:99–103.

Esposito, M., M. G. Grusovin, P. Coulthard, and H. V. Worthington. 2006. The efficacy of various bone augmentation procedures for dental implants: A Cochrane systematic review of randomized controlled clinical trials. *Int. J. Oral Maxillofac. Implants* 21(5):696–710.

Esposito, M., M. G. Grusovin, M. Willings, et al. 2007. The effectiveness of immediate, early, and conventional loading of dental implants: A Cochrane systematic review of randomized controlled clinical trials. *Int. J. Oral Maxillofac. Implants* 22(6):893–904.

Esposito, M., J. M. Hirsch, U. Lekholm, and P. Thomsen. 1998. Biological factors contributing to failures of osseointegrated oral implants: I. Success criteria and epidemiology. *Eur. J. Oral Sci.* 106:527–551.

Froum, S. J. 2005, July. Immediate placement of implants into extraction sockets: Rationale, outcomes, technique. *Alpha Omegan* 98(2):20–35.

Froum, S. J., S. C. Cho, H. Francisco, et al. 2007. Immediate implant placement and provisionalization—two case reports. *Pract. Proced. Aesthet. Dent.* 19(10):621–628.

Froum S., S. Emtiaz, M. J. Bloom, J. Scolnick, and D. P. Tarnow. 1998. The use of transitional implants for immediate fixed temporary prostheses in cases of implant restorations. *Pract. Periodontics Aesthet. Dent.* 10(6):737–746.

Fugazzotto, P. A., W. S. Lightfoot, R. Jaffin, and A. Kumar. 2007, September. Implant placement with or without simultaneous tooth extraction in patients taking oral bisphosphonates: Postoperative healing, early follow-up, and the incidence of complications in two private practices. *J. Periodontol.* 78(9):1664–1669.

Fugazzotto, P. A., and J. Vlassis. 2007. Report of 1633 implants in 814 augmented sinus areas in function for up to 180 months. *Impl. Dent.* 16(4):369–378.

Grant, B. T., C. Amenedo, K. Freeman, and R. A. Kraut. 2008. Outcomes of placing dental implants in patients taking oral bisphosphonates: A review of 115 cases. *J. Oral Maxillofac. Surg.* 66(2):223–230.

Greenstein, G., and J. Cavallaro. 2011. The clinical significance of keratinized gingiva around dental implants. *Compend. Contin. Educ. Dent.* 32(8):24–31.

Heberer, S., D. Hildebrand, and K. Nelson. 2011. Survival rate and potential influential factors for two transitional implant systems in edentulous patients: a prospective clinical study. *J. Oral Rehabil.* 38(6):447–453.

John, V., R. De Poi, and S. Blanchard. 2007, December. Socket preservation as a precursor of future implant placement: Review of the literature and case reports. *Compend. Contin. Educ. Dent.* 28(12):646–53; quiz, 654, 671.

Keith, J. D., Jr., and M. A. Salama. 2007, November. Ridge preservation and augmentation using regenerative materials to enhance implant predictability and esthetics. *Compend. Contin. Educ. Dent.* 28(11):614–21; quiz, 622–4.

Kfir, E., V. Kfir, E. Eliav, and E. Kaluski. 2007. Minimally invasive guided bone regneration. *J. Oral Implantol.* 33:205–210.

Kois, J. C. 2001. Predictable single tooth peri-implant esthetics: Five diagnostic keys. *Compend. Contin. Educ. Dent.* 3:199–206.

Lang N. P., T. Berglundh, L. J. Heitz-Mayfield, B. E. Pjetursson, G. E. Salvi, and M. Sanz. 2004. Consensus statement and recommended clinical procedures regarding implant survival and complications. *Int. J. Oral Max. Imp.* 19:150–154.

Lang, N. P., A. Mombelli, and R. Attström. 2003. Dental plaque and calculus. In *Clinical periodontology and implant dentistry*, 4th ed., 81–105. Oxford, UK: Blackwell Publishing.

Lekholm, M. 1986. Marginal tissue reactions at osseointegrated titanium fixtures. *Int. J. Oral Maxillofac. Implants* 15:53–61.

Lekholm, M., and G. A. Zarb. 1985. Patient selection. In eds. P.-I. Brånemark, G. A. Zarb, and T. Albrektsson. *Tissue integrated prosthesis. Osseointegration in clinical dentistry*, 199–209. Chicago: Quintessence.

Listgarten, M. A., N. P. Lang, H. E. Schroeder, and A. Schroeder. 1991. Periodontal tissues and their counterparts around endosseous implants. *Clin. Oral Implant Res.* 2:1–19.

Marx, R. E. 2007. *Oral and intravenous bisphsphonate-induced osteonecrosis of the jaws: History, etiology, prevention, and treatment.* Chicago, IL: Quintessence, 15.

Marx, R. E., J. E. Cillo, Jr., and J. J. Ulloa. 2007, December. Oral bisphosphonate-induced osteonecrosis: Risk factors, prediction of risk using serum CTx testing, prevention, and treatment. *J. Oral Maxillofac. Surg.* 65(12):2397–2410.

Marx, R. E., Y. Sawatari, M. Fortin, and V. Broumand. 2005. Bisphosphonate-induced exposed bone (osteonecrosis/osteopetrosis) of the jaws: Risk factors, recognition, prevention, and treatment. *J. Oral Maxillofac. Surg.* 63:1567–1575.

McAllister, B. S., and K. Haghighat. 2007. Bone augmentation techniques. *J. Periodontol.* 78:377–396.

Meffert, R., B. Langer, and M. Frutz. 1992. Dental implants: A review. *J. Periodontol.* 63:859–870.

Mengel, R., M. Stelzel, C. Hasse, and L. Flores-de-Jacoby. 1996. Osseointegrated implants in patients treated for generalized severe adult periodontitis. An interim report. *J. Periodontol.* 67:782–787.

Migani, M., and M. Esposito. 2007, May–June. Vertical ridge augmentation with autogenous bone grafts: Resorbable barriers

supported by osteosynthesis plates versus titanium-reinforced barriers. A preliminary report of a blinded, randomized controlled clinical trial. *Int. J. Oral Maxillofac. Implants* 22(3):373–382.

Mombelli, A., and N. P. Lang. 1992. Antimicrobial treatment of peri-implant infections. *Clin. Oral Implants Res.* 3:162–168.

Nemcovsky, C. E., and M. Ofer. 2002. Rotated palatal flap. A surgical approach to increase keratinized tissue width in maxillary implant uncovering: Technique and clinical evaluation. *Int. J. Periodont. Restor. Dent.* 22:607–612.

Nevins, M., and B. Langer. 1995. The successful use of osseointegrated implants for the treatment of the recalcitrant periodontal patient. *J. Periodontol.* 66:150–157.

Newman, M., and T. Flemmig. 1988. Periodontal considerations of implants and implant associated microbiota. *J. Dent. Ed.* 52:737–744.

Orton, G. S., D. L. Steele, and L. E. Wolinsky. 1987. The dental professional's role in monitoring and maintenance of tissue-integrated prosthesis. *Int. J. Oral Maxillofac. Implants* 4:305–310.

Petrungaro P. S., and N. Windmiller. 2001. Using transitional implants during the healing phase of implant reconstruction. *Gen. Dent.* 49(1):46–51.

Quirynen, M., D. van Steenberghe, R. Jacobs, A. Schotte, and P. Darius. 1991. The reliability of pocket probing around screw-type implants. *Clin. Oral Implant Res.* 2:186–192.

Sheets, C. G., and J. C. Earthman. 1993. Natural tooth intrusion and reversal in implant-assisted prostheses. *J. Prost. Dent.* 70:513–520.

Smith, D., and G. Zarb. 1989. Criteria for success of osseointegrated endosseous implants. *J. Prosthet. Dent.* 62:567–572.

Wagenberg, B., and S. J. Froum. 2006, January–February. A retrospective study of 1925 consecutively placed immediate implants from 1988 to 2004. *Int. J. Oral Maxillofac. Implants* 21(1):71–80.

Wallace, S. S., S. J. Froum, S. C. Cho, et al. 2005, December. Sinus augmentation utilizing an organic bovine bone (Bio-Oss) with absorbable and nonabsorbable membranes placed over the lateral window: Histomorphometric and clinical analyses. *Int. J. Periodont. Restor. Dent.* 25(6):551–559.

Wang, H. L., D. Weber, and L. K. McCauley. 2007. Effect of long-term oral bisphosphonates on implant wound healing: Literature review and a case report. *J. Periodontol.* 78(3):584–594.

Weinlander, M. 1991. Bone growth around dental implants. *Dent. Clin. North Am.* 35:585–601.

Case Studies

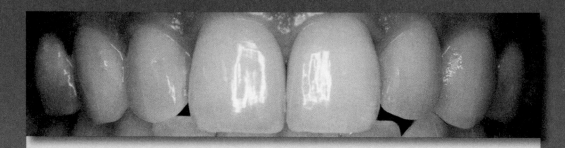

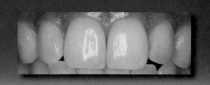

Medical History

The patient is a 31-year-old female who presents to the clinic and states that she is in perfect health. Her last physical examination was 1 year ago. The blood pressure is 125/82 and pulse is 72. She is 5 feet 4 inches tall and weighs 125 lbs (56.8 kgs). Medications: She takes Yasmin (an oral contraceptive) and a multivitamin daily.

Dental History

When she was a child, she had regular dental visits. Her "gum" problems started when she was about 12 years old. She said the dentist said she was "losing some bone around some back teeth." But she has not been to a dentist in the last 15 years. She tries to brush once a day, but if she is too busy she will not brush. She does not floss. She has a sister who also has "gum" problems. At work she has a habit of biting a pencil when under stress. She also notices that her "gums are shrinking."

Social History

The patient is married with one child. She denies smoking and consumption of alcohol.

Chief Complaint

"My teeth have spaces between them and I feel cold."

Oral Hygiene Status

The patient has poor oral hygiene. There is generalized supra/subgingival plaque and calculus.

Gingival Exam

The gingiva is red with rolled margins. The papillae are blunted, pointed, and absent. There is loss of stippling on the mandibular gingiva.

Periodontal Exam

Probing depths range up to 10 mm. The mandibular right second premolar has 5 mm of gingival recession on the direct facial surface. There is generalized bleeding on probing.

Interpretation

Patient Problem	Basis for Discussion	Questions (Q)/Answers (A)	Chapter Location
Localized bone loss started at 12 years of age.	Patient was young to have bone resorption.	Q) Why did the patient lose bone at such an early age? A) The periodontal condition is recognized as aggressive periodontitis. Initially, it was localized to the molars, and then later it became generalized. The criteria for localized (< 30% of sites) aggressive periodontitis includes clinically healthy patient, rapid attachment loss, and bone destruction and familial. Later in life, this condition became chronic periodontitis. It is not aggressive at this point because there are moderate amounts of plaque and calculus. Q) What is the cause of aggressive periodontitis? A) Bacteria and host response. Elevated levels of *Aggregatibacter actinomycetemcomitans*, and in some populations, *Porphyromonas gingivalis* may be elevated. There are also elevated levels of PGE$_2$ and IL-1β.	8
Gingival recession.	Patient is sensitive to cold and air.	Q) What is the cause of the gingival recession? A) There are many causes of gingival recession, but in this case it is caused by attachment loss where the gingival fibers are destroyed by collagenase, allowing the junctional epithelium to migrate apically onto the root surface. This is referred to as attachment loss and is the result of the disease process.	8, 16

(continued)

Interpretation (*cont.*)

Patient Problem	Basis for Discussion	Questions (Q)/Answers (A)	Chapter Location
A lot of diastemas (spaces between teeth).	The chief complaint.	Q) Why are the teeth moving and developing spaces? A) Pathologic migration due to severe bone loss. It has been documented that periodontal disease destruction of the attachment apparatus plays a major role in the development of pathological migration (abnormal movement of teeth with flaring of the anterior teeth) and is often the motivation for patients to seek periodontal care.	8, 16
Patient gets food stuck in between the teeth.	Blunting (tip of papilla is destroyed) of gingival papilla and open contacts.	Q) Why are the papillae blunted? A) There is a saying in periodontics that "gingiva follows the bone." So, with bone loss the gingiva can become blunted.	7, 15
Patient taking oral contraceptive.	May be a contributing factor to the patient's gingival condition.	Q) Do you think that the oral contraceptive is a contributing factor to the patient's periodontal condition? A) No. Also, with today's formulation of oral contraceptive less hormones are used, thus reducing the incidence of gingivitis.	6

1. Which of the following teeth exhibits a vertical defect?
   a. Maxillary right lateral incisor
   b. Maxillary left canine
   c. Maxillary right central incisor
   d. Mandibular left first molar

2. Which of the following conditions is the cause of the patient's chief complaint?
   a. Attrition
   b. Erosion
   c. Bone loss
   d. Furcation involvement
   e. Medication induced

3. The papillary condition between the mandibular right premolars and first molar is most likely to be caused by
   a. bone loss.
   b. improper flossing.
   c. overzealous toothbrushing.
   d. intrusion of opposing teeth.
   e. extrusion of mandibular teeth.

4. Which of the following factors is the cause of the condition in photo C where the arrow is pointing?
   a. Oral contraceptive
   b. Attachment loss
   c. High frenum
   d. Prominent root

5. Which of the following bacteria is most likely found in this patient?
   a. *Aggregatibacter actinomycetemcomitans*
   b. *Streptococcus mutans*
   c. *Streptococcus viridans*
   d. *Clostridium difficile*

6. Which of the following factors is the most likely cause for mobility of the mandibular incisors?
   a. Parafunctional habit
   b. Bone loss
   c. Oral contraceptive
   d. Oral biofilm

7. The amount of clinical attachment loss on the direct facial surface of the mandibular right second premolar is _____ mm.
   a. 1
   b. 2
   c. 4
   d. 5
   e. 6

8. Which of the following teeth has a hopeless prognosis?
   a. Maxillary right second premolar
   b. Maxillary left second molar
   c. Mandibular left first molar
   d. Mandibular left canine

9. Which of the following devices is best used to remove plaque in between the right mandibular lateral and canine?
   a. Dental floss
   b. Floss threader
   c. Toothpick
   d. End-tufted brush

10. Which of the following statements is correct about the right mandibular central incisor?
    a. Adequate bony support
    b. Poor crown-to-root ratio
    c. Widened periodontal ligament
    d. Extensive caries

DENTAL FINDINGS
Based upon clinical and radiographic findings
Enter / diagram radiographic findings from pg 3B

Date: _____6/15/09_____

Chart # | 5 | 6 | 7 | 1 | 4 | 1

Probe Depth 1 Date: 6/15/09	X	635	333	857	423	323	322	213	212	213	213	313	857	253	235	385
Probe Depth 2 Date: __/__/__																
	1	2	3	4	5	6	7	8	9	10	11	12	13	14	15	16

CARIES & RESTORATIVE

Missing CM RCT Ponlic Implant

TOP ROW:
Caries Scores:
EO, E1 E2, D1, D2 D3
(see legend on reverse)

BOTTOM ROW:
Fillings: color in Black
Caries: color in Red

DIAGNODENT *readings:*
Chart on reverse side as needed

Facial

Palatal

	1	2	3	4	5	6	7	8	9	10	11	12	13	14	15	16
Probe Depth 1 Date: 6/15/09	X	232	353	756	452	317	217	212	212	212	212	433	X	282	245	535
Probe Depth 2 Date: __/__/__																
Probe Depth 1 Date: 6/15/09	X	337	455	323	323	323	345	533	323	323	323	323	323	345	533	X
Probe Depth 2 Date: __/__/__																
	32	31	30	29	28	27	26	25	24	23	22	21	20	19	18	17

PERIO LEGEND

Suppuration:
5 next to crown

Free Gingival Margin -
black line

Mucogingival Line -
black line

Mobility: +1,+2,+3 *in crown*

Furcation: Class I II III

Spacing: | |

Occlusion:

Lingual

Facial

	32	31	30	29	28	27	26	25	24	23	22	21	20	19	18	17
Probe Depth 1 Date: 6/15/09	X	337	542	212	212	325	324	512	212	224	212	323	323	2310	623	X
Probe Depth 2 Date: __/__/__																

Assessment of Oral hygiene and Gingival Inflammation								Substitutions:
	Tooth #	3	9	12	19	25	28	Total	If 3, 12,19 or 28 is missing, substitute the next most posterior tooth.
	(Surface)	(B)	(B)	(B)	(L)	(L)	(L)	+ 's	
Date __/__/__	Plaque +/-								If 9 or 25 is missing, substitute the nearest incisor in the arch.
	Bleeding +/-								
Date __/__/__	Plaque +/-								If all incisors are missing from the arch, substitute a cuspid.
	Bleeding +/-								

Preliminary Clinical Findings Reviewed

Student Name/#: _____

Faculty Signature/#: _____

Final Findings Reviewed

Student Name/#: _____

Faculty Signature/#: _____

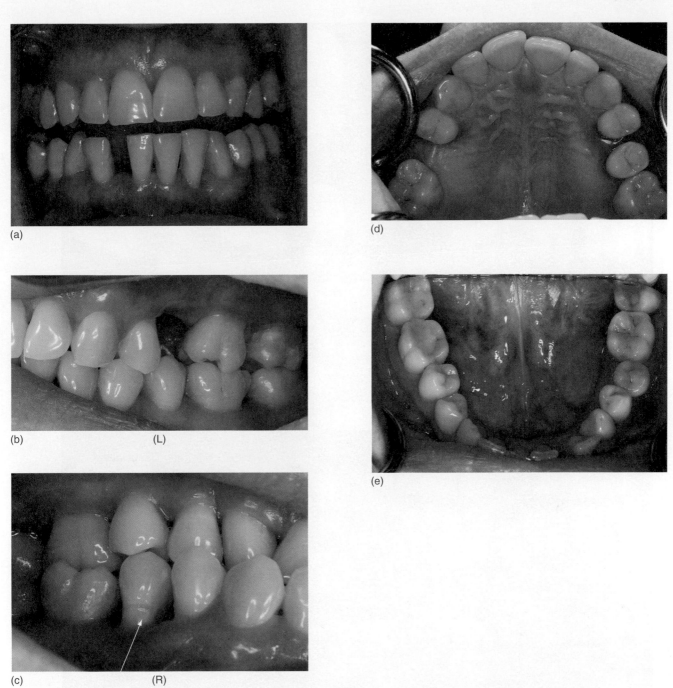

(a)

(b)   (L)

(c)   (R)

(d)

(e)

(R)

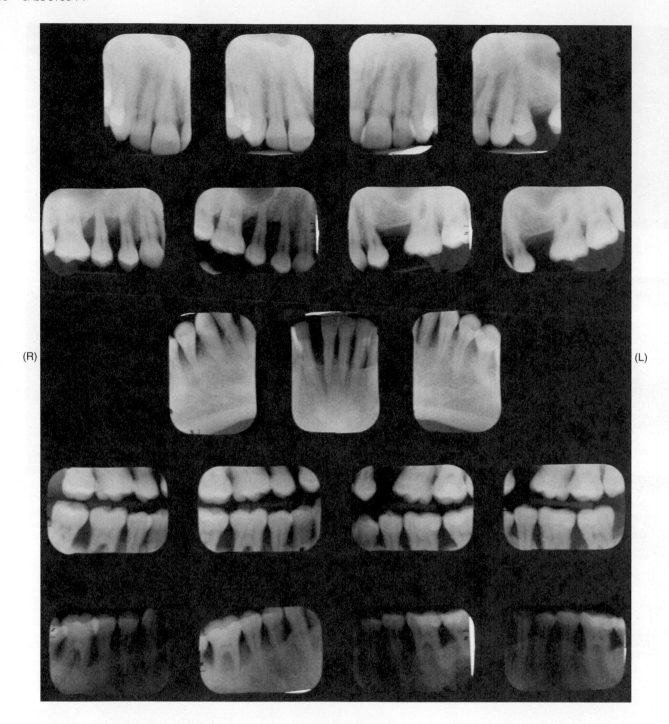

(L)

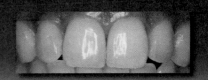

CASE STUDY II

Medical History

The patient is a 66-year-old female who presents to the dental office. She has type 2 diabetes mellitus, hypertension, and hypercholesterolnemia. She does not regularly take her blood glucose levels at home but recently it was 210. The blood pressure is 130/80 and pulse 65. She is 5 feet 7 inches tall and weighs 150 lbs (68.2 kgs). Medications: She takes amlodipine (Norvasc), metformin (Glucophage), glyburide (Diabeta), aspirin (325 mg/day), and atorvastatin (Lipitor).

Dental History

She has not been to the dentist in many years. At work she has a habit of biting a pencil when under stress.

Social History

The patient has one drink of wine every night. She denies smoking.

Chief Complaint

"My gums bleed and my teeth are getting a lot of spaces in between."

Oral Hygiene Status

The patient has poor oral hygiene. There is generalized supra/subgingival plaque and calculus.

Gingival Exam

The gingiva is red and edematous with rolled margins. The papillae are bulbous. Gingival clefts are evident.

Periodontal Exam

Probing depths are deep with numerous furcation involvements. The majority of teeth are mobile.

Interpretation

Patient Problem	Basis for Discussion	Questions (Q)/Answers (A)	Chapter Location
Patient has diabetes.	Affect of diabetes on the periodontium.	Q) Is diabetes a possible risk factor for periodontal disease? A) Yes. Diabetes (poor glycemic control) is associated with increased prevalence and severity of gingivitis and periodontitis. Periodontal destruction is worse due to hyperglycemia (increased levels of blood glucose or sugar). Poorly controlled type 2 diabetics are more likely to develop periodontal disease than well-controlled diabetics. Polymorphonuclear leukocytes (PMNs) play an important role in the maintenance of periodontal health. A reduced PMN chemotaxis (attraction of the PMN to the infection) and macrophages have been found in diabetics resulting in an increased incidence of periodontal disease and altered wound healing. Remember that the PMNs are the first line of defense when an infection is present. Also, there are both microvascular (e.g., periodontium, eyes) and macrovascular (e.g., heart, kidney) complications in diabetics, which is primarily due to an abnormal cross-linking and glycosylation of collagen (a protein) resulting in the formation of advanced glycosylated end products (AGEs). Essentially, collagen accumulates in the periodontal capillary basement membrane resulting in the membrane to thicken and gingival blood vessel walls. This causes a decrease in tissue oxygenation. In addition, any newly formed collagen is rapidly degraded by increased metabolism due to increased actions of collagenase (enzyme that breaks down collagen). Thus, diabetes is a major risk factor for periodontal diseases. Q) Is periodontal disease a possible risk factor for diabetes? A) Yes. Conversely, periodontitis may increase the risk for worsening glycemic control in diabetic patients and may increase the risk for diabetic complications.	5, 6

Patient Problem	Basis for Discussion	Questions (Q)/Answers (A)	Chapter Location
Gingiva is enlarged.	Difficult to brush.	Q) What is causing the gingival enlargement? A) The antihypertensive (amlodipine) is a calcium channel blocker and is causing gingival enlargement. Other drugs such as phenytoin (antiseizure drug) and cyclosporine (immunosuppressant drug) can also cause gingival enlargement. Q) How is the gingival enlargement managed? A) As long as the patient is taking the offending drug there will be gingival enlargement. Meticulous oral hygiene is important.	7
Teeth are mobile, and many spaces are developing.	There is a lot of bone loss.	Q) Why are the teeth mobile with development of diastemas? A) There is advanced bone loss (chronic periodontitis) with pathologic migration of the teeth.	8
Gingiva bleeds.	Inflammation is present.	Q) What is causing the bleeding? A) Bleeding is caused by vascular proliferation in the connective tissue (lamina propria). Remember that the epithelium is avascular because it does not contain any blood vessels. Bleeding on probing occurs when the sulcular epithelium becomes ulcerated, and the probe penetrates the epithelium. The enlarged blood vessels protrude from the underlying connective tissue.	7
Patient bites on pencil.	May be causing trauma and mobility of teeth.	Q) What type of occlusal trauma is seen in this patient? A) Secondary occlusal trauma occurs when even normal forces of chewing occur on teeth with compromised bone levels such as in this patient, which causes increasing tooth mobility. On the other hand, primary occlusal trauma occurs when the occlusal forces are greater than normal or outside the normal range of the chewing cycle (e.g., parafunctional habits such as bruxism, fingernail biting, or biting on pencils) on a stable and intact periodontium.	10

1. Which of the following is the most likely cause for the patient's gingival condition?
   a. Amlodipine
   b. Aspirin
   c. Alcohol
   d. Parafunctional habit
   e. Pathologic migration

2. Which of the following factors is most likely the cause for the mobility of the maxillary incisors?
   a. Secondary occlusal trauma
   b. Primary occlusal trauma
   c. Gingival enlargement
   d. Aspirin use

3. The discoloration of the gingival tissue around the left maxillary canine area in photo C is due to
   a. coffee.
   b. inflammation.
   c. lead of pencil.
   d. melanin.

4. To which of the following classifications of periodontal diseases does this patient belong?
   a. Aggressive periodontitis
   b. Ulcerative gingivitis
   c. Ulcerative periodontitis
   d. Chronic periodontitis

5. Which of the following is the arrow in Photo E pointing to?
   a. Nutrition canal
   b. Dentinal caries
   c. Root caries
   d. Supragingival calculus

6. Which of the following conditions does the arrow point to in the full-mouth-series of X-rays?
   a. Furcation defect
   b. Tooth caries
   c. Supragingival calculus
   d. Periodontal abscess

7. In Photo B, the arrow is pointing to:
   a. dental caries.
   b. endodontic abscess.
   c. furcation involvement.
   d. gingival pseudopocket.

8. Which one of the following oral hygiene devices is best for in between the mandibular central incisors?
   a. Interdental brush
   b. Tufted floss
   c. Extra soft toothbrush
   d. Toothpick-in-holder

9. From the following list, select the items associated with probable risk factors or indicators for this patient's periodontal condition.
   a. Poor oral hygiene
   b. Amlodipine (Norvasc)
   c. Atorvastatin (Lipitor)
   d. Diabetes
   e. Previous bone loss
   f. High cholesterol levels
   g. Blood pressure
   h. Host response

10. The pattern of bone loss found between the maxillary central incisors is
    a. vertical.
    b. horizontal.
    c. angular.
    d. circumferential.

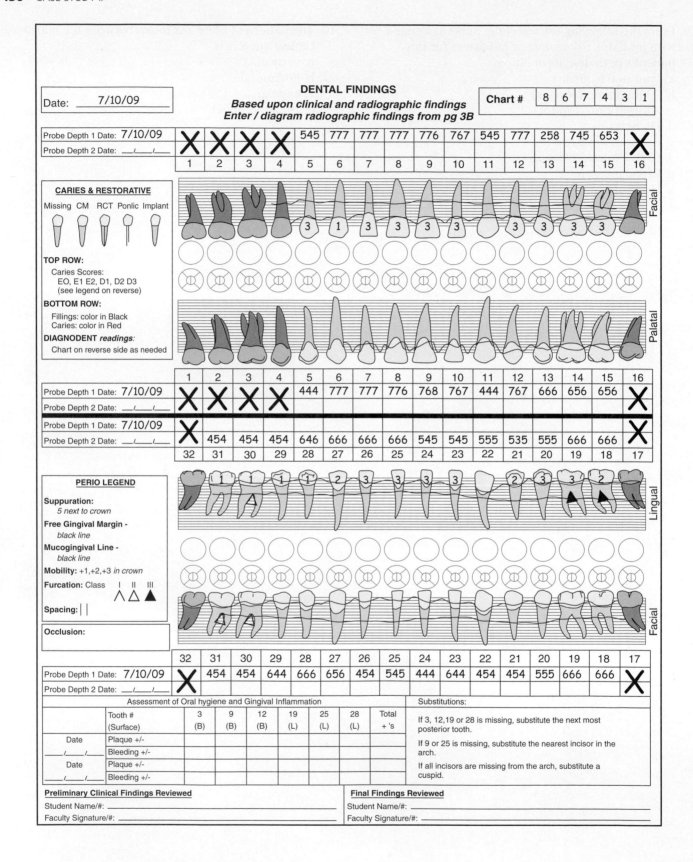

DENTAL FINDINGS
Based upon clinical and radiographic findings
Enter / diagram radiographic findings from pg 3B

Date: _7/10/09_

Chart # | 8 | 6 | 7 | 4 | 3 | 1

Probe Depth 1 Date: 7/10/09	X	X	X	X	545	777	777	777	776	767	545	777	258	745	653	X
Probe Depth 2 Date: __/__/__																
	1	2	3	4	5	6	7	8	9	10	11	12	13	14	15	16

CARIES & RESTORATIVE

Missing CM RCT Ponlic Implant

TOP ROW:
Caries Scores:
EO, E1 E2, D1, D2 D3
(see legend on reverse)

BOTTOM ROW:
Fillings: color in Black
Caries: color in Red

DIAGNODENT *readings:*
Chart on reverse side as needed

Facial / Palatal

	1	2	3	4	5	6	7	8	9	10	11	12	13	14	15	16
Probe Depth 1 Date: 7/10/09	X	X	X	X	444	777	777	776	768	767	444	767	666	656	656	X
Probe Depth 2 Date: __/__/__																
Probe Depth 1 Date: 7/10/09	X															X
Probe Depth 2 Date: __/__/__		454	454	454	646	666	666	666	545	545	555	535	555	666	666	
	32	31	30	29	28	27	26	25	24	23	22	21	20	19	18	17

PERIO LEGEND

Suppuration:
5 next to crown

Free Gingival Margin -
black line

Mucogingival Line -
black line

Mobility: +1,+2,+3 *in crown*

Furcation: Class   I   II   III

Spacing: | |

Occlusion:

Lingual / Facial

	32	31	30	29	28	27	26	25	24	23	22	21	20	19	18	17
Probe Depth 1 Date: 7/10/09	X	454	454	644	666	656	454	545	444	644	454	454	555	666	666	X
Probe Depth 2 Date: __/__/__																

Assessment of Oral hygiene and Gingival Inflammation

	Tooth # (Surface)	3 (B)	9 (B)	12 (B)	19 (L)	25 (L)	28 (L)	Total + 's
Date __/__/__	Plaque +/-							
	Bleeding +/-							
Date __/__/__	Plaque +/-							
	Bleeding +/-							

Substitutions:

If 3, 12,19 or 28 is missing, substitute the next most posterior tooth.

If 9 or 25 is missing, substitute the nearest incisor in the arch.

If all incisors are missing from the arch, substitute a cuspid.

Preliminary Clinical Findings Reviewed

Student Name/#: _____

Faculty Signature/#: _____

Final Findings Reviewed

Student Name/#: _____

Faculty Signature/#: _____

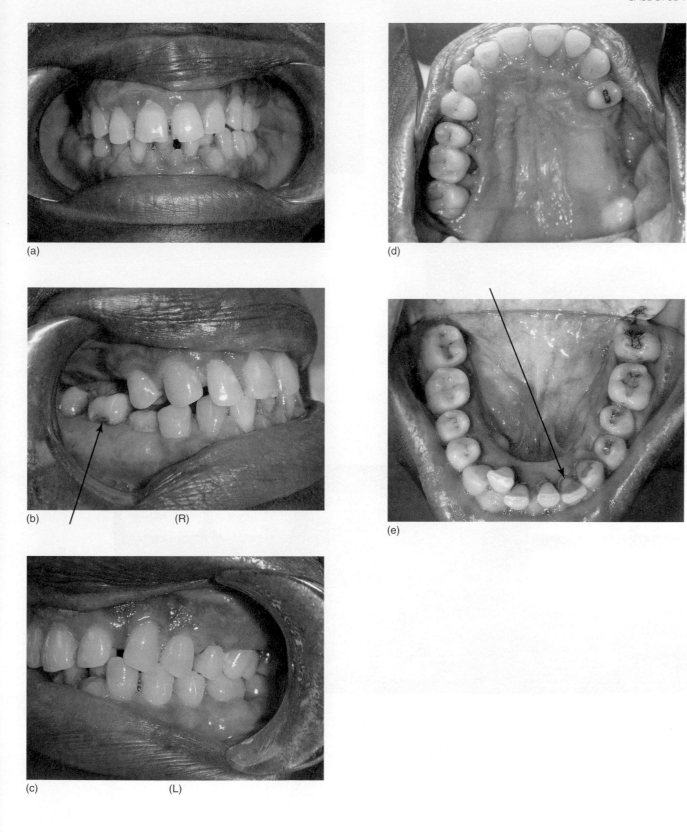

(a)

(b)   (R)

(c)   (L)

(d)

(e)

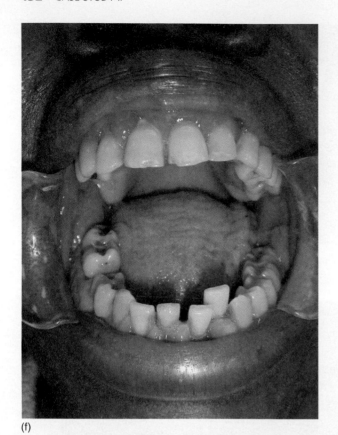

(f)

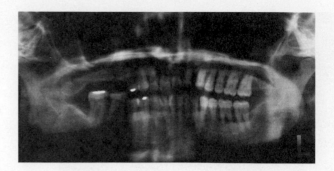

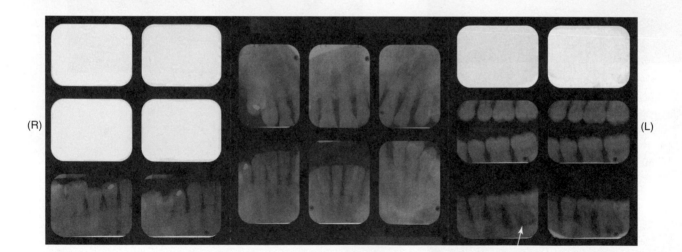

(R)

(L)

CASE STUDY III

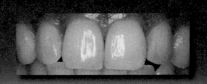

Medical History

The patient is a 29-year-old female who presents to the clinic. Her last physical examination was 1 year ago. The blood pressure is 110/70 and pulse is 68. She is 5 feet 1 inches tall and weighs 100 lbs (45.5 kgs). She has the following conditions

Heart murmur—present since birth. Asthma induced particularly by cold weather; asthma attacks about twice a year. Iron deficiency anemia. Sickle cell trait—patient has been aware of this since birth, no signs of sickle cell anemia.

Medications

The patient is taking prednisone, Singulair, Advair, and albuterol for asthma. She is also taking Claritin for allergies.

Allergies

Seasonal allergies only

Dental History

Her last dental visit was 1 year ago for adult prophylaxis. She brushes once per day and does not floss. Patient has herpes labialis outbreaks several times per year. At work she has a habit of biting a pencil when under stress.

Chief Complaint

"I have gum disease. The gum disease has led to pain, bleeding, loose teeth, and bad breath, present for a few years."

Social History

The patient is single. She is very anxious about treatment. Patient reports no drug abuse, alcohol use, or tobacco use.

Family History

Cancer and hypertension history in immediate family members.

Oral Hygiene Status

The patient's oral hygiene is poor.

Gingival Exam

The gingiva is extremely red, edematous, and painful.

Periodontal Exam

There are deep probing depths with tooth mobility. Generalized bleeding on probing.

Interpretation

Patient Problem	Basis for Discussion	Questions (Q)/Answers (A)	Chapter Location
Gingiva is red and bleeding.	Inflammation; interferes with normal function.	Q) Why is the gingiva red and bleeding? A) Vasodilation—blood vessels become dilated and engorged with blood. This is happening in the gingival connective tissue. Also, because of the microulcerations in the epithelium, the blood vessels come through, resulting in bleeding on probing.	4, 7, 8
Teeth are moving with spaces developing.	Difficult for patient to function and aesthetically unpleasing.	Q) Why are the teeth moving with development of diastemas? A) Pathologic migration.	8

Interpretation (*cont.*)

Patient Problem	Basis for Discussion	Questions (Q)/Answers (A)	Chapter Location
Severe periodontal destruction.	Prognosis of case is poor because the patient is so young.	Q) What are the underlying factors that are involved in the development of this patient's periodontal condition? A) Chronic periodontitis can occur at any age; classification is no longer based on age. It may affect a variable number of teeth, and it has variable rates of progression. The fact that the patient has asthma, has sickle cell anemia trait, and is physically challenged are not contributory to the periodontal disease. There is severe attachment loss and bone destruction. One can argue that the case may be an aggressive periodontitis because of the severe periodontal destruction in a young person. There is heavy plaque and calculus deposits. Usually in an aggressive case there are minimal deposits. But according to the American Academy of Periodontology (AAP), aggressive periodontitis has certain criteria that may not all be present, including minimal amount of deposits (this patient has heavy plaque and calculus deposits). Most likely the patient initially had aggressive periodontitis that converted into chronic periodontitis.	8, 18
Taking multiple medications.	Medications may be co-involved in changes to the periodontium.	Q) Do any of her medications affect the periodontium? A) Albuterol is an inhaler for asthma. It can cause oral candidiasis. Thus, tell the patient to rinse her mouth after every use. Systemic steroids (Advair, predisone, and Singular) have not been documented to have any influence on periodontal disease.	6

1. To which of the following classifications of periodontal diseases does this patient belong?
   a. Periodontitis associated with a genetic disorder
   b. Chronic periodontitis
   c. Periodontitis associated with systemic disease
   d. Ulcerative periodontitis

2. Which of the following factors is involved in the etiology of this patient's disease?
   a. Bacteria + immune function
   b. Medication + immune function
   c. Medical condition + medications
   d. Medical condition only

3. The periodontal condition between the maxillary right lateral and central incisor papilla is most likely due to
   a. endodontic abscess.
   b. periodontal abscess.
   c. herpetic ulcer.
   d. aphthous ulcer.

4. The arrow in Photo A is pointing to
   a. food debris.
   b. composite restoration.
   c. calculus.
   d. melanin.

5. The arrow in the posterior right mandibular periapical radiograph is pointing to
   a. furcation involvement.
   b. cervical enamel projection.
   c. enamel pearl.
   d. fremitus.

6. Considering the patient's medical history, which of the following statements is true?
   a. The systemic drugs the patient is taking for asthma contribute a lot to her disease.
   b. The patient's oral hygiene neglect is a primary cause of her disease.
   c. The patient's anemia is a secondary cause of her disease.
   d. The patient's herpes lesion is a primary cause of her disease.

7. What is the pattern of bone loss found between the maxillary central incisors?
   a. Vertical
   b. Horizontal
   c. Circumferential
   d. Hemispetal

8. The arrow in the posterior left mandibular radiograph is pointing to:
   a. furcation.
   b. palatogingival groove.
   c. calculus.
   d. radicular bone.

9. Which of the following describes the relationship of the mandibular incisors?
   a. Wide interdental septum
   b. Long, bulbous roots
   c. Crowding
   d. Close root proximity

10. The primary histological cause of the gingival condition in this patient is
    a. vasodilation.
    b. vasoconstriction.
    c. fibrosis.
    d. increased stippling.

DENTAL FINDINGS

Based upon clinical and radiographic findings
Enter / diagram radiographic findings from pg 3B

Date: 7/29/09

Chart #

7	7	6	2	3	3

Probe Depth 1 Date: ___/___/___
Probe Depth 2 Date: ___/___/___

X	538	848	746	838	537	737	737	523	523	523	523	756	745	745	X
	1	2	3	4	5	6	7	8	9	10	11	12	13	14	15	16

Facial

CARIES & RESTORATIVE

Missing CM RCT Ponlic Implant

TOP ROW:
Caries Scores:
EO, E1 E2, D1, D2 D3
(see legend on reverse)

BOTTOM ROW:
Fillings: color in Black
Caries: color in Red

DIAGNODENT *readings*:
Chart on reverse side as needed

Palatal

1	2	3	4	5	6	7	8	9	10	11	12	13	14	15	16

Probe Depth 1 Date: ___/___/___
Probe Depth 2 Date: ___/___/___

X	758	586	757	837	835	735	737	535	555	533	858	846	747	745	X

Probe Depth 1 Date: ___/___/___
Probe Depth 2 Date: ___/___/___

X	958	757	758	746	657	656	355	535	535	545	646	656	737	526	X
32	31	30	29	28	27	26	25	24	23	22	21	20	19	18	17

Lingual

PERIO LEGEND

Suppuration:
5 next to crown

Free Gingival Margin -
black line

Mucogingival Line -
black line

Mobility: +1,+2,+3 *in crown*

Furcation: Class   I   II   III
                      ∧ △ ▲

Spacing: | |

Occlusion:

Facial

32	31	30	29	28	27	26	25	24	23	22	21	20	19	18	17

Probe Depth 1 Date: ___/___/___
Probe Depth 2 Date: ___/___/___

X	768	768	857	857	755	535	555	535	556	353	636	645	747	758	X

Assessment of Oral hygiene and Gingival Inflammation

	Tooth # (Surface)	3 (B)	9 (B)	12 (B)	19 (L)	25 (L)	28 (L)	Total + 's
Date ___/___/___	Plaque +/-							
	Bleeding +/-							
Date ___/___/___	Plaque +/-							
	Bleeding +/-							

Substitutions:

If 3, 12,19 or 28 is missing, substitute the next most posterior tooth.

If 9 or 25 is missing, substitute the nearest incisor in the arch.

If all incisors are missing from the arch, substitute a cuspid.

Preliminary Clinical Findings Reviewed

Student Name/#: _____

Faculty Signature/#: _____

Final Findings Reviewed

Student Name/#: _____

Faculty Signature/#: _____

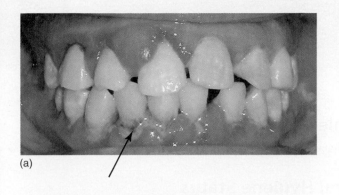

(a)

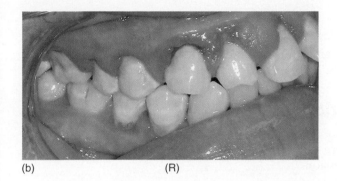

(b)   (R)

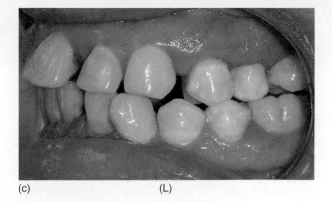

(c)   (L)

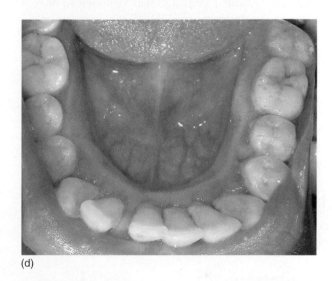

(d)

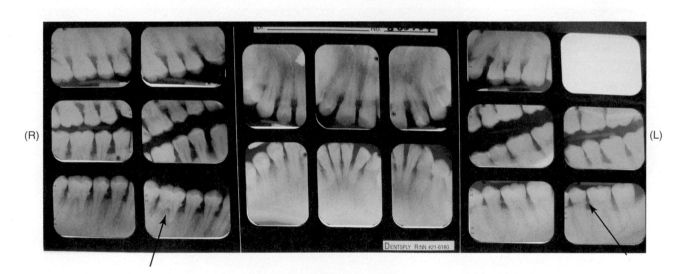

(R)   (L)

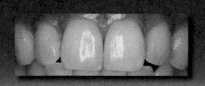

Medical History

The patient is a 66-year-old female who presents to the dental office. Her last physical examination was 6 months ago. The blood pressure is 130/82 and pulse is 72. She is 5 feet 8 inches tall and weighs 150 lbs (68.2 kgs). Medications: She takes oxybutynin (Ditropan) and previously took alendronate (Fosamax). About 1 year ago was switched to once a year intravenous zoledronic acid (Reclast).

Dental History

When she was a child, she had regular dental visits. She has not been to a dentist for the last 3 years since her regular dentist moved. She previously had periodontal surgery in only three quadrants but knows she needs more treatment. She is interested in implants. She says she tries to brush at least once a day but it does not always happen.

Social History

The patient is married with one child. She smokes three cigarettes a day.

Chief Complaint

"I have two very loose teeth on lowers."

Oral Hygiene Status

Poor oral hygiene.

Gingival Exam

The gingiva is red and fibrotic with localized edematous areas. The papillae are primarily blunted.

Periodontal Exam

There are deep probing depths with bleeding on probing. There is localized tooth mobility and generalized gingival recession.

Interpretation

Patient Problem	Basis for Discussion	Questions (Q)/Answers (A)	Chapter Location
Patient is taking bisphosphonates.	Bisphosphonates are implicating in causing osteonecrosis of the jaw (ONJ) or bisphosphonate-associated osteonecrosis (BON) or antiresorptive agent-induced osteonecrosis of the jaw (ARONJ).	Q) What is the appropriate treatment in this patient who is taking oral bisphosphonates? A) Communication between the dental clinician and physician is important. There is a higher incidence of BON in patients on IV bisphosphonates. There is still limited information concerning the risk of ONJ in patients taking oral bisphosphonates. Periodontal debridement can be performed on patients taking oral bisphosphonates, but precautions still must be taken for the development of ONJ.	6
Mandibular central incisors are mobile, and the right central incisor is supraerupted.	This is the patient's chief complaint, and it must be addressed first.	Q) Why are these teeth mobile and the central incisor supraerupted? A) Because there is advanced bone loss. The central incisor is supraerupted because of the bone loss causing pathologic migration. Because of the supraeruption there is an occlusal prematurity because the patient is biting on this tooth first before the other teeth.	8, 16
Teeth have stains.	Aesthetically unpleasing for patient.	Q) Why are the teeth stained? A) Because of smoking; nicotine staining.	14

Interpretation (*cont.*)

Patient Problem	Basis for Discussion	Questions (Q)/Answers (A)	Chapter Location
Patient wants implants.	Concern for osteonecrosis of the jaw (ONJ).	Q) Is this patient a candidate for implants? A) The patient used to take an oral bisphosphonate for osteoporosis but compliance was a problem. The oral form must be taken correctly or else the drug's absorption and effectives is reduced. Oral pills should not be taken with water and fasting. There is controversy about whether it is safe to place dental implants in a patient taking oral or intravenous (IV) bisphosphonates either for osteoporosis, cancer, or bone diseases. It has been recommended that patients taking oral bisphosphonates for < 3 years can have implants, but it is important to be aware of possible osteonecrosis of the jaw (ONJ) or BON that could still happen even if patients are taking oral bisphosphonates. Numerous references have found that even in patients taking oral bisphosphonates there is a good chance of failure for the implant to integrate. Also, there is a slight failure if patients start to take an oral bisphosphonate after a successful implant has been placed (Goss et al. 2010). The nature and frequency of bisphosphonate-associated osteonecrosis of the jaws in dental implant patients: A South Australian case series. *J. Oral Maxillofac. Surg.* 68:337–343.) Because the patient was switched to an intravenous (IV) bisphosphonate, any surgical procedure including implant placement, periodontal surgery, and extractions must be taken into consideration for the development of osteonecrosis of the jaw, and most clinicians will refrain from performing these invasive procedures.	6, 27
Left mandibular first molar has furcation involvement (Buccal II).	Surgical correction of bony defects.	Q) What type of periodontal surgery is indicated for this defect? A) Periodontal regeneration using bone graft and membranes.	26
Patient wants a mouth rinse to help her with oral hygiene.	Is a mouth rinse indicated for adjunctive therapy?	Q) Should you recommend a mouth rinse to this patient? A) Yes, mouth rinses are used as adjuncts to brushing and interdental care.	20, 21

1. Which of the following periodontal procedures is best indicated for this patient?
   a. Local antibiotics (e.g., Arestin)
   b. Systemic antibiotics
   c. Topical antimicrobial rinse (e.g., chlorhexidine)
   d. Periodontal debridement, extractions, and periodontal surgery

2. Which of the following factors is involved in the gingival recession on the mandibular left central incisor?
   a. High frenum
   b. Tooth mobility
   c. Poor toothbrushing habit
   d. Previous periodontal surgery

3. Which of the following teeth has the worst prognosis?
   a. Maxillary right first molar
   b. Maxillary right central incisor
   c. Maxillary left first premolar
   d. Mandibular right first molar

4. The patient requires multiple teeth to be extracted and periodontal surgery. Which of the following factors needs to be considered in this patient before these procedures are performed?
   a. Pulse rate
   b. Bisphosphonate use
   c. Oxybutynin use
   d. Blood pressure

5. Which of the following teeth has a periapical pathology related to an endodontic problem?
   a. Maxillary right lateral incisor
   b. Maxillary left first premolar
   c. Mandibular right first premolar
   d. Mandibular left first molar

6. To which of the following classifications of periodontal diseases does this patient belong?
   a. Chronic periodontitis
   b. Aggressive periodontitis
   c. Periodontitis associated with systemic disease
   d. Ulcerative periodontitis

7. Which of the following factors is involved in this patient's periodontal condition?
   a. Oxybutynin
   b. Alendronate
   c. Poor oral hygiene
   d. Previous periodontal surgery
   e. Bisphosphonate

8. The arrow in Photo A points to
   a. dehiscence.
   b. enamel.
   c. milky white stain.
   d. fenestration.

9. Which of the following conditions exists on the distal surface of the maxillary left first premolar?
   a. Widened periodontal ligament
   b. Infrabony defect
   c. Endodontic abscess
   d. Periodontal abscess

10. Which of the following interproximal hygiene devices is best for the area between the left maxillary lateral incisor and canine?
    a. Wooden wedge
    b. Dental floss
    c. Tufted floss
    d. Rubber-tip stimulator

Date: __8/12/09__

DENTAL FINDINGS
Based upon clinical and radiographic findings
Enter / diagram radiographic findings from pg 3B

Chart # | 8 | 9 | 3 | 1 | 3 | 1 |

Probe Depth 1 Date: 8/12/09
Probe Depth 2 Date: ___/___/___

1	2	3	4	5	6	7	8	9	10	11	12	13	14	15	16
X	X	432	314	224	322	322	313	213	213	333	333	433	X	312	X

Facial

CARIES & RESTORATIVE

Missing   CM   RCT   Ponlic   Implant

TOP ROW:
Caries Scores:
EO, E1 E2, D1, D2 D3
(see legend on reverse)

BOTTOM ROW:
Fillings: color in Black
Caries: color in Red

DIAGNODENT *readings*:
Chart on reverse side as needed

Palatal

1	2	3	4	5	6	7	8	9	10	11	12	13	14	15	16

Probe Depth 1 Date: 8/12/09
| X | X | 333 | 333 | 334 | 323 | 212 | 212 | 112 | 123 | 114 | 223 | 313 | X | 333 | X |

Probe Depth 2 Date: ___/___/___

Probe Depth 1 Date: 8/12/09
Probe Depth 2 Date: ___/___/___

32	31	30	29	28	27	26	25	24	23	22	21	20	19	18	17
X	X	X	532	557	312	212	434	434	223	223	212	223	5410	524	424

PERIO LEGEND

Suppuration:
5 next to crown

Free Gingival Magin -
black line

Mucogingival Line -
black line

Mobility: +1,+2,+3 *in crown*

Furcation: Class   I   II   III
∧ △ ▲

Spacing: | |

Occlusion:

Lingual

Facial

32	31	30	29	28	27	26	25	24	23	22	21	20	19	18	17

Probe Depth 1 Date: 8/12/09
| X | X | X | 343 | 336 | 212 | 212 | 324 | 114 | 212 | 112 | 112 | 318 | 617 | 423 | 425 |

Probe Depth 2 Date: ___/___/___

Assessment of Oral hygiene and Gingival Inflammation

	Tooth # (Surface)	3 (B)	9 (B)	12 (B)	19 (L)	25 (L)	28 (L)	Total + 's
Date ___/___/___	Plaque +/-							
	Bleeding +/-							
Date ___/___/___	Plaque +/-							
	Bleeding +/-							

Substitutions:

If 3, 12,19 or 28 is missing, substitute the next most posterior tooth.

If 9 or 25 is missing, substitute the nearest incisor in the arch.

If all incisors are missing from the arch, substitute a cuspid.

Preliminary Clinical Findings Reviewed
Student Name/#: _____
Faculty Signature/#: _____

Final Findings Reviewed
Student Name/#: _____
Faculty Signature/#: _____

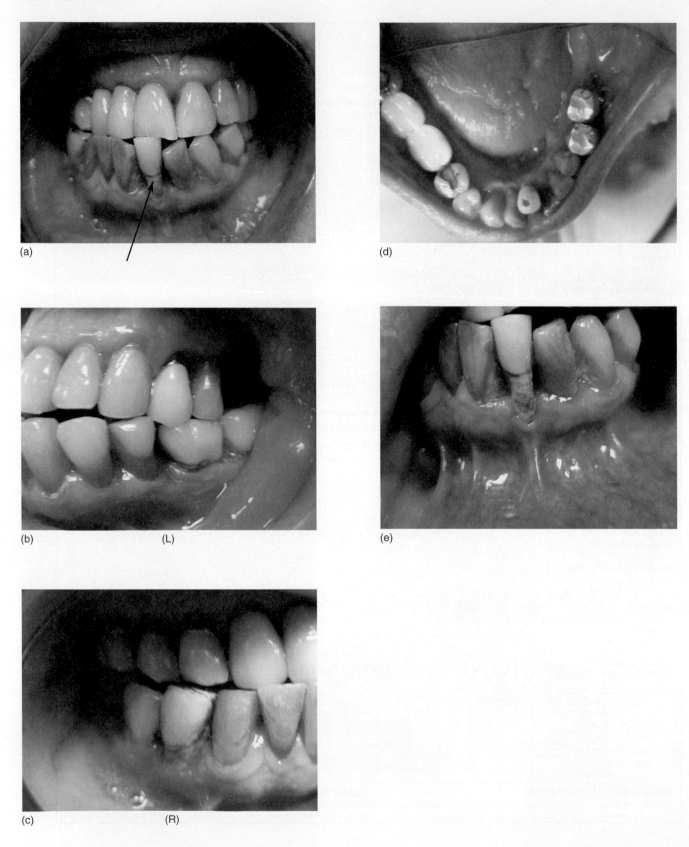

(a)

(d)

(b)   (L)

(e)

(c)   (R)

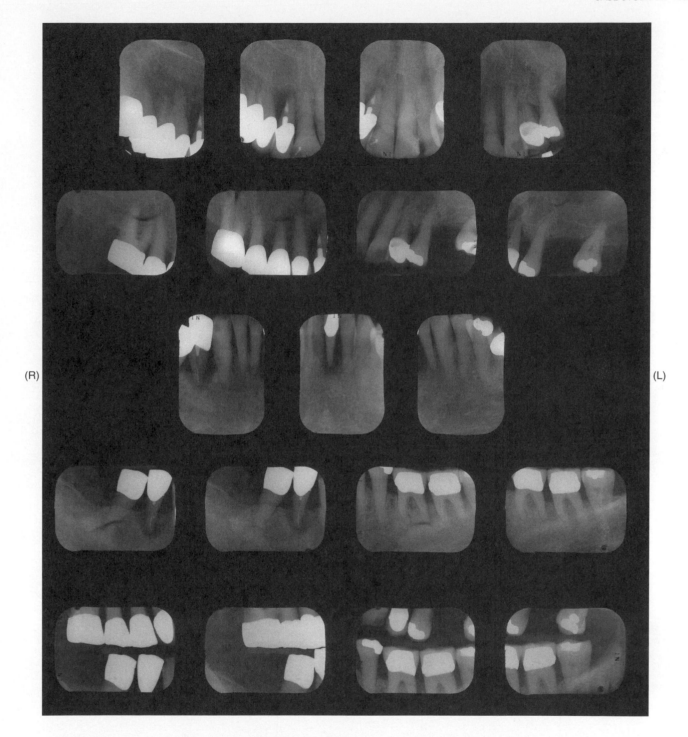

(R) (L)

Appendices

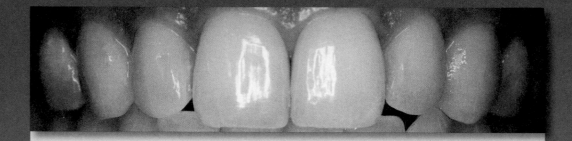

APPENDIX A
Periodontal Information Resources

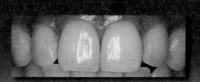

Mea A. Weinberg

A great number of scientific and clinical resources on periodontology are available from organizations and various journals. This information should be used for continuing education so that the dental hygienist can keep up with current clinical studies and product availability. The Internet provides an excellent opportunity for dental professionals and patients to obtain information related to all aspects of dental hygiene.

Publications: American Academy of Periodontology

The American Academy of Periodontology (AAP) publishes patient education brochures, practice management resources, journals, and clinical publications. The website for the American Academy of Periodontology is www.perio.org.
  The following materials are available:

1. Patient education brochures
2. *2007 Current Procedural Terminology for Periodontics and Insurance Reporting Manual*, 11th ed.
3. *2003 Practice Profile Survey: Characteristics and Trends in Private Periodontal Practice*
4. Practice management resources
   - "Designing Effective Practice Marketing Materials"
   - "Sample Periodontal Office Forms"
   - "Informed Consent for Surgical Periodontics"
5. Study club kits (binders containing slides, lecture script, consensus reports, article reprints, references)
   - "The Periodontal-Systemic Education Kit"
   - "Periodontal Maintenance for Natural Teeth and Implants Study Club Kit"
   - "Periodontal Plastic Surgery"
   - "Implant Dentistry: A Team Approach to Optimal Patient Care" presentation kit
   - "Comprehensive Insurance Workshop: Reporting Periodontal Procedures to Third Parties" (CD-ROM)
   - "Evidence-Based Periodontal Research: Set of Three Scientific Study Club Presentations"
   - "Introduction to Periodontal Surgery for Dental Hygienists" presentation kit
   - "Classification, Epidemiology and Diagnosis of Periodontal Diseases"
   - "The Role of Pharmacotherapeutics in Periodontal Diseases"
   - "Periodic Reevaluation and Supportive Periodontal Therapy"

6. Clinical publications: *Journal of Periodontology* (monthly publication)
7. *Annals of Periodontology*
   - *Annals of Periodontology* (1996 World Workshop in Periodontics), Vol. 1
   - *Annals of Periodontology* (1996 Joint Symposium on Clinical Trial Design and Analysis in Periodontics), Vol. 2
   - *Annals of Periodontology* (1997): New Directions in Periodontal Medicine, Vol. 3.
   - *Annals of Periodontology* (1999): 1999 International Workshop for a Classification of Periodontal Diseases and Conditions, Vol. 4.
   - *Annals of Periodontology* (2003): Proceedings of the Workshop on Contemporary Science in Clinical Periodontics, Vol. 8
   - *Periodontal-Systemic Links: An AAP Literature Compilation* (CD-ROM), 2003
8. *Periodontal Literature Reviews: A Summary of Current Knowledge* (1996)
9. *Periodontal Disease Management* (1993)
   - *2003 Current Procedural Terminology for Periodontics and Insurance Reporting Manual* (9th edition)
   - In-Service Exams (questions given to postgraduate students)
10. Audiotapes from past annual meetings (www.mobiltape.com or 1-800-369-5718).
11. Guidelines
    - Guidelines for the Management of Patients with Periodontal Disease (2006)
    - Guidelines for In-Office Use of Conscious Sedation in Periodontics (2001)
    - Position Statement and Guidelines for Soft Tissue Management Programs (1996)
12. Parameters of care: Various papers on the parameters of care of periodontal diseases (2000)
13. Consensus Paper/Clinical Recommendations
    - Periodontitis and Atherosclerotic Cardiovascular Disease (2009)
14. Position papers (some position papers are listed next)
    - "The Role of Supra- and Subgingival Irrigation in the Treatment of Periodontal Diseases" (2005)76:2015–2027.
    - "Periodontal Diseases of Children and Adolescents" (2003)
    - "Diagnosis of Periodontal Diseases" (2003)
    - "Oral Features of Mucocutaneous Disorders" (2003)

- "Modulation of the Host Response in Periodontal Therapy" (2002)
- "Dental Implants and Periodontal Therapy" (2000)
- "The Role of Controlled Drug Delivery for Periodontitis" (1999)
- "Tobacco Use and the Periodontal Patient" (1999)
- "The Pathogenesis of Periodontal Diseases" (1999)
- "Periodontal Disease as a Potential Risk Factor for Systemic Diseases" (1998)
- "Diabetes and Periodontal Diseases" (1999)
- "Treatment of Gingivitis and Periodontitis" (1997)
- "Epidemiology of Periodontal Diseases" (2005)
- "Implications of Genetic Technology for the Management of Periodontal Diseases" (2005)
- "Oral and Recorrective Considerations in Periodontal Therapy" (2005)
- "Periodontal Regeneration" (2005)
- "Systemic Antibiotics" (2004)
- "Drug-Associated Gingival Enlargement" (2004)

15. Product and procedure statements/Academy statements
    - Comprehensive Periodontal Therapy (2010)
      - PowerPoint Presentation and Other Resources for Sharing the Therapy Statement
    - The Efficacy of Lasers in the Non-surgical Treatment of Inflammatory Periodontal Disease (2011)
    - "Risk Assessment" (2008)
    - "Bisphosphonates" (2005)
    - "Local Delivery of Sustained or Controlled Release Antimicrobials as Adjunctive Therapy in the Treatment of Periodontitis" (2006)
    - "Periodontal Management of the Pregnant Patient" (2004)
    - "Tooth Extraction during Periodontal Therapy" (2003)
    - "The Use of Conscious Sedation by Periodontists" (2003)
    - "Gingival Curettage" (2002)
    - "Use of Moderate Sedation by Periodontists" (2013)
    - "Peri-implant Mucositis and Peri-implantitis: A Current Understanding of Their Diagnoses and Clinical Implications" (2013)
    - "Periostat® Systemically Delivered Collagenase Inhibitor of Doxycycline Hyclate" (1998)

16. AAP-Commissioned Reviews
    - Bone Augmentation Techniques (2007)
    - Diabetes Mellitus and Periodontal Disease (2006)
    - Lasers in Periodontics (2006)
    - Temporary Anchorage Devices for Tooth Movement (2006)
17. Other associations include
    - The American Dental Hygiene Association (ADHA): www.adha.org
    - The American Dental Association (ADA): www.ada.org

Journals/Bulletins

1. *Journal of Periodontology* (American Academy of Periodontology, Chicago; website: www.perio.org).
2. *Journal of Dental Hygiene* (American Dental Hygiene Association, Chicago; website: www.adha.org).
3. *Practical Periodontics and Aesthetic Dentistry* (Montage Media Corp., Mahwah, NJ; 800-899-5350).
4. *Journal of Practical Hygiene* (Montage Media Corp., Mahwah, NJ; 800-899-5350).
5. *Periodontology 2000* (Musksgaard, Copenhagen; e-mail: fsub@mail.munksgaard.dk).
6. *Journal of Clinical Periodontology* (Munksgaard, Copenhagen; e-mail: fsub@mail.munksgaard.dk).
7. *Journal of Periodontal Research* (Munksgaard, Copenhagen; e-mail: fsub@mail.munksgaard.dk).
8. *Perio Reports* (www.PerioReports.com)—research articles are reviewed (*Compendium of Current Research*).
9. *International Journal of Oral and Maxillofacial Implants* (Quintessence Publishers, Carol Stream, IL; e-mail: quintpub@aol.com; www.quintpub.com).
10. *Clinical Oral Implants Research* (Munksgaard International Publishers, ltd., Malden, MA. e-mail: fsub@mail.munksgaard.dk; www.munksgaard.dk).

Other Websites

1. www.dentalcare.com (Procter & Gamble)
2. www.colgate.com (Colgate Oral Pharmaceutical)
3. http://jeffline.tju.edu/DHNet (National Center for Dental Hygiene Research)
4. www.oralhealth.org (Oral Health Letter)

APPENDIX B
Reading the Literature

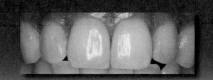

Trisha E. O'Hehir

Article Classification

- Clinical trial (in vivo)
- Laboratory study (in vitro)
- Combination studies—part clinical, part laboratory
- Case studies—reports of individual patients and their outcomes
- Epidemiology—incidence and/or prevalence of disease in a population
- Informational
- Review

Research articles include several distinct sections. Each section provides valuable information. These sections do not have to be read in the order they are printed. It depends on what information is being requested. The following is a brief summary of each section.

Abstract

- Brief overview of the entire article
- Hypothesis being tested
- Number of subjects involved
- Methods used
- Results

The last sentence of an abstract often provides the essence of the project. The last sentence is where reading of a research article should begin.

Introduction

- Lays the groundwork for the project
- Historical information on the subject area
- Past research studies are sited in this area
- Author or authors have to make a case for the project
- Controversies in the area based on previously published work
- Statement of the hypothesis

Most often, a null hypothesis is stated, which says that if the researchers do what they propose, no changes will be seen. The goal of the researchers is to then disprove the null hypothesis. Approaching the hypothesis from the other direction requires stating that the drug, tool, or therapy to be tested will have a specific effect on the test subject, which necessitates quantifying the expected result. Guessing at the outcome before the study begins can be quite difficult. Therefore, disproving a null hypothesis allows for a positive result without the need to estimate the outcome at the start.

Some researchers state their purpose rather than formulating a hypothesis. The following is an example of stating a purpose:

Thus, this study compares the amount of aerosol produced by a traditional ultrasonic scaler insert and that produced by a new focused style insert. In addition, the effect of using an aerosol reduction device with both types of inserts is evaluated. [Rivera-Hidalgo, F., Barnes, J., and Harrel, S. 1999. Aerosol and splatter production by focused spray and standard ultrasonic inserts. *J. Periodontol.*, 70:473–477]

Here is the same statement of purpose restated as a hypothesis:

The hypothesis to be tested is that no difference in aerosol spray is expected comparing traditional and focused-style ultrasonic inserts, used either alone or with an aerosol reduction device.

The goal of the researchers remains the same—to determine if there is a difference, thus disproving the null hypothesis.

Methods and Materials

This section is often divided into subsections, providing some of the following information:

- *Study population.* Collection of people, items, or observations to be studied.
- *People*
  - *Number of subjects.* Setting a desired outcome in statistical terms allows the statistician to calculate exactly how many subjects are needed.
  - *Random sample.* All subjects of a given population have an equal chance of being selected (e.g., picking names out of a hat or using a table of random numbers to select subjects).
  - *Convenience population.* Sample does not represent the population at large (e.g., dental or dental hygiene students).
  - *Volunteers or paid participants.*
  - *Subject solicitation.* Clinic patients, newspaper ads, etc.
  - *Demographics.* Age, gender, general health, oral health, dental history.

- *Location of the study.* University, clinical practice, community, etc.
- *Study design.*
  - Timeline of events, including length of the study.
  - Indices used and any modifications.
- Description of drugs, tools, or techniques to be tested
- Who the examiners were and their preparation for the study.
- Characteristics of the clinical study design.
  - *Case control.* Subjects with a certain condition are selected and compared with controls (e.g., subjects without the condition). For example, a group of subjects with oral cancer is compared with a control group without oral cancer for smoking habits over the previous 5 years.
  - *Crossover.* Each subject receives two or more treatments at different times, and end points are observed after each treatment.
  - *Cross-sectional.* End points are observed at one given point in time.
  - *Longitudinal.* End points are observed more than once over a period of time.
  - *Observational.* Subjects or objects of interest (e.g., teeth) are observed in their natural state with no intervention by researchers.
  - *Prospective.* Study subjects selected based on a certain treatment or exposure and observed for a specific outcome over a period of time (e.g., subjects selected based on smoking habits and observed for cancer development over a 5-year period).
  - *Retrospective.* Study subjects are selected based on a certain outcome, and then data are gathered on previous exposure (e.g., subjects selected based on the presence of oral cancer and studied as to smoking habits during the previous 5 years).
  - *Parallel group.* Experimental groups do not experience the same treatment or products (e.g., a control group and a test group).
  - *Randomized.* Subjects or objects of interest (e.g., teeth) are assigned to different treatments or interventions randomly.
  - *Split-mouth.* Each subject receives two or more treatments at different sites within the mouth, and outcomes are observed at a given point in time.

- *Details of laboratory tests.*
  - How specimens are collected.
  - How they are stored.
  - How the tests are run.
  - What equipment is used.
  - Who does the testing.
- *Statistical analysis.* Selection of mathematical techniques used to assist in the understanding and interpretation of data for the purpose of decision making.
- *Descriptive statistics.* Methods to simply describe data in a numerical way, such as frequency of a given parameter.
- *Inferential statistics.* Methods used to infer something about a population from a sample of observations from that population.

Results

- Factual presentation of the study data.
- Statistics. (Opinions or conclusion are left for the next section.)

Discussion

- Limitations of the study.
- Confirmation of earlier findings.
- Integration of study findings with previously published data.
- Unanswered questions.
- New questions raised by the findings.
- Interesting side findings that do not relate to this hypothesis.
- Subjective opinions of the patients who participated.
- Suggestions for future studies.
- Conclusions that can be drawn from this study.
- Significance of these findings, both statistical and clinical.

Statistical significance might be better stated as "statistical difference" because the difference actually may not be clinically significant.

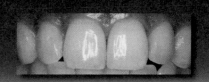

Cardiac conditions associated with the highest risk of adverse outcome from IE for which antibiotic prophylaxis is indicated (Wilson et al., 2007)

- Prosthetic cardiac valve or prosthetic material used for cardiac valve repair.
- Previous infective endocarditis.
- Congential heart disease (CHD)
  - Unrepaired cyanotic CHD, including palliative shuts and conduits.
  - Completely repaired congenital heart defect with prosthetic material or device, whether placed by surgery or by catheter intervention, during the first 6 months after the procedure.
  - Repaired CHD with residual defects at the site or adjacent to the site of a prosthetic patch or prosthetic device (which inhibit endothelialization).
- Cardiac transplantation recipients who develop cardiac valvulopathy.

Patients who have joint replacement surgery are at risk for developing infections of the implanted joints. Bacteria can enter the bloodstream and attach to implanted joints causing an infection at the prosthetic joint. In 2003, the American Academy of Orthopedic Surgeons (AAOS) and the American Dental Association (ADA) Advisory Statement recommended antibiotic prophylaxis for all patients within the first 2 years after total joint replacement surgery only. After 2 years, the recommendation for antibiotic prophylaxis was limited to high-risk or medically compromised/immunosuppressed patients that might place them at increased risk for total joint infection. In 2009, recommendations for antibiotic prophylaxis were updated by the American Academy of Orthopedic

Surgeons (AAOS). The AAOS recommends that clinicians consider antibiotic prophylaxis of all total joint replacement patients prior to any invasive procedure that may cause bacteremia. The patients should be taking antibiotic prophylaxis for their lifetime. The guideline is available at http://www.aaos.org/about/papers/advistmt/1033.asp. There is some controversy regarding the 2009 guidelines. A recent article suggests that the 2009 guidelines should not replace the 2003 guidelines until further review (Little, J. W., Jacobson, J. J., Lockhart, P. B. 2010. The dental treatment of patients with joint replacements. *JADA* 141(6):667–671). Finally, the most current guidelines where published in 2012. The American Dental Association and the American Academy of Orthopaedic Surgeons (AAOS) published the first codeveloped evidence-based guideline on the Prevention of Orthopaedic Implant Infection in Patients Undergoing Dental Procedures. This review found no direct evidence that dental procedures could cause orthopaedic implant infections. (http://www.ada.org/sections/professionalResources/pdfs/PUDP_guideline.pdf). *It is advisable to obtain a medical consult from the patient's orthopedic surgeon.*

References

Wilson, W., K. A. Taubert, M. Gewitz, et al. 2007. Prevention of infective endocarditis. Guidelines from the American Heart Association Rheumatic Fever, Endocarditis and Kawasaki Disease Committee, Council on Cardiovascular Disease in the Young, and the Council on Clinical Cardiology, Council on Cardiovascular Surgery and Anesthesia, and the Quality of Care and Outcome Research Interdisciplinary Working Group. *Circulation* 116:1736–1754.T

Prophylactic Antibiotic Regimens for Oral and Dental Procedures

Situation	Drug	Regimen (single dose taken 30 to 60 min before Dental Procedure)
Standard general prophylaxis	Amoxicillin	Adults: 2.0 g orally; Children: 50 mg/kg orally
Unable to take oral medication	Ampicillin	Adults: 2.0 g intramuscularly (IM) or intravenously (IV); Children: 50 mg/kg IM or IV
	OR	Adults: 1 g IM or IV; Children: 50 mg/kg IM or IV
	Cefazolin* or ceftriaxone*	

(continued)

Prophylactic Antibiotic Regimens for Oral and Dental Procedures (cont.)

Situation	Drug	Regimen (single dose taken 30 to 60 min before Dental Procedure)
Allergic to penicillins—oral	Cephalexin*	Adults: 2 g; children: 50 mg/kg
	OR	
	Clindamycin	Adults: 600 mg; children: 20 mg/kg
	OR	
	Azithromycin or clarithromycin	Adults: 500 mg; children: 15 mg/kg
Allergic to penicillin and unable to take oral medications	Cefazolin*	Adults: 1.0 g; children: 25 mg/kg IM or IV
	OR	
	Clindamycin	Adults: 600 mg; children: 20 mg/kg IV

*Cephalosporins should not be used in patients with immediate-type hypersensitivity reaction (urticaria, angioedema, or anaphylaxis) to penicillins.

Suggested (ADA) Antibiotic Prophylaxis Regimens in Patients at Potential Increased Risk of Hematogenous Total Joint Infection

Situation	Drug	Regimen
Standard general prophylaxis	Cephalexin or amoxicillin	2 g orally 1 h before dental procedure
Patients unable to take oral medications	Cefazolin or ampicillin	1 g IM or IV 1 h before procedure 2 g IM or IV 1 h before procedure
Allergic to penicillin	Clindamycin	600 mg orally 1 h before procedure
Allergic to penicillin and unable to take oral medications	Clindamycin	600 mg IV 1 h before procedure

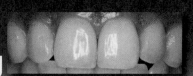

The literature supports the conclusion that smokers, especially cigarette smokers, have increased calculus, greater bone loss, and increased pocket depths but have the same levels of biofilm accumulation and the same or less gingival inflammation (American Academy of Periodontology, 1996; Haber et al., 1993). It also has been shown that surgical periodontal procedures are less effective for smokers (Bergström, Eliasson, & Preber, 1991). The amount and frequency of tobacco use are essential information when evaluating the risk factors associated with smoking (American Academy of Periodontology, 1996). Because smoking cessation may decrease the progression of periodontal diseases, it is important that the dental hygienist urge periodontal patients who smoke to stop and perhaps recommend an effective smoking-cessation program. The dental hygienist should perform periodic soft tissue evaluations and recognize any deleterious changes in the periodontium. The dental hygienist can provide assistance in guiding patients to stop smoking, yet he or she needs to realistically assess the effects of this habit on the gingival health and the resulting compromised healing. Education and continued support are beneficial factors influencing the patient's decision to stop smoking. In addition, smoking exerts a strong, chronic, and dose-dependent suppressive effect on gingival bleeding on probing (Dietrich, 2004).

Practical Steps to Smoking Cessation

Smoking-cessation programs can be made available in the dental office or patients can be referred outside. The dental office is a logical place to counsel patients on the effects of smoking on the periodontium and the importance of stopping smoking for improved long-term periodontal health and better results after periodontal treatment. Furthermore, it is important to stress to the patient that smoking cessation also can reduce the risk for other medical diseases such as cancer (Christen, McDonald, & Christen, 1991), heart disease, and respiratory disease (e.g., bronchitis). A smoking-cessation program should be a part of comprehensive preventive periodontal care. This includes behavior modification and, if necessary, medications.

The first step in establishing a smoking-cessation program is to get the office staff organized by selecting a director or coordinator such as the dental hygienist. The role of the director is to become familiar with the National Cancer Institute (NCI) manual and parts of the program, organize records and procedures, assist patients by reviewing self-help material with them, and involve the entire dental office team (Stone & Mattana, 1996).

Patients should be reassured that the entire office is going to help them. If a patient shows interest in quitting, then a program can be initiated. If a patient is not interested in quitting, do not force him or her, but rather counsel the patient and give him or her literature to take home. At the next visit ask the patient about smoking cessation again. Once the patient is enrolled in a program (yours or another one), continued maintenance or follow-up visits and communication through phone calls are important.

The role of the dental hygienist includes patient education and counseling in tobacco prevention and cessation. The patient should be informed that smoking influences periodontal conditions such as implant failure (Bain, 1996), oral cancer, and periodontal problems such as loss of clinical attachment (Grossi et al., 1994), impaired wound healing (Grossi et al., 1997; Jones & Triplett, 1992), halitosis, increased calculus formation, black-brown extrinsic staining, and bone loss (Bergström et al., 1991).

A set of guidelines is presented to the patient. Behavior modification should be part of a comprehensive smoking-cessation program. This includes talking to patients about their smoking habits and possibly incorporating hypnosis. Hypnosis has been used for many years in the treatment of habits (Weinberg, 1986). Hypnosis allows patients to be more susceptible to accepting suggestions, such as quitting smoking. This allows the patient to be in full control of the situation, and responsibility is placed on the patient not to smoke (Weinberg, 1986). Patients are put into a situation where they see themselves not smoking anymore. The dentist can perform hypnosis on the patient in the office. The patient is never asleep during this procedure. The patient also can learn self-hypnosis, which can be used anytime and anywhere.

Smoking-Cessation Program

The Smoking, Tobacco, and Cancer Program of the National Cancer Institute (1996) recommends guidelines to help patients to stop using tobacco. The 4A Program consists of the following components that are reviewed with the patient during the initial examination and periodically:

Ask. Inquire whether your patient smokes and, if so, how long he or she has been smoking and how much.
Advise. Inform the patient of the benefits of quitting and the risks associated with continuing the tobacco habit; strongly suggest that your patient should work toward a goal of complete smoking cessation.

Assist. Give the patient behavioral self-monitoring techniques and, as appropriate, pharmacologic intervention such as nicotine gum, nicotine patches, or another agent. Encourage the patient to quit smoking. Let the patient set up a quitting date or discuss different therapies.

Arrange for follow-up. Set up follow-up visits. The patient should return to the office at regular intervals to observe his or her periodontium and to reinforce his or her quitting behavior.

In addition, another "A" would be to assess for motivation to stop. Patients should be assessed for their reasons for quitting smoking and their thoughts for quitting.

Pharmacologic Agents

Table D–1 ■ reviews various types of smoking-cessation methods.

Pharmacologic agents include nicotine gum, transdermal nicotine patches, nasal sprays, and a systemic dosage form. The nicotine-replacement drugs (gum or patches) work by replacing the nicotine that is absorbed in the body while smoking and act as a substitute for the cigarette. Nicotine gum is absorbed through the buccal mucosa. The manufacturers of these products claim that they help patients quit while lessening any concomitant nicotine cravings (Stone &

Mattana, 1996). The efficacy of this method is questionable on a long-term basis. Patients must refrain from smoking while on the gum or patch because nicotine from these products is being introduced into the body. Nicotine therapy should not be used in a patient who continues to smoke. The importance of taking the gum as directed must be stressed to the patient. The gum should be placed between the cheek and gingiva and chewed slowly for about 30 minutes and then thrown away. Currently, the gum is available over the counter without a prescription. Nicotine patches are available in different doses that are worn on the skin for variable amounts of time. Indications for use of these products is for the reduction of symptoms associated with smoking cessation, including nicotine craving.

Bupropion HCl (Zyban® Sustained-Release Tablets, Glaxo Wellcome, Research Triangle Park, NC) is an oral medication prescribed by dentists or physicians to help decrease the withdrawal symptoms and the urge to smoke that accompany smoking cessation. Advantages to this form of therapy are that it is nicotine free and helps the patient to quit while still smoking. Bupropion is also used to treat depression. Adverse side effects include dry mouth (xerostomia) and insomnia (difficulty sleeping). Both nicotine gum and patches and bupropion should be used in conjunction with behavioral modification therapy.

Table D–1 Smoking-Cessation Methods: Pharmacologic Therapy

Product	Directions for Use	Supplied
Nicotine Gum		
Nicorette® gum (2 mg; 4 mg) (GlaxoSmithKline)	Usually start with 2 mg gum. Heavy smokers (more than 25 cigarettes a day) start with 4 mg gum. One piece of gum every 1–2 hours for weeks 1–6, every 2–4 hours for weeks 7–9, and every 4–8 hours for weeks 10–12. Do not eat or drink for 15 minutes before chewing a piece of gum. Alternatively chew and "park" between cheek and gingiva.	Over the counter; starter kit has 108 pieces, and refill kits have 48 pieces.
Nicotine Transdermal System (Patch)		
Habitrol® (Novartis Consumer, East Hanover, NJ)	Start each day by placing a new patch on a different part of the body between the neck and the waist. The patch is used for up to 8 weeks.	Over the counter; patch containing 7 mg of nicotine, 14 mg, and 21 mg; 7-day supply.
Nicoderm® CQ (GlaxoSmithKli ne)	Start each day by placing a new patch on a different part of the body between the neck and the waist. The patch is used for up to 8 weeks.	Over the counter; 7 mg patch, 14 mg patch, 21 mg patch; 7-day supply in 7 mg dose.

Product	Directions for Use	Supplied
Nicotine Lozenge		
Commit® (GlaxoSmithKline)	Use 2 mg if patient smokes the first cigarette of the day more than 30 minutes after awakening and 4 mg if smoke the first cigarette within 30 minutes of awakening. Allow lozenge to dissolve slowly over 20–30 min, swallow as little as possible. Up to 12 weeks. Taper after 4–6 weeks. Maximum per day is 20 lozenges. Adverse effect: xerostomia	Over the counter; 2 mg and 4 mg lozenge
Nicotine Nasal Spray		
Nicotrol® NS (McNeil Consumer Health Care, Fort Washington, PA)	Start with 2 sprays in each nostril every hour, which may be increased to 80 sprays per day (heavy smokers); maximum therapy is 6 months. Can cause nasal irritation. Up to 6 months, taper after 12 weeks.	Prescription; each spray delivers 0.5 mg nicotine; available in 10 mL bottles.
Nicotine Inhalation System		
Nicotrol® Inhaler (McNeil Consumer Health Care, Fort Washington, PA)	Reduces craving to smoke. Less nicotine per puff is released with the inhaler than with a cigarette. Best effect is achieved by frequent continuous puffing for about 20 minutes. The recommended treatment is up to 3 months and, if needed, a gradual reduction over the next 6–12 weeks. Total treatment should not exceed 6 months. Avoid in patients with reactive airway disease.	Prescription; the inhaler uses nicotine cartridges (10 mg/cartridge) that provide about 20 minutes of active puffing, or approximately 80 deep draws.
Oral Medications		
Bupropion HCl (Zyban®) Sustained-Release Tablets (Glaxo Wellcome, Research, Triangle Park, NC)	Start initial dose while the patient is still smoking to allow for higher blood levels; initial dose is 150 mg/day for 3 days. Maximum daily dose is 300 mg. Should stop smoking within 2 weeks of initiation of drug therapy. Continue drug therapy for 7–12 weeks after the patient stops smoking. Can be used with nicotine transdermal systems (nicotine patches). It is contraindicated in patients with eating disorders (anorexia, bulimia), seizure disorder, patients undergoing abrupt discontinuation of alcohol or sedatives	Prescription; 150 mg sustained-release tablets.
Varenicline (Chantrix™)	Day 1–3: 0.5 mg once daily; Days 4–7: 0.5 mg twice daily; Day 8–end of treatment: 1 mg twice daily Common adverse effects: nausea, sleep disturbance (trouble sleeping or vivid, unusual, or increased dreaming), constipation, gas, and vomiting.	Prescription: 0.5 and 1 mg tablets

References

American Academy of Periodontology. 1996. Tobacco use and the periodontal patient. *J. Periodontol.* 67:51–56.

Bain, C. A. 1996. Smoking and implant failure: Benefits of a smoking cessation protocol. *Int. J. Oral Maxillofac. Implants* 11:756–759.

Bergström, J., S. Eliasson, and H. Preber. 1991. Cigarette smoking and periodontal bone loss. *J. Periodontol.* 62:242–246.

Christen, A. G., J. L. McDonald, and J. A. Christen. 1991. *The impact of tobacco use and cessation on nonmalignant and precancerous oral and dental diseases and conditions.* Indianapolis: Indiana University School of Dentistry.

Dietrich, T. 2004. The effect of cigarette smoking on gingival bleeding. *J. Periodontol.* 75(1):16–22.

Grossi, S. G., J. J. Zambon, A. W. Ho, G. Koch, R. G. Dunford, et al. 1994. Assessment of risk for periodontal disease: I. Risk indicators for attachment loss. *J. Periodontol.* 65:260–267.

Grossi, S. G., J. Zambon, E. E. Machtei, R. Shifferle, S. Andreana, et al. 1997. Effects of smoking and smoking cessation on healing after mechanical periodontal therapy. *J. Am. Dent. Assoc.* 128:599–607.

Haber, J., J. Wattles, M. Crowby, R. Mandell, K. Joshipura, and R. L. Kent. 1993. Evidence for cigarette smoking as a major risk factor for periodontitis. *J. Periodontol.* 64:16–23.

Jones, J. K., and R. G. Triplett. 1992. The relationship of cigarette smoking to impaired intraoral wound healing: A review of evidence and implications for patient care. *J. Oral Maxillofac. Surg.* 50:237–239.

National Cancer Institute, U.S. Department of Health and Human Services. 1996. In eds. R. E. Mechlenburg, D. Greenspan, D. V. Kleinman, et al. *Tobacco effects in the mouth.* Bethesda, MD: Author.

Stone, C., and D. J. Mattana. 1996, January. The role of the dental team in helping patients stop using tobacco. *J. Mich. Dent. Assoc.* 58–66.

Weinberg, A. 1986. *Instructions in hypnosis,* unpublished findings.

GLOSSARY

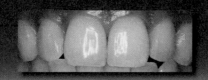

A

Abrasion Wearing away of a structure, such as a gingiva or the teeth, through an abnormal mechanical process. Examples would be gingiva or tooth abrasions due to incorrect brushing.

Abutment (tooth) A tooth or implant used for support and retention of a crown or removable partial denture.

Abutment screw A screw that secures (holds) the abutment to the implant.

Accretions Accumulation of foreign materials on the teeth, such as dental plaque, materia alba, and calculus.

Acellular Without cells.

Acellular cementum Cementum that does not contain cementocytes.

Acquired pellicle A thin film derived from salivary glycoproteins that forms over the surface of a clean tooth when it is exposed to saliva.

Adhesions Molecules on bacteria that attach to the tooth.

Adjunctive In addition to.

Aerobic Utilizing and dependent on oxygen.

Air polishing A controlled stream of sodium bicarbonate used to remove extrinsic tooth stains and dental plaque.

Allograft See Graft, osseous.

Alloplastic See Graft, osseous.

Alveolar bone See Bone, alveolar.

Alveolar crest The most coronal part of the interproximal bone.

Alveolar mucosa See Mucosa, alveolar.

Alveolar process Compact and cancellous bone that surrounds and supports the roots of the teeth.

Anaerobic Non-oxygen-utilizing. Oxygen is toxic to these organisms.

Anatomic factors Root size and shape and position of teeth in arch may influence the accumulation of biofilms.

Angle's classification of malocclusion A classification of different types of malocclusion based on the relationship of the anteroposterior relationship of the dental arches.

Class I (neutroocclusion): The mesiobuccal cusp of the maxillary first permanent molar occludes in the buccal groove of the mandibular first molar. Crowding has to be present.

Class II (distoocclusion): The mesiobuccal cusp of the maxillary first permanent molar is mesial to the mandibular first molar; the mandibular dental arch is posterior to the maxillary arch.

Class II, division 1: Labioversion of the maxillary incisors.

Class II, division 2: Linguoversion of the maxillary central incisors.

Class III (mesioocclusion): The mesiobuccal cusp of the maxillary first permanent molar is distal to the mandibular first molar; the mandibular dental arch is anterior to the maxillary arch.

Ankylosis Fusion of the tooth with the alveolar bone without an intervening periodontal ligament.

Antibiotic A soluble substance produced by microorganisms that has the capacity to inhibit the growth of or to kill other organisms.

Antibiotic prophylaxis See Prophylaxis.

Antibiotic resistence See Resistance, antibiotics.

Antibodies Serum proteins synthesized and released by plasma cells. Antibodies bind to and neutralize bacterial toxins.

Antigen A foreign substance (e.g., bacteria, bacterial toxins, and by-products) that elicits the formation of antibodies.

Antimicrobials Chemical agents that inhibit the growth of or kill a microorganism. The terms *antimicrobial* and *anti-infective* are used interchangeably.

Antiseptic An antimicrobial applied to the skin surface or oral mucosa that inhibits the growth and development of microorganisms.

Apical Refers to the apical or anatomic end of the root of a tooth.

Assessment Process of documentation.

Attachment apparatus Comprises the cementum, periodontal ligament, and alveolar and supporting bone.

Attachment level See Clinical attachment level (CAL).

Attachment loss, connective tissue (also referred to as clinical attachment loss) A pathologic process whereby the gingival collagen fibers become detached from the root surfaces with the concomitant apical migration of the apical aspect of the junctional epithelium along the root surface.

Attrition The wearing away of tooth structure by tooth-to-tooth normal or abnormal function.

Autograft See Graft, osseous.

Autoimmune disease Disease caused by the immunologic response against components of the body's own tissues.

Avascular Lacking in blood supply (e.g., tooth enamel, gingival epithelium, cementum).

B

Bacteremia Presence of bacteria in the bloodstream.

Bactericidal The ability of a drug or agent to kill bacteria.

Bacteriostatic Inhibiting the growth of bacteria.

Barrier membrane Material placed over a bone graft (in a periodontal defect) that keeps the bone graft at the site and prevents the growth of epithelial cells into the site.

Bass toothbrushing method See Toothbrushing methods.

Bifurcation The anatomic area where roots of a two-rooted tooth separate.

Biodegradable Resorbable.

Biofilm, (plaque, oral, dental) Matrix-enclosed bacterial populations adherent to each other and/or to surfaces or interfaces.

Biologic width The combined height of the gingival connective tissue (1.07 mm) and the junctional epithelium (0.97 mm) present around teeth.

Biota, oral The bacteria and other microorganisms that normally inhabit a bodily organ or part (also called oral flora).

Bisphosphonate Chemical that inhibits osteoclasts activity. Used in the treatment of osteoporosis.

Bleeding on probing Bleeding that occurs when the gingival crevice is probed.

Bone A hard type of connective tissue that contains collagen fibers, calcium phosphate, and hydroxyapatite.

Alveolar bone (also called alveolar bone proper): Compact bone that lines the tooth socket (alveolus).

Bundle bone: Alveolar bone with insertion of Sharpey's (principal) fibers.

Cancellous bone (spongy bone): Bone with trabeculae, located between the cortical plates and alveolar bone proper. It makes up the majority of a bone.

Compact bone: Bone that is hard and dense.

Cortical (plate) bone: Compact bone found on the facial and lingual aspects of the alveolar process.

Supporting bone: Surrounds and supports the alveolar bone proper. Is composed of the compact cortical plates of bone and cancellous trabecular bone.

Bone augmentation Correction of a bone defect or deficiency with the placement of a bone graft and/or bone replacement material.

Bone grafting A surgical procedure performed to reestablish bone volume. Placement of a bone graft or bone replacement material into an infrabony defect.

Bone grafts See Grafts, osseous.

Bone loss Horizontal bone loss: An equal amount of bone loss between two teeth. Vertical bone loss (also called angular bone loss): Bone destruction that does not occur on the entire thickness of the alveolar process. Bone loss affects only a portion of bone surrounding the affected tooth. Examples include one-, two-, and three-wall bony defects. See Periodontal bony defect.

Bone resorption Bone loss.

Bone substitute materials Alternative bone grafting materials to allografts and autografts. Many of these alternatives use a variety of materials, including natural and synthetic polymers, ceramics, and composites.

Bovine (as in bovine bone) Pertaining to cattle (cows).

Broad-spectrum (antibiotic) Antibiotic that affects a wide range of bacteria, including both gram-negative and gram-positive microorganisms.

Bruxism The involuntary and unconscious grinding or clenching of teeth. It is usually triggered by emotional stress, anxiety, or occlusal irregularities and usually results in abnormal wear patterns on the teeth.

Bundle bone See Bone, bundle.

C

Calculus Calcified microbial plaque. It is not viable (living bacteria) and thus is a local contributing risk factor for periodontal diseases. Bacteria embed into the porous surface.

Cancellous bone See Bone, cancellous.

Cellular immunity Immune response coordinated by T-lymphocytes that targets and kills cells infected with microorganisms such as viruses, fungi, and certain bacteria.

Cementocytes Cementoblasts from the periodontal ligament that lie close to the root and become surrounded by forming cementum.

Cementoenamel junction The area at which the enamel and cementum are united at the cervical region of the tooth.

Cementum Thin, calcified layer of connective tissue that covers the root of teeth.

Centric occlusion See Occlusion, centric.

Centric relation The most posterior or retruded position of the mandible to the maxilla from which lateral movements of the jaw can be made.

Cervical enamel projection Apical extension of the coronal enamel beyond the CEJ.

Charters' toothbrushing method See Toothbrushing methods.

Chemotaxis The process by which cells (PMNs, macrophages) are attracted toward an inflamed area, often by certain substances, including bacterial products, proteins, and interleukins.

Chemotherapeutic agents Drugs used to treat various forms of bacterial diseases and cancers.

Chemotherapeutics The prevention or treatment of a disease by medical visit.

Chief complaint Statement describing the symptom or problem that is the reason for the dental/medical visit.

Cleft, gingival A vertical-shaped slit extending from and into the gingival margin, usually due to the start of pocket formation or improper flossing.

Clinical Pertaining to the signs, symptoms, and course of a condition or disease as observed by a clinician.

Clinical attachment level (CAL) Distance measured from the cementoenamel junction to the location of the tip of the periodontal probe at the most coronal level of the attached periodontal tissues (junctional epithelium). More reliable marker for disease progression than probing depth measurements.

Clinical attachment loss See Attachment loss, connective tissue.

Clinical connective tissue attachment loss See Attachment loss.

Codestructive Another factor besides the primary factor further contributes to destruction (e.g., some believe that occlusal trauma and periodontal inflammation may act as codestructive agents in periodontal disease).

Col A valley-like depression of the interdental gingiva that connects the facial and lingual papillae. It is just below the contact area of the tooth.

Collagen The most abundant protein of skin, bone, and other connective tissues. Synthesized by fibroblasts, osteoblasts, and odontoblasts.

Collagen fibers See Fibers, collagen.

Collagenase Belongs to a family of enzymes called matrix metalloproteinases, which are responsible for the normal turnover of connective tissue and destruction of host (body's) tissue (collagen). Produced and secreted by bacteria and host cells including PMNs and fibroblasts. Collagenase produced and secreted by PMNs is responsible for the host tissue destruction. Collagenase produced and secreted by fibroblasts is responsible for the normal remodeling and turnover of collagen.

Community periodontal index of treatment needs (CPITN) An index used in population studies of periodontal disease designed by the World Health Organization to assess periodontal treatment needs.

Compact bone See Bone, compact.

Complement A sequence of serum proteins that, when activated, attempt to destroy a foreign substance.

Complement system See Complement.

Compliance The patient's ability to adhere to the appointment schedule and oral home self-care instructions given by the dental hygienist or dentist.

Computed tomographic (CT) scan Digitized tomography that results in an enhanced image that is much easier to read than a plane (conventional) tomogram. It measures the amount of energy transmission through an object. It produces a cross-sectional image of a slice of tissue (e.g., bone). Many slices are made of a given edentulous site.

Connective tissue attachment Mechanism of attachment of the connective tissue (gingival fibers) to the tooth or implant surface.

Continuing care See Periodontal maintenance.

Contributing factor Does not initiate the disease process or act independently as an etiologic agent. Helps to allow a condition to become established and/or progress.

Contributory Helping to bring about a result.

Controlled Release delivery device for an active agent dispersed in a biodegradable matrix that slowly is released from that matrix (e.g., Atridox, Arestin, and PerioChip).

Conventional radiograph X-rays taken with films.

Coronal Toward the crown of a tooth.

Cortical bone See Bone, cortical.

Crater Interdental depressions in the gingiva or bone.

C-reactive protein (CRP) A blood marker for inflammation.

Crestal Of or pertaining to the crest or most coronal portion of the alveolar bone.

Curets Area-specific curets (also called Gracey curets): Designed to be used on specific tooth surfaces of different teeth. Their design includes one cutting edge per end with a rounded back and toe.

Universal curets: Designed to be used on the mesial and distal surfaces of teeth without changing the instrument. Their design includes two cutting edges per end with a rounded back and toe.

Curettage, gingival Removal of the ulcerated soft tissue pocket wall.

Cytokines Proteins produced and secreted by host cells including macrophages and lymphocytes. These proteins signal and modify the behavior or actions of these cells and other cells. Examples are the interleukins, such as interleukin-1 (IL-1), which is responsible for bone destruction.

Cytotoxic The ability to kill cells, including human cells.

D

Debridement The removal of inflamed, devitalized, or contaminated tissue or foreign material from or adjacent to a lesion.

Dehiscence Loss of radicular bone on a root or implant extending from the crest and proceeding apically.

Dental hygiene diagnosis An analysis of the cause and nature of the periodental problem.

Dental calculus Calcified plaque.

Dental charting Provides a graphic description of the conditions in a patient's mouth, including caries and probing depths.

Dental implant An artificial (usually titanium metal) post that substitutes for a tooth root and to which a prosthesis is attached. See Endosseous implant.

Dental/medical history Account of a patient's past and present state of health.

Dental plaque Accumulations of bacteria and other microorganisms on tooth surfaces in the area of the sulcus or pocket. Referred to as plaque (dental) biofilm.

Dentifrice A powder, paste, or gel used in conjunction with a toothbrush to aid in the removal of plaque, materia alba, and stain from teeth.

Dentinal hypersensitivity The short, exaggerated, painful response elicited when exposed dentin is subjected to certain thermal, mechanical, or chemical stimuli.

Dentogingival unit Composed of two parts, the gingival connective tissue attachment and the junctional epithelium.

Deplaquing The removal of subgingival dental plaque after the completion of periodontal debridement. It is performed at the reevaluation/supportive periodontal therapy appointments.

Desensitization Reducing or eliminating dentin sensitivity.

Diagnosis Dental diagnosis: Refers to the identification and naming of a disease. Dental hygiene diagnosis: Identifies certain problems or the patient's response to the disease process that can be treated by a dental hygienist.

Diastema A space between two adjacent teeth in the same dental arch.

Digital imaging X-ray images that use a sensor to transmit the image directly to a computer via a cable link. X-ray image appears on a monitor and can be manipulated electronically to change contrast, orientation, resolution, and size of the image.

Direct digital radiography Direct conversion of transmitted x-rays into a digital image.

Disease A process characterized usually by at least two of these criteria: a recognized etiologic agent (or agents), an identifiable group of signs and symptoms, and consistent anatomic alterations.

Disease activity See Periodontal disease activity.

Disease severity See Periodontal disease severity.

Documentation The recording in a permanent format of information derived from activities.

Donor site Area in the mouth or body from which a graft (bone or soft tissue) is harvested.

Drifting Tooth migration as a result of loss of proximal contact of adjacent teeth in a healthy periodontium.

E

Edema An abnormal swelling caused by an accumulation of fluid in a tissue or part.

Edentulous Without teeth.

Enamel matrix derivative (EMD) Protein obtained from amelogenin (enamel matrix precurser of enamel) of the developing tooth. Product called Emdogain®. Indicated for bone grafting.

Endosseous implant Type of implant placed in a hole (osteotomy) drilled in the bone. See Implant, endosseous.

Embrasure The spaces that widen out from the proximal contact area. Each interdental space has four embrasures: facial embrasure, lingual embrasure, an occlusal or incisal embrasure, and a gingival embrasure. An open gingival embrasure is seen frequently in patients with periodontal disease.

Endotoxins Lipooligosaccharide (lipid) complexes formed by gram-negative bacteria. When the bacteria die and break apart (lysis), the endotoxin is released from the cell wall of the bacteria and is capable of having a toxic or harmful effect on the host tissue.

Enzyme A protein substance formed by living cells that acts to speed up metabolic processes or chemical reaction.

Epidemiology The study of the distribution and determinants of illnesses and their associated factors in the human population.

Epithelial ridges Ridge-like projections of epithelium into the underlying lamina propria.

Epithelium (oral) The tissue that lines the intraoral surfaces. It extends into the gingival crevice and adheres to the tooth at the base of the gingival crevice.

Erosion Chemical wearing away of a structure, such as a tooth.

Erythema (erythematous) Redness of the mucous membranes due to inflammation.

Evaluation Judging the value of material based on personal opinions.

Exposure time Duration of the process of exposure to radiation.

Extent The number or percent of diseased teeth or sites in an individual.

Extrusion (extrude) Overruption of a tooth from its normal occlusal position in the dental arch.

Exudate A fluid substance formed within tissues as a result of inflammation. It consists of polymorphonuclear leukocytes, degenerated tissues, dead cells, bacteria, and tissue fluid.

F

Facial Pertaining to the face. The facial surfaces of the teeth are called buccal and labial.

Failed implant A dental implant that is mobile; lost failing implant osseointegration. A dental implant that is progressively losing bone around it.

Fenestration Root or implant surface is denuded (loss) of bone but the crestal bone is intact.

Fiber A filament or thread. In periodontics, the term usually refers to collagenous or connective tissue fibers.

Collagen fibers: White fibers composed of collagen. Found within connective tissue of the gingiva and periodontal ligament arranged in bundles or haphazardly distributed. Characterized by its hydroxyproline and hydroxylysine content.

Gingival fibers: (also called gingival connective tissue or supracrestal fiber apparatus) Fibers composed primarily of collagen that radiate from the cementum or bone into the lamina propria. Includes alveogingival, circular, dentogingival, dentoperiosteal, and transseptal.

Periodontal ligament fibers (principal fibers): Collagen fibers of the periodontal ligament. Includes alveolar crest, apical, horizontal, interradicular, and oblique.

Fibroblast A cell found within connective tissue that synthesizes collagen and ground substance of connective tissue.

Fibrotic Tissue that is in a state of repair; tissue is hard and not resilient or spongy.

Filtration The use of absorbers for the selective reduction in intensity of radiation of certain wavelengths from a primary x-ray beam.

Flap A part of tissue (gingiva) separated from the underlying tissues except at its base.

Fluorosis, dental Enamel hypoplasia due to the ingestion of water containing excessive amounts of fluoride.

Food impaction The forceful wedging of food into the interproximal space by chewing pressure or tongue or cheek pressure.

Free gingival graft See Graft.

Fremitus Vibrational movement of the tooth under occlusal function.

Frenum A narrow band of alveolar mucosa radiates from a fixed part to a movable part and limits movement of that part. Example: Frenum runs from the gingiva to the lip, cheek, or under the tongue.

Frequency The number of times per second the insert tip moves back and forth during one cycle.

Full-mouth survey The production of the minimal number of radiographic examinations necessary for a radiographic interpretation.

Furcation (also called furca) Anatomic area on multirooted teeth where the root base divides.

Furcation involvement (defect) Pathologic loss of bone in the furcation of a multirooted tooth.

G

Gain in clinical attachment (also referred to as gain in periodontal attachment) A decrease in probing depths after periodontal therapy due to an increase in resistance of the periodontal probe into the tissue and maybe gingival recession. The inflamed tissue is replaced by firm collagen fibers.

Genetics Inheritance or transmission of a disease or condition from a parent to a child.

Gingiva A part of the masticatory mucosa that is attached to the teeth and alveolar process.

Attached gingiva: The portion of the gingiva that is firm, dense, and tightly bound down to the underlying periosteum, tooth, and bone.

Free (marginal) gingiva: The portion of the gingiva that is unattached and forms the wall of the gingival crevice in health. It is continuous with the attached gingiva.

Gingival abscess A localized collection of pus confined to the gingival tissue.

Gingival assessment Evaluation of the gingiva for inflammation.

Gingival crevice A shallow opening between the free gingiva and the enamel or cementum. In gingival health it is called the gingival sulcus and in disease a pocket.

Gingival crevicular fluid Fluid originating in the gingival connective tissue that seeps through the sulcular and junctional epithelium. Flow increases in the presence of inflammation.

Gingival pocket (pseudopocket) See Pocket, gingival.

Gingival recession (soft tissue recession) Apical migration of the marginal gingiva resulting in exposure of the root surface to the oral environment.

Gingival sulcus Space between the tooth and the marginal gingiva in gingival health. If bleeding is present, it is not a sulcus but a pocket.

Gingivitis Inflammation of the gingiva without involvement of the underlying bone or periodontal attachment. The following are gingival diseases listed in the new classification of periodontal diseases (American Academy of Periodontology, 1999):

Drug-influenced gingivitis: Gingivitis or gingival enlargement caused by drugs (e.g., calcium channel blockers, phenytoin, cyclosporine, and oral contraceptives).

Plaque-associated gingivitis: Gingivitis caused by dental plaque alone.

Pregnancy-associated gingivitis: Hormonally influenced inflammation and enlargement of the gingiva during pregnancy.

Puberty-associated gingivitis: Hormonally influenced inflammation of the gingiva during puberty.

Graft, osseous (bone) Allograft (allogenic graft): Bone taken from human beings (cadavers) other than the patient. Bone is bought from tissue banks. Three types: freeze-dried bone allograft (FDBA), demineralized freeze-dried bone allograft (DFDBA), and frozen.

Alloplast (alloplastic graft): Synthetic or natural bone (inorganic) substitutes.

Autograft: Tissue such as bone (osseous material; organic) taken from the patient's mouth or extraoral area such as the hip.

Graft, soft tissue Connective tissue graft: Connective tissue (donor) taken from underneath the epithelium and placed in a prepared recipient bed for the purposes of root coverage and increasing the amount of attached gingiva.

Free gingival graft: Gingiva taken from an area in the patient's mouth, usually the palate (donor), and placed in a prepared recipient bed primarily to increase the amount of attached gingiva.

Grinding See Bruxism.

Growth factors A substance that affects the growth of a cell or an organism.

Guided bone regeneration (GBR) Bone regeneration (surgical) procedure using barrier membrane to regenerate bone.

Guided tissue regeneration (GTR) Periodontal procedures performed in an attempt at regeneration. Barrier techniques are used with materials that exclude the junctional epithelium from the wound site in an attempt to allow periodontal ligament cells to populate the wound site.

H

Halitosis Bad breath.

Hemostasis Control of and stopping bleeding.

Histopathogenesis Pathologic (disease) changes within the periodontal structures at a microscopic level.

Host Referring to the body or self.

Host cells Cells normally present in the body (e.g., polymorphonuclear leukocytes [PMNs], macrophages, fibroblasts).

Host-derived enzymes Enzymes produced and secreted by cells in the human body such as neutrophils (PMNs) or fibroblasts.

Host response How the body responds to an implanted device or material.

Humoral immunity Branch of the immune-system that depends on antibodies.

Hypertrophy Increase in bulk of a part or organ not due to tumor formation.

I

Iatrogenic Factor situation caused by dental or medical treatment; abnormal condition induced by a clinician.

Immune response Mechanisms used by the body as protection against environmental agents that are foreign to the body.

Immune system Components include the lymph nodes, thymus, spleen, and bone marrow.

Immunity The organism's (or body's) capacity for successfully resisting the actions of harmful foreign substances or pathogenic (disease-producing) microorganisms such as bacteria or viruses.

Immunodeficiency A deficiency in the immune system caused by an upset in the number of lymphocytes.

Immunoglobulins Group of large glycoproteins that are secreted by plasma cells and function as antibodies in the immune system (e.g., IgA, IgG, IgM).

Implant, endosseous Dental implant placed within bone.

Implementation Carrying out a plan for doing something (e.g., developing a treatment plan and treating a patient according to the treatment plan.)

Incidence The rate of new occurrence of the disease in a population over a given period of time.

Index (plural: Indices) A screening tool designed to quantify and simplify the disease assessment in population surveys. Examples include plaque, debris, calculus, and periodontal destruction.

Infection Pathogenic invasion of the body and the body's response to these organisms.

Infective endocarditis Inflammation of the inner lining of the heart caused by a microbial infection.

Inflammation Protective response elicited by injury or destruction of tissues that attempts to destroy or wall off the injurious agent and tissue. It is also the cellular and vascular tissue reaction that occurs when tissue is injured.

Inflammatory cells Cells involved in the inflammatory response of tissues to injury or infection (e.g., PMNs, macrophages, mast cells).

Inflammatory periodontal diseases A group of inflammatory diseases of the periodontium including gingivitis and periodontitis.

Inflammatory process A localized protective reaction of tissue to irritation, injection, or injury.

Informed consent A written agreement by patients to voluntarily have treatment performed on them or to participate in a study.

Infrabony defect See Periodontal bony defects.

Interdental Between two adjacent teeth.

Interdental septum That part of the alveolar process extending between adjacent teeth.

Interproximal Pertaining to the area between two adjacent teeth. See Interdental.

Interradicular That part of the alveolar process between the roots of a multirooted tooth (e.g., molars, premolar).

Interview process A face-to-face meeting with the patient for questions and answers.

J

Junctional epithelium Epithelium that is located at the base of the gingival crevice.

K

Keratin A protein that is the main component of keratinized epithelium synthesized by keratinocytes.

Keratinocyte A cell found in the epithelium (a type of epithelial cell) that forms keratin.

L

Lamina dura A layer of compact bone forming the wall of a tooth alveolus (alveolar bone). In a radiograph, it appears as a thin radiopaque line separated from the tooth by the radiolucent image of the periodontal ligament space.

Lamina propria The gingival connective tissue layer under the epithelium.

Lipooligosaccharide Another name is endotoxin. A component of gram-negative bacteria that is released on destruction of the bacterial cell and can cause tissue and bone destruction.

Load External mechanical force applied to a tooth, implant, or prosthesis.

Lymphadenopathy Lymph nodes that are abnormal in size, consistency, or number.

Lymph nodes Small, round, or oval organs containing lymphocytes. Found in groups or chains in certain regions, often associated with large blood vessels.

Lymphocyte A type of white blood cell involved in the immune response. There are two types of lymphocytes: T cells and B cells.

M

Macrophage A large tissue cell responsible for removing damaged tissue, cells, and bacteria through phagocytosis. Increase in number in chronic inflammation.

Malocclusion Deviation from the acceptable relationship of opposing teeth. See Angle's classification of malocclusion.

Marginal Pertaining to the margin or edge.

Marginal ridge A ridge or elevation of enamel that is on the border of the occlusal surface of a tooth.

Mast cell A large tissue cell that releases inflammatory substances or mediators when damaged.

Masticatory (mastication) The process of chewing food.

Microbiota See Biota, oral.

Microflora Bacteria living in a part of the body (e.g., the mouth, intestines, nose). See also Biota, oral.

Microorganisms Organisms of microscopic size (e.g., bacteria, yeasts, simple fungi).

Migration, pathologic The movement of a tooth out of its natural position, usually as a result of advanced periodontal disease.

Mobility, tooth The degree of looseness of a tooth beyond physiologic movement. Tooth movement away from its normal position in a buccal/lingual or apical direction when slight pressure is applied.

Monitoring The act of listening or watching.

Mucogingival involvement (defect) A discrepancy in the relationship between the gingival margin and the mucogingival junction. Usually, there is minimal to no attached gingiva.

Mucogingival junction Demarcation between the attached gingiva and alveolar mucosa.

Mucosa A mucous membrane.

Alveolar mucosa: Mucosa covering part of the alveolar process and continuing into the vestibule and floor of the mouth. It is movable and loosely attached to the underlying periostium.

Masticatory mucosa: Mucosa of the gingiva and hard palate.

N

National Health and Nutrition Examination Survey (NHANES I) A national survey of adults from 1960 to 1962.

National Health and Nutrition Examination Survey (NHANES III) This is the seventh in a series, beginning in 1960, of national examination surveys of the U.S. population conducted by the National Center for Health Statistics in collaboration with the National Institute for Dental Research (NIDR). The survey was designed to collect data representative of the total U.S. civilian, non-institutionalized population age 12 months and older.

National Institute of Dental Research (NIDR) Survey A national survey of employed adults between 18 and 64 years of age conducted by the National Institute of Dental Research. It was named the National Survey of Oral Health of U.S. Adults 1985–1986. More than 15,000 people were examined, representing over 100 million working adults in the United States.

Necrotizing periodontal diseases Formerly known as acute necrotizing ulcerative gingivitis (ANUG). Because acute is a clinical descriptive term, it should not be used as a diagnostic classification. Thus the correct term is necrotizing ulcerative gingivitis (NUG). In the new classification, NUG is a type of necrotizing periodontal disease. It is an inflammation of the gingiva characterized by necrosis of the gingival margin and interdental papillae. Included in this classification is necrotizing ulcerative periodontitis (NUP), which is characterized by necrosis of gingival tissues, periodontal ligament, and alveolar bone.

Necrotizing ulcerative gingivitis (NUG) An infection of the gingiva characterized by punched out or cratered papillae, with bleeding and pain.

Necrotizing ulcerative periodontitis (NUP) An infection characterized by necrosis of the gingival periodontal ligament and alveolar bone.

Neutrophil See Polymorphonuclear leukocyte.

Nitrogenous Compounds or substance containing nitrogen.

Nonmetallic materials Non–stainless steel (e.g., plastic).

Nonnitrogenous Compounds or substances that do not contain nitrogen.

O

Objective Based on facts; not affected by personal feelings.

Objective data Signs or observations made by the clinician that can be verified by another person.

Obligate Able to survive only in a specific environment (e.g., an obligate anaerobe is only able to live in a non-oxygen environment).

Occlusal adjustment (also called selective grinding or occlusal equilibration) Reshaping the occlusal or incisal surfaces of teeth by grinding to create harmonious contact relationships between the upper and lower teeth.

Occlusal therapy A treatment to establish and maintain a stable, comfortable, and functional occlusion.

Occlusal trauma Injury to the attachment apparatus as a result of excessive occlusal forces.

Primary occlusal trauma: Excessive occlusal forces placed on a healthy periodontium that produces changes in the periodontal tissues. Examples include placement of a "high" restoration and orthodontic movement of teeth.

Secondary occlusal trauma: Normal forces of mastication on a periodontium with bone loss (periodontitis) that produce changes in the periodontal tissues.

Occlusion Contact of opposing teeth (maxillary and mandibular teeth); centric occlusion: maximum intercuspation of maxillary and mandibular teeth.

Open bite Anterior or posterior teeth do not occlude with the opposing teeth.

Operculum Gingival flap overlying the crown of an erupting tooth.

Opsonins A molecule that acts as a binding enhancer for phagocytosis (e.g., complement).

Oral biofilm See Biofilm.

Oral epitheluim Epithelium covering oral mucous membranes.

Oral hygiene self-care Removal of dental plaque with brushes, dental floss, and other oral aids.

Oral prophylaxis See Prophylaxis.

Osseointegration The biologic phenomenon by which bone grows up to and contacts the surface of implants, thereby anchoring them to the jaw bone.

Osseous Referring to bone.

Ostectomy Surgical removal of supporting bone.

Osteoblast A cell that forms bone.

Osteoclast A cell that resorbs bone.

Osteoconduction Bone growth by laying down of form from the surrounding bone. Bone material acts as a scaffolding along which bone will be laid down.

Osteointegration New bone growth from osteoprogenitor cells.

Osteonecrosis of the jaw (ONJ) A severe bone disease causing necrosis of the jaws, especially the mandible. Usually associated with bisphosphonate usage.

Osteoplasty Surgical reshaping or removal of nonsupporting bone.

Outcome measure The recording of activity or effort that can be expressed in a quantitative or qualitative manner assessing therapy completed (e.g., the outcome measure of initial therapy is periodental probing and oral hygiene assessment).

Overbite Vertical overlap of the upper incisor teeth over the lower incisor teeth.

Overdenture A removable partial or complete denture that is supported by implants or implant/tissue.

Overjet Horizontal projection of the upper teeth beyond the lower teeth.

P

Panoramic film A type of conventional radiograph showing the entire area of the mandible and maxilla.

Papillary Pertaining to the interdental papillae.

Parafunctional habit A habit characterized by abnormal (out of the normal range) function (e.g., bruxism, pencil chewing, nail biting).

Paralleling technique A technique in intraoral radiographs in which the film is positioned parallel to the long axis of the teeth.

Passive eruption Physiologic process with recession of the gingiva from the enamel apically toward the cemento-enamel junction.

Pathogenic Disease-producing.

Pathologic mobility Horizontal or vertical displacement of a tooth beyond its physiologic movement.

Patient adherence Term used to describe how well a patient is sticking to their hygiene program; compliance.

Patient education The process of informing a patient about a health (dental) matter.

Periapical film A type of conventional radiograph that shows the entire tooth, including the area around the root apex.

Periapical pathology Disease occurring around the apex of a tooth.

Pericoronitis (also termed pericoronal abscess) Inflammation of the operculum or tissue flap over a partially erupted tooth, especially a third molar.

Peri-implant Around a dental implant.

Peri-implant disease A descriptive term used to describe nonspecific inflammation around the dental implant. There are two types of peri-implant disease: peri-implantitis, which is inflammation with loss of bone surrounding a functioning implant. Peri-implantitis may show the following symptoms; bleeding on probing, increased probing pocket depth, mobility, suppuration and pain. Peri-implant mucositis is inflammation localized to the soft tissues and not involving bone. It is reversible with treatment.

Peri-implantitis Inflammation of the gingival tissues around an implant and bone loss.

Perimucosal seal Tissue tension provided by the circular fibers between the gingiva and the implant.

Periocoronal abscess See Pericoronitis.

Periodontal Occurring around a tooth.

Periodontal abscess (also called lateral periodontal abscess) Localized accumulation of pus in periodontal tissues formed by the disintegration of tissue.

Periodontal assessment Steps followed to evaluate periodontal tissues.

Periodontal bony defects A deviation from the normal form or contour of bone due to periodontal disease.

Crater (interproximal crater): A two-wall infrabony defect (facial and lingual bony walls remain).

Hemiseptum defect: The remaining interdental bone septum where the mesial or distal part has been destroyed, with one bony wall remaining (half of a septum).

Infrabony defect: A general term to describe any periodontal bony defect associated with vertical (angular) bone loss. These defects are named according to the number of bony walls remaining in the interproximal area that surround the pocket (e.g., one-wall, two-wall, and three-wall).

Intrabony defect: A type of three-wall defect with three bony walls remaining. The defect may or may not be totally lined by cortical bone and may have cancellous bone behind. Not all three-wall defects are intrabony.

Periodontal debridement The removal of a foreign material (e.g., plaque, calculus) or dead tissue from the crown, root surface, pocket space, pocket wall, and bone surface.

Periodontal diseases A bacterial infection affecting the gingiva (gingivitis) and attaching fibers and bone (periodontitis).

Periodontal disease activity (PDA) The ongoing loss of connective tissue attachment and bone at a particular point in time (e.g., at the clinical examination appointment). It is difficult to determine disease activity. A 2 to 3 mm change in clinical attachment level must occur before a site can be labeled disease active.

Periodontal disease severity The total periodontal destruction and healing that occur prior to the clinical examination. Disease severity is determined after the periodontal assessment (visual, periodontal probing, radiographs) is completed. Severity can be classified as mild, moderate, or severe.

Periodontal ligament (fibers) The connective tissue that surrounds the root surface of the tooth and attaches it to the alveolar bone.

Periodontal maintenance Also referred to as recare or continuing care. An extension of periodontal therapy. Procedures performed at selected intervals to assist the periodontal patient in maintaining oral health.

Periodontal pathogens Bacteria that cause periodontal disease.

Periodontal pocket See Pocket, periodontal.

Periodontal probing Measures the location where physical resistance of the probe is met by the junctional epithelial attachment to the tooth.

Periodontal regeneration Restoring lost supporting tissue around the tooth, including new alveolar bone, cementum, and periodontal ligament fibers.

Periodontal therapy Treatment of the periodontal lesion.

Periodontics The specialty of dentistry dealing with the prevention, diagnosis, and treatment of diseases of the tissues that surround the teeth.

Periodontist A dental practitioner who practices periodontics.

Periodontitis Inflammation of the supporting tissues of teeth where there is connective tissue attachment loss and alveolar and supporting bone loss. The following is a classification system developed by the American Academy of Periodontology (1999):

Aggressive periodontitis: Formerly known as early-onset periodontitis (e.g., juvenile periodontitis, prepubertal periodontitis, and rapidly progressive periodontitis). Except for the presence of periodontitis, patients are otherwise clinically healthy. There is rapid attachment loss and bone destruction. Patients have defects in host defense. Includes prepubesent children who have periodontal destruction without any modifying systemic conditions. The following specific features are identified:

Generalized aggressive periodontitis: Formerly known as generalized juvenile periodontitis. Usually affects persons under 30 years of age, but patients may be older. Generalized interproximal attachment loss affecting at least three permanent teeth other than first molars and incisors.

Localized aggressive periodontitis: Formerly known as localized juvenile periodontitis (LJP). Circumpubertal onset. Primarily affects the first permanent incisors and first molars. Attachment loss may progress at a rate three to five times faster than chronic periodontitis. These patients are characterized by a lack of clinical signs of inflammation, harbor *Aggregatibacter actinomycetemcomitans* in their microflora, and display an altered immune response.

Chronic periodontitis: Formerly known as adult periodontitis. A form of periodontitis that usually is prevalent in adults but can occur in children and adolescents (formerly known as prepubertal periodontitis). The amount of periodontal destruction is consistent with the presence of local factors. Bone resorption usually progresses slowly.

Necrotizing periodontal diseases: Replaces necrotizing ulcerative gingivitis (NUG) and necrotizing ulcerative periodontitis (NUP). A form of periodontitis seen in the HIV/AIDS patient. (See Necrotized periodontal diseases.)

Refractory periodontitis: Patients who do not respond to conventional periodontal therapy treatment. It is not considered a single disease entity because it can occur in all forms of periodontitis.

Periodontium Comprises the periodontal tissues that support and surround the teeth, including the gingiva, cementum, periodontal ligament, and alveolar and supporting bone.

Periodontology The scientific study of the periodontal structures in health and disease.

Periosteum Connective tissue covering the outer surface of bone.

Phagocytosis The process of destroying bacteria by devouring and digesting them by phagocytic cells such as polymorphonuclear leukocytes and macrophages.

Pharmacokinetics What the body does to a drug (e.g., absorption, distribution, metabolism, and elimination).

Phase-contrast microscopy A method of using a microscope through which the shape, size, and mobility of bacteria can be viewed.

Phenytoin An anticonvulsant drug that can cause gingival enlargement.

Plaque-associated gingivitis See Gingivitis.

Pocket Gingival pocket: A deepening of the gingival crevice due to the coronal migration of the gingival margin without apical migration of the junctional epithelium (loss of attachment) and bone loss. Examples: drug-influenced gingival enlargement, inflammation of the gingiva. Also called a pseudopocket.

Periodontal pocket: A pathologic deepening of the gingival sulcus characterized by apical migration of the junctional epithelium and alveolar bone loss. Two types of periodontal pockets: infrabony and suprabony.

Infrabony pocket: A periodontal pocket that extends apical to the adjacent alveolar crest or into an infrabony defect (a defect with a vertical pattern of bone loss). There is apical migration of the junctional epithelium and bone loss; the base of the pocket is apical to the crest of alveolar bone.

Suprabony pocket: A periodontal pocket that extends coronal to the alveolar crest or into a suprabony defect with a horizontal pattern of bone loss. The base of the pocket is coronal to the crest of alveolar bone.

Polishing The removal of acquired pellicle, bacterial plaque, and stain from the external tooth surface through mechanical means and an abrasive agent.

Polymorphonuclear leukocyte (PMN) The major mobile phagocytic white blood cell involved in engulfing, killing, and digesting microorganisms. The first cell to migrate to the acute inflammatory site. Impairment in their function is related to the pathogenesis of aggressive periodontitis.

Population survey A statistical term used to evaluate representative samples of individuals within a study population to assess the true risk for disease and quantify how many individuals are or will be affected by disease.

Prevalence The proportion of individuals in a population having periodontal disease or the number of individuals expected to have periodontal disease in a specific time.

Primary herpetic gingivostomatitis An initial oral infection caused by herpes simplex type 1 in young children.

They are at risk for developing extensive oropharyngeal vesicular eruptions when first infected with the virus.

Primary occlusal trauma See Occlusal trauma, primary.

Primary prevention Action performed to preclude or prevent the development of a disease (e.g., use of fluorides to prevent caries).

Probing See Periodontal probing.

Probing depth The distance from the soft tissue (gingiva or alveolar mucosa) margin to the tip of the periodontal probe. The health of the attachment apparatus can affect the measurement.

Problem-based In reference to learning. Learning that is driven by a question or problem and uses various methods of inquiry research to address the question or problem.

Prognosis A prediction or forecast of the course and outcome of a disease.

Prophylaxis Prevention of disease.

Antibiotic prophylaxis: Antibiotic coverage necessary before invasive dental procedures that cause bleeding to prevent a bacteremia that ultimately could cause infective endocarditis or serious infections.

Oral prophylaxis: The removal of plaque, calculus, and stains from the exposed and unexposed surfaces of the teeth by scaling and polishing as a preventive measure for the control of local irritational factors.

Proximal Surface of a tooth next to another tooth.

Pseudocleft Slit or fissure of the gingiva associated with severe gingival inflammation or certain medications causing the papillae to enlarge and approach each other and not due to pocket formation.

Pseudopocket See Pocket, gingival or Pocket, pseudo.

Pus See Suppuration.

R

Radicular Pertaining to the root.

Recession See Gingival recession.

Recurrent When signs of disease return.

Reevaluation Pertaining to evaluating the results of therapy a second time (e.g., evaluating the results of initial or surgical therapy).

Regeneration, periodontal Formation of new alveolar and supporting bone, cementum, and periodontal ligament on a previously diseased root surface.

Resistance, antibiotic An antimicrobial agent no longer is effective in killing or inhibiting growth of microorganisms.

Rete pegs See Epithelial ridges.

Retreatment After active periodontal therapy more treatment is needed to get the disease under control.

Rheumatic heart disease A disease of the heart resulting from rheumatic fever, chiefly manifested by abnormalities of the valves.

Risk assessment Pertaining to periodontal risk assessment. Is a test tool to help you understand whether you are at a risk for developing a periodontal disease.

Risk factors Characteristics that have been shown to directly cause periodontal disease (e.g., dental plaque, diabetes mellitus, tobacco smoking).

Risk indicators Behavioral and socioeconomic characteristics that are associated with periodontal diseases but are not considered to cause the disease (e.g., aging). Risk factors are not causal—just puts an individual more at risk.

Root planing A treatment procedure designed to remove cementum or surface dentin that is rough, impregnated with calculus, or contaminated with toxins or microorganisms.

S

Saccharolytic Bacteria that can break down a sugar molecule.

Scaler A periodontal instrument that is designed to scale primarily supragingival tooth surfaces.

Sonic: Produces mechanical vibrations by means of air pressure rather than electrical energy. The operating frequency is between 3,000 and 8,000 cycles per second.

Ultrasonic: Devices operating at frequencies between 18,000 and 50,000 cycles per second. They use electrical energy to produce mechanical vibrations that will remove calculus.

Magnetostrictive ultrasonic: Produces mechanical movement using a low-voltage magnetic signal. The operating frequency is between 18,000 and 45,000 cycles per second. The handpiece contains coils that activate the interchangeable inserts, causing them to vibrate. The working ends can be used on all sides, providing better adaptation to the tooth surfaces.

Piezoelectric ultrasonic: Produces mechanical movement using a high-voltage magnetic signal. The operating frequency is between 25,000 and 50,000 cycles per second. Only two sides of the working end are adapted to the tooth surface.

Scaling The removal of dental plaque, calculus, and stains from the crown and root surfaces.

Screening A single examination to separate periodontally healthy from diseased patients and to determine the patient's dental needs. It does not make a specific dental hygiene diagnosis or tell the type of treatment to be given. It simply requires probing depth measurements and conventional radiographs.

Secondary occlusal trauma See Occlusal trauma, secondary.

Secondary prevention Activities are aimed at early disease detection, thereby increasing opportunities for interventions to prevent progression of the disease and development of symptoms (e.g., removal of all calculus and dental biofilms while performing root debridement).

Selective grinding See Occlusal adjustment.

Severity Degree of disease involvement, quantifying the amount of attachment loss or probing depth. May be expressed as mild or slight, moderate, and severe.

Sign Any abnormality indicative of disease, discoverable by the clinician at the evaluation of a patient.

Single-stage implant An implant placed in a one-stage surgery.

Smoking cessation A means to quit smoking.

Soft-tissue healing Natural process by which the body repairs itself after periodontal debridement or surgery.

Sonic See Scaler, sonic.

Stem cells Cells from which all the blood cells "stem" or come.

Stillman's toothbrushing method See Toothbrushing methods.

Stippling The "orange peel" appearance (depressions) on the attached gingiva. Stippling is not present on the free gingiva.

Subgingival (submarginal) Beneath the gingiva or gingival margin; into the crevice.

Subgingival debridement Other term: subgingival scaling. Removal of plaque and calculus apical to the gingival margin.

Subjective As described in an individual's words or opinions rather than facts.

Subjective data Those facts that are observable and measurable by the clinician. Personal feeling entering into the testing method or result analysis (e.g., patient's description of pain).

Substantivity Ability of a substance to absorb or bind to a surface such as the tooth root, tissues, bacterial plaque, or enamel and slowly released over time in its active form.

Sulcular epithelium Epithelium that lines the gingival crevice.

Sulcus See Gingival sulcus.

Supporting bone See Bone, supporting.

Suppuration The formation of pus. An inflammatory or purulent exudate formed within the tissues. It consists of neutrophils, bacteria, degenerated and liquefied cells, and tissue fluids that form within the tissues in disease and escape through the ulcerated pocket epithelium into the oral cavity.

Supragingival Coronal (above) to the free gingival margin.

Supragingival debridement Other term: supragingival scaling. Removal of plaque and calculus coronal to the gingival margin.

Surface texture The tactile quality of a material or tissue; the arrangement of parts of the tissue as it affects the appearance or feel of the surface.

Surgery The act and art of treating injuries or disease by manual operations.

Mucogingival surgery: Periodontal surgery involving the soft tissue (gingival) aspects such as root coverage or increasing the height and width of the alveolar ridge.

Osseous surgery: Periodontal surgery involving the addition or resection (removal) of bone.

Symptom A departure from the normal in function, appearance, or sensation experienced by a patient. A subjective sign.

Syndrome The aggregate of signs and symptoms associated with any morbid process and constituting together the picture of the disease.

Systemic Affecting or pertaining to the whole body.

Systemic disease A disease that affects the entire body instead of a specific organ.

Systemic drug delivery Administration of a drug by mouth (oral) or parenterally (e.g., intravenous, intramuscular, subcutaneous).

T

Temporomandibular joint The connecting sliding hinge mechanism between the mandible (lower jaw) and the base of the skull (temporal bone).

Therapeutic levels (of a drug) Concentration of a drug in body fluids that causes a pharmacologic effect.

Toothbrushing methods

Bass bristles of toothbrush are placed at a 45-degree angle into the gingival sulcus and a vibratory motion in used. When using a modified version the bristles are moved down toward the occlusal/incisal part of the tooth. The occlusal surfaces of the teeth are brushed with a back and forth motion.

Charters' bristles of toothbrush are placed parallel to the long axis of the tooth and pointed incisally. The bristles are placed at a 45-degree angle, and the brush is shimmied back and forth until the bristles engage the gingival tissues and interproximal area.

Stillman The brush is placed against the buccal or lingual aspects of the tooth with the bristles pointing toward the gingival margin. The sides of the bristles should extend about 3 to 4 mm onto the attached gingival but should not extend beyond the mucogingival junction. The bristles are placed at a 45-degree angle and the brush is shimmied in a mesiodistal direction while moving it toward the occlusal/incisal edge.

Tooth mobility Referring to pathologic mobility. Loosening of a tooth or teeth. Mobility is an important diagnostic sign.

Tooth wear Loss of tooth structure (e.g., abrasion, erosion, attrition).

Topical delivery Referring to the administration of a drug or agent as a rinse or into the gingival crevice.

Toxin Substance that is harmful to the body (e.g., endotoxin).

Treatment plan List of treatment that the patient needs.

Treatment planning The act of making a list of treatment that the patient needs.

Trifurcation Anatomic area where roots diverge in a three-rooted tooth.

U

Ultrasonic See Scaler, ultrasonic.

V

Vascular Refers to blood.

W

Wear facet A flattened, highly polished worn spot on the occlusal or incisal surface of a tooth (usually seen on the side of a cusp). It may be a clinical sign of attrition.

World Health Organization A specialized agency of the United Nations with primary responsibility for international health matters and public health.

X

Xerostomia Dryness of the mouth due to inadequate salivary secretion as a result of aging, salivary gland conditions, or medications.

ANSWERS
to Self-Quiz Questions

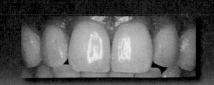

Chapter 1
1. a, b, c, d
2. c
3. c
4. c
5. b
6. c, d
7. 1. b; 2. a; 3. c; 4. d; 5. e
8. c, e, f, g
9. d
10. d

Chapter 2
1. b
2. b
3. a
4. b
5. c
6. a
7. c
8. a
9. b
10. a

Chapter 3
1. a, c, e
2. d
3. a, b
4. d
5. b
6. b
7. d
8. c
9. a
10. c

Chapter 4
1. c
2. a, c, e
3. a
4. a
5. a
6. a, c
7. e
8. b
9. d
10. 1. c; 2. a; 3. b; 4. d

Chapter 5
1. b
2. d
3. a
4. c
5. c

Chapter 6
1. b
2. c
3. c
4. a
5. b
6. c
7. b
8. a, b
9. c
10. a

Chapter 7
1. c, f
2. c
3. a
4. b
5. c
6. a
7. a
8. c
9. b
10. a

Chapter 8
1. 1. f
   2. c, f
   3. c, f
   4. a, b, d, e, g
2. a
3. d
4. d
5. 1. c
   2. b
   3. a
6. 1. c
   2. a
   3. b
   4. d
   5. e

7. d
8. a
9. d
10. 1. c
   2. d
   3. a
   4. b

Chapter 9
1. c
2. a
3. b
4. a
5. b
6. a, b, c, e, f, h
7. b
8. a
9. b
10. 1. d; 2. b; 3. a; 4. c; 5. e

Chapter 10
1. c
2. b
3. a, b, c
4. a, f, g, h
5. c
6. b
7. a, b, e
8. b
9. b
10. d

Chapter 11
1. b
2. c, d
3. a, e
4. 1. c
   2. d
   3. c
   4. a, c
   5. d
   6. a
   7. a, b, c, d
5. c
6. a
7. a, b, c, e
8. c

9. a, b, c, d, e
10. a, b, c

Chapter 12
1. b
2. c
3. a
4. d
5. b

Chapter 13
1. a
2. a, d, e
3. b, c
4. d
5. d

Chapter 14
1. b
2. a
3. b
4. 1. b
   2. c
   3. a
   4. d
5. e

Chapter 15
1. d
2. a
3. a
4. a, b, d, g, h, i
5. e
6. c
7. a
8. b
9. a
10. b

Chapter 16
1. b
2. a, c, e
3. a
4. c
5. c
6. c
7. c

8. b
9. a
10. a

Chapter 17
1. a
2. c
3. d
4. c
5. c
6. b
7. a
8. c
9. a
10. c

Chapter 18
1. b, f
2. d
3. b
4. c
5. b
6. b
7. c
8. b
9. c
10. c

Chapter 19
1. a
2. c
3. b
4. e
5. a
6. c
7. a
8. b
9. a
10. a

Chapter 20
1. c
2. b
3. c
4. d
5. a, b, d, e
6. b, c, d
7. b

8. 1. b, c
   2. b, c
   3. b, c
   4. a
9. c
10. c

Chapter 21
1. c
2. d
3. c
4. d
5. a

Chapter 22
1. a, b, c
2. a
3. a, b, c
4. b
5. d
6. b
7. a, b, d
8. c
9. c
10. a, b, c, d

Chapter 23
1. d
2. a, b, c, d
3. c
4. d
5. a

Chapter 24
1. a, b, c
2. c
3. a, c, d, e
4. b
5. c, e
6. d
7. a, c, d, e, f, g
8. c
9. a
10. b

Chapter 25
1. a
2. c

3. b
4. e
5. d
6. b
7. d
8. a
9. d
10. e

Chapter 26
1. 1. a
   2. b
   3. f
   4. d
   5. e
   6. c
2. a
3. a
4. a
5. b
6. b
7. b
8. 1. b
   2. c
   3. a
9. b
10. b, c, d

Chapter 27
1. b
2. c
3. b
4. a
5. a
6. c
7. b
8. c
9. d
10. e

Case Studies
Case I
1. d
2. c
3. a
4. b
5. a
6. b

7. e
8. a
9. d
10. b

Case II
1. a
2. a
3. d
4. d
5. d
6. a
7. a
8. a
9. a, b, d, e, h
10. b

Case III
1. b
2. a
3. b
4. c
5. a
6. b
7. b
8. c
9. d
10. a

Case IV
1. d
2. a
3. c
4. a
5. a
6. a
7. c
8. a
9. b
10. a

INDEX

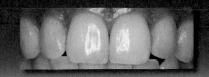

Page numbers with f indicate figures; those with t indicate tables.